Fundamentals of
Geriatric Medicine

Fundamentals of Geriatric Medicine
A Case-Based Approach

Editor

Rainier P. Soriano, MD

Assistant Professor and Director of Medical Student Education, Brookdale Department of Geriatrics and Adult Development, Mount Sinai School of Medicine, New York, New York

Associate Editors

Helen M. Fernandez, MD

Assistant Professor and Fellowship Director, Brookdale Department of Geriatrics and Adult Development, Mount Sinai School of Medicine, New York, New York

Christine K. Cassel, MD, MACP

President and CEO, ABIM Foundation and American Board of Internal Medicine, Philadelphia, Pennsylvania

Rosanne M. Leipzig, MD, PhD

Professor and Vice Chair of Education, Brookdale Department of Geriatrics and Adult Development, Mount Sinai School of Medicine, New York, New York

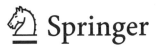 Springer

Editor:

Rainier P. Soriano, MD, Assistant Professor and Director of Medical Student Education, Brookdale Department of Geriatrics and Adult Development, Mount Sinai School of Medicine, New York, NY 10029, USA

Associate Editors:

Helen M. Fernandez, MD, Assistant Professor and Fellowship Director, Brookdale Department of Geriatrics and Adult Development, Mount Sinai School of Medicine, New York, NY 10029, USA

Christine K. Cassel, MD, MACP, President and CEO, ABIM Foundation and American Board of Internal Medicine, Philadelphia, PA 19106, USA

Rosanne M. Leipzig, MD, PhD, Professor and Vice Chair of Education, Brookdale Department of Geriatrics and Adult Development, Mount Sinai School of Medicine, New York, NY 10029, USA

Material in this book is based as noted on Cassel CK, Leipzig RM, Cohen HJ, Larson EB, Meier DE, eds. Managing editor Capello CF. *Geriatric Medicine: An Evidence-Based Approach*, 4th Ed. New York: Springer, 2003. ISBN 0-387-95514-3

Library of Congress Control Number: 2006920314

ISBN-10: 0-387-32324-4   eISBN-10: 0-387-32326-0
ISBN-13: 978-0-387-32324-4   eISBN-13: 978-0-387-32326-8

Printed on acid-free paper.

For our students: past, present, future . . .

Foreword

Prior to the evolution of modern medicine, with its superabundance of diagnostic and therapeutic medical technology and the rise of the litigious society, the value of clinical skills was evident in both history taking and the physical examination. Even today, physicians can make a correct diagnosis solely by utilizing their clinical skills in about 90% of patient encounters. Furthermore, in the past physicians understood their role as a "psychologist" and were more apt to be familiar with the social context of their patients. House calls were common. The doctor was also a "placebo" who, at his best, inspired hope and probably sped recovery.

Geriatricians use both clinical skills and take advantage of modern technology sparingly, for they know they are dealing with the most challenging and frail of patients—older patients who so often present with multiple, complex, interacting behavioral, social, and physical problems. In contrast to medicine for young people, working with the older patient is much more demanding. Furthermore, the complex issue of societal attitudes toward old people can come into play, specifically the physician's need to deal with natural fears of aging, dependency, depression, dementia, and death. Ageism is the enemy of effective medical treatment.

At its best, geriatrics exemplifies ways that medical care for all ages can become more humane, problem-oriented, and holistic.

Fundamentals of Geriatric Medicine: A Case-Based Approach discusses 32 core topics of geriatric medicine. Its case-based approach focuses ultimately upon the challenge of decision making. Soriano et al. have given us all a distinctive book that will further catalyze the emerging field of geriatric medicine.

Robert N. Butler, MD
President and CEO
International Longevity Center, USA

Preface

Fundamentals of Geriatric Medicine: A Case-Based Approach is intended as a practical educational companion to *Geriatric Medicine*, 4th edition, by Christine K. Cassel et al. (New York: Springer, 2003). This book covers a broad range of knowledge and skills students need for approaching the problems frequently encountered when caring for older adults. The book encompasses the continuum of care in various clinical settings, and highlights the geriatric syndromes, common acute and chronic illnesses, as well as other pertinent topics (such as polypharmacy and palliative care). The book also emphasizes the importance of geriatric interdisciplinary team members, including nurses, social workers, advanced practice nurses, therapists, and how these different disciplines intersect in the older adult's care.

The smaller scope of this companion text makes it easier for students to immediately integrate knowledge into clinical application. Cross-referencing will help them find more detailed information in *Geriatric Medicine*, 4th edition, and aid in fostering self-directed learning. Finally, it is our hope that this companion book's case-based instructional approach will help students become familiar with a methodology for dissecting the complexity of disease prevention, presentation, and treatment in older adults. This also gives them a clinical frame of reference in the medical decision-making process and prioritization of diagnostic problems that are so common in the care of older adults.

We are truly indebted to the contributors to *Fundamentals of Geriatric Medicine* and to the authors of the original chapters of *Geriatric Medicine*, 4th edition. We also acknowledge the mentorship and assistance from the associate editors, Rosanne M. Leipzig, MD, PhD, and Christine K. Cassel, MD, MACP, whose original work in *Geriatric Medicine*, 4th edition, made this companion book possible. We are eternally grateful to the John A. Hartford Foundation, Inc. and most especially, to William T. Comfort, Jr., trustee, for their invaluable support and vision for this book. Lastly, we also thank James O'Sullivan, Robert Albano, Sadie Forrester, Barbara Chernow, Suzy Goldhirsch, Sarah Panepinto, Jennifer Reyes, Gerard

Murphy, John Mark Hopkins, Renz Andrew Rafal, and Drs. Reena Karani, Audrey Chun, and Emily Chai, and our respective families, who, in various capacities, provided much needed assistance toward the realization of this book.

Rainier P. Soriano, MD
Helen M. Fernandez, MD

Contents

Contributors

Olusegun A. Apoeso, MD
Assistant Professor, Department of Medicine, University of Connecticut Health Center, Director of Outpatient Services, Hebrew Health Care, West Hartford, CT 06117, USA

R. Morgan Bain, MD
Assistant Professor and Medical Director, Palliative Care Unit, Department of Medicine, Wake Forest University School of Medicine, Winston-Salem, NC 27157, USA

Kenneth S. Boockvar, MD, MS
Geriatric Research, Education, and Clinical Center, James J. Peters Veterans Affairs Medical Center, Bronx, NY 10468, Assistant Professor, Brookdale Department of Geriatrics and Adult Development, Mount Sinai School of Medicine, New York, NY 10029, USA

Eileen H. Callahan, MD
Associate Professor, Brookdale Department of Geriatrics and Adult Development, Mount Sinai School of Medicine, New York, NY 10029, USA

Emily J. Chai, MD
Assistant Professor and Medical Director, Hertzberg Palliative Care Institute, Brookdale Department of Geriatrics and Adult Development, Mount Sinai School of Medicine, New York, NY 10029, USA

Rengena E. Chan-Ting, DO
Attending Physician, Care Level Management, Woodland Hills, CA 91367, USA

Audrey K. Chun, MD
Assistant Professor and Director, Coffey Geriatrics Practice, Brookdale Department of Geriatrics and Adult Development, Mount Sinai School of Medicine, New York, NY 10029, USA

Helen M. Fernandez, MD
Assistant Professor and Fellowship Director, Brookdale Department of Geriatrics and Adult Development, Mount Sinai School of Medicine, New York, NY 10029, USA

Jennifer M. Hensley, MD
Clinical Instructor and Geriatrics Hospitalist, Department of Medicine, Stony Brook University School of Medicine, Stony Brook, NY 11794, USA

Judith L. Howe, PhD
Associate Professor, Brookdale Department of Geriatrics and Adult Development, Mount Sinai School of Medicine, New York, NY 10029, Associate Director/Education, Bronx-New York Harbor Geriatrics Research, Education, and Clinical Center, James J. Peters Veterans Affairs Medical Center, Bronx, NY 10468, USA

Reena Karani, MD
Assistant Professor and Director, Geriatrics Consultation and Liaison Service, Brookdale Department of Geriatrics and Adult Development, Mount Sinai School of Medicine, New York, NY 10029, USA

Rosanne M. Leipzig, MD, PhD
Professor and Vice Chair of Education, Brookdale Department of Geriatrics and Adult Development, Mount Sinai School of Medicine, New York, NY 10029, USA

Hannah I. Lipman, MD, MS
Assistant Professor, Department of Medicine, Divisions of Geriatrics/Cardiology, Montefiore Medical Center, Bronx, NY 10467, USA

Anna U. Loengard, MD
Assistant Professor, Brookdale Department of Geriatrics and Adult Development, Mount Sinai School of Medicine, New York, NY 10029, USA

S. Brent Ridge, MD, MBA
Assistant Professor and Director of Clinical Strategies, Brookdale Department of Geriatrics and Adult Development, Mount Sinai School of Medicine, New York, NY 10029, USA

Sandra E. Sanchez-Reilly, MD
Assistant Professor and Palliative Care Fellowship Director, Division of Geriatrics, Department of Medicine, University of Texas Health Science Center, San Antonio, Texas 78229, USA

Rainier P. Soriano, MD
Assistant Professor and Director of Medical Student Education, Brookdale Department of Geriatrics and Adult Development, Mount Sinai School of Medicine, New York, NY 10029, USA

Kathleen R. Srock, MD
Clinical Instructor, University of Colorado Health Sciences Center, Denver, CO 80262, USA

Hans L. Stöhrer, MD
Assistant Attending, Department of Emergency Medicine, Coney Island Hospital, New York City Health and Hospitals Corporation, Brooklyn, NY 11235, USA

Daniel E. Wollman, MD, PhD
Director, Center for Comprehensive Care, Shelton, CT 06484, USA

Introduction

Modern educators understand that adults learn in many different ways. Perhaps the least effective is to plough through large, densely packed scholarly textbooks. And, yet, these large textbooks remain the standard of collecting state-of-the-art information for the education of medical students, residents, fellows, and physicians in practice. They are not books to be read through, but books to be used as references. Soriano has created a book that exemplifies a modern approach to adult education. Based on the reference text, it is, importantly, case-based and includes just in time learning and brings together related areas. The case-based nature is what really captures medical learners. Physicians in practice are said to be able to incorporate information much more easily if it is directly related to a patient they are currently seeing. The same, of course, is true for medical students and residents. What this book offers are realistic, clinically based cases that draw the reader into the practical realities of patient management and then provide state-of-the-art, evidence-based information that can contribute to learning about how to care for that kind of patient. In addition, instead of taking each pathophysiologic or organ-system condition on a one-by-one basis as is traditional in scholarly textbooks, Soriano has pulled together related areas that often come together clinically; for example, delirium, dementia, and depression. These three would be separate chapters in a major scholarly textbook, and yet often are overlapping and connected in clinical practice.

In addition to providing clinically relevant information in a way that is engaging and easy to absorb, Soriano has recognized that there are new ways of delivering medical care, especially for the geriatric patient. That is to say, it is not just the physician—certainly not just the geriatrician—whose expertise is relative to the care of the geriatric patient. The geriatrician, other primary care physicians, medical and surgical specialists, nonphysician providers, nurses, nurse practitioners, physical therapists, social workers, pharmacists, and many others have direct contact with patient care. All of those professionals will find this book accessible and relevant to the work they do and to the learning necessary to provide the best care for their patients. In addition to clinical knowledge, Soriano has added a heavy dose of tips on interpersonal and communication skills: one of the most challenging aspects of geriatric medicine. In addition to managing multiple complex chronic illnesses, often with acute illnesses superimposed, and multiple interacting medications and the complications of hospitalizations and procedures, there are also complex family and personal issues around health care decision making. *Fundamentals of Geriatric Medicine* walks the student or the practitioner through these kinds of challenging communication situations in an educational mode that is as effective as their conveying of clinical information.

Why is this book so different from other textbooks? One of the reasons is that Rainier Soriano is a clinician who has extensive experience taking care of patients who present with complex illnesses and need continuity of care. He has taken that experience and applied it to a textbook that is eminently practical in the teaching of medical students, residents, fellows, and physicians in practice.

This may be a new model of textbooks for the future; and if so, it is a good one.

Christine K. Cassel, MD, MACP
President and CEO
ABIM Foundation and American Board of Internal Medicine
Philadelphia, Pennsylvania, USA

1
Approach to the Older Adult Patient

Rainier P. Soriano

Learning Objectives

Upon completion of the chapter, the student will be able to:

1. Identify the different components of the history and physical examination and how these differ in older adults compared to younger adults.
2. Identify and understand the potential challenges in caring for older adults and ways to overcome them.
3. Enumerate the changes that occur with normal aging and contrast them with changes that occur secondary to disease.

Case (Part 1)

You are working with Dr. Hopkins, a primary care physician in the community. He has a very busy practice and most of the patients are older adults. You meet him in his office. Upon entering, you notice how brightly lit the entire space is. Large signs hang around the office space. You also noticed that the patient information handouts have a print size that is unusually large, and the print is in black and on white paper. You think it is a little plain compared to the multicolored patient information handouts with fancy fonts on glossy paper you saw at the pediatrics practice you were in last week.

Dr. Hopkins meets you and brings you over to the examining room where a patient is waiting.

Material in this chapter is based on the following chapters in Cassel CK, Leipzig RM, Cohen HJ, Larson EB, Meier DE, eds. Geriatric Medicine: An Evidence-Based Approach, 4th ed. New York: Springer, 2003: Taffet GE, Physiology of Aging, pp. 27–35. Tangarorang GL, Kerins GJ, Besdine RW. Clinical Approach to the Older Patient: An Overview, pp. 149–162. Koretz B, Reuben DB. Instruments to Assess Functional Status, pp. 185–194. Reuben DB. Comprehensive Geriatric Assessment and Systems Approaches to Geriatric Care, pp. 195–204. Selections edited by Rainier P. Soriano.

General Considerations

The initial evaluation of older patients with multiple disorders and treatments is generally prolonged, as compared with the time needed for younger persons. Brief screening questions, rather than elaborate instruments, are appropriate for first encounters (1); more detailed assessment should be reserved for patients with demonstrated deficits (2). Dividing the new patient assessment into two sessions can spare both patient and physician an exhausting and inefficient 2-hour encounter. Other office personnel can collect much information by questionnaire before the visit, from previous records, and from patient and family prior to the physician's contact. It is essential that good care, fully informed by current geriatrics knowledge, be delivered within a reasonable time allocation consistent with contemporary patterns of primary care. One hour for a new visit and 30 minutes for a follow-up are an absolute maximum in most environments.

Completing a home visit may also provide valuable insight into a patient's environment and daily functional status. How mobility may affect function in a particular environment, nutrition, medication use and compliance, and social interactions and support can all be assessed quickly by a home visit. Comprehensive geriatric evaluation and management by an interdisciplinary team in selected populations may improve overall health outcomes, maintain function, and possibly reduce health care utilization (3,4).

Sites of Care

Ambulatory Office Setting

The common occurrence of physical frailty among older persons demands particular attention to providing both a comfortable and safe environment for evaluation. Autonomic dysfunction is commonly encountered in older persons and increases vulnerability to excessively cool or warm settings, especially when the patient is dressed appropriate to the outside temperature. Accordingly, examining rooms should be kept between 70° and 80°F. Brighter lighting is required for adequate perception of the physician's facial expression and gestures by the older patient, whose lenses admit less than half the light they did in youth, due to cross-linking of lens proteins.

Presbycusis (present in >50% of older persons) makes background noise more distracting and interferes with the patient's hearing. Even in a quiet setting, the high-tone loss of presbycusis makes consonants most difficult to discriminate; speaking in a lower-than-usual pitch helps the patient hear, and facing the patient directly improves communication by allowing lip reading. The patient's eyeglasses, dentures, and hearing aid should always be brought to and used at the physician visit. Chairs with a higher-than-standard seat or a mechanical lift to assist in arising are useful for frail older persons with quadriceps weakness, and a broad-based step stool with handrail can make mounting and dismounting the examining table safe. Drapes for the patient should not exceed ankle length so as not to be a risk for tripping and falling.

Acute Hospital or Nursing Home Setting

The patient room is commonly the site of evaluation for the nursing home resident or hospitalized older adult. There is little difference in evaluating older persons in the hospital; the patient is usually confined to bed, so that safety and comfort are dictated by hospital amenities. All other considerations relevant in the ambulatory setting apply. Respect demands either drawing the privacy curtain or, in the nursing home, asking a roommate to leave, if possible. Privacy and identification of the nursing home room as a living space rather than a medical-care space are important issues for the nursing home resident and staff.

Case (Part 2)

Dr. Hopkins introduces you to Mrs. Bauer, a 78-year-old woman with hypertension and osteoarthritis. Dr. Hopkins tells Mrs. Bauer that you will be taking her history while he finishes up with another patient in another room. As soon as Dr. Hopkins leaves the room, Mrs. Bauer turns to you and remarks how she is amazed how young you look. She even comments that you remind her so much of her grandchild. You smile back at Mrs. Bauer and as you take a deep breath, you then proceed to take Mrs. Bauer's history.

The History

Although it is important to discover the patient's reliability as soon as possible, one should not simply dismiss patients with dementia as unreliable and confine data collection to other informants or previous records (1). Beginning history-taking with questions whose answers will illuminate mental status (e.g., time and place orientation, reasons for the visit, previous health care contacts, biographical data, problem solving) can quickly establish the credibility of responses. Even in cases of severe impairment, questions concerning current symptoms may still give useful information (5), and interaction at any level is an essential part of conveying a caring and respectful attitude.

Regardless of mental status, it is common for older patients to be accompanied by family members. Always give the patient the option of being interviewed and examined alone; including family members or companions during the visit should only occur at the patient's request. Certain older adults may be more comfortable meeting the physician with others present, but this decision should be left to the patient.

Generally, it is best to ask if the patient wants a relative or other concerned person present for the history or physical examination; getting some time alone with the patient is essential for the patient to communicate any information he or she regards as confidential for the physician (6). If the relative is present during the history, it is critical to make clear that the patient is to answer all questions; the relative should answer only if the physician asks for clarification. In cases of cognitive impairment or a long and complex history, family members, previous medical records, and other providers can provide supplementary data.

The Chief Complaint

A single or chief complaint is less common among older patients; more often, multiple diseases and problems have multiple symptoms and complaints associated with them. Accordingly, trying to structure the history in the standard format of chief complaint, history of present illness, and past medical history usually results in frustration for the clinician. More useful is the enumeration of a comprehensive problem list, followed by complaints, recent and interval history, and remote information for each of the active problems being considered at a visit. The first evaluation, regardless of setting, requires creating a complete database; its future utility justifies the initial time allocation. It may be easiest to commence the history with an open-ended question, such as, "What do you feel interferes most with your day-to-day activities?" Such a question is usually very helpful in focusing the clinical evaluation.

Another common finding in older patients is that the *law of parsimony*, or *Occam's razor*, is not valid—multiple complaints and abnormal findings arise from multiple diseases; discovering a diagnosis that unifies multiple signs, symptoms, and laboratory data is uncommon and, although welcome in patients of any age, should not be expected in older persons. The classic paradigm in which clinical findings lead directly to a unifying diagnosis has been found to operate in fewer than half of older patients studied (7).

Case (Part 3)

As you proceed with Mrs. Bauer's interview, you start asking her about her medications. She says that she takes enalapril 5 mg daily and acetaminophen 325 mg every 6 hours as needed for her joint pains. She start to bring out her bottles of medications and you notice that she had two of the same medication in two separate bottles. Mrs. Bauer also says that she takes several vitamins and minerals but did not bother to bring them since, according to her, they are "not medications" anyway.

Medication History

The importance of collecting and inquiring about each and every medication taken by or in the possession of the older patient cannot be overemphasized (8). Older adults often take duplicate, overlapping, and conflicting drugs (9), usually acquired from multiple prescribing physicians and over-the-counter sources. All drugs owned by the patient, including supplements, herbals, vitamins, laxatives, sleeping pills, and cold preparations, should be gathered from the bathroom cabinet, bedside table, purse, kitchen drawer, and relatives, and brought to the office visit. Ask patients specifically about food and vitamin supplements and the use of any other alternative medications or remedies they may take. Also, a sizable number of people who are taking alternative medicines fail to inform the clinician, which emphasizes the need for the clinician to specifically inquire about nonprescription drug use (10). All containers should be placed on a table and the patient asked how often each drug is taken and for what, if any, symptomatic indication (8). Consider review of all types of medications every 3 months. Ascertaining pneumococcal, influenza, and tetanus vaccination status can be conveniently done as part of the medication history.

In the hospital, caution should be exercised in ordering all drugs that have been prescribed; toxic accumulation of one or several agents is common, usually because the patient has not been taking prescribed medications as instructed. Self-protective nonadherence to the regimen, often in response to adverse reactions when drugs were taken as ordered, has led to reduction in dosage or frequency by the patient. Return to the originally prescribed schedules produces toxicity.

In the nursing home, the major additional caution concerns the continued administration of unnecessary drugs that were initiated for transient problems arising during hospitalization. Sedative, antipsychotic, diuretic, antiarrhythmic, and antiinfective drugs are often continued indefinitely at the nursing home on the incorrect assumption that they are needed (11). Careful winnowing of the medication list is indicated at least every 3 months and following any hospitalization.

Social History

Crucial information for developing a coherent and feasible care plan at home includes any change in living arrangements, who is available at home or in the local community, and what plans if any exist for coverage in times of illness or functional decline. Although a home visit is the best way to evaluate risks or limitations, inquiring about stairs, rugs, thresholds, bathing facilities, heating, and neighborhood crime can increase the care plan's utility. Stable and durable plans for care at home fulfill both the patient's goal to remain at home and the system's goal to control costs of institutional care. Extent of social relationships is a powerful predictor of functional status and mortality for older adults (12); accordingly, determining the patient's friendship network and recommending ideas for increased socialization can be an appropriate clinical role. Encouraging older persons to become involved with local senior center activities may be one mechanism to enhance social relationships, reduce isolation, and improve daily functioning.

Nutrition History

Although independent elders in the community are generally adequately nourished, the prevalence of under- and overnutrition increases in older persons. Undernutrition is most often unrecognized (13). Most of the undernutrition occurs in those with chronic diseases that directly or indirectly interfere with nutrition. Oral or gastrointestinal disorders, drug effects on appetite, systemic illness, and psychiatric disease increase the risk of undernutrition. Screening questions include a diet history (within the past few days), pattern of weight during recent years, and shopping and food preparation habits (14). Other questions should include any recent intentional efforts to gain or lose weight or any history of eating disorders. Sites of eating, companionship, and skipped meals are also relevant. Serum albumin is a good marker of nutritional status over the preceding 3 months and is correlated with mortality rates (15). The prealbumin reflects nutrition over the past 20 days.

Though not strictly part of the nutritional history, this is a convenient time to inquire about alcohol and tobacco use. Alcohol misuse by older persons is often overlooked in all but florid situations, in part because symptoms and signs are often attributed to other problems common in older persons (16). The CAGE (*cut* down, *a*nnoyed, *g*uilty feelings, *eye*-opener) questionnaire has been validated in older persons (17). It is more useful than the MAST-G (Michigan Alcoholism Screening Test–geriatric version) as it requires only four easily memorized questions (18) and has comparable sensitivity and specificity (70% and 81%, respectively, for MAST-G score ≥5 and 63% and 82%, respectively, for CAGE score ≥2). A positive response to two of four questions has traditionally been considered a positive screen. However, in a patient population with high prevalence of drinking problems, even a score of 1 should trigger appropriate investigation (19).

Family History

Although causes of mortality among relatives are usually irrelevant, history of Alzheimer's disease or nonspecified dementia appears to be important. Likewise, certain psychiatric disorders, such as depression and dysthymia, appear to cluster within families. From a mental health perspective, the medical family history also can identify caregiving by the older person.

Caregiving of a disabled spouse and its attendant stress confers substantial mortality risk for the caregiver. Persons who were providing care and who were experiencing strain have a 50% greater risk of dying within 4 years, compared to noncaregiving controls (20).

Sexual History

Older persons continue to be sexually active unless inhibited by the absence of a partner or the occurrence of a disease that reduces libido, makes intercourse painful, or prevents it mechanically (21). Discomfort or awkwardness may result from physician rather than patient attitudes; a simple open-ended question, such as "Tell me about your sex life" or "Are you satisfied with sex?" may encourage the older person to give information not spontaneously reported.

Miscellaneous History

Routine questions should be asked regarding driving habits, seatbelt use, recreational activities, and gambling history.

Case (Part 4)

Mrs. Bauer says that she is able to care for herself. In fact, one of her sons actually moved back in with her. She even gets up early in the morning to cook hot cereal for him. She says that she often does his laundry as well as her own. She cleans up her own apartment but only if her joints are not hurting that much. She regularly swims at a local YMCA but has to take a short bus ride downtown to get there.

Self-Reported Functional Status

The patient should be asked screening questions about independence and self-care—ability to get out of bed, dress, shop, and cook (22,23). Any reported or observed difficulty should provoke more elaborate questions concerning dependence in basic activities of daily living (ADLs), that is, mobility, bathing, transferring, toileting, continence, dressing, hygiene, and feeding (24) and in instrumental activities of daily living (IADLs), that is, shopping, cooking, cleaning, managing money, telephoning, doing laundry, and traveling out of the house (25). Questions should also be asked about vision, hearing, continence, and depression; deficits should be followed up.

Values History (Preferences for Care)

It is wise to take a values history—the patient's beliefs about technological interventions to prolong life, what defines life quality for the patient as an individual, and with what decrements the patient would still think life were worth living. Documenting discussions, executing a living will, and designating a proxy decision maker and durable power of attorney for health care are part of this process of helping the patient have a voice in decisions that may need to be made when the patient, by reason of illness, cannot participate (26).

Physical Examination

General Appearance

General appearance of the older patient should include any noteworthy features; vitality, markedly youthful or aged appearance, and any indicators of frailty or clinical problems (e.g., odor of urine or stool; signs of abuse, neglect, or poverty; hygiene and grooming) warrant mention. Merely observing how long it takes for the patient to get ready for the examination and the extent and nature of help that may be required remains a useful and reliable tool to measure functional capacity (Table 1.1).

Vital Signs

Vital signs do not change with age. Hypothermia is more common, and reliable low-reading thermometers are essential, especially for emergency room and wintertime use. Blood pressure should be taken with the patient in the supine position after at least 10 minutes' rest, and immediately and 3 minutes after standing. Orthostatic hypotension defined as either a 20mmHg drop in systolic pressure or any drop accompanied by typical symptoms occurs in 11% to 28% of individuals older than 65 years (27,28). In acute moderate blood loss, postural hypotension is a fairly specific but poorly sensitive sign of hypovolemia (29). Blunting of the baroreflex mechanism with age makes cardioacceleration with the upright position a late and unreliable sign of volume depletion in older persons.

Tachypnea at a rate of more than 25 per minute is a reliable sign of lower respiratory infection, even in very elderly patients (30). Weight is the most reliable measure of undernutrition in older outpatients and should be carefully recorded under comparable conditions at each visit. Specific assessment of general or localized pain should be considered as the *fifth vital sign* and should be recorded using a uniform scale (e.g., 0 to 10) (31).

TABLE 1.1. Major changes in systems

Endocrine system	Impaired glucose tolerance (fasting glucose increased 1 mg/dL/decade; postprandial increased 10 mg/dL/decade)
	Increased serum insulin and increased hemoglobin ($HgbA_{1C}$)
	Nocturnal growth hormone peaks lost; decreased insulin-like growth factor 1 (IGF-1)
	Marked decrease in dehydroepiandrosterone (DHEA)
	Decreased free and bioavailable testosterone
	Decreased triiodothyronine (T_3)
	Increase parathyroid hormone (PTH)
	Decreased production of vitamin D by skin
	Ovarian failure, decreased ovarian hormones
	Increased serum homocysteine levels
Cardiovascular	Unchanged resting heart rate (HR); decreased maximum HR
	Impaired left ventricular filling
	Marked dropout of pacemaker cells in sinoatrial (SA) node
	Increased contribution of atrial systole to ventricular filling
	Left atrial hypertrophy
	Prolonged contraction and relaxation of left ventricle
	Decreased inotropic, chronotropic, lusitropic response to β-adrenergic stimulation
	Decreased maximum cardiac output
	Decreased hypertrophy in response to volume or pressure overload
	Increased serum atrial natriuretic peptide
	Large arteries increase in wall thickness, lumen, and length, and become less distensible and compliance decreases
	Subendothelial layer thickened with connective tissue
	Irregularities in size and shape of endothelial cells
	Fragmentation of elastin in media of arterial wall
	Peripheral vascular resistance increases
Blood pressure (BP)	Increased systolic BP, unchanged diastolic BP
	β-Adrenergic–mediated vasodilatation decreased; α-adrenergic–mediated vasoconstriction unchanged
	Brain autoregulation of perfusion impaired
Pulmonary	Decreased forced expiratory volume at 1 second (FEV_1) and forced vital capacity (FVC)
	Increased residual volume
	Cough less effective
	Ciliary action less effective
	Ventilation-perfusion mismatching causes PaO_2 to decrease with age: 100 − (0.32 × age)
	Trachea and central airways increase in diameter
	Enlarged alveolar ducts due to lost elastic lung parenchyma structural support result in decreased surface area
	Decreased lung mass
	Expansion of thorax
	Maximum inspiratory and expiratory pressures decrease
	Decreased respiratory muscle strength
	Chest wall stiffens
	Diffusion of CO decreased
	Decreased ventilatory response to hypercapnia
Hematologic	Bone marrow reserves decreased response to high demand
	Attenuated reticulocytosis to erythropoietin administration
Renal	Decreased creatinine clearance and glomerular filtration rate (GFR) 10 mL/decade

TABLE 1.1. *Continued*

	25% decrease in renal mass mostly from cortex with a relative increased perfusion of juxtamedullary nephrons
	Decreased sodium excretion and conservation
	Decreased potassium excretion and conservation
	Decreased concentrating and diluting capacity
	Impaired secretion of acid load
	Decreased serum renin and aldosterone
	Accentuated antidiuretic hormone (ADH) release in response to dehydration
	Decreased nitric oxide production
	Increased dependence of renal prostaglandins to maintain perfusion
	Decreased vitamin D activation
Genitourinary	Prolonged refractory period for erections for men
	Reduced intensity of orgasm for men and women
	Incomplete bladder emptying and increased postvoid residuals
	Decreased prostatic secretions in urine
	Decreased concentrations of antiadherence factor Tamm-Horsfall protein
Temperature regulation	Impaired shivering
	Decreased cutaneous vasoconstriction and vasodilation
	Decreased sweat production
	Increased core temperature to start sweating
Muscle	Marked decrease in muscle mass (sarcopenia) due to loss of muscle fibers
	Aging effects smallest in diaphragm (role of activity), more in legs than arms
	Decreased myosin heavy chain synthesis
	Small if any decrease in specific force
	Decreased innervation, increased number of myofibrils per motor unit
	Infiltration of fat into muscle bundles
	Increased fatigability
	Decrease in basal metabolic rate (decrease 4%/decade after age 50) parallels loss of muscle
Bone	Slower healing of fractures
	Decreasing bone mass in men and women both trabecular and cortical bone
	Decreased osteoclast bone formation
Joints	Disordered cartilage matrix
	Modified proteoglycans and glycosaminoglycans
Peripheral nervous system	Loss of spinal motor neurons
	Decreased vibratory sensation especially in feet
	Decreased thermal sensitivity (warm and cool)
	Decreased sensory nerve action potential amplitude
	Decreased size of large myelinated fibers
	Increased heterogeneity of axon myelin sheaths
Central nervous system	Small decrease in brain mass
	Decreased brain blood flow and impaired autoregulation of perfusion
	Nonrandom loss of neurons to modest extent
	Proliferation of astrocytes
	Decreased density of dendritic connections
	Increased numbers of scattered neurofibrillary tangles
	Increased numbers of scattered senile plaques
	Decreased myelin and total brain lipid
	Altered neurotransmitters including dopamine and serotonin
	Increased monoamine oxidase activity
	Decrease in hippocampal glucocorticoid receptors

TABLE 1.1. *Continued*

	Decline in fluid intelligence
	Slowed central processing and reaction time
Gastrointestinal	Decreased liver size and blood flow
	Impaired clearance by liver of drugs that require extensive phase I metabolism
	Reduced inducibility of liver mixed-function oxidase enzymes
	Mild decrease in bilirubin
	Hepatocytes accumulate secondary lysosomes, residual bodies, and lipofuscin
	Mild decrease in stomach acid production, probably due to nonautoimmune loss of parietal cells
	Impaired response to gastric mucosal injury
	Decreased pancreatic mass and enzymatic reserves
	Decrease in effective colonic contractions
	Decreased calcium absorption
	Decrease in gut-associated lymphoid tissue
Vision	Impaired dark adaptation
	Yellowing of lens
	Inability to focus on near items (presbyopia)
	Minimal decrease in static acuity, profound decrease in dynamic acuity (moving target)
	Decreased contrast sensitivity
	Decreased lacrimation
Smell	Detection decreased by 50%
Thirst	Decreased thirst drive
	Impaired control of thirst by endorphins
Balance	Increased threshold vestibular responses
	Reduced number of organ of Corti hair cells
Audition	Bilateral loss of high frequency tones
	Central processing deficit
	Difficulty discriminating source of sound
	Impaired discrimination of target from noise
Adipose	Increased aromatase activity
	Increased tendency to lipolysis
Immune system	Decreased cell-mediated immunity
	Lower affinity antibody production
	Increased autoantibodies
	Facilitated production of antiidiotype antibodies
	Increased occurrence of monoclonal gammopathy of unknown significance (MGUS)
	More nonresponders to vaccines
	Decreased delayed type hypersensitivity
	Impaired macrophage function [interferon-γ, transforming growth factor-β (TGF-β), tumor necrosis factor (TNF), interleukin-6 (IL-6), IL-1 release increased with age]
	Decreased cell proliferative response to mitogens
	Atrophy of thymus and loss of thymic hormones
	Accumulation of memory T cells (CD-45+)
	Increased circulating IL-6
	Decreased IL-2 release and IL-2 responsiveness
	Decreased production of B cells by bone marrow

Source: Taffet GE. Physiology of aging. In: Cassel CK, Leipzig RM, Cohen HJ, et al., eds. Geriatric Medicine, 4th ed. New York: Springer, 2003.

Integument

Skin undergoes many changes with age, including dehydration, thinning, and loss of elastic tissue. Wrinkling is more powerfully predicted by sun exposure and cigarette smoking than by age. Most proliferative lesions, benign and malignant, are related to sun exposure; accordingly, basal and squamous cell cancers and melanomas should be most aggressively hunted on exposed skin. Because of skin aging, turgor is not a reliable sign of hydration status. All skin should be examined, exposed to sun or not, for evidence of established or incipient (nonblanching redness) pressure sores. Ecchymoses should also be noted, whether due to purpura of thin old skin or trauma; the possibility of abuse should be considered.

Head and Neck

Head and neck examination begins with careful observation of sun-exposed areas for premalignant and malignant lesions. Palpation of temporal arteries for pain, nodularity, and pulse is recommended, but asymptomatic temporal or giant cell arteritis or polymyalgia rheumatica is not common (32), and palpation is an insensitive test. Arcus ocularis, or cornealis, a white-to-yellow deposit at the outer edge of the iris, along with xanthelasma, predicts premature coronary disease in young adults. Beyond age 60, it does not identify increased risk.

Visual acuity and hearing screening are necessary, given the high prevalence of impaired vision and auditory acuity among older persons. For most clinical situations, a pocket Snellen chart, held 14 inches from the eye, is more practical than a wall-mounted chart. The whispered voice is as sensitive as an audioscope for detection of hearing loss (33,34), but the latter is, to date, the best objective measurement of hearing and more accurate at following changes over time. Inspecting the ear canals and drums using an otoscope is especially necessary if hearing loss is detected; removing impacted cerumen is a common quick-fix intervention for many older patients.

Oral examination for denture sores, tooth and gum health, and oral cancers is essential and should include inspection and palpation with dentures out (35). The earliest detectable malignant oral lesion is red and painless; if persistent beyond 2 weeks, biopsy is mandatory. Although on the decline, oral cancers are most common in older persons with longstanding alcohol or tobacco use or poor hygiene.

Vascular sounds in the neck usually arise from vessels other than the carotid artery (36); true carotid bruits confer more risk for coronary events and contralateral stroke than for ipsilateral stroke, and may cease unpredictably (37).

Breast Examination

Breast examination is generally simpler in older women. Fat diminishes, making breast tissue and the tumors that arise from it more easily palpable. Routine screening mammograms annually or every other year should be continued lifelong or until a decision is reached that a discovered cancer would not be treated (38); age-specific breast cancer incidence increases at least until age 85, and no evidence indicates that treatment is not effective in older women (39,40). Current recommendations for breast cancer screening suggest yearly mammography until age 69, but there has been much discussion about revising the age to 74 or 79, or removing an upper age limit entirely. Routine screening mammography annually is part of Medicare benefit, and age cutoffs or stopping screening on the basis of age alone is controversial. Accordingly, discussions as to how the information will be utilized should take place before testing is initiated.

Case (Part 5)

After your thorough history taking, you asked Mrs. Bauer to change to a hospital gown in preparation for her physical examination. Her blood pressure (BP) = 150/75 mmHg; heart rate (HR) = 62/min; respiration rate (RR) = 12/min; and temperature = 36.7 C. Her head and neck exam is unremarkable. Her lungs are clear to auscultation and percussion. There is a systolic murmur present at the aortic area on exam without any radiation to the neck. Her abdomen and extremities examination are normal.

Heart and Lung Examination

Lung examination is little different in the older patient. Rales are abnormal at any age; evanescent crackles of atelectasis are the most common cause of rales in the absence of pathology.

Cardiac examination has several special features in aged patients. Both atrial and ventricular ectopy are common at baseline without symptoms or ominous prognosis (41,42). Although S_4 is common among older persons free of cardiac disease, S_3 is associated with congestive heart failure. The ubiquitous systolic ejection murmur is less reliable as a sign of hemodynamically significant aortic stenosis in older individuals. A loud murmur (>2/6), diminution of the aortic component of S_2, narrowed pulse pressure, and dampening of the carotid upstroke suggest aortic stenosis, but each may be absent and be falsely reassuring (43). In the absence of typical symptoms, a systolic ejection murmur lacking any of the features of stenosis may be followed without cardiac imaging. Although for decades aortic sclerosis was considered benign, it has recently been associated with increased risk for myocardial infarction, congestive heart failure, stroke, and death from cardiovascular causes, even without evidence of significant outflow tract obstruction (44).

Abdominal and Rectal Examination

Abdominal and rectal examination have few additional or special components for the older patient. Unsuspected fecal impaction is common and, despite no complaint of constipation, should be treated with a bowel regimen that includes fiber and scheduled toileting. Evidence of fecal or urinary incontinence is usually obvious to the alert examiner. A chronically overfilled and distended bladder should be suspected in men who are incontinent. Although part of the screen for prostate cancer, prostatic masses detected on digital rectal examination may also reflect granuloma, calcification, or hyperplasia, and benign causes outnumber malignant ones; differentiation by imaging is thought not to be reliable unless calcification is present. Prostatic enlargement of benign hyperplasia (since cell proliferation occurs, hypertrophy is an incorrect term) correlates poorly with both urethral obstruction and symptoms of prostatism; anterior periurethral encroachment causes symptoms, but it is the posterolateral portions of the gland that are accessible on digital examination. The need for and utility of screening for fecal occult blood in the early detection and reduction of mortality and morbidity of colon cancer is established in patients of all ages (45,46).

Musculoskeletal Examination

Examination of the musculoskeletal system, which is often a source of abundant complaints and pathology in older adults, begins with simple screening. In the absence of complaints or loss of function, brief tests of function are adequate to reveal unsuspected limitations. For the upper extremity, asking the patient to "touch the back of your head with your hands" and "pick up the spoon" are sensitive and specific (1). Gait and mobility can be assessed by the timed "up-and-go" test (arise from a chair, walk 3 meters, turn, walk back, and sit down) (47); requiring that each foot be off the floor in the up-and-go test makes the test a better predictor of functional deficits than a standard detailed neuromuscular examination (48). Neuromuscular abnormalities may not identify persons with mobility deficits and demonstrable difficulties in the up-and-go test. When deficits are detected in any screening test, more detailed evaluation, including neuromuscular exam and longer standard objective tests (2,49), and likely inclusion of a physical therapist in evaluation and treatment are indicated.

Pelvic Examination

Pelvic examination in older women often is neglected. Atrophic vaginitis, with associated urinary incontinence, or itching or dyspareunia, is remarkably easy and gratifying to treat. Ovaries or uterus palpable more than 10 years beyond menopause usually indicate pathology, often tumor. Any adnexal mass in a woman over 50 years is considered malignant until proven otherwise (50). If arthritis or frailty make stirrups uncomfortable for the patient, examination in bed or on a table with the patient positioned on her side with knees drawn up will allow speculum exam and Papanicolaou smear. The bimanual exam can be done with the patient supine, again avoiding use of stirrups. Signs of abuse may only be apparent on pelvic examination.

Neurologic Examination

The most important principle is that although abnormalities are common in the neurologic examination of the older patient, one-third to one-half the abnormal findings have no identifiable disease causing them. Abnormalities are classified as (1) attributable to a disease or an isolated abnormality, and (2) more common with increasing age or not. Abnormalities occurring in the absence of detectable disease and more common with increasing age are the best current definition of changes of aging in the nervous system. Abnormalities attributable to disease and more common with increasing age simply reflect diseases that are more common in older persons and have nervous system findings. Abnormalities occurring in the absence of detectable disease but not more common with increasing age are most likely individual variations not attributable to aging; the unlikely possibility also exists that lack of progression occurs following changes that developed before age 65.

The considerable prevalence of neurologic abnormalities in older persons carefully evaluated and found to have no disease explaining the finding demands even greater caution in attributing predictive significance to the abnormality. For example, *frontal release signs* (also called primitive reflexes)—snout, palmomental, root, suck, grasp, glabellar tap—have been reported to identify patients with dementia (51–53) or with Parkinson's disease. Because these signs appear in 10% to 35% of older adults screened to exclude disease (54–56), it is difficult to accept reports of these signs as identifiers of disease, at least in older persons. Ankle jerks, reported to be absent among many otherwise healthy older persons, turn out to be just a bit more difficult to elicit. Using a high-quality, round neurologic hammer rather than a lightweight, red triangulated hammer, and striking briskly will improve accuracy. It appears that reports of loss of ankle jerk with age may be a result of the care and expertise with which the reflex is elicited, rather than an aging effect (54,57).

General Considerations

- Health and disease behavior in older adults refers both to differences in the way diseases behave when occurring in older persons and to differences in the way older persons behave when afflicted with disease.
- Self-perception of health is heavily influenced by an individual's disease burden and its current activity as well as the norms and expectations of the group against which one measures health and dependence.
- Although older adults have the highest levels of health-promoting behavior, they are also least likely to take action in response to symptoms of serious illness. They most often attributed symptoms to aging and reacted to those symptoms by (1) waiting and watching, (2) accepting symptoms, (3) denying danger, or (4) delaying or rejecting medical care.
- Multiple pathology, or concurrence of diseases, is common among older persons and poses multiple hazards to older patients and their health care providers. The first hazard is that active medical problems frequently interact with one another to the detriment of the patient—disease–disease interactions. A second risk is that unidentified multiple pathologies can interact with diagnostic studies or treatment undertaken to manage a diagnosed problem and produce iatrogenic harm—disease–treatment interaction.

Suggested Readings

Koretz B, Reuben DB. Instruments to assess functional status. In: Cassel CK, Leipzig RM, Cohen HJ, et al., eds. Geriatric Medicine, 4th ed. New York: Springer, 2003:185–194.

Reuben DB. Comprehensive geriatric assessment and systems approaches to geriatric care. In: Cassel CK, Leipzig RM, Cohen HJ, et al., eds. Geriatric Medicine, 4th ed. New York: Springer, 2003:195–204.

Taffet GE. Physiology of aging. In: Cassel CK, Leipzig RM, Cohen HJ, et al., eds. Geriatric Medicine, 4th ed. New York: Springer, 2003:27–35.

Tangarorang GL, Kerins GJ, Besdine RW. Clinical approach to the older patient: an overview. In: Cassel CK, Leipzig RM, Cohen HJ, et al., eds. Geriatric Medicine, 4th ed. New York: Springer, 2003:149–162.

References

1. Lachs M, Feinstein A, Cooney L, et al. A simple procedure for general screening of functional disability in elderly patients. Ann Intern Med 1990;112: 699–706.

2. Applegate WB, Blass JP, Williams TF. Instruments for the functional assessment of older patients. N Engl J Med 1990;322:1207–1214.
3. Burns R, Nichols LO, Martindale-Adams J, et al. Interdisciplinary geriatric primary care evaluation and management: two year outcomes. J Am Geriatr Soc 2000;48(1):8–13.
4. Stuck AE, Siu AL, Wieland GD, et al. Comprehensive geriatric assessment: a meta-analysis of controlled trials. Lancet 1993;342:1032–1036.
5. Davis PB, Robins LN. History-taking in the elderly with and without cognitive impairment. J Am Geriatr Soc 1989;255:237–249.
6. Greene MG, Majerovitz SD, Adelman RD, Rizzo C. The effects of the presence of a third person on the physician-older patient medical interview. J Am Geriatr Soc 1994;42:413–419.
7. Fried LP, et al. Diagnosis of illness presentation in the elderly. J Am Geriatr Soc 1991;39:117–123.
8. Nolan L, O'Malley K. Prescribing for the elderly, Part I: sensitivity of the elderly to adverse drug reactions. J Am Geriatr Soc 1988;36:142–149.
9. Montamat SC, Cusack BJ, Vestal RE. Management of drug therapy in the elderly. N Engl J Med 1989;321:303–309.
10. Eisenberg DM, Davis RB, Ettner SL, et al. Trends in alternative medicine use in the United States, 1990—results of a follow-up national survey. JAMA 1998;280(18):1569–1575.
11. Beers MH, Ouslander JG, Fingold SF, et al. Inappropriate medication prescribing in skilled-nursing facilities. Ann Intern Med 1992;117:684–689.
12. Berkman LF. Social networks, support, and health: taking the next step forward. Am J Epidemiol 1986;123:559.
13. Morley JE. Why do physicians fail to recognize and treat malnutrition in older persons? J Am Geriatr Soc 1991;39:1139–1140.
14. Detsky AS, Smalley PS, Chang J. Is this patient malnourished? JAMA 1994;271:54–58.
15. Corti M-C, Guralnik JM, Salive ME, et al. Serum albumin level and physical disability as predictors of mortality in older persons. JAMA 1994;272:1036–1042.
16. Graham K. Identifying and measuring alcohol abuse among the elderly: serious problems with existing instrumentation. J Stud Alcohol 1986;47:322–325.
17. Buchsbaum DG, Buchanan RG, Welsh J, et al. Screening for drinking disorders in the elderly using the cage questionnaire. J Am Geriatr Soc 1992;40:662–665.
18. Morton JL, Jones TV, Manganaro MA. Performance of alcoholism screening questionnaires in elderly veterans. Am J Med 1996;101(2):153–159.
19. Buchsbaum DG, Buchanan RG, Welsh J, et al. Screening for drinking disorders in the elderly using the CAGE questionnaire. J Am Geriatr Soc 1992;40:662–665.
20. Schulz R, Beach SR. Caregiving as a risk factor for mortality: the caregiver health effects study. JAMA 1999;282:2215–2219.
21. Bretschneider JG, McCoy NL. Sexual interest and behavior in healthy 80 to 102 year olds. Arch Sex Behav 1988;17:109–129.
22. Guralnik JM, Simonsick EM, Ferrucci L, et al. A short physical performance battery assessing lower extremity function: association with self-reported

disability and prediction of mortality and nursing home admission. J Gerontol 1994;49:M85–M94.

23. Reuben DB, Siu AL, Kimpau S. The predictive validity of self-report and performance-based measures of function and health. J Gerontol 1992;47: M106–M110.

24. Katz S, Ford AB, Moskowitz RW, et al. Studies of illness in the aged: the index of ADL: a standardized measure of biological and psychosocial function. JAMA 1963;185:914–919.

25. Wilson LA, et al. Multiple disorders in the elderly. Lancet 1962;2:841.

26. Cassell EJ. Art of medicine. In: Reich Warret T, ed. Encyclopedia of Bioethics, III. New York: Simon & Schuster Macmillan, 1995:1674–1679.

27. Oowi WL, Barrett S, Hossain M, et al. Patterns of orthostatic blood pressure change and their clinical correlates in a frail elderly population. JAMA 1997;277:1299–1304.

28. Raiha I, Luntonen S, Piha J, et al. Prevalence, predisposing factors and prognostic importance of postural hypotension. Arch Intern Med 1995;155: 930–935.

29. Witting MD, Wears RL, Li S. Defining the positive tilt test: a study of healthy adults with moderate acute blood loss. Ann Emerg Med 1994; 23(6):1320–1323.

30. McFadden JP, Price RC, Eastwood HD, et al. Raised respiratory rate in elderly patients: a valuable physical sign. Br Med J 1982;284:626–627.

31. AGS Panel on Chronic Pain in Older Persons. American Geriatrics Society. The management of chronic pain in older persons. J Am Geriatr Soc 1998; 46(5):635–651.

32. Hunder G, Bloch DA, Michel BA, et al. The American College of Rheumatology 1990 criteria for the classification of giant cell arteritis. Arthritis Rheum 1990;33:1122–1128.

33. Reuben DB, Mui S, Damesyn M, et al. The prognostic value of sensory impairment in older persons. J Am Geriatr Soc 1999;47(8):930–935.

34. Swan IRC, Browning GG. The whispered voice as a screening test for hearing impairment. J R Coll Gen Pract 1985;35:197.

35. Lichtenstein MJ, Bess FH, Logan SA. Validation of screening tools for identifying hearing-impaired elderly in primary care. JAMA 1988;259: 2875–2878.

36. Ruiswyk JV, Noble H, Sigmann P. The natural history of carotid bruits in elderly persons. Ann Intern Med 1990;112:340–343.

37. Heyman A, et al. Risk of stroke in asymptomatic persons with cervical arterial bruits. N Engl J Med 1980;302:838.

38. Mandelblatt JS, Wheat ME, Monane M, et al. Breast cancer screening for elderly women with and without comorbid conditions. Ann Intern Med 1992;116:722–730.

39. Horm JW, Asire AJ, Young JL, et al. SEER Program: Cancer Incidence and Mortality in the US, 1973–1981. NIH publication 85–1837. Bethesda, MD: Department of Health and Human Services, 1985.

40. Yancik R, Ries LG, Yates JW. Breast cancer in aging women. Cancer 1989;63:976–981.

41. Fleg JL, Kennedy HL. Long-term prognostic significance of ambulatory electrocardiographic findings in apparently healthy subjects >60 years of age. Am J Cardiol 1992;70:748–751.

42. Aronow WS, Mercando AD, Epstein S. Prevalence of arrhythmias detected by 24–hour ambulatory electrocardiography and value of antiarrhythmic therapy in elderly patients with unexplained syncope. Am J Cardiol 1992; 70:408–410.

43. Lembo NJ, Dell Italia LJ, Crawford MH, et al. Bedside diagnosis of systolic murmurs. N Engl J Med 1988;318:1572–1578.

44. Otto CM, Lind BK, Kitzman DW, et al. Association of aortic valve sclerosis with cardiovascular mortality and morbidity in the elderly. N Engl J Med 1999;341:142–147.

45. Mandel JS, Bond JH, Church TR, et al. Reducing mortality from colorectal cancer by screening for fecal occult blood. N Engl J Med 1993;328:1365–1371. (Also see editorial, Winawer SJ. Colorectal cancer screening comes of age. N Engl J Med 1993;328:1416–1417.)

46. Winawer SJ, Zauber AG, Ho MN, et al. Prevention of colorectal cancer by colonoscopic polypectomy. N Engl J Med 1993;329:1977–1981.

47. Podsiadlo D, Richardson S. The timed "up and go": a test of basic functional mobility for frail elderly persons. J Am Geriatr Soc 1991;39:142–148.

48. Tinetti ME, Ginter SF. Identifying mobility dysfunctions in elderly patients: standard neuromuscular examination or direct assessment? JAMA 1988; 259:1190–1193.

49. Reuben DB, Siu AL. An objective measure of physical function of elderly outpatients, the physical performance test. J Am Geriatr Soc 1990;38:1105–1112.

50. Dumesic DA. Pelvic examination: what to focus on in menopausal women. Consultant 1996;36:39–46.

51. Thomas RJ. Blinking and the release reflexes: are they clinically useful? J Am Geriatr Soc 1994;42:609–613.

52. Forstl H, Burns A, Levy R, et al. Neurologic signs in Alzheimer's disease. Results of a prospective clinical and neuropathological study. Arch Neurol 1992;49:1038–1042.

53. Backine S, Lacomblez L, Palisson E, et al. Relationship between primitive reflexes, extra-pyramidal signs, reflective apraxia and severity of cognitive impairment in dementia of the Alzheimer's type. Acta Neurol Scand 1989; 79:38–46.

54. Odenheimer G, Funkenstein H, Beckett L, et al. Comparison of neurologic changes in "successfully aging" persons vs the total aging population. Arch Neurol 1994;51:573–580.

55. Jenkyn LR, Reeves AG, Warren T, et al. Neurologic signs in senescence. Arch Neurol 1985;42:1154–1157.

56. Forgotten symptoms and primitive signs (editorial). Lancet 1987;1(8537): 841–842.

57. Impallomeni M, Kenny RA, Flynn MD, et al. The elderly and their ankle jerks. Lancet 1984;1(8378):670–672.

2
The Comprehensive Geriatric Assessment

RAINIER P. SORIANO

Learning Objectives

Upon completion of the chapter, the student will be able to:

1. Explain the rationale behind the comprehensive geriatric assessment (CGA).
2. Enumerate the components of the CGA and the process of care.
3. Identify the members of the CGA team and understand their corresponding roles in the team.
4. Identify the various assessment instruments used to evaluate the different components or dimensions of the CGA.

Case (Part 1)

An 84-year-old African-American woman comes to your office accompanied by her niece. You begin your history by asking the patient why she came to see you. She replied: "I don't know why I'm here!" Her niece then interjects: "She has problems with memory."

General Considerations

Geriatric assessment refers to an overall evaluation of the health status of the elderly patient. The well-being of any person is the result of the interactions among a number of factors, only some of which are medical. Thus, an overall functional assessment is more holistic than the traditional medical

---

Material in this chapter is based on the following chapters in Cassel CK, Leipzig RM, Cohen HJ, Larson EB, Meier DE, eds. Geriatric Medicine: An Evidence-Based Approach, 4th ed. New York: Springer, 2003: Koretz B, Reuben DB. Instruments to Assess Functional Status, pp. 185–194. Reuben DB. Comprehensive Geriatric Assessment and Systems Approaches to Geriatric Care, pp. 195–204. Selections edited by Rainier P. Soriano.

evaluation. The ultimate goal of these evaluations is to improve or maintain function.

Conceptually, comprehensive geriatric assessment is a three-step process: (1) screening or targeting of appropriate patients; (2) assessment and development of recommendations; and (3) implementation of recommendations, including physician and patient adherence with recommendations. Each of these steps is essential if the process is to be successful at achieving health and functional benefits.

Frequently, assessment instruments are used in geriatric assessments to evaluate the various components of patients' lives that contribute to their overall well-being. These components, or domains, include cognitive function, affective disorders, sensory impairment, functional status, nutrition, mobility, social support, physical environment, caregiver burden, health-related quality of life, and spirituality. The results from an individual geriatric assessment can be used to establish a baseline for future comparisons, form diagnoses, monitor the course of treatment, provide prognostic information, and screen for occult conditions. A list of some suggested instruments appears in Table 2.1.

Screening and Selection of Appropriate Patients

Most CGA programs have used some type of identification of high risk (targeting) as a criterion for inclusion in the program. The purpose of such selection is to match health care resources to patient need. For example, it would be wasteful to have multiple health care professionals conduct assessments on older persons who are in good health and have only needs for preventive services. Rather the intensive (and expensive) resources needed to conduct CGA should be reserved for those who are at high risk of incurring adverse outcomes. Such targeting criteria have included chronological age, functional impairment, geriatric syndromes (e.g., falls, depressive symptoms, urinary incontinence, functional impairment), specific medical conditions (e.g., congestive heart failure), and expected high health care utilization.

Each of these criteria has been shown to be effective in identifying patients who may benefit from some type of geriatric assessment and management. However, none of these criteria are effective in identifying patients who would benefit from all geriatric assessment and management programs. Accordingly, the specific targeting criteria should be matched to the type of assessment and intervention that is being implemented.

Assessment and Development of Recommendations

Once patients have been identified as being appropriate for CGA, the traditional model of CGA invokes a team approach to assessment. Such teams are intended to improve quality and efficiency of care of needy older

TABLE 2.1. Suggested brief geriatric assessment instruments

Domain	Instrument	Sensitivity (%)	Specificity (%)	Time (min)	Cut point	Comments
Cognition Dementia	MMSE (3)	79–100[a]	46–100	9	<24[b]	Widely studied and accepted
	Timed Time and Change Test (8)	94–100	37–46	<2	<3sec for time and <10sec for change	Sensitive and quick
Delirium	CAM (12)	94–100	90–95	<5		Sensitive and easy to apply
Affective disorders	GDS 5 Question form (17)	97	85	1	2	Rapid screen
Visual impairment	Snellen chart (62)	Gold standard	Gold standard	2	Inability to read at 20/40 line 50% correct	Universally used
Hearing impairment	Whispered voice (23,62)	80–90	70–89	0.5		No special equipment needed
	Pure tone audiometry (23,25)	94–100	70–94	<5	Inability to hear ≥2 of 4 40-dB tones (0.5, 1, 2, and 3 kHz)	Can be performed by trained office staff
Dental health	DENTAL (28)	82	90	<2 (estimated)	Score of ≥2	
Nutritional status	Weight loss of >10lb in 6 months or weight <100lb (63)	65–70	87–88		Yes to either	
Gait and balance	Timed up-and-go test (46,63)	88	94	<1	>20 seconds	Requires no special equipment

[a] While some studies gave lower sensitivities, most studies of dementia subjects fall in this range (3).
[b] Cutoff is dependent on a number of variables including age, education, and racial or ethnic background (3).
Source: Koretz B, Reuben DB. Instruments to assess functional status. In: Cassel CK, Leipzig RM, Cohen HJ, et al, eds. Geriatric Medicine, 4th ed. New York: Springer, 2003.

persons by delegating responsibility to the health professionals who are most appropriate to provide each aspect of care. Appropriateness in this case indicates both special expertise (e.g., social workers have unique knowledge about community resources) and costs of providing care (e.g., a nurse may be able to conduct some medical assessments as well as a physician). Such team care requires a set of operating principles and governance. Otherwise, it can result in uncoordinated, redundant, or dysfunctional care.

Implementing Recommendations from the Comprehensive Geriatric Assessment

In inpatient settings where the assessment team has primary care of the patient, generally implementation of recommendations is not a problem, provided that there are adequate resources. However, patients may refuse to participate in diagnostic or therapeutic plans. When the CGA team is providing consultative services, the link between recommendations and implementation is less certain. In outpatient settings, the implementation of CGA recommendations is particularly tenuous because the process can fail at several points including lack of implementation of CGA recommendations by primary care physicians and poor adherence to CGA recommendations by patients. Successful strategies to increase adherence to CGA recommendations have included telephone calls from the primary care provider to the referring physician with follow-up patient-specific recommendations by mail, and patient and family education including empowerment techniques. Newer technologies, including fax and e-mail, are increasingly being used to communicate recommendations. Even when primary care physicians and patients are in agreement with CGA recommendations, access barriers to receiving indicated services may limit the effectiveness of outpatient CGA. These access barriers include lack of transportation, fragmented services, and gaps in insurance coverage. A potential solution to some of these obstacles is use of home health agencies, which can provide a wide range of services to those who are homebound.

The Comprehensive Geriatric Assessment Team

The composition of the CGA team has traditionally included core and extended team members. Core members evaluate all patients, whereas extended team members are enlisted to evaluate patients on an as-needed basis. Most frequently, the core team consists of a physician (usually a geriatrician), a nurse (nurse practitioner or nurse clinical specialist), and a social worker.

The extended members of the team include a variety of rehabilitation therapists (e.g., physical, occupational, speech therapy), psychologists or psychiatrists, dietitians, pharmacists, and other health professionals (e.g., dentists, podiatrists).

Regardless of the composition of the team, a key element is the training of the team (1) to ensure that team members have an adequate understanding of the CGA process; (2) to raise the level of expertise of team members in their specific contribution to the team; (3) to develop standard approaches to problems that are commonly identified through CGA; (4) to define areas of responsibility of individual team members; and (5) to learn to work effectively as a team.

Components of the Process of Care in the CGA

If CGA is to be effective, the following six components of the process of care must be addressed: (1) data gathering, (2) discussion among team members, (3) development of a treatment plan, (4) implementation of the treatment plan, (5) monitoring response to the treatment plan, (6) revising the treatment plan as necessary.

With increased flexibility in team structure and scheduling, team discussions in outpatient and home settings are increasingly changing from face-to-face meetings to conference calls or via Internet conferencing. In this manner, discussions can occur at convenient times, even though team members may be in geographically disparate locations. However, in inpatient settings, where discharge planning is an exceptionally important role for the team, most meetings still occur face-to-face.

Case (Part 2)

The patient's niece starts telling you her aunt's history. She says, "She lives alone. She shops and prepares food herself. However, last week she started to boil some water and completely forgot it was on the stove. The plastic cover was completely melted. When I asked her about this she said she just forgot. She often forgets where she has placed things. This has been going on for many years but has gotten worse just recently. Also, at one time she has fallen at home at night after tripping on a rug. She did not break anything, but bruised her shoulder and forehead. She also used to go to church almost every day but rarely goes now. She hardly socializes and prefers to stay at home and watch TV. She does not have any kids and we're her closest relatives. You also have to shout, she's very hard of hearing. She has the hearing aids but she doesn't like wearing them."

What dimensions of the comprehensive geriatric assessment need to be addressed in the patient?

Dimensions of Geriatric Assessment

Cognitive Function

Assessment of the cognition of elderly patients generally focuses on detection of dementia and delirium. Although these two conditions can be distinguished by time course, pathophysiology, and clinical features, they may coexist. In fact, the presence of dementia is a risk factor for the development of delirium in elderly hospitalized patients (1).

Cognitive Impairment

The prevalence of dementia, an acquired, progressive impairment of multiple cognitive domains, is age dependent. Therefore, the yield of screening for cognitive impairment increases as the population ages. Because the initial phases of impairment can be quite subtle, it can be difficult for a clinician to make the incidental discovery of cognitive impairment. Structured examination techniques may be helpful in detecting early dementia.

The most widely used assessment tool for cognitive status is the *Mini–Mental State Examination* (MMSE) (2). Originally developed to detect delirium, dementia, and affective disorders in inpatient settings, it has since been validated in a number of other settings (3). In a 5- to 10-minute period of time, the MMSE tests a number of cognitive domains: orientation, registration, attention and calculation, language, recall, and visual-spatial orientation. It is easy to apply and interpret. In fact, the instrument can be given by office staff after minimal training. The *Short Portable Mental Status Questionnaire* (4) is similar in design but has a more narrow focus. It requires that the patient answer many of the same orientation questions as the MMSE, but also asks for the name of the current and past president, the patient's mother's maiden name, and his or her birthday, address, and phone number. As the questionnaire is shorter, it takes less time to administer. A disadvantage to both of these performance tests is that they measure functions that are not particularly relevant in everyday life, such as drawing intersecting pentagons and performing serial subtraction.

Other useful and rapidly administered performance-based tests are the clock drawing task and the *Time and Change Test*. Several clock drawing tests and clock completions tests have currently been validated and they assess executive functioning and visuospatial skills. There are standardized scoring methods for the drawing (5), and one of these tests has been shown to have a high negative predictive value for Alzheimer's disease (6). The Time and Change Test is a brief performance-based test in which a patient must read a clock face set at 11:10 and separate one dollar in change from a collection of coins totaling $1.80 (7,8). It has been shown to be accurate for both inpatient and outpatient populations (7,8). To improve sensitivity, time thresholds may be applied; taking longer than 3 seconds to correctly tell the time and longer than 10 seconds to correctly make change indicates the need for further evaluation.

A very different type of cognitive assessment is the *Set Test* (9). As originally described, the patients are given four categories (colors, fruit, towns, and animals) and an unlimited amount of time to list as many members of that category as possible. The maximum score in each category is 10. A score under 5 is considered abnormal (10). This test examines a number of cognitive domains including language, executive function, and memory. Unimpaired older persons should be able to generate a list of 10 items within 1 minute. (See Chapter 13: Depression, Dementia, Delirium, page 216.)

Delirium

Delirium is an acute, fluctuating alteration in level of consciousness and attention. It is a common occurrence, particularly in hospitalized elderly patients. Because its manifestations can be variable, it is often overlooked. Delirium is associated with increased morbidity and cost of care.

Several assessment instruments can facilitate the detection of delirium (11). The most commonly used is the *confusion assessment method* (CAM) (12). When using it, the examiner diagnoses delirium based on the demonstration of (1) an altered mental status with an acute onset and fluctuating course, (2) impaired attention, and (3) either disorganized thinking or a change in level of consciousness. Its high sensitivity and brevity make the confusion assessment method a clinically useful instrument. Clinical tests of attention, such as digit span or stating the months of the year backward, may also help detect delirium at an early stage. Because of the temporal variability that is the hallmark of delirium, a patient may seem entirely lucid at the time of evaluation. (See Chapter 13: Depression, Dementia, Delirium, page 236.)

Case (Part 3)

The patient says, "I don't know why I'm here. Oh, I remember that time when I left the pot on the stove. Well I just forgot. Do you know how old I am? I'm 84 years old and my memory is not what it used to be. I go to the shop myself when my knees don't hurt. Usually I just eat whatever is left over in my refrigerator when I don't get to the store. I also fell one time, I think. I had to go to the bathroom and I fell. I hit my head but it wasn't bad. I didn't break any bones or anything. I don't go out much. I'm alone most of the time. I love going to church but I couldn't hear what my minister is saying. I also couldn't read the program. Well I'm 84 years old and it comes with age. I have a hearing aid but they don't work. I take my medicines but I don't remember what they are but I do take them!"

What additional dimensions of the geriatric assessment need to be addressed based on the patient's story?

Affective Disorders

Depression is one of the most common psychiatric disorders affecting older persons. It is associated with significant morbidity and mortality (13). The earliest depression scales relied heavily on the presence of somatic symptoms (14,15). Hence, the scales may be less useful for geriatric populations with a high prevalence of such symptoms due to other comorbid medical illness (16). The *Geriatric Depression Scale* (GDS) was specifically designed for elderly patients (17). Initially validated in a 30-question format, a 15-question version also has been validated, and a five-item version has been described (18,19). The threshold scores for a positive depression screen are 15, 5, and 2, respectively (17–19). An even more concise approach, a single-question screen, "Do you ever feel sad or depressed?" has been validated (20). The single question may be as accurate in identifying depression as the 30-item GDS (21), although this technique identifies too many false positives to be useful as a screening instrument (22). (See Chapter 13: Depression, Dementia, Delirium, page 227.)

Visual Impairment

The leading causes of visual loss in older adults—cataract, glaucoma, age-related macular degeneration, and diabetic retinopathy—are prevalent and treatable. One accepted method of screening is having patients read the letters from the handheld Jaeger card at a distance of 14 inches from their eyes. Decreased visual acuity is defined as the patient being unable to read the 20/40 line. The wall-mounted Snellen chart, generally considered to be the gold standard, can be similarly used. Visual acuity tests do not assess the functional impact of visual impairment. Self-report instruments such as the Activities of Daily Vision Scale (23), the Visual Function (VF-14) (24), and the National Eye Institute Visual Function Questionnaire (25) assess patients' perceptions of impairments of their visual function. (See Chapter 9: Vision and Hearing Impairment, page 143.)

Case (Part 4)

On your examination, the patient is in no distress. Her blood pressure (BP) = 170/80mmHg, heart rate (HR) = 72/min, respiration rate (RR) = 18/min afebrile. She has cataracts on both eyes with the left lens more opaque than the right. On otoscopy, she has impacted cerumen in both ears, thus the tympanic membranes were not visualized. The rest of her exam are unremarkable.

Hearing Impairment

Hearing impairment can result in social isolation, depression, and decreased functional status. Treatment by amplification with a hearing aid has been demonstrated to improve quality of life. Analogous to the visual impairments screens, both performance-based and self-reported measuring tools are used to determine hearing loss.

Performance tests include the whispered voice, finger rub, and tuning forks. Of these, the *whispered voice test* has been shown to have acceptable sensitivity and specificity to be useful as a screen (26). The examiner performs it by initially asking the patient to repeat a series of words. Then the examiner stands out of sight of the patient, occludes one of the patient's ears, and whispers one of the previously spoken words at a minimum of 6 cm from the patient's ear. A passing score is the ability to correctly repeat at least 50% of the whispered words. Screening can also be accomplished with the audioscope, a hand-held otoscope with a built-in audiometer capable of delivering a 40-dB tone at 500, 1000, 2000, and 4000 Hz frequencies. Patients fail the screen if they are unable to hear at least two of the four tones. Compared to pure tone audiometry, the audioscope has a sensitivity of 94% and a specificity of 72% for detecting hearing impairment. Its positive predictive value is 60% (27). (See Chapter 9: Vision and Hearing Impairment, page 152.)

Dental Health

Dental disease, like visual or hearing impairment, requires a specialist for management. Nevertheless, primary care providers should recognize dental problems and the resulting functional impact so that they can make appropriate referrals. Two of the assessment instruments available are the *Geriatric Oral Health Assessment Index* (GOHAI) and the *DENTAL instrument*. The GOHAI (28) is a 12-item self-report measure that assesses the impact of oral disease in three domains: physical function, psychosocial function, and discomfort. It is sensitive to the change of function and symptoms that occur after the subject receives dental care (29). The DENTAL instrument, on the other hand, is used for screening purposes and to provide dental referrals from primary care practices (30). It is composed of a list of six conditions: dry mouth, oral pain, oral lesions, difficulty eating, altered food selection, and no recent dental care. The presence of one of the first three or two of the latter three conditions should trigger a dental referral.

Case (Part 5)

On your assessment, the patient has a MMSE of 24/30, a 15-item GDS score of 7, and a timed Up and Go Test of >20 seconds. She says that she rarely socializes due to fear of embarrassment. The patient says that she is independent on all activities of daily living (ADLs) and most instrumental activities of daily living (IADLs). She needs assistance with her housework, medication management, and money matters.

Functional Status

Functional status has been defined as "a person's ability to perform tasks and fulfill social roles associated with daily living across a broad range of complexity" (31). Measures of functional status are used for a wide variety of purposes. Clinicians apply them to establish baselines, to monitor the course of treatment, or for prognostic purposes.

Examinations of function may be divided into three levels: *basic* activities of daily living (BADL) (32), *instrumental* activities of daily living (IADL) (33), and *advanced* activities of daily living (AADL) (34). Basic activities of daily living refer to those functions that are necessary, but not sufficient, for maintaining an independent living status. Katz et al. (32) describe basic functional tasks: feeding, maintaining continence, transferring, toileting, dressing, and bathing. Individuals with multiple dysfunctions at this level require significant in-home support, such as 24-hour care, or nursing home admission.

Instrumental activities of daily living are more complicated levels of activity that are necessary to maintain an independent household. These include tasks such as paying bills, taking medications, shopping, and preparing food. People with several deficiencies in these areas usually require an assisted living, extensive community services, or some in-home support. At this level, opportunity and motivation are important contributors to maintaining function (35).

The highest level of activity is represented by the AADL. These are tasks such as working, attending religious services, volunteering, and maintaining hobbies. These are the most complex and require the highest level of multiple abilities to complete and thus the most sensitive to changes in health status.

Performance-based measures of functional status provide useful prognostic information. Several instruments have been developed including those that focus on lower extremity function (e.g., standing balance, gait speed, and rising from a chair) (36) and those that include upper extremity function (37). These instruments predict functional decline, institutionalization, and mortality.

Nutritional Status

Malnutrition occurs frequently among elderly patients, particularly those residing in nursing facilities. It has been associated with increased mortality, morbidity, and admission to nursing homes (38).

Nutritional status can be evaluated by self-report screens, biochemical markers, and anthropometric measures. The most widely used self-report screen is the 10-question, self-administered checklist portion of the *Nutrition Screening Initiative* (39,40). A score of six or more indicates that a patient is at risk for malnutrition. If patients score at this level, they are prompted to see health care providers for more in-depth evaluations. Checklist scores can predict future disability and identify persons at high risk for hospitalization (41).

Biochemical markers, though not specific for malnutrition, can be used as prognostic indicators. The most studied serum marker is the *serum albumin*. It predicts morbidity and mortality in community-dwelling, hospitalized, and institutionalized patients (42). Hypocholesterolemia is also associated with increased mortality (43). The combination of hypoalbuminemia and hypocholesterolemia can be used to predict long-term mortality and functional decline (44).

Anthropometric tools have been used to assess nutrition. The easiest one for the primary practitioner to employ is the *body mass index* (BMI). It is calculated by dividing the body weight in kilograms by the square of the height in meters. A BMI of less than 22 indicates undernutrition and predicts future mortality (45). Measurements of skin folds assess nutritional status. However, these measurements require specialized equipment and training and may not be reliable in elderly patients. (See Chapter 11: Nutrition, page 177.)

Gait and Balance Impairment

Falls are a major cause of morbidity and mortality in geriatric patients. Assessments of gait and balance impairment should begin with the clinician asking patients about their histories of falls, including frequency, resulting injury, and circumstances surrounding each incident. However, because many patients do not recall previous falls (46), self-report measures alone may not be sufficient. Performance-based assessment instruments can be more useful. For example, the *Performance-Oriented Assessment of Mobility* (47) employs a series of simple tasks: sitting and standing balance, turning, standing without the use of upper extremities for a push-off, and gait. Five other common maneuvers—head turning, reaching, bending over, back extension, and standing on one leg—can be added for a further assessment of balance. All of these simulate real-life situations in which the patient may be at increased risk for falls. While impairment in these activities is not diagnostic of a particular pathologic process, clinicians can use this information to identify those in need of further diagnostic evaluation.

Other screening instruments include the *Timed Up-and-Go Test* (48) and *functional reach* (49). In the Timed Up-and-Go Test, patients arise from a seated position, walk 3 meters, turn around, return to the chair, and sit down. A healthy, elderly individual should be able to complete this task in less than 10 seconds; any result greater than 20 seconds should prompt a more in-depth evaluation. This test may also be useful to follow patients over time for functional decline.

Although falls themselves create disability, even the fear of falling can produce functional limitation. The Survey of Activities and Fear of Falling in the Elderly is an instrument designed to evaluate how this fear contributes to the restriction of physical activity (50). (See Chapter 20: Instability and Falls, page 356.)

Social Support

There is a strong association between patients' social functioning and health status. Clinicians should be familiar with their patients' levels of social interaction. During times of physical or emotional stress, these social networks may mean the difference between remaining independent in the community or requiring nursing home care. As part of the social history, the health care provider should ask about who lives with the patient, who provides meals and transportation if the patient is unable to do so, and if the patient provides care for anyone else. These questions are particularly important because any subsequent absence of a caregiver, if present, would have major implications for the patient's well-being. (See Chapter 6: Psychosocial Influences in Health in Late Life, page 80.)

Environment

Although physicians rarely perform home safety evaluations themselves, many home health providers are trained to do so. These evaluations are covered by Medicare for those who are eligible for home health services. Environmental hazards that may lead to falls are common in community-based housing and in retirement communities (51). The most common hazards are poor lighting, pathways that are not clear, and loose rugs or other slip and trip threats. (See Chapter 20: Instability and Falls, page 366.)

Case (Part 6)

The patient's niece adds, "She has been followed-up at the medical clinic for more than 10 years but she has had sporadic visits. She was hospitalized before for blood clots in the legs that actually went to her lungs. She had a colonoscopy 2 years ago and they found this growth. They did a biopsy and they said it wasn't cancer. I have all of her medicines with me. She has glaucoma and she takes these eye drops on both eyes. She also has this 'water pill' that she takes for her high blood pressure. She also has a cane to help her but she doesn't use it outside the house. She says it's 'too obvious.'" The patient's niece was almost tearful when she was telling you all of this. She says that she feels frustrated. She is a mother of four children herself.

Caregiver Burden

Because dementia and other chronic illnesses affecting the elderly are prevalent, older persons are frequently caregivers for their spouses or other relatives. The psychological, physical, and economic burden associated with caregiving can be substantial. Moreover, such stress also has effects on patients who are recipients of care. Increased caregiver burden independently predicts use of medical services and nursing home placement (52). Interventions to decrease the stress of caregivers may delay nursing home placement (53).

Scales to assess caregiver burden are primarily used for research (54), but some may have clinical applications. The *Screen for Caregiver Burden* (55) evaluates spouse caregivers of patients with Alzheimer's disease. It is a 25-item self-administered questionnaire that is sensitive to changes over time. The *Caregiving Hassles Scale* also evaluates the stress experienced by the caregivers of family members with Alzheimer's disease (56). This 42-item self-administered instrument focuses on the minor irritations associated with providing care on a daily basis.

Quality of Life

Many elderly patients have chronic diseases that result in discomfort and disability. As it is impossible to cure these problems, the goal is to ameliorate suffering and improve patients' perceptions of their lives. Measurements of health-related quality of life provide feedback to researchers and clinicians so they can better target their efforts. Unfortunately, there is not yet any brief, widely accepted quality-of-life scale specifically targeting the geriatric population.

Spirituality

For many older patients, spiritual beliefs are very important components of quality of life. Furthermore, attendance at religious services has been associated with decreased mortality (57). The SPIRIT mnemonic provides a structure for taking a patient's spiritual history (58). The interview covers *S*piritual belief system, *P*ersonal spirituality, *I*ntegration within a spiritual community, *R*itualized practices and restrictions, *I*mplications for medical care, and *T*erminal events planning. These issues may be particularly important for patients who are approaching death. As with problems in other domains, clinicians should not hesitate to involve specialists. Clergy members can be helpful, especially during times of health crisis.

Strengths and Weaknesses of Instruments

Assessment instruments are simply tools to begin an evaluation process. It is easy to overestimate their value and make their application an end unto itself. The crucial step in the use of assessment instruments is the interpretation of their findings. Knowing how to proceed based on positive or negative results is one of the most important duties of the clinician.

The choice of which assessment instrument to use is based on a careful consideration of its relative strengths and weaknesses as they apply to a given clinical situation. For instance, comprehensive but lengthy interview-based questionnaires may be appropriate for research settings but not in clinical practice. Patients are usually unwilling to submit to prolonged interviews, and practitioners are unlikely to have enough time to conduct them. Thus, clinically useful assessment instruments must be concise.

An element to consider is the contrast between measures of capacity and those of performance. There are advantages and disadvantages to each approach. *Capacity* refers to what patients report they are able to do. As the task or skill at issue is not actually performed in an observed setting, the rating process can be completed quickly. Similarly, there is no need for any special equipment. The chief disadvantage of capacity assessment is the reliance on patients' subjective estimates of their abilities. Thus, clinicians frequently ask what patients actually do instead of what they can do. Because some patients function substantially below their capacity, this approach may underestimate their functional ability.

Performance-based measures are direct observations of particular actions. Advantages include an increase in objectivity as patients' biases and those of their proxies are minimized. Disadvantages include the need to train the observer and the costs for specialized equipment to create the task being observed—an audiometer to create a tone, stairs to climb, etc. Some tasks (e.g., role functions), however, cannot be measured in clinical settings. Patient factors may also affect the performance of the instrument in clinical settings. These include educational level, social background, gender, and ethnicity (59–61). An additional element—patient fatigue—can affect scores on cognitive or performance-based measures.

Finally, each test has a limited range in which it is sensitive. These are commonly referred to as ceiling and floor effects. A *ceiling effect* describes limited usefulness of an instrument because virtually everyone scores at the top. Conversely, a *floor effect* is when everyone scores at the bottom of the scales. For example, in a population of healthy community-dwelling older persons, the ceiling effect would apply if one measured BADL. Almost all of the patients are able to complete all of the relevant tasks. Similarly, in a nursing-home population, almost all patients will be dependent in all items of the IADL scale; thus the instrument does not capture a range of function—a floor effect.

Incorporating Assessment Instruments

The biggest challenge for clinicians with regard to assessment instruments is incorporating them into a busy practice. The particular combination of self-reported and performance instruments that results in the best yield, highest accuracy, and most efficient use of time varies from practice to practice. Similarly, how to best utilize trained ancillary staff to maximize the amount of useful information obtained during each office visit depends on the patient populations and resources of each practitioner. Finally, assessment instruments are valuable only if the practitioner can respond to abnormal findings. Hence, clinicians should be knowledgeable and skilled in the management of the conditions detected, including having referral resources available.

General Principles

- Geriatric assessment refers to an overall evaluation of the health status of the elderly patient. It is a three-step process: (1) screening or targeting of appropriate patients; (2) assessment and development of recommendations; and (3) implementation of recommendations, including physician and patient adherence with recommendations.
- Assessment instruments are used in geriatric assessments to evaluate the various components of patients' lives that contribute to their overall well-being. These components, or dimensions, include cognitive function, affective disorders, sensory impairment, functional status, nutrition, mobility, social support, physical environment, caregiver burden, health-related quality of life, and spirituality.
- Assessment instruments are simply tools to begin an evaluation process. It is easy to overestimate their value and make their application an end unto itself.

Suggested Readings

Koretz B, Reuben DB. Instruments to assess functional status. In: Cassel CK, Leipzig RM, Cohen HJ, et al., eds. Geriatric Medicine, 4th ed. New York: Springer, 2003:185–194.

Reuben DB. Comprehensive geriatric assessment and systems approaches to geriatric care. In: Cassel CK, Leipzig RM, Cohen HJ, et al., eds. Geriatric Medicine, 4th ed. New York: Springer, 2003:195–204.

Report of the U.S. Preventive Services Task Force. Guide to Clinical Preventive Services, 2nd ed. Alexandria, VA: International Medical Publishing, 1996. *A comprehensive review and guide to preventive care.*

References

1. Elie M, Cole MG, Pimeau FJ, et al. Delirium risk factors in elderly hospitalized patients. J Gen Intern Med 1998;13:204–212.
2. Folstein MF, Folstein SE, McHugh PR. Mini-mental state: a practical method for grading the cognitive state of patients for the clinician. J Psychiatr Res 1975;12:189–198.
3. Tombaugh TN, McIntyre NJ. The mini-mental state examination: a comprehensive review. J Am Geriatr Soc 1992;40:922–935.
4. Smyer MA, Hofland BF, Jonas EA. Validity study of the short portable mental status questionnaire for the elderly. J Am Geriatr Soc 1979;27: 263–269.
5. Sunderland T, Hill JL, Mellow AM, et al. Clock drawing in Alzheimer's disease: a novel measure of dementia severity. J Am Geriatr Soc 1989; 37:725–729.
6. Esteban-Santillan C, Praditsuwan R, Ueda H, et al. Clock drawing test in very mild Alzheimer's disease. J Am Geriatr Soc 1998;46:1266–1269.
7. Inouye SK, Robinson JR, Froehlich TE, et al. The time and change test: a simple screening test for dementia. J Gerontol 1998;53A:M281–286.
8. Froehlich TE, Robinson J, Inouye S. Screening for Dementia in the outpatient setting: the time and change test. J Am Geriatr Soc 1998;46:1506–1511.
9. Isaacs B, Akhtar AJ. The set test: a rapid test of mental function in old people. Age Ageing 1972;1:222–226.
10. Isaacs B, Kennie AT. The set test as an aid to the detection of dementia in old people. Br J Psychiatry 1973;123:467–470.
11. Trzepacz P. A review of delirium assessment instruments. Gen Hosp Psychiatry 1994;16:397–405.
12. Inouye SK, van Dyck CH, Alessi C, et al. Clarifying confusion: the confusion assessment method. Ann Intern Med 1990;113:941–948.
13. NIH consensus conference: diagnosis and treatment of depression in late life. JAMA 1992;268:1018–1024.
14. Beck AT, Ward CH, Mendelson M, et al. An inventory for measuring depression. Arch General Psychiatry 1961;4:561–571.
15. Zung WWK. A self-rating depression scale. Arch General Psychiatry 1965;12:63–70.

16. Van Gorp WG, Cummings JL, as cited by Applegate W, Blass JP, Williams TF. Instruments for the functional assessment of older patients. N Engl J Med 1990;322:1207–1213.
17. Yesavage JA, Brink TL. Development and validation of a geriatric depression screening scale: a preliminary report. J Psychiatr Res 1983;17:37–49.
18. Sheikh JI, Yesavage JA. Geriatric depression scale (gds): recent evidence and development of a shorter version. In: Brink TL, eds. Clinical Gerontology: A Guide to Assessment and Intervention. New York: Haworth, 1986.
19. Hoyl MT, Alessi CA, Harker JO, et al. Development and testing of a five-item version of the geriatric depression scale. J Am Geriatr Soc 1999;47:873–878.
20. Lachs M, Feinstein AR, Conney LM, et al. A simple procedure for general screening for functional disability in elderly patients. Ann Intern Med 1990;112:699–706.
21. Mahoney J, Drinka TJK, Abler R, et al. Screening for depression: single question versus GDS. J Am Geriatr Soc 1994;42:1006–1008.
22. Maly RC, Hirsch SH, Reuben DB. The performance of simple instruments in detecting geriatric conditions and selecting community-dwelling older people for geriatric assessment. Age Ageing 1997;26:223–231.
23. Mangione CM, Phillips RS, Seddon JM, et al. Development of the activities of daily vision scale. Med Care 1992;30:1111–1126.
24. Steinberg EP, Tielsch JM, Schein OD, et al. The vf-14 an index of functional impairment in patients with cataracts. Arch Ophthalmol 1994;112:630–638.
25. Mangione CM, Lee PP, Pitts J, et al. Psychometric properties of the national eye institute visual function questionnaire. Arch Ophthalmol 1998;116:1496–1504.
26. Uhlmann RF, Rees TS, Psaty BM, et al. Validity and reliability of auditory screening tests in demented and non-demented older adults. J Gen Intern Med 1989;4:90–96.
27. Lichtenstein MJ, Bess FH, Logan S. Validation of screening tools for identifying hearing impaired elderly in primary care. JAMA 1988;259:2875–2878.
28. Atchinson KA, Dolan TA. Development of the geriatric oral health assessment index. J Dental Educ 1990;11:680–687.
29. Dolan TA. The sensitivity of the geriatric oral health assessment index to dental care. J Dental Educ 1997;61:37–46.
30. Bush LA, Horenkamp N, Morley JE, et al. D-e-n-t-a-l: a rapid self-administered screening instrument to promote referrals for further evaluation in older adults. J Am Geriatr Soc 1996;44:979–981.
31. Reuben DB, Wieland DL, Rubensein LZ. Functional status assessment of older persons: concepts and implications. Facts Res Gerontol 1993;7:232.
32. Katz S, Downs TD, Crash H, et al. Progress in development of the index of ADL. Gerontologist 1970;10:20–30.
33. Lawton MP, Brody EM. Assessment of older people: self-maintaining and instrumental activities of daily living. Gerontologist 1969;9:179–186.
34. Reuben DB, Solomon DH. Assessment in geriatrics of caveats and names. J Am Geriatr Soc 1989;37:570–572.
35. Feinstein AR, Josephy BR, Wells CK. Scientific and clinical problems in indexes of functional disability. Ann Intern Med 1986;105:413–420.
36. Guralnik JM, Simonsick EM, Ferrucci L, et al. A short physical performance battery assessing lower extremity function: association with self-reported dis-

ability and prediction of mortality and nursing home admission. J Gerontol Med Sci 1994;49:M85–94.

37. Reuben DB, Siu AL. An objective measure of physical function of elderly patients: the physical performance test. J Am Geriatr Soc 1990;38:1105–1112.

38. Covinsky KE, Martin GE, Beyth RJ, et al. The relationship between clinical assessments of nutritional status and adverse outcomes in older hospitalized medical patients. J Am Geriatr Soc 1999;74:532–538.

39. White JV, Dwyer JT, Posner BM, et al. Nutrition screening initiative: development and implementation of the public awarness checklist and screening tools. J Am Diet Assoc 1992;92:163–167.

40. Lipshitz DA, Ham RJ, White JV. An approach to nutritional screening for older Americans. Am Fam Physician 1992;45:601–608.

41. Boult C, Krinke UB, Urdangarin CF, et al. The validity of nutritional status as a marker for future disability and depressive symptoms among high-risk older adults. J Am Geriatr Soc 1999;47:995–999.

42. Committee of Nutrition Services for Medicare Beneficiaries. Undernutrition. In: The Role of Nutrition in Maintaining Health in the Nation's Elderly. Evaluating Coverage of Nutrition Services for Medicare Beneficiaries. Washington DC: National Academy Press, 2000.

43. Harris T, Feldman JJ, Kleinman JC, et al. The low cholesterol-mortality association in a national cohort. J Clin Epidemiol 1992;45:595–601.

44. Reuben DB, Ix JH, Greendale GA, et al. The predictive value of combined hypoalbuminemia and hypocholesterolemia in high functioning community-dwelling older persons: MacArthur studies of successful aging. J Am Geriatr Soc 1999;47:402–406.

45. Landi F, Zuccali G, Gambassi G, et al. Body mass index and mortality among people living in the community. J Am Geriatr Soc 1995;47:1072–1076.

46. Cummings SR, Nevitt ML, Kidd S. Forgetting falls: the limited accuracy of recall of falls in the elderly. J Am Geriatr Soc 1988;36:613–616.

47. Tinetti ME. Performance-oriented assessment of mobility problems in elderly patients. J Am Geriatr Soc 1986;34:119–126.

48. Podsiadlo D, Richardson J. The timed "up and go": a test of basic functional mobility for frail elderly persons. J Am Geriatr Soc 1996;39:142–148.

49. Duncan PW, Weiner DK, Chandler J, et al. Functional reach: a new clinical measure of balance. J Gerontol Med Sci 1990;45:M192–M197.

50. Lachman ME, Howland J, Tennstedt S, et al. Fear of falling and activity restriction: the survey of activities and fear of falling in the elderly (safe). J Gerontol Pyschol Sci 1998;53:P43–P50.

51. Gill TM, Willimas CS, Robinson JT, et al. A population-based study of environmental hazards in the homes of older persons. Am J Public Health 1999;89:553–6.

52. Brown LJ, Potter JF, Foster BG. Caregiver burden should be evaluated during geriatric assessment. J Am Geriatr Soc 1990;38:455–460.

53. Mittelman MS, Ferris SH, Shulman E, et al. A family intervention to delay nursing home placement of patients with Alzheimer disease. JAMA 1996;276:1725–1731.

54. Vitaliano PP, Young HM, Russo J. Burden: a review of measures used among caregivers of individuals with dementia. Gerontologist 1991;31:67–75.

55. Vitaliano PP, Russo J, Young HM, et al. The screen for caregiver burden. Gerontologist 1991;31:76–83.
56. Kinney JM, Stephens MAP. Caregiving hassles scale: assessing the daily hassles of caring for a family member with dementia. Gerontologist 1989;29: 328–332.
57. Oman D, Reed D. Religion and mortality among the community dwelling elderly. Am J Public Health 1998;88:1469–1475.
58. Marrgans TA. The spiritual history. Arch Fam Med 1996;5:11–16.
59. O'Connor DW, et al. The influence of education, social class and sex on mini-mental state scores. Psychol Med 1989;19:771–776.
60. Tombaugh T, McIntyre N. The mini-mental state examination: a comprehensive review. J Am Geriatr Soc 1992;40:922–935.
61. Weiss B, Reed R, Kligman E, et al. Literacy and performance on the mini-mental state examination. J Am Geriatr Soc 1995;43:807–810.
62. Miller DK, Brunworth D, Brunworth, DS, et al. Efficiency of geriatric case finding in a private practitioner's office. J Am Geriatr Soc 1995;43:533–537.
63. Moore A, Siu A. Screening for common problems in ambulatory elderly: clinical confirmation of a screening instrument. Am J Med 1996;100:438–443.

3
Geriatric Pharmacology and Drug Prescribing for Older Adults

ROSANNE M. LEIPZIG

Learning Objectives

Upon completion of the chapter, the student will be able to:

1. Describe age-associated changes in pharmacokinetics and pharmacodynamics.
2. Describe common adverse drug effects and drug-disease interactions in older adults.
3. Identify methods for enhancing older patients' ability to manage their medications.

General Considerations

The proper use of medications represents one of the most crucial ways in which the practice of geriatric medicine differs from conventional medical care. Pharmacotherapy is probably the single most important medical intervention in the care of elderly patients, and its appropriate implementation requires a special understanding of the unique pharmacologic properties of drugs in this population, as well as a grasp of the clinical, epidemiologic, sociocultural, economic, and regulatory aspects of medication use in aging.

Material in this chapter is based on the following chapters in Cassel CK, Leipzig RM, Cohen HJ, Larson EB, Meier DE, eds. Geriatric Medicine: An Evidence-Based Approach, 4th ed. New York: Springer, 2003: Avorn J, Gurwitz JH, Rochon P. Principles of Pharmacology, pp. 65–81. Beizer JL. Clinical Strategies of Prescribing for Older Adults, pp. 83–89. Selections edited by Rosanne M. Leipzig.

Case A

You are seeing Ms. Clark for the first time. She is an 88-year-old woman who lives alone. She has long-standing hypertension, bipolar disorder, and a seizure disorder, all of which have been well controlled for years with verapamil 80 mg po three times a day, lithium 300 mg po three times a day, and phenytoin 300 mg nightly.

Over the past few years she has been eating poorly. Recently she has been feeling drowsy and woozy, a bit confused, with increased urination, nausea, and difficulty walking. She fell yesterday without loss of consciousness or head trauma.

Ms. Clark's exam is remarkable for a weight of 89 lb (40 kg), blood pressure of 110/60 mmHg lying down and 90/60 mmHg standing, nystagmus, an ataxic gait, and fine hand tremors. Laboratory results are all within normal limits except for blood urea nitrogen of 6 mg/dL, an albumin of 2.5 g/dL, and a white blood count (WBC) of 11,000. Creatinine is 1.0 mg/dL. Urine reveals no evidence of urinary tract infection (UTI). Lithium level is 1.5 (target 0.6 to 1.2 mEq/L) and phenytoin level is 15 (target 10–20).

• Is it possible that Ms. Clark's symptoms are due to her medications, even though she is taking them as prescribed?
• Does Ms. Clark appear to be clinically phenytoin toxic? Is her blood drug level above normal? How about her free drug level?
• Which of the medications Ms. Clark is taking has much greater bioavailability in older than younger adults? How would this affect the serum levels of the drug and the patient's response to the drug?
• Which of these medications is primarily renally excreted? What is Ms. Clark's estimated creatinine clearance?

Age-Associated Changes in Pharmacokinetics and Pharmacodynamics

Pharmacokinetics

Of the four traditional components of pharmacokinetics—*absorption, distribution, metabolism,* and *excretion*—only the last three are meaningfully affected by age. In the absence of malabsorptive syndromes, traditional oral formulations of drugs are absorbed as well in old age as in youth. The well-reported changes in gastric motility and blood flow to the gut with aging do not appear to alter meaningfully the efficiency with which medications move from the gastrointestinal tract into the systemic circulation

(1,2). However, data on the kinetics of slow-release, transdermal, transbuccal, and transbronchial drug administration in the elderly are too limited to allow conclusions regarding age-related changes in drug absorption via those routes (3), even though the elderly are among the most prominent users of such drug-delivery systems.

One aspect of drug distribution that varies importantly with age is the volume of distribution. This is the theoretical space in a given patient that a particular drug occupies. The volume of distribution is heavily influenced by the relative proportions of lean body mass versus fat. Because the latter increases in the elderly at the expense of the former, lipid-soluble drugs (such as some benzodiazepines) have a greater volume of distribution in an older patient, and water-soluble drugs (such as lithium) have a smaller volume of distribution (4). Combined with changes in clearance, these alterations in body composition can have important implications for both the half-life and the steady-state concentration of many medications. Women comprise an increasingly large majority of the aging population, making it important to also consider gender differences in drug distribution and effects. Women have a lower lean body mass compared with men at all ages, and there may also be gender differences in other pharmacokinetic and pharmacodynamic functions (5).

Drug Levels

An aspect of drug distribution that is not affected by normal aging is the binding of drugs to carrier proteins such as serum albumin (6,7). Despite these observations on serum proteins in healthy aging, it is crucial to consider that serum albumin levels may be markedly decreased in older patients suffering from malnutrition or severe chronic disease (8,9), with important consequences for drug binding.

Many assays measure the total amount of drug that is present in serum, both protein-bound and unbound ("free"). The unbound concentration is more clinically relevant than the total concentration because only unbound drug is pharmacologically active. For a patient with hypoalbuminemia or another deficiency in binding protein, any given serum drug level reflects a greater concentration of unbound drug than the same level would signify in a patient with normal protein-binding capacity. A hypoalbuminemic patient with a normal total serum drug concentration may actually have an unbound drug concentration that is unacceptably high. By contrast, the same patient with a slightly lower than normal total serum concentration may have an unbound drug concentration that is in a reasonable range. For extensively protein-bound drugs whose binding is reduced due to hypoproteinemia, clinicians should expect both therapeutic and toxic events at lower total serum concentrations (10). Phenytoin, which is highly bound to albumin, is one example of a drug for which the interpretation of serum levels reflecting total drug concentration (rather than the "free" drug concentration) can be difficult in malnourished or chronically ill elderly patients.

In evaluating serum drug levels in the older patient, it is also important to recall that the therapeutic range routinely reported on such assays may not be an accurate guide to either efficacy or toxicity in the geriatric patient. Such ranges have typically been defined in nonelderly subjects, and cannot take into account pharmacodynamic differences (see below) or idiosyncratic aspects of specific patients.

Drug Clearance and Aging

The liver represents the major site of metabolism for many medications. Normal aging is associated with a reduction in the liver mass, as well as in hepatic blood flow. These changes are likely responsible for the reduction in hepatic metabolism of drugs, which can be as large as 25% over the life span (11,12). Autopsy and ultrasound studies have found a progressive decrease in liver mass after age 50. Regional blood flow to the liver at age 65 is reduced by 40% to 45% relative to that in a 25-year-old; this observation may partially reflect a fall in cardiac output with advancing age. Such changes can also result in reduced clearance rates for drugs exhibiting flow-dependent clearance characteristics ("first-pass" effects) (13), such as verapamil, lidocaine, and labetalol. Interindividual variation in hepatic metabolizing capacity is substantial (14), suggesting that genetic, environmental, and other patient-specific factors often have a greater impact on hepatic drug metabolism than the aging process itself.

Renal Excretion

Several commonly used drugs are excreted primarily by the kidney, including digoxin, lithium, ranitidine, and the aminoglycoside antibiotics (15). Early cross-sectional studies of renal function in aging suggested that there is a linear decrease in renal function between young adulthood and old age, amounting on average to a reduction in glomerular filtration rate (GFR) by nearly a third (16). Although this is true in the aggregate, longitudinal studies indicate that some subjects evidence no changes or only small changes in creatinine clearance with advancing age; another subgroup showed a linear decrease with age; still others appeared to show some improvement in renal function as they got older (17). Thus, although the aggregate findings have been enshrined in conventional gerontologic wisdom and in nomograms used to calculate drug dosing with age, these longitudinal studies make it clear that the effect of age on renal function (and therefore on the excretion of many drugs) can be quite variable. Here, too, differences among patients often will be as important as the changes attributed to the aging process itself.

Although blood urea nitrogen (BUN) and serum creatinine levels may be useful (albeit crude) markers of renal function, it must be remembered that each is susceptible in its own way to perturbations that can occur with aging but have nothing to do with renal function itself. For example, the BUN reflects the concentration of urea in the blood. However, the origin of much of this urea is ingested protein, so that a malnourished older patient may not consume enough nitrogen to produce an appropriate rise in BUN, even in the face of renal impairment. Similarly, serum creatinine is produced by muscle, and if a patient has a markedly diminished muscle mass, whether due to chronic illness or any other cause, he or she may not produce enough creatinine to reflect a change in the ability of the kidney to excrete this substance. Thus, overreliance on a normal-appearing BUN and creatinine in older patients can severely underestimate the degree of renal impairment.

The *Cockcroft-Gault* formula (18) is sometimes used to estimate renal function in older patients who are to receive potentially nephrotoxic drugs (e.g., aminoglycosides) or drugs that are primarily excreted by the kidneys (e.g., digoxin):

$$\text{Estimated creatinine clearace} = \frac{(140 - \text{age}) \times (\text{body weight in kg})}{\text{Serum creatinine} \times 72}$$

For women, multiply the result by 0.85.

It should be emphasized that these estimates are valid only in patients whose renal function is in steady state and who are not taking medications that directly alter renal function or affect creatinine excretion. Although the formula has some utility in assessing renal function in healthy ambulatory individuals, it has limited utility and can be misleading in severely ill, clinically unstable, elderly patients (19).

Pharmacodynamics

Pharmacodynamic changes with aging (i.e., end-organ effects) have been more difficult to define than pharmacokinetic changes. The study of this phenomenon is complicated by the fact that the effect of many drugs is magnified in the elderly because of reduced drug clearance, resulting in higher serum level (20). Therefore, in studying the effects of aging on pharmacodynamics, one must control for the age-related changes in pharmacokinetics discussed above. Age-related changes in pharmacodynamics can result in greater therapeutic effect as well as an increased potential for toxicity. Increases in medication sensitivity with age have also been suggested for a number of other medications, including warfarin (21–23) and the opioids.

Case B

Ms. Abramson is a 75-year-old woman who lives alone in a second-story apartment. You are her primary care physician and treat her for hypertension, diabetes, and chronic obstructive pulmonary disease (COPD). Over the last year her blood pressure and hemoglobin A_{1c} have been out of control despite increases and changes in medication. She has had three hospitalizations for COPD exacerbations, which always respond to a prednisone burst and taper. Her current medications are: losartan 50 mg po twice a day, verapamil 80 mg po three times a day, pioglitazone (Actos) 45 mg po daily, metformin 1000 mg po twice a day, flunisolide (AeroBid) inhaler 2 puffs twice a day, ipratropium bromide (Atrovent) inhaler 2 to 3 puffs 3–4 times daily, esomeprazole (Nexium) 40 mg po daily.

- How can you determine if this medication regimen is accurate?
- How can you determine if Ms. Abramson is complying with this medication regimen?
- What might contribute to Ms. Abramson being noncompliant with this medication regimen?
- What is the monthly cost of this medication regimen? Yearly cost?

Clinical Strategies for Prescribing for Older Adults

Before even considering any of the issues involving drug therapy in a given patient, it is essential that the prescriber know exactly what medications the patient is taking. This can be achieved by taking a thorough and accurate medication history, as detailed in Table 3.1.

TABLE 3.1. Taking an accurate and thorough medication history

1. Specifically ask about:
   a. Prescription medications
   b. Over-the-counter (OTC) products
   c. As needed (prn) medications
   d. Vitamins and minerals
   e. Herbal products
   f. Home remedies
   g. Other health care providers seen since the patient's last visit with you
2. How to be thorough:
   a. Ask by category of product (pills, patches, injections, suppositories)
   b. Ask by review of symptoms (anything for your eyes, ears, etc?)
   c. Have patient bring in all medications and medicinal products
3. End with: "Do you do anything else for your health?"

Source: Leipzig RM. Prescribing: keys to maximizing benefit while avoiding adverse drug effects. Geriatrics 2001 Feb;56(2):30–34, with permission.

Minimizing Overmedication

One of the most crucial elements of geriatric pharmacotherapy is not to overmedicate the patient. *Polypharmacy*, the use of many medications, is a major cause of noncompliance, adverse effects, and drug interactions. Before adding a new medication to a patient's regimen, current therapy should be assessed. Questions that should be addressed include: Is the new symptom a side effect of an existing medication? Can the problem be handled by adjusting the dose of current medications or discontinuing a medication? An important point to remember is that it is usually easier not to start a medication that may not be necessary than it is to stop a current medication.

When choosing the dose of a medication for an older patient, the motto has always been "start low, go slow." The other half of that statement should be "but don't stop too soon." Although doses of medications used for the elderly should be held to a minimum, the right dose for an elderly patient is the dose that is both effective and well tolerated. Initially, doses should be modified based on pharmacokinetic predictions, but actual pharmacodynamic responses to the medication should then be used to adjust the dose. When pharmacokinetic data are not available, doses can be initiated at one-half the usual adult dose, whenever practical. This can be achieved by splitting tablets or by extending the dosing interval. Some manufacturers, realizing the need for smaller doses in the elderly, have marketed smaller dosage forms or liquid formulations to facilitate dosing.

When withdrawing medications thought to be unnecessary, it is crucial to monitor the patient for recurrence of symptoms. The most common medications associated with adverse drug withdrawal events (ADWEs) were cardiovascular, central nervous system, and gastrointestinal drugs.

Maximizing Compliance

Noncompliance can be defined as a patient's intentional or unintentional deviation from the medication regimen prescribed or recommended by the health care professional. Noncompliance includes omitting doses, adding doses, taking doses at the wrong time, and incorrectly administering the medication, to name only a few noncompliant behaviors.

Studies reporting compliance rates in elderly patients have found that the adherence rate ranges from 26% to 59%. In the elderly, there are numerous causes of noncompliance or barriers to good compliance with medication regimens. Attitudes about illness, aging, and even the medications themselves can impair compliance. Medications may be a reminder of illness and growing older, and the patient may resist or ignore the medications. Living alone, with no support system to remind the patient to take the medication, may also lead to noncompliance.

Studies on compliance measures have shown that no one intervention is universally better than another. Rather, as in Table 3.2, a compliance plan should be individualized to the needs of the patient and should include a combination of interventions focusing on behavioral as well as educational interventions.

Medication Administration Skills and Compliance Aids

Changes in functional and cognitive status are some of the key causes of noncompliance, and creative solutions are sometimes needed to overcome these barriers. One of the simplest ways to assess compliance is to watch the patient take the medication. Assessment of elderly patients' functional ability to take medication has been reported in several studies. Tablet splitters and crushers can be used for those patients who have difficulty swallowing tablets. Before splitting or crushing a tablet, the patient or prescriber should check with the pharmacist or the manufacturer's information to make sure that the medication will not be affected by breaking the tablet. Sustained-release formulations and enteric-coated medications should not be split or crushed.

Patients with difficulties with special dosage forms should be referred to their pharmacist, who can recommend compliance aids. For example, for diabetics, there are magnifiers that fit onto the insulin syringes. For liquid

TABLE 3.2. Maximizing compliance

1. Simplify the number of medications and doses per day.
2. Discuss with the patient whether they can open child-resistant caps.
3. Prescribe generics when available. Know differences in costs between drugs in the same class.
4. Provide the patient and family/caregiver with written information containing:
   a. The name of the medication and its indication
   b. Dose and schedule of the medication and how long to take it
   c. What to avoid while on the medication
   d. Major adverse effects and what to do if they occur
5. Use patient education materials modified for elders:
   a. Reading materials that use a large font size and have a reading level not greater than 6th grade
   b. Black print on non-glare white or yellow paper to ease the readability
6. Watch the patient administer the medication.
   a. Have the patient open the vial, count out the correct number of tablets or capsules, and swallow them.
   b. As needed, check technique for using inhalers, instilling ophthalmic preparations, injecting insulin, measuring liquids or applying a transdermal patch or creams and ointments.
7. Refer to pharmacist for compliance aids.
8. Suggest reminder aids such as a calendars, medication boxes

Source: Leipzig RM. Prescribing: keys to maximizing benefit while avoiding adverse drug effects. Geriatrics 2001 Feb;56(2):30–34, with permission.

medications, there are a variety of dosing spoons, cups, and oral syringes. Even transdermal patches can present a problem. An elderly patient with visual problems or arthritis may have difficulty peeling off the protective backing on the patch. Very small vials may be difficult to manage for a patient with severely arthritic hands or who has hemiplegia. In these cases, a larger vial may be easier to grasp.

Specific dosage forms may be particularly difficult for the older patient to manage. Seventy percent of patients in one study could not adequately instill an ophthalmic preparation into their eyes. Eye drop guides, which fit onto the eye drop bottle, can help steady the hand and direct the drop into the eye. When using the guide, the percent of people who could instill a drop on the first try increased from 20% to 87%.

In all patients, difficulties in properly using a metered-dose inhaler (MDI) can impair the effectiveness of the medication. Newer versions of MDIs are breath-activated, making it easier for older patients who may not be able to coordinate their breathing with pressing down on the canister. Additionally, there are a variety of devices that can adapt MDIs for patients with arthritis, making it easier to press down on the canister. There are various inhalation aids and spacer devices, such as the InspirEase® and Aerochamber®, which can improve the delivery of the medication to the airways.

Even child-resistant caps, which have been required on prescription medications in the United States since 1970, can be barriers to compliance in the older patient. It is the responsibility of the prescriber and the pharmacist to ask elderly patients if they need a non–child-resistant cap. The prescriber can note it on the prescription or the patient can tell the pharmacist directly. The pharmacist should document this information on the individual's patient profile for further prescriptions.

Visual problems can affect patients' ability to read the medication label or patient education material and may even impair their ability to discriminate between colors of tablets. Decreased hearing can make patient counseling challenging for the health professional. When interacting with sensory-impaired patients, it is important to ensure that they are accurately receiving the information.

If despite compliance aids the patient is still having difficulty administering the medication, alternative dosage forms may be necessary. For example, a patient having difficulty with a transdermal nitroglycerin patch may be better managed on isosorbide mononitrate once a day. In other cases, a family member or caregiver may need to be trained to help with the medications.

Other Methods for Reducing Noncompliance

Table 3.2 describes ways that prescribers can maximize compliance. The first step to improve compliance should be to simplify the regimen. The minimum number of medications and doses per day should be the goal. It is advisable to avoid medications that need to be given more than twice a day. The use of sustained-release dosage forms or taking advantage of prolonged elimination half-lives in the elderly can decrease the number of doses per day. For example, ciprofloxacin can often be dosed once a day in elderly patients. Scheduling is also important as to the time of day. Medications that can cause drowsiness should be dosed at bedtime.

Financial issues can force patients to compromise their compliance. Many elderly patients do not have prescription coverage. As the cost of medication soars, elderly patients on fixed incomes may have difficulty affording their drug therapy. Prescribers need to learn the costs of medications, specifically the cost of 30 days at a geriatric dose. It is also useful to be familiar with therapeutic alternatives, and which one is most cost effective. For example, one angiotensin-converting enzyme (ACE) inhibitor may be less expensive than another.

It is also important to be aware of which medications are available generically. There are little data on the use of generic medications in the elderly and whether any significant pharmacokinetic or pharmacodynamic changes are evident. For verapamil, even though a significant amount of variability is seen in the maximum serum concentration and the area under the curve in older adults, no clinically significant differences were found. A study comparing generic warfarin and the brand Coumadin found no significant difference between the two products in respect to their average international normalized ratio (INR) values. The median age of that study population was 79 years (range 42–96). Patient education about the safety and appropriateness of generics may help improve their acceptance.

Simply remembering to take the medication can be difficult for the cognitively impaired patient. There are a variety of reminder aids that can be used to help patients remember to take their medications. The simplest method is to design a calendar that lists the medications and the time of day to take them. The calendar can be posted on the refrigerator or other prominent place in the home. Weekly or monthly calendar cards with boxes to check off each dose can be used and correlated with tablet counts to assess level of compliance.

There are commercially available medication boxes that can aid in compliance. These boxes hold one day or one week of medication and some have compartments for up to four dosing times per day. There are electronic aids that have been developed. These devices can be set to beep at the correct times and some even provide a warning if a dose has been missed. Some systems are locked and tamper-proof and will actually dispense the medication only at the correct time.

For more severely impaired patients, actions requiring judgment, such as recognizing adverse events or self-monitoring their therapy, may be impossible. Simplifying the regimen, reminder aids, and family or caregiver involvement are the best methods to improve compliance in these patients. One of the medication noncompliance problems that is often overlooked is the reasons for family caregiver difficulties has with (1) giving medications to a confused or uncooperative person, (2) working the medication schedule into the care routines, and (3) recognizing adverse or toxic effects. Thus, family caregivers must be given proper instructions on how to administer medications and be educated about the medications themselves.

Case C

Mr. Thompson, a 77-year-old man, has been having problems sleeping due to extreme anxiety. Dr. Reed, his 32-year-old doctor, concerned about the unintentional consequences of medications in older adults, read that lorazepam is one of the best benzodiazepines to use in the elderly because the pharmacokinetics and the percentage decline in memory are the same as in younger adults. Having taken the medication himself previously, Dr. Reed felt he experienced few, if any, memory changes with the drug. He therefore prescribed Mr. Thompson loraze-pam, 1.0 mg po nightly. Three weeks later the patient's family members reported that they had considerable concerns that Mr. Thompson was developing dementia, as his short-term memory was getting much worse.

- Could the lorazepam be causing impairment in short-term memory?
- What is the mechanism for this concerning symptom?.

Adverse Drug Effects Associated with Commonly Used Drug Therapies

The diagnosis of drug-induced illness in elderly patients is further compli-cated by the lack of awareness of the physiology of normal aging, and by the tendency of patients, families, and even physicians to mislabel many symptoms as signs of "just growing old." As a result, drug-induced incon-tinence, confusion, fatigue, depression, and many other problems may be attributed to the human condition, when they may well be amenable to appropriate diagnosis and therapeutic action. A useful antidote to these problems is a very high index of suspicion for drug-induced illness in elderly patients. An overstatement that is of great clinical use and forms a good starting point for clinical evaluation can be stated as follows: *Any symptom in an elderly patient may be a drug side effect until proved otherwise.*

Psychoactive Drugs

Psychotropic drugs have been associated with the occurrence of hip fracture in a number of epidemiologic studies. One study examining risk for hip fracture in older patients exposed to psychotropic medications indicated that a significantly increased risk was associated with use of hypnotic-anxiolytics with long (>24 hour) elimination half-lives, tricyclic antidepressants, and neuroleptics (24). The long-elimination half-life hypnotics-anxiolytics included flurazepam, diazepam, and chlordiazepoxide. More recent studies have suggested that it is the dose of benzodiazepine rather than the drug's half-life that is the most important risk factor for drug-induced accidents (25,26). Until this issue is resolved, it is prudent to avoid both long-acting drugs and high doses of any benzodiazepine in older patients, unless there is a compelling reason to do otherwise.

The tricyclic antidepressants most often implicated in drug-induced injury in the elderly include the older tertiary amines amitriptyline, doxepin, and imipramine. However, more recent findings suggest that risk of falls and fractures is seen as well with selective serotonin reuptake inhibitors (SSRIs) as well as with the older heterocyclic antidepressants (27,28). Indeed, one study found that depressed older patients appeared to be at increased risk of falls even before antidepressant therapy had been started.

Anticoagulants

Long-term oral anticoagulant therapy with warfarin is essential for the management or prevention of many thromboembolic and vascular disorders whose prevalence is increased in elderly patients (29). In fact, anticoagulation in patients with chronic nonrheumatic atrial fibrillation can reduce the risk of stroke by more than two thirds. However, willingness to initiate anticoagulant therapy in an older patient is often tempered by concerns about the risk of bleeding, despite the fact that these patients may have the most to gain from anticoagulant therapy. The extent of anticoagulation, as reflected by the INR, is the dominant risk factor for hemorrhagic complications (31). Several studies have presented conflicting findings on whether there is a greater risk of anticoagulant-induced hemorrhage in elderly patients. This may be explained to a large extent by differences in treatment setting and in the attention given to monitoring (31,32). Specialized anticoagulation consultation services and clinics can assess risks for bleeding, monitor closely for potential warfarin-drug interactions, and pay close attention to target therapeutic ranges. Risk of anticoagulant-related bleeding appears to be reduced when expert consultation is provided at the start of anticoagulant therapy and when patients are monitored in specialized anticoagulation clinics (33,34). Careful assessment of the appropriate indications for anticoagulant therapy, the optimal target INR, and the use of potentially interacting medications are the most important strategies for reducing the risk of bleeding complications in older patients.

Nonsteroidal Antiinflammatory Drugs

The elderly are among the most frequent users of nonsteroidal antiinflammatory drugs (NSAIDs). The NSAIDs inhibit cyclooxygenase, a major enzyme in the synthesis of prostaglandins. Prostaglandins also mediate a variety of important protective physiologic effects. For example, prostaglandins maintain renal blood flow and glomerular filtration when the effective or actual circulatory volume decreases (e.g., congestive heart failure, cirrhosis with ascites, volume depletion due to diuretic therapy, and hemorrhage with hypotension). Under such conditions, vasodilatory renal prostaglandins mitigate vasoconstrictive effects on renal blood flow, maintaining renal perfusion and preventing prerenal azotemia and eventual ischemic damage to the kidney. When this prostaglandin-mediated compensatory mechanism is suppressed by NSAID therapy, impairment in renal function can result. A prospective study of elderly residents of a large long-term care facility who were newly treated with NSAID therapy demonstrated that 13% developed azotemia over a short course of therapy (35). Risk factors associated with this adverse effect included higher NSAID dosage and concomitant loop diuretic therapy.

Prostaglandins also mediate a range of effects that protect the mucosa of the stomach and duodenum from injury. These include the inhibition of acid secretion, an increase in mucus secretion and bicarbonate, and enhancement of mucosal blood flow. When the biosynthesis of prostaglandins is impaired by NSAIDs, this can lead to impaired mucosal defense; acid and peptic activity can then produce ulcers. A meta-analysis of epidemiologic studies investigating the association between NSAIDs and severe upper gastrointestinal tract disease indicated that old age was associated with a higher risk of gastrointestinal toxicity (36).

To limit the occurrence of side effects, NSAID therapy should be limited to those clinical situations where it is absolutely required. The lowest feasible dose should be prescribed for the shortest time necessary to achieve the desired therapeutic effect. Because of the iatrogenic nature of these disorders, the best treatment for NSAID-associated nephrotoxicity or gastropathy is discontinuation of the NSAID. Alternative analgesic therapies are available and effective for many patients. For example, nonacetylated salicylates may be a safer alternative to NSAIDs. Another effective analgesic choice is acetaminophen. One study comparing the analgesic effects of acetaminophen (4 g per day) to ibuprofen (1.2 g per day and 2.4 g per day) in patients with osteoarthritis found no difference in pain relief in patients treated with acetaminophen compared to those given NSAID therapy (37). Although acetaminophen is free of NSAID-related side effects, its use should not exceed 4 g per day in most patients; its toxicity is increased in the presence of hepatic insufficiency, heavy alcohol intake, or fasting (38).

Cyclooxygenase-2 receptors (COX-2 inhibitors) are similar to nonselective NSAIDs in terms of efficacy. Relative to nonselective NSAIDs, COX-2 inhibitors are less likely to produce gastrointestinal ulcers, although ulcers do occur and this complication can be serious and even fatal. The COX-2 inhibitors have a similar effect as NSAIDs on renal function in older adults, decreasing GFR (40). In addition, due to cardiovascular side effects (myocardial infarction and stroke), some of these medications have been withdrawn from the market, which has led to the overall decrease in utilization of this class of medications. These findings indicate the need for caution when prescribing COX-2 inhibitors to older adults.

General Principles

- Of the four components of pharmacokinetics—absorption, distribution, metabolism and secretion—only the last three are meaningfully affected by age.
- Dosages for older adults: start low, go slow . . . BUT don't stop too soon!
- Any symptom in an elderly patient may be a drug side effect until proven otherwise.
- A normal serum creatinine does NOT mean normal GFR in an older person. Estimate creatinine clearance before prescribing a renally excreted drug to an older person.

Suggested Readings

Avorn J, Gurwitz JH, Rochon P. Principles of pharmacology. In: Cassel CK, Leipzig RM, Cohen HJ, et al., eds. Geriatric Medicine, 4th ed. New York: Springer, 2003:65–82.

Beizer JL. Clinical strategies of prescribing for older adults. In: Cassel CK, Leipzig RM, Cohen HJ, et al., eds. Geriatric Medicine, 4th ed. New York: Springer, 2003:83–89.

Leipzig RM. Prescribing. Keys to maximizing benefit while avoiding adverse drug effects. Geriatrics 2001;56(2):30–34. *A practical guideline on drug prescribing for older adults. Includes a very useful table on what drugs to avoid in older adults.*

References

1. Schmucker DL. Aging and drug disposition: an update. Pharmacol Rev 1985;37:133–148.

2. Castleden CM, et al. The effect of ageing on drug absorption from the gut. Age Ageing 1977;6:138–143.

3. Schwartz JB. Clinical pharmacology. In: Hazzard WR, Bierman EL, Blass JP, Ettinger WH Jr, Halter JB, eds. Principles of Geriatric Medicine and Gerontology, 3rd edition. New York: McGraw-Hill, 1994.

4. Frontera WR, Hughes VA, Lutz KJ, Evans WJ. A cross-sectional study of muscle strength and mass in 45- to 78-yr-old men and women. J Appl Physiol 1991;71:644–650.

5. Thurmann PA, Hompesch BC. Influence of gender on the pharmacokinetics and pharmacodynamics of drugs. Int J Clin Pharmacol Ther 1998;36:586–590.

6. Campion EW, deLabry LO, Glynn RJ. The effect of age on serum albumin in healthy males: report from the Normative Aging Study. J Gerontol 1988;43:M18–M20.

7. Grandiston MK, Boudinot FD. Age-related changes in protein binding of drugs: implications for therapy. Clinical Pharmacokinetics 2000;38:271–290.

8. MacLennan WJ, Martin P, Mason BJ. Protein intake and serum albumin levels in the elderly. Gerontology 1977;23:360–367.

9. Conti MC, Goralnik JH, Salive ME, Sarkin JD. Serum albumin level and physical disability as predictors of mortality in older persons. JAMA 1994;272:1036–1042.

10. Greenblatt DJ, Sellers EM, Koch-Weser J. Importance of protein binding for the interpretation of serum or plasma drug concentrations. J Clin Pharmacol 1982;22:259–263.

11. Vestal RE. Aging and pharmacology. Cancer 1997;80:1302–1310.

12. Kinirons MT, Crome P. Clinical pharmacokinetic considerations in the elderly. Clin Pharmacokinet 1997;33:302–312.

13. Mooney H, Roberts R, Cooksley WGE, et al. Alterations in the liver with aging. Clin Gastroenterol 1985;14:757–771.

14. Vestal RE, Norris AH, Tobin JD, et al. Antipyrine metabolism in man: influence of age, alcohol, caffeine, and smoking. Clin Pharmacol Ther 1975;18:425–432.

15. Muhlberg W, Platt D. Age-dependent changes of the kidneys: pharmacological implications. Gerontology 1999;45:243–253.

16. Rowe JW, Andres R, Tobin JD, et al. The effect of age on creatinine clearance in man. J Gerontol 1976;31:155–163.

17. Lindeman RD, Tobin JD, Shock NW. Longitudinal studies on the rate of decline in renal function with age. J Am Geriatr Soc 1985;33:278–285.

18. Cockcroft DW, Gault MH. Prediction of creatinine clearance from serum creatinine. Nephron 1976;16:31–41.

19. Friedman JR, Norman DC, Yoshikawa TT. Correlation of estimated renal function parameters versus 24-hour creatinine clearance in ambulatory elderly. J Am Geriatr Soc 1989;37:145–149.

20. Greenblatt DJ, Harmatz JS, Shapiro L, Engelhardt N, Gouthro TA, Shader RI. Sensitivity to triazolam in the elderly. N Engl J Med 1991;324:1691–1698.

21. O'Malley K, Stevenson IH, Ward CA, et al. Determinants of anticoagulant control in patients receiving warfarin. Br J Clin Pharmacol 1977;4:309–314.

22. Shephard AMM, Hewick DS, Moreland TA. Age as a determinant of sensitivity to warfarin. Br J Clin Pharmacol 1977;4:315–320.
23. Gurwitz JH, Avorn J, Ross-Degnan D, Choodnovskiy I, Ansell J. Aging and the anticoagulant response to warfarin. Ann Intern Med 1992;116: 901–904.
24. Ray WA, Griffin MR, Schaffner W, Baugh DK, Melton LJ 3rd. Psychotropic drug use and the risk of hip fracture. N Engl J Med 1987;316:363–369.
25. Wang PS, Bohn RL, Glynn RJ, Mogun H, Avorn J. Hazardous benzodiazepine regimens in the elderly: effects of half-life, dosage, and duration on risk of hip fracture. Am J Psychiatry 2001;158(6):892–898.
26. Herings RMC, Stricker BCLARK, de Boer A, Bakker A, Sturmans A. Benzodiazepines and the risk of falling leading to femur fractures. Arch Intern Med 1995;155:1801–1807.
27. Liu B, Anderson G, Mittmann N, To T, Axcell T, Shear N. Use of selective serotonin-reputake inhibitors of tricyclic antidepressants and risk of hip fractures in elderly people. Lancet 1998;351:1303–1307.
28. Thapa PB, Gideon P, Cost TW, Milam AB, Ray WA. Antidepressants and the risk of falls among nursing home residents. N Engl J Med 1998;339:875–882.
29. Fifth ACCP Consensus Conference on antithrombotic therapy (1998): summary recommendations. Chest 1998;114(suppl):439S–769S.
30. Hylek EM, Singer DE. Risk factors for intracranial hemorrhage in outpatients taking warfarin. Ann Intern Med 1994;120:897–902.
31. Fihn SD, McDonell M, Martin D, Henikoff J, Vermes D, Kent D, White RH. Risk factors for complications of chronic anticoagulation: a multicenter study. Warfarin Optimized Outpatient Follow-up Study Group. Ann Intern Med 1993;118:511–520.
32. Kalish S, Gurwitz JH, Avorn J. Anticoagulant therapy in the elderly. Primary Cardiology 1993;7:34–42.
33. Landefeld CS, Anderson PA. Guideline-based consultation to prevent anticoagulant-related bleeding. A randomized, controlled trial in a teaching hospital. An Intern Med 1992;116:829–837.
34. Poller L, Shiach CR, MacCallum PK, et al. Multicentre randomised study of computerised anticoagulant dosage. European Concerted Action on Anticoagulation. Lancet 1998;352:1505–1509.
35. Gurwitz JH, Avorn J, Ross-Degnan D, Lipsitz LA. Nonsteroidal anti-inflammatory drug-associated azotemia in the very old. JAMA 1990;264: 471–475.
36. Bollini P, Garcia Rodriguez LA, Perez Gutthann S, Walker AM. The impact of research quality and study design on epidemiologic estimates of the effect of nonsteroidal anti-inflammatory drugs on upper gastrointestinal tract disease. Arch Intern Med 1992;152:1289–1295.
37. Bradley JD, Brandt KD, Katz BP, Kalasinski LA, Ryan SI. Comparison of an antiinflammatory dose of ibuprofen, an analgesic dose of ibuprofen, and acetaminophen in the treatment of patients with osteoarthritis of the knee. N Engl J Med 1991;325:87–91.
38. Whitcomb DC, Block GD. Association of acetaminophen hepatotoxicity with fasting and ethanol use. JAMA 1994;272:1845–1850.

39. Feldman M, McMahon AT. Do cyclooxygenase-2 inhibitors provide benefits similar to those of traditional nonsteroidal anti-inflammatory drugs, with less gastrointestinal toxicity? Ann Intern Med 2000;132:134–143.
40. Swan SK, Rudy DW, Lasseter KC, et al. Effect of cyclooxygenase-2 inhibition on renal function in elderly persons receiving a low-salt diet. Ann Intern Med 2000;133:1–9.

4
Sites of Care for Older Adults

KENNETH S. BOOCKVAR

Learning Objectives

Upon completion of the chapter, the student will be able to:

1. Weigh the likelihood of benefit and harm when deciding whether to hospitalize an older adult.
2. Anticipate hazards of hospitalization for older adults and take measures to prevent them.
3. Discuss the advantages and disadvantages of different sites for post-acute care with patients and families.
4. Understand the mechanisms for provision of long-term care in the United States and how they are financed.
5. Optimize continuity of care during patient relocation.

General Considerations

Geriatric medicine is characterized by multiple levels or contexts of care. The geriatrician and his/her team typically care for elderly patients along a continuum of these contexts, stretching from hospitalization for an acute problem, such as a stroke, to rehabilitation on a subacute ward, to convalescence in a nursing home, to continued care at home via a home care program, and finally to a return to primary care in the office. Each of these contexts of care has its own scope of purpose, its own rationale, its own teams of care professionals, and its own financial considerations and incen-

---

Material in this chapter is based on the following chapters in Cassel CK, Leipzig RM, Cohen HJ, Larson EB, Meier DE, eds. Geriatric Medicine: An Evidence-Based Approach, 4th ed. New York: Springer, 2003: Rubenstein LZ. Contexts of Care, pp. 93–97. Kane RL. The Long and the Short of Long-Term Care, pp. 99–111. Levine SA, Barry PP. Home Care, pp. 121–131. Palmer RM. Acute Hospital Care, pp. 133–145. Selections edited by Kenneth S. Boockvar.

tives, all of which are actively evolving along with changes in the overall health care system and larger society. Proper geriatric care requires familiarity with all these contexts and an understanding of how best to manage patients within them.

Case (Part 1)

Ms. K. is an 87-year-old woman with mild cognitive impairment, occasional urge incontinence, and hypothyroidism whom you have cared for 3 years as an outpatient. Ms. K's daughter brings her into the office before her scheduled appointment because over 2 days ago she developed a cough, low-grade fever, and dyspnea. Chest examination reveals inspiratory rhonchi and expiratory wheezes on the left side. You make the diagnosis of lower respiratory tract infection, order a chest x-ray, and are now considering whether to hospitalize Ms. K.

Epidemiology of Hospitalization

Although rates of hospitalization have declined in the past two decades for all age groups, the proportion of hospitalized patients who are age 65 years and older is increasing. In nonfederal acute hospitals, elderly patients account for 37% of all discharges and 47% of inpatient days of care (1). Among noninstitutionalized adults, patients age 75 years and over have the highest rates of hospitalization, with nearly 15% being hospitalized yearly and 5.3% hospitalized two or more times per year (2). In addition, older patients have longer hospitalizations, higher mortality rates, and higher rates of nursing home placement after hospitalization (1). In-hospital mortality rates increase from 5% among those 65 to 74 years of age to 10% in those 85 years of age and older. Risk factors among older adults for 2-year mortality after hospitalization include weight loss, cognitive dysfunction, impaired functional status, greater chronic disease burden, and worse severity of acute disease (3).

Hazards of Hospitalization

For older patients, hospitalization is a two-edged sword. Although hospitalization for acute illness offers older patients the hope of relief of symptoms and cure of disease, it also exposes them to the adverse risks of hospitalization: functional decline, iatrogenic illness, and possible institutionalization (Table 4.1).

Prospective cohort studies found that 20% to 32% of patients admitted to general medical units lose independence in their ability to perform one or more basic activities of daily living (ADLs) by the time of discharge

TABLE 4.1. Iatrogenic problems in hospitalized older adults and keys to prevention

Iatrogenic problem	Common reasons	Keys to prevention
Adverse drug effects	Polypharmacy; drug–drug interactions; altered drug disposition and tissue sensitivity with aging	Rational drug prescribing: review all medications taken prior to admission; use lower than usual maintenance doses when geriatric dose is unknown; limit use of psycho-active drugs; avoid drugs that affect cytochrome P450 metabolism or are highly albumin-bound
Falls/immobility	Weakness of leg muscles; postural hypotension; deconditioning due to prolonged bed rest; cognitive impairment; sensory impairment	Assess falls risk at admission (chronic disease burden, cognitive dysfunction, neuromuscular dysfunction, sensory impairment); avoid physical restraints; order physical therapy for transfer-dependent and gait-impaired patients; prescribe assistive devices (e.g., canes, walkers); modify environment (e.g., add handrails, grab bars to rooms); prescribe prophylactic subcutaneous heparin to immobile patients to prevent deep venous thrombosis
Pressure ulcers	Immobility; sustained point pressure over bones; excess moisture, friction and shearing forces	Pressure ulcer risk assessment: paresis, cognitive dysfunction, incontinence, malnutrition; turn patients at least every two hours; lubricate skin; optimize nutrition; order pressurized bed mattresses
Dehydration/undernutrition	Chronic disease predisposing to protein-calorie malnutrition; poor oral intake due to acute illness; anorexia; preparation for diagnostic studies	Assess nutritional status at admission: body weight; muscle wasting; serum albumin, cholesterol, hemoglobin; monitor calorie and fluid intake; obtain dietitian consult; give IV fluids when oral intake is inadequate or prohibited; consider enteral alimentation or peripheral hyperalimentation when oral intake is inadequate or contraindicated
Nosocomial infection	Transmission of resistant/opportunistic microorganisms by providers; use of broad-spectrum antibiotics; instrumentation (e.g., urethral catheters); pulmonary aspiration	Hand-washing; sterilization of medical equipment; use narrow-spectrum antibiotics when feasible; aspiration precautions in high risk patients; disinfection of patient's skin prior to insertion of intravenous or intraarterial line; urethral catheterization intermittently rather than continuously when indicated
Contrast-associated nephropathy	Hypertonic contrast agents given intravenously for diagnostic studies; dehydration; renal disease; myeloma	Avoid contrast studies, especially with renal diseases, dehydration, or multiple myeloma; substitute noncontrast studies; maintain adequate hydration before and after study

Source: Palmer RM. Acute hospital care. In: Cassel CK, Leipzig RM, Cohen HJ, et al., eds. Geriatric Medicine, 4th ed. New York: Springer, 2003.

(4–6). The loss of independent functioning during hospitalization is associated with serious sequelae, including prolonged hospital stay, nursing home placement, and mortality. Studies have also identified risk factors for functional decline in hospitalized elderly patients which include age ≥75 years old; presence of disability in the performance of instrumental activities of daily living (IADLs) prior to admission; low mental status scores on admission; presence of pressure ulcers; low social activity level; delirium; and presence of depressive symptoms (4,5,7).

Immobility

Immobility is associated with functional decline, increased risk of nursing home placement after discharge, medical complications (including deep venous thrombosis, urinary incontinence, pressure sores, joint contractures, cardiac deconditioning and muscle weakness), and falls (8). Cardiac and muscular deconditioning occur within days of sustained bed rest. When in the hospital, patients should be allowed free movement, and may need encouragement to sit up or to get out of bed even when they prefer bed rest (8).

Malnutrition

Undernutrition and protein-energy malnutrition are common in hospitalized older patients and are linked to increased hospital and posthospital mortality (9). Acutely ill patients have greater nutritional requirements than well elderly patients. Nutritional consultation and appropriately prescribed nutritional supplements are warranted for patients at risk for malnutrition (10,11). Patients often have orders for nothing by mouth (NPO), and nutritional supplements are often not consumed. Therefore, in the hospital, food and fluids should be prescribed and monitored daily (See Chapter 11: Nutrition, pages 177, 178, 180, 187).

Delirium

Delirium, an acute disorder of attention and cognition, occurs in 20% to 30% of elderly patients admitted with an acute medical diagnosis. Delirium may be precipitated by processes of hospital care, including immobilization of the patient, use of an indwelling bladder catheter, use of physical restraints, dehydration, malnutrition, iatrogenic complications, and psychosocial factors (12). Delirium prolongs hospital length of stay, increases costs of care, and increases the risk of nursing home placement or death (13). Delirium is best approached by preventive multicomponent interventions, since if it occurs, delirium can be difficult to treat (see Chapter 13: Depression, Dementia, Delirium, pages 236, 237, 242).

Iatrogenesis

Iatrogenic illness is any illness that results from a diagnostic procedure or therapeutic intervention and that is not a natural consequence of the patient's disease (14). Of iatrogenic events, adverse drug events are common in hospitalized patients and are associated with significantly prolonged length of stay, higher costs of care, and increased risk of death. Virtually any class of medication can cause an adverse event, but antibiotics and cardiovascular drugs have been most commonly implicated in studies of hospitalized patients. The increased risk for adverse drug events in older adults is partly attributable to alterations in drug disposition and tissue sensitivity associated with usual aging and to drug–drug interactions.

Nosocomial (hospital-acquired) infection is another common iatrogenic complication of hospitalization, commonly involving the urinary tract, respiratory tract and blood stream (due to intravascular catheters). Colonization or infection with resistant or opportunistic infections may complicate hospitalization (15).

Depression

Depression and depressive symptoms are present in 20% to 25% of medically ill elderly patients in the hospital (7). Environmental changes (e.g., a brighter room), physical and occupational therapy, increased frequency of family visits, and psychological counseling may be of immediate benefit to the depressed patient. (See Chapter 13: Depression, Dementia, Delirium, page 227.)

Improving Outcomes of Hospitalization

In light of the known hazards of hospitalization, the alternatives for an older patient should be considered, such as home care for patients with acute but non–life-threatening illnesses, hospice or palliative care for patients with terminal illness, or direct admissions to a skilled nursing facility. Prior to hospitalization, the personal values and priorities of patients and the wishes of their families should be addressed. The patient's advance directive should be reviewed with the appropriate family member or power of attorney for health care. A review of the objectives of hospitalization, the diagnostic evaluation, and probable outcome should be discussed before or early in hospitalization (see Chapter 7: Medicolegal Aspects of Older Adult Care, pages 94, 96, 98).

If the decision is to hospitalize, personal comfort should be addressed throughout hospitalization. Privacy and quiet at night are important. Family members should be encouraged to visit patients. A normal bowel and bladder regimen is maintained with a toileting schedule, and a bedside commode or urinal for men. Fiber supplements or hyperosmolar laxatives are helpful to prevent fecal impaction in immobilized patients or those taking opiates or anticholinergic agents.

In addition, models of care designed to enhance patient functioning during hospitalization or immediately postdischarge have emerged in the past decade, and include acute care of elders (ACE) units (5,16,17), the Geriatric Care Program (18), and the Elder Life Program (19). These models should be taken advantage of. The objectives of these interventions are to improve functional outcomes of hospitalization, reduce hospital lengths of stay, prevent nursing home admissions, or prevent rehospitalization. They offer hope that the adverse consequences of hospitalization can be attenuated through comprehensive assessment, special units, and comprehensive discharge planning.

Case (Part 2)

Ms. K. is admitted to the hospital and is prescribed intravenous antibiotics. Her symptoms of infection and dyspnea improve, and she is medically stable for discharge on hospital day 4. However, she has become deconditioned from lying in bed and nurses have observed her performing unsafe maneuvers while ambulating in her room. She agrees to undertake rehabilitative treatment, and you need to help her decide on a post–acute care location.

Post-Acute Care

Post-acute care refers to medical, nursing, and rehabilitative care provided to patients following acute illness and hospitalization. Formerly, this phase of care took place in the hospital, during extended hospital stays. However, currently, because of financial incentives to reduce hospital length of stay, almost all post-acute care occurs outside the hospital. Thirty eight percent of all Medicare-covered hospital discharges in 1995 received one or more forms of post-acute care. The dominant model was home health care, accounting for over half of all the post-acute care usage. Other sites of post-acute care are nursing home and hospital rehabilitation units. However, hospital-based rehabilitation is available only to a small number of individuals who can adhere to a rigorous (at least 3 hours a day) regimen of rehabilitative therapy, leaving most patients and caregivers of older adults with a choice of home or nursing home-based care (see Chapter 10: Exercise and Rehabilitation, pages 168, 171, 172).

Medicare covers 100 days of post-acute care after hospitalization, and only fully covers the first 20 days, with a substantial co-pay (20%) after that; thus, many courses of rehabilitation are less than 20 days. Medicare coverage can only be invoked for skilled services, for example, parenteral therapy (not including insulin), complex wound care, or daily physical,

TABLE 4.2. Advantages (+) and disadvantages (−) of post-acute care sites

	Home	Nursing home	Hospital
Ease of placement	+/−	+/−	−
Recovery of physical function	+	−	+
Return to community living	+	−	+
Around-the-clock custodial care	−	+	+
Comfort and autonomy	+	−	−
High out-of-pocket and informal costs	−	+	+

occupational, or speech therapy. Daily compliance and consistent medical or functional improvement is necessary to retain the benefit. If patients cannot meet these requirements, the Medicare benefit is terminated (see Chapter 5: Medicare and Medicaid, pages 73–75).

Compared with other sites of post-acute care (e.g., home with home care, hospital rehabilitation units), nursing homes may be at a disadvantage in providing the necessary services (Table 4.2). Many nursing homes do not have the nursing staff, especially professional nurses, to meet the needs of patients just discharged from the hospital. In addition, doctors are less inclined to do rounds in the nursing home as frequently as they do in the hospital, in part because Medicare is less likely to pay for frequent visits. Likewise, nursing homes may not be able to provide the rehabilitative services needed. Some homes have physical therapists on staff; others contract for such care. Nursing homes with subacute or rehabilitative units are more likely to have the full range of rehabilitation services and team members (Table 4.3).

Case (Part 3)

Ms. K. enters a subacute unit at a local nursing home and undergoes 15 days of gait training and strength exercise therapy. She recovers most of her strength and is discharged home with a walker. Her daughter arranges for 4 hours of home assistance daily and takes over Ms. K.'s bill paying. In the subsequent months you see Ms. K. as an outpatient at regular intervals. Ms. K. experiences a slow decline in memory, which impedes her ability to perform instrumental activities of daily living such as medication management, shopping, and cooking. She also begins to experience more frequent episodes of urge incontinence, despite treatment. Her daughter schedules an appointment with you to discuss options for Ms. K.'s long-term care.

Long-Term Care

Long-term care is defined as assistance given over a sustained period of time to individuals with disabilities. Most long-term-care recipients also need active medical care, because their disability is often a result of one or more chronic diseases. The definition of long-term care does not imply care given at a particular site. In fact, the backbone of long-term care is informal care provided by family and others. Only about 8% of care provided to persons living in the community comes from paid sources. Another 28% is provided by a combination of formal and informal care; and almost two thirds comes solely from informal sources (20). Even with the substantial amount of informal care being provided, many older people still do not receive the help they need.

Medicare and Medicaid together account for about 60% of formal long-term-care expenditures and about the same proportion of nursing home expenditures. Taken individually, Medicaid plays a much larger role in nursing home care, whereas Medicare is major funder of home care. Until now, long-term care has been largely a state responsibility because of the heavy role Medicaid has played, resulting in a wide variety of programs and quality of care. Recent efforts to measure quality of long-term care have focused on clinical outcomes such as physical functional change, maintenance of weight, and skin condition (i.e., avoidance of pressure sores). An outcomes focus allows comparisons across modalities of care. By shifting the emphasis away from structure and methods of care to accountability for outcomes, it is possible to preserve flexibility in choice of site of care while assuring accountability.

Nursing Home

The nursing home has served as the touchstone for long-term care. Other forms of long-term care are usually considered in relation to the nursing home. The nursing home has a mixed heritage, descended from the almshouse on one side and the hospital on the other. Because nursing home care has been closely associated with Medicaid, a welfare program, it carries the welfare stigmata. At the same time, early federal regulations used small hospitals as the template for nursing home standards.

The hospital model of multiple persons in a room, fixed hours for eating and being awake, limited choice of food, and an overarching therapeutic philosophy does not provide a normal living environment. These practices were developed to make care more efficient, but they rob patients of their identity and dignity. The plight of the nursing home has been made more serious by its efforts to provide services to many different types of patients, including those with physical frailty, cognitive impairment, terminal illness, and those with temporary disability. Trying to fill multiple needs makes it more difficult to achieve good results.

Care providers should be aware of the experience of entering a nursing home from the patient's perspective. It is a depressing and distressing event, a concrete marker of debility and disease, in which one joins with others in the same condition. The admission process to the nursing home is also highly regulated. It is a prolonged process involving paperwork and discussions of illness, code status, funeral home choice, relinquishment of belongings, and adaptation to the unfamiliar. Emotional and functional adaptation to the nursing home sometimes takes 6 months. The physical and emotional tolls are equaled by the financial toll. Nearly half of nursing home care is paid for out of private funds. Typical daily cost for nursing home care ranges from $150 to $300 per day.

Medical care in nursing homes is evolving. Nurse practitioners have been shown to improve quality of primary care in nursing homes (21,22), and, in conjunction with the emergence of managed care, teams of physicians and nurse practitioners have been effectively used to follow nursing home residents (23,24). Special managed care programs directed specifically at nursing home residents have been created with the hypothesis that aggressive primary care can avert hospitalizations (25), which are frequent events during a nursing home stay.

Assisted Living

An emerging form of long-term care is assisted living. Although there is no consistent definition of this style of care, most people agree that it includes an opportunity to live alone with quarters that provide one's own toilet and bathing facilities and some means to preserve and prepare food. At the heart of this concept is the idea that people are first seen as inhabitants of their space with control over their lives. Services are provided as conditions dictate. Some may be offered as a part of an overall package (e.g., congregate dining, a minimum number of service hours per week); others can be purchased as needed.

Assisted living is providing new competition to nursing homes. Private paying clients especially are attracted to the idea of being able to live in more commodious settings, often at lower costs. A few vanguard states, like Oregon and Washington, have made deliberate efforts to redirect Medicaid expenditures from nursing homes to community care, including institutional options like assisted living. But most states have been hesitant or unable to make such a shift.

Home Care

Home care recipients are community-dwelling individuals who depend on the assistance of others to perform ADLs. In the absence of this help, they would be at high risk of nursing home placement. Thus, the term *home care* includes all health and social services that may be provided in the home, ranging from homemaker, chore, and meal services to nursing and physician care (Table 4.3). Nationwide, some 9.5 million people older than 50 receive help with at least one basic ADL (bathing, dressing, eating, toileting, continence, transferring, and ambulating) or IADLs (management of finances, use of the telephone, organizing transportation, meal planning and cooking, shopping, taking medications) (26). Of people receiving home health services in 1996, 72% were aged 65 or older, 67% were female, 65% were white, 29% were married, and 35% were widowed (27).

In 1990, the American Medical Association suggested that medical care at home could be (1) preventive, including home safety evaluation, patient education, provision of assistive equipment, or monitoring; (2) diagnostic, including home assessment, comprehensive geriatric assessment, or evaluation of functional capacity and the environment; (3) therapeutic, from "high tech" to hospice; (4) rehabilitative, especially with family involvement; and (5) long-term maintenance for chronically ill and disabled patients, with supportive care by formal and informal caregivers (28).

TABLE 4.3. Services available in the home

Professional	Ancillary/supportive	Diagnostics	Medical equipment
• Physician	• Home health aides	• Phlebotomy	• Intravenous infusion for hydration, chemotherapy, blood transfusion, antibiotics, total parenteral nutrition, pain management and other medications
• Nurse	• Personal care assistants	• X-rays	
• Dentist		• Electrocardiograms	
• Podiatrist	• Homemakers	• Holter monitoring	
• Optometrist	• Chore aides	• Oximetry	
• Rehabilitation therapists: occupational physical speech respiratory	• Volunteers	• Blood cultures	
	• Home-delivered meals		
• Psychologist			• Mechanical ventilators
• Dietitian			• Dialysis
• Pharmacist			• Medical alert devices
• Social worker			• Glucometers

Source: Levine SA, Barry PP. Home care. In: Cassel CK, Leipzig RM, Cohen HJ, et al., eds. Geriatric Medicine, 4th ed. New York: Springer, 2003.

Situations in which a home visit by the physician may be required include ambiguities in reports of the patient's status, acute declines in health or function in frail patients, unexplained failure to thrive, unexplained failure of the care plan, request for physician evaluation in the home by another team member, need for a patient/family meeting to make an important decision, and routine medical care for the patient who cannot leave home (29).

The vast majority of care provided in the home is unpaid, nonmedical, informal care; 72% of caregivers are female, mostly wives and daughters, and over one third of all caregivers are 65 or older. One-third of caregivers themselves are in fair or poor health and most are poor or nearly poor (31%) or low to middle income (57%). Due to the competing demands of elder caregiving with childcare or employment, 9% have left work and 20% have reduced work hours (30).

Funding for home care services comes from a variety of public and private sources. Medicare is the largest single payer of home care services, accounting for 31.6% of total estimated home care expenditures in 2002, followed by private out-of-pocket spending (18.0%) and Medicaid (13.3%) (31). Medicare covers services deemed to be "reasonable and necessary for the treatment of an illness or injury," and therefore is not intended to cover long-term care provided by an individual or a nursing home. However, long-term home care recipients require active medical care because, like other long-term-care recipients, their disability is a result of one or more chronic diseases. Such medical care, as well as post-acute care after hospitalization, is covered at home by Medicare. Services that are 100% covered under Medicare Part A include skilled nursing, skilled therapy, home health aide services, and social services. It is important to be aware of exclusions in Medicare coverage, including homemaker services, long-term-care nursing, home-delivered meals, transportation that is nonemergent, all bathroom equipment, and patient care for those who do not require skilled nursing services. From 1997 to 2003, Medicare home care expenditures increased from $3.9 billion to $12.2 billion.

Medicaid funding for long-term home care services is provided jointly by the federal and state governments. The regulations are federal, but eligibility is determined on a state-by-state basis. Coverage is designed for those who not only meet state income eligibility guidelines but also are blind or disabled. The majority of states cover nursing and home health aide services, durable medical equipment, and medical supplies. Coverage for diagnostics, medication, transportation, adult day care, social work, personal care, and physical, speech, or occupational therapy varies from state to state. Medicaid payments for home health services fall into three main categories: the traditional home health benefit, which is a mandatory benefit provided by all states, and two optional programs: the personal care option and home and community-based waivers. Medicaid spending for home health services has grown enormously in the last two decades, from $70 million in 1975 to $24.3 billion in 2000. Home care services made up 14.4% of Medicaid payments in 2000 (31).

An interdisciplinary-team approach and the use of a home care coordinator for case management are essential in implementing complex plans that may include numerous referrals and services as well as education for the patient and family. This approach also allows continuous assessment of outcomes over time so that the plan can be revised as the patient's needs and health status change. The collaborative nature of this practice requires communication among the varied disciplines that provide services in the home. The role of physicians in home care may include authorization of services; communication with providers, patients, and families; and home visits. Advantages of house calls include patient convenience, support, and reassurance, and the availability of assessment information. Disadvantages of house calls are that they are time-consuming, inefficient, and poorly reimbursed, with concerns about safety and lack of equipment (32). In small practices where the physician does not have the luxury of an interdisciplinary team, the physician must act as the case manager in concert with a visiting nurse.

Case (Part 4)

Ms. K., at her daughter's suggestion, opts to enter a nearby assisted living facility, where she can have her meals prepared and medications administered. In the next 12 months Ms. K. has a recurrent episode of pneumonia that requires hospitalization. After this illness she returns to the nursing home subacute care unit where she stayed previously for rehabilitative treatment. After completing this course of rehabilitation she still needs help transferring, toileting, and dressing. At this point she and her daughter decide that the best option for her is to move to another floor in the nursing home permanently for long-term care.

Optimizing Continuity of Care

As portrayed in this chapter's unfolding case, older adults often find themselves transferred to and from different levels of care in a collection of institutions. Each of these transitions causes discontinuity in care. This includes the change in physician and nursing staff and change in environment that can be disruptive to care and hazardous to patients. Coordination of care between sites of care is important to avoid duplication of work and provider errors. Optimally a single provider follows the patient throughout their medical course. In the absence of a single provider, continuity of care depends on communication between providers at different sites. Often the plan for communication between sites of care is a transfer of paper documents that occurs with, or just following, the physical transfer of a patient. Several authors have proposed standards for what type of information should be included in transfer documents (33–36). Because older adults have a high prevalence of complex medical histories, long medication lists, disability, and surrogate decision makers, most authors recommend including these classes of information, as each is crucial for providing health care to an individual (Table 4.4).

When transfer documents do not include all the information that a provider needs, or there is some question as to their accuracy, other methods of interinstitutional communication should be employed, such as telephone communication between providers or sharing of electronic data. In U.S. Veterans Affairs Medical Centers, providers in the hospital, nursing home, and outpatient practice can look at the complete medical record from medical encounters anywhere in the system, because all records are carried electronically on a common server. To optimize the transfer process, efforts should be made by providers at different sites to contact one another by phone to communicate more detailed information, especially for patients who cannot provide a medical history due to communicative impairments. This can occur at all levels (e.g., between physicians, nurses, social workers, physical therapists), and can be useful well after the transfer to help troubleshoot unanticipated changes in patients' conditions. In addition, primary care providers, especially physicians and physician extenders, should visit patients in the hospital and other sites (including post-acute care sites, nursing home, and home) whenever possible. This allows primary care providers to get updates on the individual's condition and to give suggestions on the plan of care to providers at each site.

TABLE 4.4. Checklist of items to be included in transfer documents

Physician contact information
Family contact information
Clinical course
Advance directives
History of adverse drug reactions
Chronic conditions
Vital signs
Recent laboratory results
Assistive devices
Physical function
Sensory function
Cognitive function
Medications

General Principles

- Because the hospital exposes older adults to significant risk of iatrogenic harm, one should routinely consider appropriate alternatives to hospitalization for ill older adults (e.g., outpatient workup, treatment in the nursing home).
- When older adults are hospitalized, interventions should be implemented that have been shown to reduce the risk of inpatient adverse events such as delirium and functional decline.
- When deciding among sites for post-acute care, one should consider results of studies that have suggested that individuals who receive post-acute care at home or in acute rehabilitation units have better physical function outcomes than those who receive post-acute care in nursing homes.
- Long-term care should be provided in the least restrictive environment possible that ensures the health and safety of individuals (i.e., consider home with home care or assisted living prior to nursing home placement).
- Providers who discharge and admit geriatric patients to/from new sites of care are responsible for complete and accurate communication of medical information, and for communication of the plan of care with patients and their surrogates. Reliance on written transfer forms may be inadequate.

Suggested Readings

American Medical Association. Medical Management of the Home Care Patient: Guidelines for Physicians. Chicago, IL: AMA, 1998. *An invaluable guide to practitioners in the home care setting.*

Inouye SK, Bogardus ST Jr, Charpentier PA, et al. A multicomponent intervention to prevent delirium in hospitalized older patients. N Engl J Med 1999;340:669–676. *The first large-scale trial proving that modifiable risk factors for delirium could be identified and addressed to prevent delirium among hospitalized patients.*

Kane RL. The long and the short of long-term care. In: Cassel CK, Leipzig RM, Cohen HJ, et al., eds. Geriatric Medicine, 4th ed. New York: Springer, 2003: 99–112.

Kane RL, Chen Q, Finch M, Blewett L, Burns R, Moskowitz M. The optimal outcomes of post-hospital care under Medicare. Health Serv Res 2000;35:615–661. *This study estimated the differences in functional outcomes attributable to discharge to one of four different sites for posthospital care. It found that nursing homes are generally associated with poorer outcomes and higher costs than the other posthospital care modalities.*

Levine SA, Barry PP. Home care. In: Cassel CK, Leipzig RM, Cohen HJ, et al., eds. Geriatric Medicine, 4th ed. New York: Springer, 2003:121–132.
Palmer RM. Acute hospital care. In: Cassel CK, Leipzig RM, Cohen HJ, et al., eds. Geriatric Medicine, 4th ed. New York: Springer, 2003:133–148.
Rubenstein LZ. Contexts of care. In: Cassel CK, Leipzig RM, Cohen HJ, et al., eds. Geriatric Medicine, 4th ed. New York: Springer, 2003:93–98.

References

1. Graves EJ, Gillum BS. National hospital discharge survey: annual summary, 1994. Vital Health Stat 13 1997;i–v:1–50.
2. Benson V, Marano MA. Current estimates from the National Health Interview Survey, 1995. Vital Health Stat 10 1998:1–428.
3. Teno JM, Harrell FE Jr, Knaus W, et al. Prediction of survival for older hospitalized patients: the HELP survival model. Hospitalized Elderly Longitudinal Project. J Am Geriatr Soc 2000;48:S16–S24.
4. Sager MA, Rudberg MA. Functional decline associated with hospitalization for acute illness. Clin Geriatr Med 1998;14:669–679.
5. Landefeld CS, Palmer RM, Kresevic DM, Fortinsky RH, Kowal J. A randomized trial of care in a hospital medical unit especially designed to improve the functional outcomes of acutely ill older patients. N Engl J Med 1995;332:1338–1344.
6. Inouye SK, Wagner DR, Acampora D, et al. A predictive index for functional decline in hospitalized elderly medical patients. J Gen Intern Med 1993;8:645–652.
7. Covinsky KE, Fortinsky RH, Palmer RM et al. Relation between symtoms of depression and healthy status outcomes in acutely ill hospitalized older persons. Ann Intern Med 1997;126(6):417–425.
8. Mahoney JE. Immobility and falls. Clin Geriatr Med 1998;14:699–726.
9. Sullivan DH, Sun S, Walls RC. Protein-energy undernutrition among elderly hospitalized patients: a prospective study. JAMA 1999;281:2013–2019.
10. Woo J, Ho SC, Mak YT, Law LK, Cheung A. Nutritional status of elderly patients during recovery from chest infection and the role of nutritional supplementation assessed by a prospective randomized single-blind trial. Age Ageing 1994;23:40–48.
11. Delmi M, Rapin CH, Bengoa JM, Delmas PD, Vasey H, Bonjour JP. Dietary supplementation in elderly patients with fractured neck of the femur. Lancet 1990;335:1013–1016.
12. Inouye SK, Viscoli CM, Horwitz RI, Hurst LD, Tinetti ME. A predictive model for delirium in hospitalized elderly medical patients based on admission characteristics. Ann Intern Med 1993;119:474–481.
13. Inouye SK, Rushing JT, Foreman MD, Palmer RM, Pompei P. Does delirium contribute to poor hospital outcomes? A three-site epidemiologic study. J Gen Intern Med 1998;13:234–242.
14. Steel K, Gertman PM, Crescenzi C, Anderson J. Iatrogenic illness on a general medical service at a university hospital. N Engl J Med 1981;304:638–642.

15. Riedinger JL, Robbins LJ. Prevention of iatrogenic illness: adverse drug reactions and nosocomial infections in hospitalized older adults. Clin Geriatr Med 1998;14:681–698.
16. Palmer RM. Acute hospital care: Future directions. In: Yoshikawa TT, Norman DC, eds. Acute Emergencies and Critical Care of the Geriatric Patient. New York: Marcel Dekker, 2000:461–486.
17. Palmer RM, Landefeld CS, Kresevic D, Kowal J. A medical unit for the acute care of the elderly. J Am Geriatr Soc 1994;42:545–552.
18. Inouye SK, Wagner DR, Acampora D, Horwitz RI, Cooney LM Jr, Tinetii ME. A controlled trial of a nursing-centered intervention in hospitalized elderly medical patients: the Yale Geriatric Care Program. J Am Geriatr Soc 1993;41:1353–1360.
19. Inouye SK, Bogardus ST Jr, Charpentier PA, et al. A multicomponent intervention to prevent delirium in hospitalized older patients. N Engl J Med 1999; 340:669–676.
20. Gage B. Impact of the BBA on post-acute utilization. Health Care Financ Rev 1999;20:103–126.
21. Kane RL, Jorgensen LA, Teteberg B, Kuwahara J. Is good nursing-home care feasible? JAMA 1976;235:516–519.
22. Kane RL, Garrard J, Buchanan JL, Rosenfeld A, Skay C, McDermott S. Improving primary care in nursing homes. J Am Geriatr Soc 1991;39: 359–367.
23. Reuben DB, Schnelle JF, Buchanan JL, et al. Primary care of long-stay nursing home residents: approaches of three health maintenance organizations. J Am Geriatr Soc 1999;47:131–138.
24. Farley DO, Zellman G, Ouslander JG, Reuben DB. Use of primary care teams by HMOs for care of long-stay nursing home residents. J Am Geriatr Soc 1999;47:139–144.
25. Kane RL, Huck S. The implementation of the Evercare Demonstration Project. J Am Geriatr Soc 2000;48:218–223.
26. Kassner E, Bectel RW. Midlife and Older Americans with Disabilities: Who Gets Help? A chartbook. Washington, DC: Public Policy Institute, American Association of Retired Persons, 1998.
27. Haupt BJ. An overview of home health and hospice care patients: 1996 National Home and Hospice Care Survey. Adv Data 1998;16:1–35.
28. Council on Scientific Affairs. Home care in the 1990s. JAMA 1990;263: 1241–1244.
29. American Medical Association. Medical Management of the Home Care Patient: Guidelines for Physicians. Chicago, IL: AMA, 1998.
30. Stone R, Cafferata GL, Sangl J. Caregivers of the frail elderly: a national profile. Gerontologist 1987;27:616–626.
31. National Health Expeditures Projections: 1990–2012. Washington, DC: Health Care Finance Administration, Office of the Actuary, 2004.
32. Campion EW. Can house calls survive? N Engl J Med 1997;337:1840–1841.
33. Conger SA, Snider LF. Is there a gap in communication between acute care facilities and nursing homes? Health Soc Work 1982;7:274–282.
34. Jones JS, Dwyer PR, White LJ, Firman R. Patient transfer from nursing home to emergency department: outcomes and policy implications. Acad Emerg Med 1997;4:908–915.

35. Madden C, Garrett J, Busby-Whitehead J. The interface between nursing homes and emergency departments: a community effort to improve transfer of information. Acad Emerg Med 1998;5:1123–1126.
36. Tangalos EG, Freeman PI. Assessment of geriatric patients—spreading the word. Mayo Clin Proc 1988;63:305–307.

5
Medicare and Medicaid

S. BRENT RIDGE

Learning Objectives

Upon completion of the chapter, the student will be able to:

1. Distinguish between Medicare and Medicaid.
2. Know the significance of Medicare Parts A, B, C, and D and the coverage provided by each.
3. Identify who is eligible for Medicare and how it is obtained.
4. Understand the role of Medicare Supplemental Insurance Plans and Medicare Health Maintenance Organization (HMO).

Case (Part 1)

Ms. C. is a 69-year-old woman who had not seen a doctor during most of her adult life. One month ago, she was admitted to the hospital after presenting to the emergency room (ER) with left-sided weakness. Head computed tomography (CT) revealed a small internal capsule infarct on the right. During her hospitalization, she was also diagnosed with high blood pressure and was started on medications for treatment. After a 1-month stay in a subacute rehabilitation center, she comes to see you as a new patient and is accompanied by her daughter. After determining that her blood pressure is well controlled and her physical examination otherwise stable, you ask if the patient or the daughter have any further questions. Both are concerned about the cost of the recent hospitalization and rehabilitation. The patient has a small amount of savings and is worried that she will not be able to cover her basic expenses if she now has medical bills to pay. They want to know how much of their hospital bill will be covered by Medicare and want to know what it takes to be on Medicaid.

Material in this chapter is based on the following chapter in Cassel CK, Leipzig RM, Cohen HJ, Larson EB, Meier DE, eds. Geriatric Medicine: An Evidence-Based Approach, 4th ed. New York: Springer, 2003: Vladeck BC. Mechanisms of Paying for Health Care, pp. 1201–1211.

TABLE 5.1. Medicare eligibility

- 65 years old or older
- U.S. citizen or permanent legal resident for 5 continuous years
- Disabled and have had Social Security for at least 2 years (regardless of age)
- Kidney failure and require continuous dialysis or need a kidney transplant (regardless of age)
- Amyotrophic lateral sclerosis (regardless of age)

Medicare vs. Medicaid

Medicare is a universal, federally managed health insurance provided to Americans 65 years old and older (Table 5.1) (1). It is a compulsory social insurance program financed by payroll taxes on all wage and salary earners. Traditionally, there are two parts to Medicare, Part A and Part B (Table 5.2) (2). Medicare Advantage Part C (formerly known as the Medicare + Choice) and the Prescription Drug Plan (Part D) are recent optional features provided for beneficiaries by the program.

Medicaid is a state-administered, federal-state health insurance program for the poor. Patients older than 65 who get Medicare benefits may also qualify for and receive Medicaid benefits if their income is lower than the number established by the state in which they live. In most states, the income must be below $600/month. There are no age restrictions on Medicaid.

Medicare Part A covers:

1. Inpatient hospitalization:
   a. $812 deductible per benefit period that the patient or his/her supplemental insurance must pay
   b. After deductible, full coverage for days 1 to 60 of hospitalization
   c. After day 60, co-insurance or patient must pay.
   d. A "benefit period" begins the day a patient enters the hospital or nursing home and ends only when the patient has been out of the

TABLE 5.2. Services covered by Medicare

Part A (no copayment)	Part B (20% copayment)
• Home health aide • Visiting nurse: RN observation/ assessment, management and evaluation of care plan • Social service • Physical therapy, occupational therapy, speech therapy	• Physician visit • Certain durable medical equipment • Some diagnostic labs, electrocardiography, and x-rays

Source: Levine SA, Barry PP. Home care. In: Cassel CK, Leipzig RM, Cohen HJ, et al., eds. Geriatric Medicine, 4th ed. New York: Springer, 2003.

nursing home or hospital for 60 continuous days. Readmission prior to the end of the benefit period is cumulative. If a patient was hospitalized for 14 days, discharged, and returned 2 weeks later, the first day of the second hospitalization would be counted as day 15, meaning that the 60-day period of full Medicare coverage could be reached very quickly if frequent hospitalizations are necessary.

2. Skilled nursing facility
   a. No deductible
   b. Full coverage for days 1 to 20
   c. From day 21 to 100, pays all but $101.50
   d. Medicare does not offer coverage after day 100. Nursing home stays greater than 100 days must be paid for by the patient. Nursing home care remains self-pay until the patient's assets are depleted and they then become available for Medicaid benefits.
3. Home health and hospice care
   a. No deductible
   b. Time limited

Medicare Part B covers:

1. 80% of the fees for outpatient doctor's services, laboratory and x-ray services, durable medical equipment (hospital beds, walkers, wheelchairs, etc.), ambulance services, outpatient hospital care, home health care and blood and medical supplies, chiropractor and physical therapy services.

2. The remainder 20% is covered by co-insurance if the patient has it or directly out-of-pocket. There is a $100 yearly deductible in addition to the monthly fee.

Medicare *does not* cover private duty nursing, custodial care, cosmetic surgery, care outside of the United States, acupuncture, eyeglasses, or dental care (3–7).

Medicare Advantage (Part C)

Medicare Part C, formerly known as Medicare+Choice, is now known as Medicare Advantage. If beneficiaries are entitled to Medicare Part A and enrolled in Part B, they are eligible to switch to a Medicare Advantage plan, provided they reside in the plan's service area. Medicare Advantage provides for coordinated care plans (the Balanced Budget Act of 1997's umbrella term for managed care plans) with the following options:

1. Health Maintenance Organization (HMO) plans emphasize preventive care but without coverage for providers or facilities outside the HMO network. They almost always require a network primary care physician referral to access a network specialist; they usually offer drug benefits.

2. Point of Service (POS) plans offer a network of preferred providers, like HMO plans, but also provide reduced benefits for providers or

facilities outside the HMO network. They typically require a referral from a network primary care physician to access a network specialist; they sometimes offer drug benefits.

3. Regionally expanded Preferred Provider Organization (PPO) plans are similar to POS plans but have broader geographic access to network providers in a larger service area, and with reduced benefits outside the PPO network. They do not typically require a referral from a network primary care physician to access network specialists. They may or may not offer drug benefits.

4. Provider-Sponsored Organization (PSO) plans are similar to the POS plans but are usually organized with physicians that practice in a regional or community hospital. There may or may not be coverage for providers or facilities outside the PSO network, depending on the plan designs offered. They may require a referral from a network primary care physician to access network specialists. They typically offer drug benefits.

5. Medical savings accounts set up in conjunction with private fee-for-service plans provide at least the same benefit coverage levels as Medicare Parts A and B or high deductible coverage.

Medicare Prescription Drug Plan (Part D)

The Medicare Prescription Drug, Improvement and Modernization Act of 2003 added Part D. Medicare beneficiaries purchasing optional part D are able to get drug coverage through a separate drug insurance policy. If they are covered by a privately operated health plan that includes a prescription drug benefit, they would be ineligible for Part D (7).

The government guarantees drug coverage in any region that does not have at least one stand-alone drug plan and one private health plan. Employers that offer equivalent drug coverage for retirees would receive tax-free subsidies. Employers could also offer premium subsidies and cost-sharing assistance for retirees who enroll in Medicare drug plans.

Enrolling in Medicare

If patients are getting Social Security when they turn 65, they will be automatically enrolled in Medicare Part A and Part B on the first day of the month in which they turn 65. A card will be mailed to them. If patients are not receiving Social Security, they should go to the local Social Security office to enroll in Medicare 3 months before their 65th birthday. They have 4 months after their birthday to enroll without penalty. Regardless of privately held insurance, *all* patients turning 65 should enroll in the Medicare program. People can sign up for Social Security retirement benefits at the age of 62. They cannot sign up for Medicare until turning 65 unless one of the special medical circumstances cited above applies.

Medicare Fee

Medicare Part A is free. Medicare Part B has a monthly premium of approximately $88.50 (2006), and this amount is generally deducted from the monthly Social Security check. Patients can decide not to take this benefit. Medicare Part D has a monthly premium of approximately $35 (2006).

Case (Part 2)

Ms. C. does have Medicare Part A and B but is worried about paying the deductible. You tell her and her daughter that the local Medicaid office would be able to determine if she qualified for this program. You also mention that she and her daughter may want to explore supplemental insurance to cover the health-related expenses not paid by Medicare.

Medicare Supplemental Insurance

There are supplemental insurance packages offered by private companies and organizations like the American Association of Retired Persons (AARP). These are often referred to as "Medigap" policies. While the characteristics of the Medigap market differ dramatically from one state to the next, premiums for these plans have been rising dramatically in most of the nation in the last decade.

Medicare Health Maintenance Organizations

Medicare HMOs are private companies paid by the federal government to provide Medicare-covered health care. Patients interested in an HMO must have Part A and Part B. Unlike regular Medicare, a Medicare HMO will dictate which doctor the patient may or may not see, and although some HMOs cover prescription medications, they may cover only certain drugs of a particular class and not the one that the physician prescribed (8–10). Medicare HMOs are not available everywhere. The social worker in your clinic or hospital should be able to tell you what programs exist in your community.

There are also Medicare assistance programs funded by the state governments that offer varying degrees of coverage for the health expenditures not covered by Medicare and/or will pay for the Medicare Part B premium (11,12). Enrollment in these programs is based on income and assets. These programs are meant to aid those individuals who do not qualify for Medicaid. Income limitations vary by state. There are four such programs: Qualified Medicare Beneficiary (QMB), Specified Low-Income Medicare Beneficiary

(SLMB), Qualifying Individuals (QI-1), and QI-2. The local Medicaid office can help patients determine whether they qualify for assistance.

Medicare Reimbursement

Doctors can choose to opt out of the Medicare program and accept only patients with private insurance coverage or patients able to self-pay for medical care. Since 1992, Medicare has prepared a physician fee schedule that dictates how much each procedure or exam is worth. When doctors agree to "accept assignment" for Medicare claims, they are willing to take the amount Medicare approves for a payment in full. Again, Medicare usually covers 80% of the amount, and the patient or Medigap plan pays the remaining 20%. If a doctor does not accept assignment, federal law mandates that he/she can only charge up to 15% over the amount Medicare approves. The patient or Medigap plan would then be responsible for payment of the fee.

General Principles

- Every American over age 65 has access to Medicare coverage.
- Medicare Part A covers inpatient care and is universal.
- Medicare Part B covers outpatient care. Patients who opt for this coverage must pay a monthly fee.
- Medicare Part C, formerly known as Medicare + Choice, is now known as Medicare Advantage and provides the option for coordinated care plans and medical saving accounts.
- Medicare Part D is the Medicare Drug Prescription Plan and has a $35-per-month premium.
- Medicaid is an insurance program for the poor. Medicare patients can qualify for Medicaid if they meet the income requirement. Medicaid provides coverage for prescription medications. Medicare does not.
- Medicare HMOs are private companies paid by the federal government to provide Medicare-covered health care. Medicare HMOs are not available in all geographic locations and may vary in cost and extent of services provided.

Suggested Readings

Center for Medicare and Medicaid Services web page: http://www.cms.gov. *This Web site answers all questions regarding both Medicare and Medicaid. The site is divided into sections for the public and for providers.*

Gallagher P, Smith S. Medicare: The Physician's Guide, 2002. Chicago: American Medical Association, 2002. *An excellent resource for the practicing physician, this guide offers detailed explanations of the billing and reimbursement process.*
Vladeck BC. Sounding board: plenty of nothing—a report from the Medicare Commission. N Engl J Med 1999;340:1503–1506.
Vladeck BC. The storm before the calm before the storm: Medicare home care in the wake of the Balanced Budget Act. Care Manage J 2000;2(4):232–237.
Vladeck BC. Mechanisms of paying for health care. In: Cassel CK, Leipzig RM, Cohen HJ, et al., eds. Geriatric Medicine, 4th ed. New York: Springer, 2003: 1201–1212.

References

1. Medicare Payment Advisory Commission. Report to the Congress: Medicare Payment Policy. Washington, DC: Government Printing Office, March 2000.
2. Manton KG, Vaupel JW. Survival after the age of 80 in the United States, Sweden, France, England and Japan. N Engl J Med 1995;333(18):1232–1235.
3. Medicare Payment Advisory Commission. Report to the Congress: Selected Medicare Issues. Washington: Government Printing Office, June 2000.
4. Medicare Payment Advisory Commission. Health Care Spending and the Medicare Program: A Data Book. Washington: MedPAC, July 1998.
5. Physician Payment Review Commission. Annual Report to the Congress. Washington, DC: Government Printing Office, 1997.
6. Iezzoni LI. The demand for documentation for Medicare payment. N Engl J Med 1999;341(5):365–367.
7. The Medicare Program: Medicare and Prescription Drugs. Henry J. Kaiser Family Foundation, April 2003 Menlo Park, CA.
8. Luft HS. Medicare and managed care. Annu Rev Public Health 1998;19: 459–475.
9. Medicare 2000: 35 years of Improving Americans' Health and Security. Washington: Health Care Financing Administration, July 2000.
10. Physician Payment Review Commission. Annual Report to the Congress. Washington: Government Printing Office, 1997.
11. Annual Report of the Board of Trustees of the Federal Hospital Insurance Trust Fund. Washington, DC: Government Printing Office, April 24, 1997.
12. Annual Report of The Board of Trustees of the Federal Hospital Insurance Trust Fund (corrected). Washington, DC: Government Printing Office, April 20, 2000.

6
Psychosocial Influences on Health in Later Life

JUDITH L. HOWE

Learning Objectives

Upon completion of the chapter, the student will be able to:

1. Explain key psychosocial domains to consider in an assessment of an older patient.
2. Describe the standardized assessment tools available in conducting a comprehensive assessment, with a focus on psychological, emotional, environmental, spiritual, and social domains.
3. Articulate the role of a social worker in maintaining and enhancing the quality of life of older people.
4. Describe the tools to ensure culturally competent assessment and care.
5. Articulate the prevalent problem of elder mistreatment and neglect.
6. Describe issues related to caregiving and caregiving burden.
7. Delineate several ways that the clinician can work with older patients to maximize independence, productivity and quality of life.

Case (Part 1)

Mrs. Gomez is a 72-year-old Hispanic woman who was recently widowed. She has a history of hypertension, treated with an angiotensin-converting enzyme inhibitor and a mild diuretic, and osteoarthritis, especially of the lower back, treated intermittently with a nonsteroidal antiinflammatory drug. She lives alone in an apartment in a suburb of a large city. Her daughter, Helen, 48 years old, works as an office manager, is married with two teenage children, and lives in another suburb that is a 30-minute drive from her mother's. She visits on the

---

Material in this chapter is based on the following chapter in Cassel CK, Leipzig RM, Cohen HJ, Larson EB, Meier DE, eds. Geriatric Medicine: An Evidence-Based Approach, 4th ed. New York: Springer, 2003: Clipp EC, Steinhauser KE. Psychosocial Influences on Health in Later Life, pp. 53–63. Selections edited by Judith L. Howe.

weekends to run errands and do some light housekeeping. An unmarried son lives in a city about 150 miles away.

Since her husband died 4 months ago, Mrs. Gomez, who does not drive, has been socially isolated, especially because she is unable to participate in her usual activities, such as church meetings and arts and crafts at the local senior center. Her daughter is quite concerned because of her mother's lack of appetite and neglect of personal care. On questioning, Mrs. Gomez admits to early morning awakening, lack of appetite, weight loss, and crying spells. There is no prior history of depression, but she is thought to be depressed as part of her grief reaction.

General Considerations

The relationship between psychosocial factors and health and well-being in later life has been demonstrated in several areas. First, psychosocial and cultural factors influence differences in illness behavior between older and younger patients. Second, these differences in illness behavior interact with age-related physiologic organ change, leading to delayed or altered disease presentation and multiple concurrent pathology. Third, variation in disease presentation and comorbidity profiles gives rise to different trajectories of recovery and clinical outcomes. These observations anticipated the introduction of nonmedical supports as important to clinicians' goals of maintaining and improving patient outcomes. Geriatric assessment often includes patients' emotional tone and lifelong habits. Geriatrics is an interdisciplinary area of practice, and hence the psychosocial domains of a patient's well-being (including the psychological, emotional, social, spiritual, financial, and environmental areas of assessment and care) must be addressed in a comprehensive assessment and subsequent plan of care. The physician caring for an older adult needs to feel comfortable in gathering information in these areas and to be aware of issues and conditions signaling the need for a more comprehensive social work assessment. In settings specializing in geriatrics, there is often an interdisciplinary geriatrics team composed of a physician, social worker, nurse, and often other professionals such as a pharmacist, nutritionist, psychologist, rehabilitation specialist, and audiologist. The social worker is qualified to expand the psychosocial history of the initial assessment to include areas such as social interaction and support systems, environmental conditions, spiritual beliefs, and community and financial resources—all factors likely to influence patients' future functioning and disability management in the community.

If psychosocial needs go unmet through misdiagnosis, lack of detection, lack of treatment, or lack of follow-up, older people are at risk of further health problems that can lead to physical deterioration, reduced independence, and the need for more intensive and expensive care (1). Inattention

TABLE 6.1. Instruments to measure functioning in psychosocial domains (11)

Assessment domain	Assessment tool
Physical health	See Chapter 2: The Comprehensive Geriatric Assessment
Psychological and emotional well-being	Geriatric Depression Scale; Mini–Mental Status Examination
Social functioning	Norbeck Social Support Questionnaire; Lubben Social Network Scale
Competence in activities of daily living	Activities of Daily Living and Instrumental Activities of Daily Living Scales
Spirituality	Hatch's Spiritual Involvement and Belief Scale
Community and financial resources	Economic Resources Assessment Scale of Older Americans Resources and Services Multidimensional Functional Assessment Questionnaire
Environmental safety	The Environmental Checklist

Source: Gallo JJ, Fulmer T, Paveza GJ, Reichel W. Handbook of Geriatric Assessment, 3rd ed., 2000: Jones and Bartlett Publishers, Sudbury, MA. www.jbpub.com. Reprinted with permission.

to psychosocial assessment can also lead to inappropriate placement in nursing homes or other long-term care settings. The systematic, interdisciplinary approach to comprehensive geriatric assessment is significantly broader than other medical specialties. In managed care environments, performing comprehensive assessment is a formidable task within the shorter encounter time frames of most practices (1). In geriatric assessment, in addition to physical health, the principal psychosocial domains are psychological and emotional well-being, social functioning, competence in activities of daily living, spirituality, financial resources, and environmental safety. A number of instruments have been developed in recent years to measure functioning in these psychosocial domains, as listed in Table 6.1. The physician treating an older adult should be knowledgeable about these instruments and comfortable in administering them (2). However, if the physician is a member of an interdisciplinary team, another team member such as a social worker, nurse, nurse practitioner, chaplain or occupational therapist can also administer these instruments.

Role of the Social Worker

A social worker can follow up with identified problems in the psychosocial domains. The physician caring for older adults should be aware of the unique and multiple roles of the social worker on the geriatrics interdisciplinary team for appropriate referral and inclusion of the social worker's knowledge and skills on a team. Social workers are trained to be knowledgeable in assessing and providing care in psychological, social, environmental, spiritual, emotional, financial, and social areas and in the specific techniques outlined in Table 6.2.

TABLE 6.2. The role of the social worker in interdisciplinary geriatric teams (12)

The role of the social worker on an interdisciplinary team includes but is not limited to the following:

The Distinctive Role of Geriatric Social Work

Geriatric social workers conduct holistic biopsychosocial geriatric assessments, which attempt to untangle interconnected physical, psychological, and social factors that affect health and well-being; are skilled in crisis and work with family systems; resolve barriers to service utilization; monitor the effectiveness and appropriateness of services; and assist the elderly in resource development.

Interdisciplinary Teams and Social Work

The social work profession's emphasis on advocacy, and its knowledge of delivery systems in both public and private sectors, enables social workers to take leadership in promoting interdisciplinary practice, facilitating the coordination of services and avoiding duplication, and providing potentially preventive approaches. A social worker has multiple roles within teams including team leader, convener, facilitator, and expert.

Social Work's Multiple Roles on Interdisciplinary Teams

Social workers with their training in interpersonal relationships, group work and interdisciplinary team skills play a vital role in the development and functioning of the interdisciplinary team unit and in all major phases of its work, including assessment and care planning, and monitoring/evaluation. The primary roles of social workers are as follows:

1. Assessor: The social work assessment is based on the biopsychosocial approach and takes into consideration the strengths and weaknesses of the patient (and caregiver) in six areas: physical, psychological, social, cultural, environmental, and spiritual. The social worker assists the patient/family in developing a treatment plan with goals based on this assessment.
2. Care manager: Equally referred to as case manager, the social worker identifies problems, links patient/family with resources, and coordinates resources.
3. Counselor: Individual psychosocial counseling is intended to assist patients and families to adjust to major life transitions and stressors, such as illness, disability, institutionalization, and loss, as well as to empower the client.
4. Group work facilitators: Group work modalities such as supportive psychoeducational groups are designed to help patients, families, or caregivers cope with illness and other events.
5. Liaison: The social worker serves as a vital link between the patient/family and the professional community.
6. Advocate: Social workers serves as representatives for patients/families, working on their behalf to obtain needed services and rights.
7. Community resource expert: Social workers use their extensive knowledge of community resources to match patients with appropriate services.

Source: Mellor MJ, Lindeman D. The role of the social worker in interdisciplinary geriatric teams. J Gerontol Social Work 1998;30(3/4):3–7. Adapted with permission of The Haworth Press, Inc.

Cultural Competency

In the future, the percentage of minority elders will increase substantially, making it important that the physician caring for an older person be sensitive to the culture of the client. *Culture* can be defined as "the shared values, traditions, norms, customs, arts, history, folklore, and institutions of a group of people" (3). A culturally competent physician is able to provide health care in ways that are acceptable and useful to older persons and congruent with their cultural background and expectations (4). It is essential that physicians be aware of their own values and attitudes when interacting with older patients, particularly those from different cultural or racial backgrounds.

Flexibility and skill in responding and adapting to different cultural contexts and circumstances enhances patient care. Table 6.3 provides an overview of issues that the physician should be aware of in the patient–provider relationship to avoid misunderstandings and lack of compliance (4).

Cultural competency also calls for consideration of the historical experiences of older ethnic populations. Cohort analysis helps us to understand the impact of these experiences on elders of varying ethnic groups and to thus take appropriate social histories (5). For instance, when working with older individuals of any ethnicity, it is important to gain information about their experiences during their earlier years. Cohort analysis also helps us to take appropriate social histories and to understand the influences on the older client's trust and attitudes about health care. Table 6.4 provides a brief overview of some of the key cohort experiences of today's minority elders.

TABLE 6.3. Cultural considerations for the physician to be aware when treating an older adult

Language and cultural barriers between providers, patients, and patients' families
Explanatory models of illness
Dietary habits
Medication compliance
Alternative (non-Western) practices (e.g., herbal medicines) or belief in existence of nonbiomedical illnesses or in the efficacy of scientific treatments
Role of religion, with ethical dilemmas of life-sustaining interventions conflicting with religious beliefs
Cultural attitude of some communities and families concerning expectations that patients should be cared for at home
Western emphasis on "independence" as a goal of therapy
Unrealistic expectations
Different expectations as to entitlement to good medical care
Difficulty establishing trusting relationships
Ignorance of how the American medical system works and lack of skills in navigating it
Patient is unable to verbalize his or her symptoms in detail

TABLE 6.4. Selected minority group cohort experiences of today's elders (born between 1900 and 1940)

Minority group	Cohort experiences
African American	Urban migration, Ku Klux Klan active, World War I, Depression, Jesse Owens, and Joe Lewis
American Indian	Reservations, laws banning spiritual practices, forced boarding schools, loss of land by allotment system, forced assimilation
Chinese American	Immigration laws excluding Asians, urbanization, families emerge in Chinatowns
Mexican Americans	Mexican Revolution, massive immigration, depression, repatriation

Source: Adapted from Yeo G, Hikoyeda N, McBride M, Chin S-Y, Edmonds M, Hendrix L. Cohort Analysis as a Tool in Ethnogeriatrics: Historical Profiles of Elders from Eight Ethnic Populations in the United States. Stanford Geriatric Education Center, Working Paper #12. Stanford, CA: Stanford GEC, 1998, with permission.

Case (Part 2)

Helen was able to rearrange her schedule in order to provide transportation to the senior center and to church. Counseling has been arranged to help Mrs. Gomez cope with the grieving process. Overall, these efforts mitigated some of her feelings of depression, and she improved considerably over the next several months.

Mrs. Gomez remained at the same functional level, receiving assistance from her daughter, with her son keeping in touch by phone and helping out financially, until, at age 77, Mrs. Gomez sustained a hip fracture after slipping on the ice on the way to her mailbox. She was hospitalized with a fracture of the left femoral neck and made a good recovery after insertion of a pin to stabilize her hip. She spent two months in a nursing home, receiving physical therapy and rehabilitation and kept her spirits up with the thought of returning home. She was discharged to her home where she ambulates with a walker. To accommodate her, the bedroom is moved downstairs, a commode is placed at her bedside, and a ramp is installed to eliminate the need for stairs to the outside. Her movement, however, is more severely limited than previously. Her daughter continues to provide help with shopping and housework and enlisted the help of the postal carrier as a daily check on Mrs. Gomez's well-being. She continues to feel isolated, lonely, and misses her social activities. Her two best friends from the senior center have died within the last 2 years and she misses their conversations.

Elder Mistreatment and Neglect

Caregiving relationships sometimes exacerbate physical violence or other forms of elder mistreatment including verbal, financial, sexual, or emotional abuse, abandonment, or intentional neglect. Primary care physicians taking care of older adults hold key positions in detecting such abuse because of the frequency with which they interface with older patients and their family members and are required by statutes in most states to report suspected abuse to adult protective services. Among caregivers of elderly persons with dementing disorders, abuse by spouses is more common than abuse by children. Pillemer and Finkelhor (6) suggest that elder mistreatment is more likely to occur when a potential perpetrator has problems, such as mental illness or substance abuse, when the recipient of the abuse is financially or otherwise dependent on the abuser, in socially isolated environments, and in the presence of external stress.

In assessing elder mistreatment, it is important to ask, in separate sessions, the caregiver and the patient about their relationships with each other. This provides an opportunity for each to speak privately and frankly. Physicians suspecting mistreatment or neglect need to consider the safety of sending the older patient back home, the services that may be available to reduce caregiver stress, and the need for closer than usual follow-up. Fortunately, most home care situations involving caregivers and elderly care recipients do not involve abuse. Most informal caregivers are deeply committed to the health and well-being of their care recipients and work to help them age as successfully as possible.

Table 6.5 contains some tips on assessing the patient and caregiver for elder mistreatment or neglect.

Case (Part 3)

Three years later, Mrs. Gomez is now 80 years old. Her daughter, at age 56, is hospitalized for a myocardial infarction and is unable to keep up the same level of help. At least temporarily, she will no longer be available to assist her mother in shopping, housekeeping, laundry, meal planning and preparation, and bathing, or to provide emotional support. Mrs. Gomez is now homebound with no arrangements to the senior center or church. Her house is becoming increasingly untidy and she is eating sporadically. She refuses to participate in the Meals on Wheels program because she does not like the food—it is not what she is used to.

When her son visits, he is surprised and a little angry at the condition his mother is in, although he keeps it to himself, considering his sister's recent heart attack. He is unable to provide the same level of support that his sister did given the fact that he lives 150 miles away and is a single with a full-time job. He believes his mother should be placed immediately in a protective environment. Because Mrs. Gomez is adamant about staying home, her son makes a compromise agreement with her to allow a live-in housekeeper. Although he tries to find a satisfactory live-in helper, he cannot find one who is satisfactory to both Mrs. Gomez and him.

Because her son must return to work, and Helen is unable to care for her mother, Mrs. Gomez reluctantly agrees to nursing home placement in an intermediate care facility, at least on a trial basis.

TABLE 6.5. Patient and caregiver assessment of elder abuse or neglect

Assessing the patient
First, get the history from the patient: include direct questions about mistreatments and look for indications of unusual confinement, sudden withdrawals or closing of bank accounts, excessive weight gain or loss, insomnia or excessive sleeping

Physical indicators of mistreatment
New and inadequately explained injuries such as welts, bruises, lacerations, fractures, rope marks or burns, pressure ulcers
Dehydrated or malnourished appearance
Lack of cleanliness, grooming, personal hygiene
Presence of head injury, hair loss, or hemorrhaging beneath scalp
Signs of possible sexual abuse: discharges, bruising, bleeding, or trauma around the genitalia or rectum, unexplained venereal disease or genital infections
Laboratory findings indicating medication overdose or undermedication

Environmental indicators of mistreatment
Social isolation of older person: lack of involvement of family and friends
Inadequate housing or unsafe conditions in home

Behavior of the patient indicating mistreatment
Acts overly medicated or overly sedated
Fear of speaking for oneself in the presence of caretaker; anxious to please
Anxiety, confusion, withdrawal, depression
Shame, fear, embarrassment
Little or no eye contact or communication
Explanation is not consistent with the medical findings

Assessing the caregiver
Threatening remarks and/or behavior
Conflicting stories
Insults, aggressive behavior
Withholding of attention, security, affection
Attitude of indifference or anger toward older person
Unusual fatigue, depression
Obvious absence of assistance or attendance
Problems with alcohol or drugs
Previous history of abusive behavior
Contradictory and/or inconsistent explanations given by the patient and the caregiver
History of violence in family
Financial or family problems
Appears emotionally and/cognitively "stressed out"

Source: Adapted from Howe JL, Sherman DW, Amato N, Banc T. 2002. Geriatrics, Palliative Care, and Interprofessional Teamwork: An Interdisciplinary Curriculum. Bronx-New York Harbor VA GRECC, www.nygrecc.org.

Caregiver Issues

Many older patients presenting to physicians for evaluation or follow-up are accompanied by their informal caregivers. These providers are most often related to the older patient, such as a spouse or adult child, but also may be a close personal friend. In many instances, it would be impossible for the older person to continue to live in the community without the occasional or routine assistance provider by caregivers. Caregivers provide the critical support that compensates for the older person's limitations caused by chronic illness, disability, or physical or mental frailty.

Who are the caregivers? It is estimated that in one in four U.S. households a person over the age of 18 had provided care to someone over age 50 at some point during the previous year. The Assets and Health Dynamics Among the Oldest Old (AHEAD) study found that about 8.5 million individuals over age 70 are impaired in activities of daily living (ADLs; e.g., using the toilet, eating) or instrumental activities of daily living (IADLs; e.g., taking medications, making phone calls), thus requiring some level of assistance to function in the community (7). By 2030, this number may be as high as 21 million. For the practicing clinician, this translates to approximately two out of five older patients in one's practice who need assistance with one or more of these routine activities. The data suggest that most caregivers are family members (72%), the majority of whom are adult children (42%) and spouses (25%), and identifies significant ethnic variation in typical caregiving arrangements. For example, Caucasian older patients tend to receive help from spouses, Hispanics from adult children, and blacks from informal providers outside the family. Most of the caregivers surveyed provide daily care; about 21% assist several times a week. The large majority (80%) allocates up to 5 hours of assistance per day, and a small group, approximately 7%, provides care 24 hours a day.

Caregiving is often time-consuming, labor-intensive, and stressful. Further, there may be a substantial financial impact on the caregivers. A study of families of seriously ill patients found that in 20% of cases a family member had to quit work or make another life change in order to provide care for the patient. Further, almost one third of families reported the loss of most or all of the family savings (7). In shouldering this burden, caregivers often experience substantial levels of emotional distress and physical exhaustion. Caring for an older person with physical impairment involves organizing ADLs and orchestrating medical and home care arrangements. Caring for an older adult with cognitive impairment requires this same organization of ADLs and health services, plus additional burdens associated with progressive memory loss, complex decisions about health care, legal arrangements and finances, personal control and autonomy issues, challenging behavior problems and communication deficits, and anticipatory grief.

Overall, about 15% of caregivers in the AHEAD study reported experiencing a physical or mental health problem because of their caregiving responsibilities. Among caregivers of dementia patients, links have been found between caregiving and anxiety and depression symptomatology, psychotropic drug use, lower ratings of self-rated health, less optimum health-related behaviors such as getting enough exercise or sleep, and changes in immune function (8). Perhaps the most provocative research to date, from a population-based cohort, suggests that being an elderly spousal caregiver under mental or emotional strain is an independent risk factor for mortality (9).

All caregivers, but especially those caring for patients with progressive dementia disorders or those caring for individuals at the end of life, constitute a vulnerable population at high risk for adverse health consequences, including death. Physicians need to be able to identify caregivers in their practices who may be at risk for adverse health outcomes. Data indicate that being female, of low means, and caring for a patient with problem behaviors or a patient with cognitive impairment are risk factors for negative health consequences for the caregiver (8). The wealth of data identifying health risks associated with informal care provision underscores the importance of family assessment in geriatric patient evaluations. Clinicians should inquire about the level (unskilled vs. skilled) and intensity (occasional, daily, round-the-clock) of care, and caregivers' needs for additional assistance or services. By identifying at-risk caregivers and referring them to appropriate community resources or to other health care professionals before irreversible health problems arise, geriatricians increase the likelihood that dedicated caregivers can continue to provide care and that elderly impaired patients are able to age in place. As most clinicians are acutely aware, however, not all presumably supportive relationships are, in fact, supportive. Some compromise or seriously threaten elderly patients' health and well-being.

Successful Aging

The most significant articulation of the successful aging concept occurred with the publication of results from the MacArthur Foundation successful aging studies by Rowe and Kahn (10), entitled *Successful Aging*. The authors merged their perspectives from geriatrics and social science, rejected the established approach of studying aging in terms of decline, and used data to show that lifestyle choices rather than genetic inheritance are key factors that determine how successfully people age. Rowe and Kahn point to three tightly interrelated critical components of successful aging: (1) avoidance of disease, (2) lifestyle choices, and (3) engagement with life. Obviously, the avoidance of acute and chronic disease is critical. However, equally important are certain lifestyle choices that maintain or improve physical and mental function and social engagement with life.

More specifically, the MacArthur studies showed that one of the most statistically significant predictors of maintaining cognitive functioning with age was the older patient's sense of *self-efficacy*, or the belief in one's own ability to handle various situations. Rowe and Kahn (10) call self-efficacy the "can-do factor." Other predictors were physical exercise, education, and lung function. People demonstrating this can-do attitude also demonstrated higher levels of productivity (e.g., gardening, homemaking, volunteering). Physical functioning was more dependent on an elderly person's level of social support, specifically emotional support as opposed to instrumental support or tangible assistance. Elderly people with higher levels of emotional support (i.e., expressions of affection, respect, love, encouragement) were more likely to engage in physical activity, such as brisk walking and substantial housework, whereas instrumental support (direct, hand-on assistance, provision of resources) was associated with lower physical performance. These data suggest the importance of providing adequate emotional support to older persons, but at the same time not limiting their autonomy by doing things that they are able to do themselves.

Perhaps the most exciting conclusion of these studies is that lifestyle factors and choices, such as adopting a positive attitude about meeting challenges (i.e., self-efficacy), engaging in routine exercise, and seeking opportunities to engage others, are modifiable. With this knowledge, more geriatricians currently are shifting their goals from identifying and managing disease to preventing or delaying disease and promoting health. Because many older individuals have multiple comorbid illnesses, delaying the onset of one condition through lifestyle changes may also reduce risks associated with the development of other medical problems as well. More aggressive attempts to modify risk in elderly patients through exercise, diet, and efforts to detect and prevent disease are important. However, recent data on successful aging suggest that in order to reduce the total period of disability for any one patient, efforts should be made to enhance patients' self-efficacy by promoting their beliefs that challenges can be met and by encouraging close relationships with others. Clinicians should make their older patients aware that they are more responsible than anyone else for their own health in later life.

General Principles

- The psychosocial domains (Table 6.6) of an older patient's well-being must be addressed in an interdisciplinary, comprehensive assessment and care plan.
- If psychosocial needs go unmet through misdiagnosis or lack of detection, treatment, or follow-up, the older patient is at risk of further health problems that can lead to physical deterioration, reduced independence, and the need for more extensive and expensive care.
- Social workers are uniquely qualified in terms of knowledge and skills in assessment and provision of care in psychological, social, environmental, spiritual, emotional, financial, and social areas.
- Working on teams, social workers can provide biopsychosocial assessments, case management, individual and group counseling, liaison with the professional community, advocacy, and the identification of services and programs.

- Physicians who are flexible and skilled in adapting to different cultural contexts will deliver more effective and sensitive care.
- Elder abuse and neglect is common, underdiagnosed, and refers not only to physical but also to emotional, financial, verbal, and sexual abuse. Physicians are key in the detection of abuse through assessment of the patient and caregiver.
- Caregivers who provide the critical support necessary for some older persons to remain in the community are at risk for physical and psychological problems due to the multiple demands of caregiving; physicians need to be sensitive to the factors associated with caregiver stress.
- The three key correlates of successful aging are avoidance of disease, a healthy lifestyle, and a positive, "can-do" attitude about life.

TABLE 6.6. Guiding questions in assessing psychosocial domains

Gender, ethnicity, and socioeconomic status

- Observe gender and inquire about education or years of formal schooling. Assess level of knowledge; do not assume. For example, older patients with lower levels of education have been shown to confuse the concept of living will with a legal/financial document.
- In the absence of financial information (e.g., income, assets), geriatricians can probe their patients' *perceived* adequacy of financial resources, often a more powerful predictor of well-being than objective income. "Are your bills difficult to meet? Does your money take care of your needs? Can you afford to buy those little "extras"—that is, those small luxuries?" Such questions may open doors for discussion of unmet needs.

Cohort

- "Were you born in the United States?" If not, were the circumstances of immigration likely to be traumatic (e.g., Holocaust, revolution)?
- "Are you a veteran? Which war? Did you experience combat?"
- If yes, probe into the meaning of that experience in day-to-day life. Consider potential links between chronic stress and coronary artery disease (CAD). If patient mentions posttraumatic stress disorder (PTSD) symptoms (e.g., nightmares, flashbacks, or reexperiencing), make appropriate referral.

Social relationships

- The structure of patients' social networks can be appreciated by asking about the people with whom the patient interacts and the assistance, if any, provided by those persons. For example, "With whom do you live?" One of the strongest predictors of noninstitutionalization is the presence of a spouse. "How many people are in your support network? What kinds of things do they do for you? Do you receive help with shopping? Housework? Transportation? How often?" Is the patient involved in organized groups, such as a senior center or recreation club?
- The adequacy of emotional support can be probed by such questions as the following: "Do you feel supported by and close to those around you? Do you feel the need for more assistance than you are currently receiving? Is there someone in your life with whom you can discuss your deepest concerns and feelings?"
- "Who would you contact if you needed help?"

(Continued)

TABLE 6.6. *Continued*

Spirituality

- "What role does faith or spirituality play in your life?" This brief question may help the clinician understand for whom spiritual activity (including formal religious participation and private practices) is a critical component in coping with illness, decision making, and general well-being.

Caregiving

- Determine caregiver status by asking patient or family member if they are providing care for anyone on a routine basis.
- If the answer is yes, ask about the intensity of care provision (primary vs. secondary provider, daily basis or less often) and type of care (personal management, household, physical care).
- Identify potential stressors (use of alcohol or drugs to cope) and feelings of helplessness and hopelessness that could lead the caregiver to mistreat the patient.
- Ask about caregivers' needs for assistance—what would help caregiver most (e.g., support group, respite, in-home care, sitter service, chore worker).

Elder mistreatment

- Ask the patient if problem behavior exists in the family, such as acts of violence or excessive force. "Has anyone tried to hurt or hit you? Has anyone made you do things that you did not want to do? Has anyone taken your things?"
- The next steps may involve notifying Adult Protective Services or other state-specific agencies and creating a safety plan for the patient.

Successful aging

- Are measures being taken to avoid disease and maintain optimal cognitive and physical function (e.g., scheduling regular checkups, eating a nutritious diet, engaging in regular, moderate physical activity, and avoiding high-risk behaviors such as smoking)?
- Does the patient cope well with setbacks?
- In general, does the patient have a positive attitude?
- Is the patient socially connected and engaged with life?

Source: Adapted from Clipp EC, Steinhauser KE. Psychosocial Influences on Health in Later Life. In: Cassel CK, Leipzig RM, Cohen HJ, et al., eds. Geriatric Medicine, 4th ed. New York: Springer, 2003.

Suggested Readings

Butler RN, Lewis M, Sunderland T. Aging and Mental Health: Positive Psychoso-cial and Biomedical Approaches, 4th ed. New York: Macmillan, 1991. *This seminal book provides an extensive overview to health professionals in the diagnosis, treatment and prevention of psychological and mental problems and disorders, such as depression and anxiety. It also details successful therapies and interventions to assist older people and their caregivers.*

Clipp EC, Steinhauser KE. Psychosocial influences on health in later life. In: Cassel CK, Leipzig RM, Cohen HJ, et al., eds. Geriatric Medicine, 4th ed. New York: Springer, 2003:53–63.

Howe JK, ed. Older People and Their Caregivers Across The Spectrum of Care. Binghamton, NY: Haworth, 2003. *This book focuses on issues related to care across the continuum and the key role of social work assessment in care of older adults. The need for sensitive and appropriate assessment is emphasized in a variety of settings, including community and long term care settings, as well as*

populations, such as veterans, victims of elder abuse, and those suffering from HIV/AIDS.
Rowe JW, Kahn RL. Successful Aging. New York: Pantheon, 1998. *Based on the results of the groundbreaking MacArthur Foundation Study on Aging in America, this book discusses the factors that enable older persons to preserve or even improve their physical and mental vitality in late life. The researchers found that lifestyle choices, more than genes, determined how we age, and outline those choices, such as diet, exercise, and self-efficacy in practical terms.*

References

1. Berkman B, Maramaldi P, Breon E, Howe JL. Social work gerontological assessment revisited. J Gerontol Social Work 2002;40:1–14.
2. Reuben DB, Herr KA, Pacala JT, et al. Geriatrics at Your Fingertips: 2005, 7th ed. American Geriatrics Society, New York, 2005.
3. U.S. Department of Health and Human Services, Administration on Aging. Profile of Older Americans 2000, http://www.aoa.org.
4. Howe JL, Sherman DS, Banc TE, eds. Geriatrics, Palliative Care and Interdisciplinary Teamwork: An Interdisciplinary Curriculum, Module 17. Developed by the Bronx VAMC GRECC Program, 2002.
5. Yeo G, et al. Core Curriculum in Ethnogeriatrics, 2nd ed. Stanford, CA: Stanford University, 2000.
6. Pillemer K, Finkelhor D. Causes of elder abuse: caregiver stress versus problem relatives. Am J Orthopsychiatry 1989;59:179–187.
7. Shirley L, Summer L. Caregiving: Helping the Elderly with Activity Limitations. Washington, DC: National Academy on an Aging Society Series, vol 7, 2000.
8. Schultz R. Handbook on Dementia Caregiving. New York: Springer, 2000.
9. Schultz R, Beach S. Caregiving as a risk factor for mortality: the caregiver health effects study. JAMA 1999;282:2215–2219.
10. Rowe JW, Kahn RL. Successful Aging. New York: Pantheon, 1998.
11. Gallo JJ, Fulmer T, Paveza GJ, Reichel W. Handbook of Geriatric Assessment, 3rd ed. Gaithersburg, MD: Aspen, 2000:162–166.
12. Mellor MJ, Lindeman D. The role of the social worker in interdisciplinary geriatric teams. J Gerontol Social Work 1998;30(3/4):3–7.

7
Medicolegal Aspects of the Care of Older Adults

OLUSEGUN A. APOESO

Learning Objectives

Upon completion of the chapter, the student will be able to:
1. Understand the concept of informed consent.
2. Enumerate the components of an informed consent.
3. Appreciate the importance of advance care planning.
4. Differentiate between competency and decision-making capacity and describe the steps in assessing these in older adults.

General Considerations

Older patients enter into relationships with physicians and other members of the health care team in order to obtain medical care. These relationships can be characterized as both *contractual* (i.e., based on a mutual exchange of explicit or implicit promises) and *fiduciary* (i.e., based on the trust the dependent patient must invest in relying on the more knowledgeable and powerful health care provider). Within either of these frameworks, the resulting relationships implicate a variety of legally enforceable obligations on the part of the physician. Thus, some familiarity with treatment-related legal requirements and associated potential liabilities is essential.

Informed Consent

The fundamental ethical principle of autonomy or self-determination is embodied in the legal doctrine of *informed consent*. There are three essential elements that must be present in order for patient's choices about

Material in this chapter is based on the following chapters in Cassel CK, Leipzig RM, Cohen HJ, Larson EB, Meier DE, eds. Geriatric Medicine: An Evidence-Based Approach, 4th ed. New York: Springer, 2003: Kapp MB. Medical Treatment and the Physician's Legal Duties, pp. 1221–1231. Bottrell MM, Cassel CK, Felzenberg ER. Ethical and Policy Issues in End-of-Life Care, pp. 1243–1251. Karlawish JHT, Pearlman RA. Determination of Decision-Making Capacity, pp. 1233–1242. Selections edited by Olusegun A. Apoeso.

treatment to be considered legally valid. First, the patient's participation in the decision-making process and the ultimate decision must be voluntary; that is, the person giving or withholding consent must be able to exercise free power of choice without the intervention of any element of force, fraud, deceit, duress, overreaching, or other ulterior form of constraint or coercion. It means simply that the person must be free to reject participation in the proposed intervention.

Second, the patient's agreement must be sufficiently informed. The informed consent doctrine commands that the health care provider, before undertaking an intervention, must disclose certain information to the person who is the subject of the proposed intervention (or that person's authorized surrogate). The adequacy of disclosure is judged against the amount and type of information that a reasonable, prudent physician would have disclosed under similar circumstances. The patient's age may affect what information is material to that person's decision-making calculations. For instance, a likely side effect that will not manifest itself for another 20 years may not be very important to an older person. However, the probability that a particular intervention will be accompanied by a great amount of physical pain or discomfort may make quite a difference to an old, frail individual. Physicians always should take into account the physical and mental effects of aging, among numerous other factors, when deciding what information regarding an intervention might be material to the specific person and how to communicate that information most usefully.

Third, the patient must be mentally able to engage in a rational decision-making process. When the patient lacks sufficient present cognitive and emotional capacity to make medical choices, a proxy or surrogate decision maker must be involved.

Case (Part 1)

You enter the hospital room of a 76-year-old woman before morning rounds to obtain informed consent for a diagnostic procedure. You find the patient to be somewhat confused. Her Mini–Mental State Examination score is 24/30.

The patient has had a 30-lb unintentional weight loss over the last 3 months, associated with iron-deficiency anemia. She is currently admitted for a colonic carcinoma workup. She is widowed with two children, a 45-year-old daughter and a 40-year-old son. Both of them live out of state. She lives alone independently, requiring occasional assistance with the payment of her bills. She had been able to make health-related decisions prior to this hospitalization.

What necessary steps will you take in order to obtain an informed consent for the diagnostic procedure?

Surrogate Decision Making

Physicians involved in the diagnosis and treatment of older patients frequently must deal with substitute decision makers responsible for intervening on behalf of patients whose cognitive or emotional deficits are so severe that they prevent the patient from personally making and communicating autonomous choices (1). The topic of surrogate decision making by third parties acting for the incapacitated patient is a complex and legally inexact one.

There are several alternative ways to delegate legally what would ordinarily be the patient's authority to make decisions, in order for the proxy or surrogate to exercise that power on behalf of the incapacitated patient: (1) delegation of authority beforehand by the patient, through methods of advance planning; (2) delegation of authority by operation of statute, regulation, or broad judicial precedent; (3) informal delegation of authority by custom; and (4) delegation of authority by a court order in the specific case.

Advance Care Planning

The two most important current devices for advance health care planning are the living will (in some jurisdictions called a declaration) and the durable power of attorney for health care (2). The Patient Self-Determination Act (PSDA) passed by Congress as part of the Omnibus Budget Reconciliation Act (OBRA) of 1990 (3), in the aftermath of the United States Supreme Court's decision in *Cruzan v. Director, Missouri Department of Health* (4), imposes a number of requirements on hospitals, nursing homes, health maintenance organizations, preferred provider organizations, hospices, and home health agencies that participate in the Medicare and Medicaid programs. Among these are mandates that the provider create and distribute to new patients or their surrogates a written policy on advance directives, consistent with applicable state law; the provider inquire at the time of admission or enrollment whether the patient has previously executed an advance directive; and, if no advance directive has been executed previously and the patient currently retains sufficient decisional capacity, the provider inquire whether the patient wishes to execute such a directive now (5,6).

Statutory, Regulatory, and Judicial Guidelines

In some circumstances, particular facets of decision-making authority may devolve or pass from the patient to someone else by operation of a statute, regulation, or judicial precedent. It is in the area of decision making about care of the critically ill patient that statutory, regulatory, and judicial guidance about substitute decision making is clearest. Statutes in 27 states and the District of Columbia empower designated relatives, and sometimes others, to make particular kinds of medical decisions on behalf of incapacitated persons who have not executed a living will or durable power of attorney (7). In addition, courts in many jurisdictions have formally recognized the family's authority to exercise an incapacitated person's rights on his or her behalf and for families to act in future cases without the need for prior court authorization in individual cases.

In the absence of a specific statute, regulation, or court order delegating authority to a substitute decision maker, or a court order naming a person to act as guardian or conservator, neither the family as a whole nor any of its individual members have any automatic legal authority to make decisions on behalf of a patient who cannot speak for himself. Nevertheless, it has long been a widely known and implicitly accepted medical custom or convention to rely on families as decision makers for incompetent persons, even in the absence of express legal power. Even when there is no explicit judicial or legislative authorization in one's own state, the legal risk for a physician or health care institution for a good faith treatment decision made in conjunction with an incompetent patient's family is very slight. In fact, the few courts that have been presented with the question in the context of litigation have virtually unanimously ratified the family's authority.

Guardianship

In some cases, however, informal substitute decision making by the physician and family members may not work satisfactorily. The family members may disagree among themselves. They may make decisions that seem to be at odds with the earlier expressed or implied preferences of the patient or that clearly appear not to be in the patient's best interests (e.g., a family's financially or psychologically driven selfish choices). The family may request a course of conduct that seriously contradicts the physician's or facility's own sense of ethical integrity.

When such situations occur, judicial appointment of a guardian or conservator empowered to make decisions on behalf of an incompetent ward may be practically and legally advisable (8). Guardianship usually entails an extensive deprivation of the individual's basic rights and may be imposed in the absence of meaningful procedural safeguards. It also involves substantial financial, time, and emotional costs. Thus, it should be pursued only as a last resort when less formal mechanisms of substitute decision making have failed or are unavailable.

> **Case (Part 2)**
>
> After further history is obtained from the daughter, who has been somewhat involved with the patient's health care, it is noted that the patient does have a living will and a Do Not Resuscitate (DNR) order. She, however, does not have a designated durable power of attorney for health care.
>
> What is a "living will," a "DNR," and a designated durable power of attorney for health care?
>
> What are the medicolegal implications of having, or not having, advance care planning?

"Do Not" Orders

"Do Not" orders from the attending physician to other members of the health care team mostly involve decisions to withdraw or withhold certain types of medical interventions from specified patients. Most attention has been devoted, especially in the acute hospital environment, to Do Not Resuscitate (DNR) orders (also called No Codes), or instructions by the physician to refrain from attempts at cardiopulmonary resuscitation (CPR) in the event of a cardiac arrest. Other kinds of "Do Not" orders are also important, particularly in the long-term-care environment (e.g., "Do Not Hospitalize" and "Do Not Intubate" orders).

The Competent Adult

A competent adult patient has the constitutional, common law, and (in many states) statutory right to voluntarily and knowingly refuse basic (e.g., CPR) or advanced cardiac life support or any of its specific components, hospitalization, or any other form of medical intervention and to demand a precisely written "Do Not" order. Courts have not ordered competent elderly patients to endure medical interventions over their stated objections. The wishes of close family members should be considered by the physician but should never be permitted to override the decision of a competent patient.

When a capable patient has made a "Do Not" decision, he or she must be able to reevaluate and reconsider that decision continually in light of any change in physical or mental condition that might really make a difference in the possible benefits and burdens of different treatment alternatives. A "Do Not" decision can be revoked or modified at any time. It is part of the physician's duty to continually update the patient with new information pertinent to "Do Not" decisions.

The Mentally Incapacitated Patient

For the mentally incapacitated patient, clarification of respective rights and responsibilities may be available from the patient's advance directive or from the designated proxy. Even in the absence of a valid advance directive or explicitly legally authorized proxy, "Do Not" orders are still permissible for incapacitated patients according to the same general legal principles governing other kinds of decisions about life-sustaining medical treatment, that is, balancing the likely benefits and burdens of the particular intervention from the perspective of the patient. The only pertinent distinction between "Do Not" orders and other decisions to limit the use of life-prolonging medical interventions lies in the prospective nature of the former.

The physician's and health care institution's responsibility to adopt, educate about, and communicate concerning a clear policy on "Do Not" orders applies with full force when presently incapacitated patients are involved. When a patient is not presently capable of participating fully in decision making, the communication and negotiation about potential "Do Not" management strategies must encompass available, interested family members. The family has the same legal authority to make "Do Not" decisions for an incapacitated relative as to make other types of medical decisions. Even in the absence of specific legal authorization, it is the medical custom or convention to involve families in "Do Not" decisions. From a practical risk management perspective, extensive interaction with family members concerning such decisions is a prudent, protective practice. A communication and negotiation process that is marked by compassion, clarity, and patience should resolve family/physician disagreement peacefully in the vast majority of situations. When serious disagreement between physician and family or among family members themselves does surface and persist, consultation with an ethics committee may be advisable (9). During the communications process, the family should be informed that the continuing propriety of a "Do Not" order will be reevaluated regularly and that it can be rescinded or modified if prognosis or other factors materially change.

Documentation and Communication

The wishes of the patient (if ascertainable), the family, and significant others should all be recorded. The judgments of involved health care professionals, as well as the reasoning underlying those judgments, should be documented completely and candidly, as well as any attempts to change the minds of the patient or family. Honesty and accuracy in record keeping is the best defense for the physician and health care facility against any subsequent allegations of negligence or malevolent intent. Failure to put decisions and orders in writing not only exposes the physician to greater legal risk, but also engenders possible inappropriate responses by other team members based on the mixed and confused signals that are given.

Along with documentation, there is the need for communication among appropriate health care team members and institutions once a "Do Not" order has been written. A decision to refrain from certain interventions needs to be made known to those responsible for carrying out the order because, in the absence of such an order, the health care team normally is obligated to treat the patient with the full medical arsenal available.

Finally, decisions to limit specific elements of treatment should not signify total disregard or the writing off of an older person. Alleviating suffering is a basic goal of medical care and a part of the standard of care legally and ethically owed by health care professionals, even when cure of underlying disease is no longer possible. Management goals should consist of the following: remaining in physical and emotional contact with the dying person; relieving terminal symptoms (such as pain, confusion, anxiety, or restlessness); providing nourishment and hydration as long as they are palliative; skin care, bowel and bladder care, and personal grooming; and supporting the family through the period of dying, death, and bereavement. Appropriate high-dose opioids and sedatives can be used as long as the therapeutic intention is to control the symptoms of human suffering, not to precipitate an earlier death.

Case (Part 3)

After establishing her mother's DNR status, the daughter inquires about the possibility of just "ending it all." She is concerned about the burden versus the benefits of going through a battery of tests in view of the presumptive diagnosis of colonic carcinoma.

What is physician-assisted suicide and how would you differentiate it from euthanasia?

Physician-Assisted Suicide and Euthanasia

Current U.S. law is unambiguous in the condemnation of health care providers engaging in *active euthanasia* (i.e., actively and intentionally doing something to hasten the death of a patient). In addition, almost all states explicitly condemn *physician-assisted suicide* (i.e., actively helping a patient to purposely take his or her own life), through either a specific statute on the subject or judicial interpretations of their general homicide statutes. In 1997, the U.S. Supreme Court unanimously upheld the validity of state laws making it criminal for physicians or other health care professionals to assist a patient to commit suicide. In these decisions, the Court rejected the notion of any federal constitutional right to physician-assisted suicide (10,11). Although the U.S. Constitution does not require it, the door is open legally for particular states to choose, as a matter of their own respective public policies and politics, to decriminalize physician-assisted suicide or even active euthanasia. Thus far, Oregon is the only state that has accepted this invitation (12–14), and in 2006 the U.S. Supreme Court upheld Oregon's physician-assisted suicide law.

Adult Protective Services

Every state has assembled an array of programs under the general title of adult protective services (APS). It is a system of preventive, supportive, and surrogate services provided to adults living in the community, enabling them to maximize independence and to avoid abuse and exploitation. APS are characterized by two elements: (1) the coordinated delivery of services to adults at risk, and (2) the actual or potential authority to provide substitute decision making concerning these services.

The services component consists of an assortment of health, housing, and social services, such as homemaker, house repair, friendly visits, and meals. Ideally, these services are coordinated by a caseworker who is responsible for assessing an older individual's needs and bringing together the available responses. Many state APS statutes mandate that social service agencies undertake both casework coordination and delivery of services.

The second component of an APS system is authority to intervene on behalf of the client. Ordinarily, the patient (if capable of making autonomous decisions), with the encouragement of his physician, will consent to a proposed service plan. Alternatively, he/she may delegate decision-making authority to someone else through a durable power of attorney instrument. However, if the patient refuses offered assistance but some form(s) of intervention appears necessary, the legal system may be invoked to authorize appointment of a surrogate decision maker over the person's objections.

As noted, it frequently is best for APS interventions to be accepted voluntarily by older persons who need help to maximize self-control over their lives. The physician has a duty to counsel patients about available long-term-care alternatives—both institutional and home and community-based—and their relative advantages and disadvantages, or at least to direct patients to appropriate information sources. The ultimate goal is not simply to obtain protective services, whether on a voluntary or involuntary basis. Rather, the key is to assure the quality and appropriateness of the services actually provided for the older individual involved.

Confidentiality

Physicians have the duty to hold in confidence all personal patient information entrusted to them. This obligation is embodied in virtually all state professional practice acts and implementing regulations. State medical practice acts provide that violation of the duty of confidentiality is a potential ground for revoking, denying, or suspending a physician's license to practice medicine. Detailed federal regulations (15,16) are being developed to safeguard the privacy of medical records, based on a mandate in the Health Insurance Portability and Accountability Act of 1996 (HIPAA) (17). The patient's reasonable expectation of privacy extends to all members of the health care team.

Exceptions to the Rule of Confidentiality

The first exception to the usual rule of confidentiality is that a patient may waive, or give up, the right to confidentiality if this is done in a voluntary, competent, and informed manner. The physician has an obligation to cooperate fully in the patient-requested release and transfer of medical information. The patient's waiver of confidentiality and request for release of information should be honored only if it has been documented thoroughly in writing. Further, the identity and legitimate authority of the record seeker should be verified satisfactorily.

Second, when the rights of innocent third parties are jeopardized, the general requirement of confidentiality may yield. For instance, the expressed threat of a dangerous psychiatric patient to kill a specific victim, coupled with the patient's apparent present ability and intent to make good on the threat, arguably should be reported to the intended victim and to law enforcement officials (18).

Third, the patient's expectation of confidentiality must yield when the physician is mandated by state law to report to specified public health authorities the existence of certain enumerated conditions reasonably suspected in a patient. Such requirements may be based on the state's inherent police power to protect the health, safety, and welfare of society as a whole. This rationale would support, for example, reporting requirements concerning infectious diseases or vital statistics (e.g., birth and death).

Finally, the physician may be compelled to reveal otherwise confidential patient information by a judge's issuance of a court order requiring such release. This is a possibility in any type of lawsuit where the patient's physical or mental condition is in dispute.

Within these standards of disclosure, the following informational items have usually been enumerated as essential components of the ideal informed consent process: (1) diagnosis; (2) the general nature and purpose of the proposed intervention; (3) the reasonably foreseeable risks, consequences, and perils of the intervention; (4) the probability of success; (5)

reasonable alternatives; (6) the result anticipated if nothing is done; (7) limitations on the professional or health care facility; and (8) advice (i.e., the physician's recommendation).

Case (Part 3)

You reevaluate the patient the next day. She is still somewhat confused but conversant. You want to determine her capacity to make appropriate health care decisions.

What is the difference between competency and decision-making capacity?

What are the steps taken to determine capacity?

The Concepts of Competency and Decision-Making Capacity

Decision-making capacity describes a person's abilities to make a decision, whereas *competency* describes the judgment that a person's decision-making capacity is adequate to make a particular decision. The former is a condition of a person, whereas the latter is a judgment that integrates information that describes a person's capacities and the context and consequences of the decision (19).

Competency and decision-making capacity are distinct concepts. It is entirely possible that a physician could determine that a person lacks decision-making capacity but is competent to make a decision. For example, a patient who agrees to take hypertension treatment may fail to understand certain facts about that treatment ("the pills work because they reduce stress."). But although this misunderstanding represents impaired decision-making capacity, it has harms that are essentially nil. Hence, given the context and consequences, any reasonable practitioner (or judge) would conclude that the person is competent to take the medication.

The Importance of Assessing Decision-Making Capacity

The essential attributes that a person needs to make a decision are cognitive skills and a set of values that allow the person to categorize and weigh the importance of information. A number of medical diseases and geriatric syndromes can impair these attributes. These diseases include neurodegenerative dementias such as Alzheimer's disease and frontotemporal dementia, psychiatric diseases such as major depression and anxiety, and medical illnesses that precipitate the common clinical syndrome of delirium. Also, an affective disorder such as depression can affect decision-making capacity.

The importance of assessing a patient's decision-making capacity rests in the need to balance two simultaneous ethical commitments to adult patients: to respect an adult person's autonomy, and to promote that person's health and well-being. It is also important to assess decision-making capacity because it serves as a means to balance a physician's simultaneous commitments to respecting a patient's autonomy and promoting her well-being. Having assessed a patient's decision-making capacity, a physician then judges whether the patient is competent to make the decision.

How to Assess Decision-Making Capacity

The standards of decision-making capacity provide structure to the physician's assessment. The physician uses the results of the assessment to decide what degree of performance on which of the standards is adequate to decide that a patient has decision-making capacity. General rules to assess decision-making capacity are to use open-ended questions that allow the patient to think aloud, to use silent pauses rather than a battery of questions, and to sit face-to-face with a patient rather than at unequal postures such as standing at the foot of the patient's bed.

To begin an assessment it is sensible to inform the patient of the purpose of the questions that will follow. A useful opening script might be: "I'd like to take some time to go over the options of treating your breast cancer. One of my roles as doctor is as teacher. I'm a doctor of medicine, so my responsibility is to teach you about your health and options for taking care of it." To then focus on the issue of assessing decision-making capacity, a physician might say: "I'd like to go over the decision you face. Can we talk about what you see as your medical problems and the options for taking care of them?" Assessing the abilities to make a choice and a reasonable choice are relatively straightforward. Little skill is needed to assess these standards beyond giving the patient the opportunity to actually make a choice. As simple as this is, in the conduct of a busy office practice, a physician can forget to ask the patient the simple questions listed in Table 7.1.

The assessment of decision-making capacity occurs throughout the daily practice of medicine. When a patient participates in the decision and agrees to a recommended treatment that has benefits and minimal risk compared with alternative treatments, it is reasonable for the physician to presume that the patient has decision-making capacity. This describes much of outpatient practice. Conversely, when a patient is comatose, delirious, severely demented, or severely psychotic, it is reasonable for the physician to either observe that the patient does not have the capacity to make decisions or decide that further simple questions are needed to assess decision-making capacity.

TABLE 7.1. The Standards for Assessing Decision-Making Capacity (20)

- The ability to make a choice:
  - "So those are the options. What would you like to do?"
- The ability to make a reasonable choice:
  - Same as ability to make a choice. Physician judges whether the decision is "reasonable."
- The ability to appreciate:
  - Appreciate illness: "Can you tell me in your own words what you see as your problem?"
  - Appreciate treatments: "Can you tell me in your own words what you see as your options for your problem?"
- The ability to reason:
  - Comparative reasoning: "Regardless of whether you want to try surgery or medicine, how would taking the medicine be different than having the surgery?"
  - Consequential reasoning: "Regardless of whether you want to try surgery or medicine, how would having the surgery affect your daily life? What about the medicine?"
- The ability to understand:
  - "Can you tell me in your own words what I told you about the reasons for and against having the stress test?"

Source: Adapted from Grisso T, Appelbaum PS. Abilities related to competence. In: Assessing Competence to Consent to Treatment: A Guide for Physicians and Other Health Professionals. New York: Oxford University Press, 1998:31–60. By permission of Oxford University Press, Inc. Reprinted as appears in Karlawish JHT, Pearlman RA. Determination of Decision-Making Capacity, pp. 1233–1242. In: Cassel CK, Leipzig RM, Cohen HJ, et al., eds. Geriatric Medicine, 4th ed. New York; Springer, 2003.

The Five Standards for Assessing Decision-Making Capacity

At least one of five standards constitutes decision-making capacity (20). These standards were developed in the law and in bioethics and they are intuitively sensible elements of how a rational person ought to make a decision. They provide the foundation for the judgment of a patient's competence. The physician assesses the patient's performance on each standard and then uses the results of these assessments to decide whether a patient's decision-making capacity is inadequate to make the decision.

In theory, the five standards exist along a continuum from the simplest (communicating a choice) to the hardest (understanding). The significance of this is that the physician cannot simply rely upon the hardest standard as a screen for decision-making capacity. Instead, a physician can consider these standards as generally falling into two categories: the first two standards are simpler and the last three are more stringent.

Ability to Communicate a Choice

This describes a patient's ability to consistently state a choice ("I do not want the surgery."). Unlike the other standards, this standard makes no claim upon the patient's reasons. In a sense, it is the simplest standard. A physician assesses this by asking the patient, "What would you like to do?" Much of the day-to-day practice of clinical medicine relies on this standard or even a weaker version of it, namely a patient's nonverbal acquiescence to an intervention such as checking a blood pressure. Diseases that can impair a patient's ability to fulfill this standard include communication disorders and extreme states of anxiety that cause a patient to rapidly change choices.

Ability to Make a Reasonable Choice

Like the first, this standard is quite simple but unlike the first it introduces content to the choice. The content is the "reasonableness" of the choice where reasonableness is not necessarily defined by the patient's values but the values a "reasonable person" has. This is obviously a blunt standard to apply. For example, a physician who solely relies on this standard would likely find that an otherwise healthy patient who refuses a low-risk and likely beneficial intervention such as surgery for a noninvasive breast cancer would have impaired decision-making capacity. Hence, adherence to this standard alone risks a paternalistic practice of medical decision making. Diseases that can impair a patient's ability to fulfill this standard include those that cause delusions and marked deficits in judgment such as dementia and schizophrenia.

Appreciation

Standards three through five are more substantive than the first two because they require the physician to assess the patient's functional cognition. The third standard describes a patient's ability to recognize that, regardless of her choice, the facts of the decision apply to her. These facts include the diagnosis ("I know you said I have cancer and that's what this is") and the options for treatment ("I can leave it alone or have the surgery"). This standard requires that the patient recognize the relevance of the facts regardless of how the patient values those facts. Diseases that cause delusions or disassociation are likely to impair a patient's ability to fulfill this standard.

Reasoning

The ability to reason describes a patient's ability to generate consequences and compare them ("If I have the surgery, I will have given up on my faith in my ability to heal myself. If I do not have the surgery, I'll take a chance the cancer could spread"). To fulfill this standard a patient has to recognize the different options, generate consequences of each, and compare them. The ability to achieve this standard is impaired by conditions that reduce executive function, which means the ability to attend to and compare more than one concept. Diseases that impair attention such as delirium and frontal dementia can impair a patient's ability to fulfill this standard.

Understanding

This is the patient's ability to paraphrase the meaning of the information that the physician disclosed to her ("A surgery will involve cutting into my skin, removal of my gallbladder, and a 3-week period of recovery"). To fulfill this standard a patient has to "say back" or paraphrase the information the physician disclosed. In doing this, the patient demonstrates that he or she grasps the meaning of the information. Obviously, the more facts the physician discloses, the more difficult it becomes for the patient to achieve understanding. Indeed, a physician could set the fact content so complex that even a colleague would "fail." Clearly, a judgment is required as to what facts are essential for making the decision. Understanding is most dependent on a patient's memory and language. Hence, diseases that impair memory and language such as Alzheimer's disease and aphasias can significantly impair a patient's ability to fulfill this standard.

General Principles

- The fundamental ethical principle of autonomy or self-determination is embodied in the legal doctrine of informed consent.
- There are three essential elements, which must be present in order for patient's choices about treatment to be considered legally valid: (1) the patient's participation in the decision-making process and the ultimate decision must be voluntary; (2) the patient's agreement must be sufficiently informed; and (3) the patient must be mentally able to engage in a rational decision-making process.
- There are several alternative ways for the proxy or surrogate to exercise that power on behalf of the incapacitated patient: (1) delegation of authority beforehand by the patient, through methods of advance planning; (2) delegation of authority by operation of statute, regulation, or broad judicial precedent; (3) informal delegation of authority by custom; and (4) delegation of authority by a court order in the specific case.
- The two most important current devices for advance health care planning are the living will and the durable power of attorney for health care.
- A competent adult patient has the constitutional, common law, and statutory right to voluntarily and knowingly refuse basic or advanced cardiac life support or any of its specific components, hospitalization, or any other form of medical intervention and to demand a precisely written "Do Not" order.
- The five standards for assessing decision-making capacity: the ability to make a choice; the ability to make a reasonable choice; the ability to appreciate; the ability to reason; and the ability to understand.

Suggested Readings

Bottrell MM, Cassel CK, Felzenberg ER. Ethical and Policy Issues in End-of-Life Care. In: Cassel CK, Leipzig RM, Cohen HJ, et al., eds. Geriatric Medicine, 4th ed. New York: Springer, 2003:1243–1251.

Kapp MB. Medical treatment and the physician's legal duties. In: Cassel CK, Leipzig RM, Cohen HJ, et al., eds. Geriatric Medicine, 4th ed. New York: Springer, 2003:1221–1232.

Karlawish JHT, Pearlman RA. Determination of decision-making capacity. In: Cassel CK, Leipzig RM, Cohen HJ, et al., eds. Geriatric Medicine, 4th ed. New York: Springer, 2003:1233–1242.

References

1. Dubler NN, symposium editor. Symposium: the doctor-proxy relationship. J Leg Med Ethics 1999;27:5–86.
2. King NMP. Making Sense of Advance Directives, rev. ed. Washington, DC: Georgetown University Press, 1996.
3. Public Law 101–508, 4206, 4751.
4. 110 S.Ct. 2841 (1990).
5. Bradley EH, Blechner BB, Walker LC, et al. Institutional efforts to promote advance care planning in nursing homes: challenges and opportunities. J Leg Med Ethics 1997;25:150–159.
6. Molloy DW, Guyatt GH, Russo R, et al. Systematic implementation of an advance directive program in nursing homes: a randomized controlled trial. JAMA 2000;283:1437–1444.
7. Sabatino CP. The legal and functional status of the medical proxy: suggestions for statutory reform. J Leg Med Ethics 1999;27:52–68.
8. Zimny GH, Grossberg GT. Guardianship of the Elderly: Psychiatric and Judicial Aspects. New York: Springer, 1998.
9. Zuckerman C. Looking beyond the law to improve end-of-life care. Generations 1999;13:30–35.
10. Vacco v. Quill, 117 S.Ct. 2293 (1997).
11. Washington v. Glucksberg, 117 S.Ct. 2302 (1997).
12. Or. Rev. Stat. 127.800–897.
13. Chin AE, Hedberg K, Higginson GK, et al. Legalized physician-assisted suicide in Oregon: the first year's experience. N Engl J Med 1999;340:577–583.
14. Ganzini L, Nelson HD, Schmidt TA, et al. Physicians' experiences with the Oregon Death With Dignity Act. N Engl J Med 2000;342:557–563.
15. Federal Register 59,918 (November 3, 1999).
16. United States Code 1320d through 1320d-8.
17. Public Law No. 104–191, 110 Stat. 1936 (1996).
18. Tarasoff v. Regents of the University of California, 17 Cal.3d 425, 551 P.2d 334, 131 Cal.Rptr. 14 (1976).
19. White BC. Current confusion surrounding the concept of competence. In: White BC, ed. Competence to Consent. Washington, DC: Georgetown University Press, 1994:44–81.
20. Grisso T, Appelbaum PS. Abilities related to competence. In: Assessing Competence to Consent to Treatment: A Guide for Physicians and Other Health Professionals. New York: Oxford University Press, 1998:31–60.

8
Prevention and Chemoprophylaxis in the Elderly

EMILY J. CHAI

Learning Objectives

Upon completion of the chapter, the student will be able to:

1. Identify the important factors involved in deciding whether primary or secondary prevention interventions should be applied to a specific disease process.
2. Recognize screening guidelines that are important to the geriatrics population.
3. Provide age-appropriate preventive recommendations and lifestyle counseling.

General Considerations

Disease prevention and health promotion are important aspects of health for older individuals. Between 40% and 70% of all diseases are partially or totally preventable through lifestyle modification, risk factor management, and primary or secondary preventive practices (1–3). Despite a lack of definitive data regarding preventive interventions for a number of diseases and occasional disagreements among organizations publishing preventive guidelines, there is a consensus on the value of many preventive measures. Yet the underutilization of recommended preventive services remains a major challenge in medicine, including geriatric medicine.

Primary, secondary, and tertiary prevention are all important. *Primary prevention* is the avoidance of a disease before it can begin (e.g., annual influenza vaccine). *Secondary prevention*, or screening for occult disease, entails looking for early markers of a disease before it becomes symptomatic

Material in this chapter is based on the following chapter in Cassel CK, Leipzig RM, Cohen HJ, Larson EB, Meier DE, eds. Geriatric Medicine: An Evidence-Based Approach, 4th ed. New York: Springer, 2003: Bloom HG. Prevention, pp. 169–184. Selections edited by Emily J. Chai.

and then intervening early enough to positively affect outcomes (e.g., Pap smears, hypertension and cholesterol screening). *Tertiary prevention* emphasizes rigorously treating established disease to prevent adverse outcomes and complications from the natural course of that disease (e.g., aspirin for prevention of second myocardial infarction or ischemic strokes).

Important criteria for deciding on which diseases to apply primary and/ or secondary preventive interventions are addressed below and apply to all age groups, including individuals 65 and over (Table 8.1). Additionally, life expectancy and quality of life are especially important considerations for older individuals when deciding on preventive interventions.

Case A

Mrs. S. is a 75-year-old woman who has just moved into town to be closer to her newborn granddaughter. She is here today for a complete physical examination. She tells you that she had not seen a provider in 5 years because she has no medical problems and is in good health. She lives with her husband who is sick at home with the flu. She wants to know if she can continue to visit the baby. She has not been to her daughter's home since her husband got sick 2 days ago because she did not want to give her granddaughter the flu. She tells you that she was given all her vaccinations the last time she saw her physician, including the flu vaccine, which made her very sick.

Immunizations

Vaccines recommended for older individuals include influenza, pneumococcal, and tetanus. Influenza A and B and pneumococcal disease are common diseases frequently associated with significant morbidity and mortality. Tetanus, while rare, is a serious disease often resulting in death.

Influenza Vaccination

Yearly vaccination against influenza is one of the most important primary preventive practices readily available for older individuals. Influenza and pneumonia together rank as the sixth leading cause of death in persons aged 65 to 74, the fifth leading cause in persons aged 75 to 84, and the fourth leading cause in persons 85 years of age or older (4).

Inactivated influenza virus vaccine is strongly recommended for all persons 65 and older (5). Vaccination is safe and cost-effective, particularly for individuals at high risk for influenza infection, and leads to a 58% reduction in relative risk of clinically and serologically confirmed influenza infection for those who received an annual influenza vaccination compared to those receiving a placebo (6,7). Medicare covers the cost of the vaccine

TABLE 8.1. Criteria for screening tests

1. *The disease must have a significant effect on the quality and quantity of a patient's life.* Screening for common warts, for example, may be simple and inexpensive, but there are no adverse health effects from their presence and hence no reason to screen.

2. *Acceptable methods of treatment must be available.* Discovering a potentially serious condition at an early stage via screening is only useful if there is a treatment available to cure or significantly decrease morbidity from that condition. If effective treatment doesn't exist or if any individual is unable to access treatment after screening, screening is not indicated.

3. *Early treatment should yield a therapeutic result superior to that obtained by delaying treatment.* If early treatment does not lead to a better outcome, detecting a condition earlier by screening is not warranted.

4. *The disease must have an asymptomatic period during which detection and treatment significantly reduce morbidity and/or mortality.* By definition, screening is performed on individuals asymptomatic for the condition. If symptoms are present, any testing is diagnostic. Not only must an asymptomatic period exist, but finding and treating the condition at that earlier time must significantly reduce morbidity and/or mortality.

5. *Tests must be available at a reasonable cost to detect the condition in the asymptomatic period.* This criterion is more of an administrative or policy consideration. An individual may be willing to pay for a screening test that her/his insurance company won't cover. Before Medicare covered screening mammography, women had to pay for the test. More recently, some groups have advocated utilizing helical computed tomography to screen for lung cancer in smokers. The test is costly and to date there is only limited evidence of its efficacy as a screening tool.

6. *The incidence of the condition must be sufficient to justify the cost of screening.* This is also an administrative consideration. A physician may decide that if a patient can afford it, screening for a condition with an extremely low incidence is worthwhile. Conversely, the medical director of a health center, managing a limited budget, would likely not want to spend scant resources screening for a condition that would very likely never occur in that health center's population.

Source: Adapted from Bloom HG, Prevention. In: Cassel CK, Leipzig RM, Cohen HJ, et al., eds. Geriatric Medicine, 4th ed. New York: Springer, 2003:169–184.

and its administration. The vaccine needs to be given annually because of antigenic drift (variation in infectious strains) and antibody levels that wane with time (8,9). October to mid-November is usually the best time to administer influenza vaccine, but any time from September to the end of flu season (early March) is appropriate. An intranasal live-attenuated influenza vaccine has been approved by the Food and Drug Administration (FDA), but is recommended only for persons aged 18 to 49 years (10). Like the inactivated vaccine, it is used for the prevention of influenzas A and B.

Staff vaccination in long-term-care facilities provides additional protection to older institutionalized patients, and is associated with a 40% reduction in relative risk for patient mortality (11,12). During institutional influenza outbreaks, chemoprophylaxis in combination with timely annual influenza vaccination has been shown to be highly effective in preventing influenza complications in small cohort studies (13,14). M2-

channel inhibitors (amantadine or rimantadine) and neuraminidase inhibitors (oseltamivir or zanamivir) are approved for chemoprophylaxis in older adults with known or anticipated influenza A exposure. For influenza B prophylaxis, only neuraminidase inhibitors are effective. Unfortunately, there are very few randomized trials assessing the efficacy of these agents in older adults, and the data are hampered by limited population size and low influenza incidence in control groups. Zanamivir, an inhaled neuraminidase inhibitor, has demonstrated a nonsignificant trend toward efficacy against clinical and laboratory-confirmed influenza in a nonblinded randomized nursing home trial (15). Persons with underlying airway diseases should not be given zanamivir.

Chronically ill or immunodeficient older persons, those who have not received the yearly influenza vaccination or received it too late to be of use in an active outbreak, and those who received a vaccine poorly matched to the outbreak antigen are particularly likely to benefit from chemoprophylaxis during influenza outbreaks. In institutional outbreaks, 14-day chemoprophylaxis for residents (with dosage adjusted for renal function) and staff is warranted, continuing at least 7 days past the onset of the last case (16). For community-dwelling older patients and their close personal contacts, 10-day prophylaxis is usually sufficient. Drug resistance is a concern with the M2-channel inhibitors, and the side effect profile of these agents appears slightly worse than the neuraminidase inhibitors. Both drug classes are effective in reducing the duration of symptoms by 1 day in the treatment of acute influenza infection if begun within 48 hours of symptom onset.

Pneumococcal Vaccination

The 23-valent pneumococcal vaccine is between 50% and 80% effective in preventing invasive pneumococcal disease, not necessarily pneumococcal infection or pneumonia, in older adults who are immune competent (17–20).

The vaccine is safe, inexpensive, covered by Medicare, and associated with minimal serious adverse effects. The vaccine can be administered at any time during the year, even simultaneously with the influenza vaccine but in a different extremity. Although its efficacy in high-risk groups, particularly immunocompromised patients (21–24), is questionable, the United States Preventive Service Task Force and the Centers for Disease Control and Prevention (CDC)'s Advisory Committee on Immunization Practices recommends its use in this population because of the low risk of harm. There are no definitive data on whether the vaccine should be given only once in a lifetime or repeated every 5 to 6 years. Some have suggested that a one-time booster dose be given 5 to 6 years after the initial vaccination to those at extremely high risk (asplenic), those with rapidly declining titers (nephrotic syndrome, renal failure, HIV, leukemia, lymphoma, multiple myeloma, transplant, and those on immunosuppressive medications), those with chronic illnesses (diabetes mellitus and cardiopulmonary diseases), and healthy older adults who have received the primary vaccine before age 65.

Tetanus Vaccination

Although tetanus is rare in the United States, it is a serious disease and more than 60% of tetanus infections occur in older individuals (25,26). Current recommendations call for booster vaccinations every 10 years, although 15- to 30-year intervals are probably adequate in the U.S. for those properly vaccinated in childhood. If never previously vaccinated, older adults can be given a primary series that includes doses at 0, 2, and 8 to 14 months (27). The vaccine is safe, effective, and covered by Medicare.

Case B

Mrs. A. is a 67-year-old woman with a history of hypertension and diabetes, both of which have been very well controlled. She is in your office today with her husband for the results of her annual fecal occult blood test (FOBT). You tell her that the results were negative. She asks, "That means that I do not have cancer, right?" You explain to her that you cannot tell her for sure with just the results of the FOBT, and recommend additional screening for colorectal cancer since she's never had it before. She becomes alarmed and asks you, "Do you think I have cancer? But you just told me that the stool cards were negative. If you can't tell for sure why did you give them to me?" Her husband tells you that her cousin was recently diagnosed with colon cancer and they've heard that it can be hereditary. They have read that calcium, aspirin, and ibuprofen are helpful in the prevention of colorectal cancer and were wondering how much they should take. On their way out of the office, her husband pulls you aside to tell you that she started to smoke and drink again when her cousin's diagnosis was made.

Colorectal Cancer Screening and Prevention

Over 55,000 deaths annually with 140,000 new cases per year place colorectal cancer as the second most common form of cancer, as well as the cancer with the second highest mortality rate, in the United States. Both the incidence of invasive colorectal cancer and the mortality rates increase sharply with advancing age.

Early detection in the asymptomatic period is associated with better prognosis. For patients at average risk of colon cancer, the American Cancer Society (ACS) recommends screening with FOBT annually in combination with flexible sigmoidoscopy (FSIG) every 5 years (either test alone is sufficient, but the ACS prefers the combination), or a total colon exam with either a double-contrast barium enema every 5 years or colonoscopy every 10 years. As with other cancers, older adults at higher risk for colorectal cancer (e.g., those with inflammatory bowel disease or a strong family history of colorectal cancer, adenomatous polyposis, and nonpolyposis colorectal cancer) should be screened more frequently than the general older population (28). The ACS does not impose an upper age limit at which to discontinue screening, suggesting instead that continued screening is of benefit to older patients with continued good health.

The most frequently studied form of screening, FOBT, has been shown to significantly reduce the rate of death from colorectal cancer (29–31). There is also evidence that if done annually, it reduces the actual incidence of colorectal cancer by detecting premalignant adenomatous polyps (32). Adding FOBT to sigmoidoscopy improves the sensitivity of sigmoidoscopy, although recent studies suggest that the combination may miss as many as 50% to 60% of advanced proximal lesions (33,34). Double-contrast barium enemas are less useful in older adults, due to uninterpretable results because many patients can't move as required while on the radiography table (35,36) and biopsy cannot be done at the time of the exam, making a second bowel prep necessary. Colonoscopy is the most accurate of the available tests and is becoming the modality of choice for many physicians (37–39). "*Virtual colonoscopy*," which is three-dimensional computed tomographic colography, is a new technique requiring no sedation and less time, thus promising fewer complications than endoscopic colonoscopy. However, a number of improvements and more controlled studies are necessary before it can be recommended for population-based routine screening (40). Although very uncommon, serious complications do occur with screening sigmoidoscopy and colonoscopy, making the choice of screening tests, especially for older persons, an individual choice as much as a clinician preference (37).

Primary prevention of colorectal cancer with diet remains controversial. Observational data have yielded conflicting results (41,42), and there are no randomized controlled trials (RCTs) on the efficacy of fiber in primary prevention of colon cancer. Neither a wheat-bran supplemented diet nor a low-fat, high fruit and vegetable diet was found to affect the incidence of new colorectal adenomas (which can then progress to cancers) (43–45). It is important, however, to encourage measures to reduce known risk factors for colorectal cancer through weight control, smoking cessation, regular exercise, and less red meat intake (46).

Case C

Mrs. L. is a 70-year-old wheelchair-bound woman with a history of severe osteoarthritis of her knees, hypertension, and chronic stable angina who has been doing very well under your care without any complaints. In her chart, you noted that her last Papanicolaou smear and mammogram, done 3 years ago, were both negative. At that time, you had a discussion with the patient and her daughter about the appropriate frequency of these tests, and together you had decided that the patient did not need cervical cancer screening anymore since she was no longer sexually active and had a history of negative Pap smears. Getting a mammogram every 2 to 3 years would be appropriate since she had no family history of breast cancer and had not been on prolonged hormone replacement therapy. You remind the patient that she is due for a mammogram now. She asks you if mammograms are really necessary at her age.

Screening for Breast Cancer

Approximately one in eight women will develop breast cancer during her lifetime. There are over 176,000 new cases of breast cancer yearly, making it the most common cancer in women and the second leading cause of cancer death in women (47). Advanced age is an important risk factor both for developing breast cancer and for death from breast cancer (48).

The use of screening mammography has been highly recommended for women aged 50 to 69, with a decrease in the rate of late-stage disease detection correlating well with an increase in the use of mammography (49,50). A Cochrane review of the randomized controlled trials on which these recommendations are based strongly questioned the validity of five of the seven trials, only accepting two, which together suggested that mammography does not save lives (51). The National Cancer Institute's independent panel of experts, the Physician Data Query (PDQ), reviewed this evidence and concurred. Most completed clinical trials have not included women over age 70, and therefore it is not known how effective screening mammography is in women in that age group.

Additionally, mortality is not the only endpoint of interest to women who may develop breast cancer. The effect of breast cancer diagnosis at a later stage on function and quality of life is not known. There is some evidence from a retrospective cohort study that screening mammography is effective in women at least up to age 79 (52). In fact, if women 70 and older are cognitively and functionally intact with a life expectancy of 5 or more years, there is little reason to exclude routine mammography at any age in spite of there being no definitive evidence yet that this decreases breast cancer mortality. The American Geriatrics Society recommends annual or biennial screening mammography until age 75, and every 1 to 3 years after that with no upper age limit for nondemented women with life expectancies of at least 4 years (53). For women with family history of breast cancer or ongoing or previous long-term exposure to hormone replacement therapy, screening should be more frequent.

Other modalities used to screen for breast cancer include clinician breast exam and breast self-examination. There is insufficient evidence at this time in favor of or against including these in periodic screening exams (54). Nevertheless, longstanding clinical practice habits usually include periodic breast exams, and there is little reason to exclude the performance of these exams.

Regarding primary prevention of breast cancer, raloxifene and the antiestrogen tamoxifen have been recommended for women at increased risk of developing breast cancer, but not for the general risk population (55). In a large RCT in which 30% of the participants were over age 65, tamoxifen was associated with as much as a 50% reduction in invasive breast cancer incidence, particularly estrogen-receptor positive cancers, compared to placebo. Use of the drug in older women, however, was associated with an elevated risk of endometrial cancer, with a relative risk (RR) of 4.01 (56).

Screening for Cervical Cancer

Positive Pap smears are more often associated with invasive disease in older women (57,58). A significant percentage of women over age 65 have never had a Pap smear. There is some debate as to what age to discontinue Pap screening. For women who have a cervix, the United States Preventive Service finds no solid evidence to impose an upper age limit, but suggests testing be discontinued after age 65 for those who have had regular and normal screenings up until that time (59). For women at higher risk of cervical cancer (including older patients with a personal or family history of cervical cancer, previous abnormal smears, or high-risk sexual behavior), testing should continue annually (60). Medicare covers annual cervical cancer screening for women at higher risk for cervical cancer; screening for all other female beneficiaries is covered every three years.

Case D

Mr. M is a 79-year-old man with history of hypertension, hypercholesterolemia, and mild benign prostate hyperplasia who comes to you asking for prostate cancer screening. He said that his friend got a blood test and was told that he had prostate cancer. The patient wants the same test. The patient lives with his wife, is independent on activities of daily living (ADLs) and instrumental activities of daily living (IADLs), and has no family history of prostate cancer.

Screening for Prostate Cancer

Routine screening for prostate cancer using prostate-specific antigen (PSA) remains very controversial in older men. Although prostate cancer is common in older men and it can be aggressive and lethal, there are currently no reliable ways to distinguish small early cancers that will become aggressive from those that are slow-growing and non–life-threatening even if left untreated. Additionally, false-positive PSA tests are frequent and treatment is associated with the potential for significant complications (61,62). For these reasons, a number of organizations advise that an individual patient be educated about the potential benefits and risks of routine screening PSA testing followed by diagnostic confirmation and treatment and decide for himself whether to pursue testing or not.

Digital rectal exam by itself is not effective as a screening test for prostate cancer (63). In one study, the most valid screening results were obtained when suspicious digital rectal exam was combined with PSA values >4ng/mL (sensitivity 95%, positive predictive value 62%) (64). Medicare covers annual digital rectal exams as well as annual PSA screening tests without deductibles or co-insurance payments for male beneficiaries ages 50 and over (65).

Screening for Other Cancers

There are currently no reliable screening modalities for cancers of the lung, ovary, thyroid, kidneys, brain, skin, pancreas, or hematologic system.

Case E

A 72-year-old man is brought in by his son for an initial exam. His son tells you that the patient is visiting from Florida and had just run out of his medications today. The patient has diabetes and asthma. His medications include glyburide 10mg twice a day and an albuterol inhaler that he uses about once a day. He is feeling fine, denies polyuria, polyphagia, and polydipsia. He just wants to get some medications to hold him over until he returns to Florida in 3 months.

On examination, the patient's blood pressure was 145/85mmHg, heart rate of 82/min, fingerstick glucose of 180mg/dL. You repeated the blood pressure on the other arm and the reading was the same. The rest of his exam was unremarkable. Upon noting the blood pressure you asked him if he has ever had a problem with his blood pressure. He said that he did when he was younger. However, after he lost some weight, his doctor at home had told him that he didn't need medications anymore.

You give him his prescriptions, send off the lab work, and ask him to return the following week. When he returns, his blood pressure remains elevated at 148/86 mmHg, his HbgA$_{1C}$ is 7.0%, and his low-density lipoprotein cholesterol (LDL-C) is 130 mg/dL, with a high-density lipoprotein cholesterol (HDL-C) of 45 mg/dL.

Screening for High Blood Pressure

Hypertension is a chronic, highly prevalent, generally asymptomatic condition that is safely and effectively treatable in older adults. Treatment of hypertension in older persons has played a key role in leading to a significant reduction in morbidity and mortality from congestive heart failure, myocardial infarction, and stroke (66–68). Controlling hypertension can also decrease the risk for renal disease, retinopathy, and ruptured aortic aneurysm (69).

All forms of hypertension, including isolated systolic, isolated diastolic, and mixed systolic/diastolic, should be screened for at least every 2 years and treated (70). Annual screening is appropriate for patients whose most recent diastolic blood pressure is between 85 and 89 mmHg or whose systolic blood pressure is between 130 and 139; higher measurements should provoke more immediate evaluation (71). Proper cuff size and technique are especially important in older individuals, and, as with younger adults, hypertension should be diagnosed only if present at more than one reading on three separate visits (72) (see Chapter 22: Hypertension, page 386).

Screening for Lipid Disorders

Whether or not to routinely screen older individuals for high cholesterol and other lipid abnormalities remains controversial. The American College of Physicians guidelines neither recommend nor discourage cholesterol screening in patients 65 to 75 years of age, and find it unnecessary in patients older than 75 years with no evidence of coronary disease. However, the evidence upon which these recommendations were based—previous studies showing no association between coronary heart disease (CHD) mortality and high cholesterol in old age—may have been confounded by inclusion of frail elderly persons with low cholesterol. A study of 4066 older persons, after adjustment for frailty, found an association between total cholesterol and increased risk for CHD mortality (73). Older age (>45 males, >55 females) is itself an accepted risk factor for coronary artery disease.

After reviewing evidence on whether identification and treatment of asymptomatic people with abnormal lipid levels can substantially reduce the risk of CHD, the U.S. Preventive Services Task Force recently extended its recommendations to include routine lipid screening for older and middle-aged persons. Neither an optimal screening interval for older adults nor an upper age limit at which to discontinue screening has been set, but the task force has suggested that repeated screening may be less important in older people because lipid levels are less likely to increase after age 65 years. Five-year intervals have been suggested as a benchmark for the general U.S. population, with longer or shorter intervals dictated by patient risk—intervals longer than 5 years may be sufficient for older persons who have had low-risk results on previous lipid tests, whereas elderly patients showing higher-risk lipid levels should be screened more frequently. Older individuals who have never been screened should be screened (74).

The U.S. Preventive Services Task Force strongly recommends measurement of total cholesterol (TC) and HDL-C, but finds insufficient evidence to recommend for or against triglyceride measurement. The American College of Physicians has set ranges it considers to be associated with high risk for CHD: total cholesterol (>240 mg/dL), LDL-C ($\geq$160 mg/dL), and triglycerides (>400 mg/dL). The National Cholesterol Education Program sets a high-risk range for HDL-C levels—<40 mg/dL (75–79).

Case F

Mrs. K. is an 80-year-old woman with history of hypertension on a diuretic who is in your office for her semiannual follow-up. Her blood pressure was well controlled at 125/82 mmHg. She is concerned that she may have diabetes because she is thirsty all the time and she is urinating a lot, the same symptoms that her sister had when she was diagnosed with diabetes. She wants you to check her for diabetes.

She is 65 inches tall and weighed 190 lb 3 months ago. She now weighs 195 lb. She leads a very sedentary lifestyle. Her only outings are to the doctor's office or to her son's apartment downstairs.

Screening for Diabetes

Diabetes mellitus type 2 (DM-2) is an increasingly common disease in older adults. Weight loss and increased physical activity are simple lifestyle changes that significantly reduce the risk of diabetes. For screening purposes, the American Diabetes Association lowered its normal fasting glucose level for adults over age 45 to <126 mg/dL, and suggested screening occur every 3 years (80,81).

Although the value of rigorous glucose control in older diabetics to prevent end-organ damage (tertiary prevention) has not been definitively demonstrated, consensus expert opinion believes it will be equally beneficial in older as well as younger (insulin-dependent) individuals (82–84). Medicare covers home glucose monitoring kits for its beneficiaries (see Chapter 24: Diabetes Mellitus, page 437).

Case G

Mrs. C. is a thin, 68-year-old Asian woman with asthma who presented for follow-up after her recent hospitalization for pneumonia. She says that she is doing better and that today she took her last 5-mg pill of prednisone. She feels more or less back to her baseline and is using her albuterol inhaler only once a day. She is also back on her fluticasone inhaler twice a day. She had given up smoking last year after a severe asthma attack that required intubation. Although she is an active woman, caring for her sick husband and occasionally baby-sitting her grandchildren, she does not leave the house very often. She has lactose intolerance and never took hormone replacement therapy because her sister had breast cancer. She is taking one calcium tablet a day and asks you if this is sufficient at her age and if there is anything else she can do to prevent the degree of kyphosis that her mother had.

Prevention of and Screening for Osteoporosis

Even in asymptomatic older women, the prevalence of low bone mineral density (BMD) is widespread. The National Osteoporosis Risk Assessment study, a longitudinal observation of 200,160 postmenopausal women offered BMD screening at primary care sites, revealed previously undiagnosed osteoporosis in 7.2% of those screened and a further 36.9% with undiagnosed osteopenia. The consequences of undiagnosed low BMD in the year following testing, compared to those with normal BMDs, were a fourfold greater incidence of fracture with osteoporosis and a 1.8-fold greater rate of fracture with osteopenia (85,86). History of smoking or cortisone use was associated with significantly elevated risk of fracture.

As a primary preventive measure, discussing and offering hormone prophylaxis to perimenopausal and postmenopausal women has been recommended. However, two large randomized studies published in 2002 have radically changed our concepts of the effects of hormone replacement therapy (87,88). The Heart and Estrogen/Progestin Replacement Study (HERS) is a randomized, blinded, placebo-controlled trial on the effects of a combination of estrogen and progestin on CHD event risk among 2763 postmenopausal women with established CHD. This 6- to 8-year study found that hormone replacement therapy did not reduce the risk of cardiovascular events in women with CHD (88). The Women's Health Initiative (WHI) trial enrolled 161,809 postmenopausal women (ages 50 to 79) in a trial of hormone replacement therapy (HRT). The trial was stopped early when health risks were noted to exceed benefits over a follow-up of 5.2 years. The rate of coronary events, most of which were nonfatal myocardial infarctions, increased by 29% in patients receiving estrogen plus progestin when compared with patients receiving placebo. Lifestyle changes are viable alternatives to HRT in the prevention of bone loss for most older women, and include adequate calcium intake, routine exercise, and cessation of smoking (89,90). Adequate intake of vitamin D is also prudent.

Bone densitometry to screen for osteopenia in asymptomatic women at risk for osteoporosis is recommended, and if osteopenia is present, prophylactic treatment to avert frank osteoporosis should be recommended utilizing bisphosphonates (91). National Osteoporosis Foundation guidelines, issued in 2003, recommend testing for women over age 65 regardless of risk factors (see Chapter 19: Osteoporosis, page 340). Although the efficacy of osteoporosis screening in men is unproven, longevity is a risk factor in itself, and a one-time screening can establish which men need preventive treatment.

Malnutrition

Obesity, malnourishment, and failure to maintain adequate fluid intake are all common, significant problems in older adults, associated with increased mortality and morbidity, including cognitive dysfunction, depression, and delayed wound healing. Up to 15% of elderly community-living elders may be considered malnourished if the term is defined as a decrease in nutrient reserves (92). Among hospitalized or institutionalized patients the prevalence is much higher. Chronically ill persons, cognitively impaired elderly, and those with excessive alcohol intake are particularly prone to malnourishment (93); malnourishment can in turn exacerbate these same problems. Vitamin D deficiency is common in elderly populations with limited exposure to sunlight. Protein-energy malnourishment is common among older persons following elective surgical procedures or minor infections. Clinicians should maintain a high index of suspicion for nutritional deficiencies in these patients, as well as in patients with low incomes, social isolation, multiple medication use, malabsorption syndromes, or chronic myocardial, renal, or pulmonary illnesses.

The U.S. Preventive Services Task Force recommends that all patients, regardless of age, be administered periodic height and weight measurements. Body mass index (BMI) is the recommended gauge, although obtaining accurate height measurements may be difficult in bed-bound elders. A BMI below 22 or above 29 should raise red flags. Use of the single question: "Have you lost 10 pounds over the last 6 months without trying to do so?" in combination with measurement of BMI or use of height/weight charts is an effective and simple screen for malnourishment. Persons weighing less than 100 lb (45.5 kg) are more likely to be malnourished, and involuntary weight loss may indicate elevated risk of death. Older patients of normal weight or who are overweight can also be malnourished. The Nutrition Screening Initiative Checklist, with 10 yes/no questions, can also help physicians identify older persons at risk for malnourishment. Scores of 6 points or higher warrant concern. Nearly one quarter of a noninstitutionalized Medicare population surveyed with this tool was found to be at risk (94). A thorough clinician assessment of patient access to nutritious foods with counseling on daily multivitamin use and adequate water intake can prevent or alleviate many problems (see Chapter 11: Nutrition, page 177).

Case H

Mrs. W. is a 73-year-old woman who has been seeing you for the last 3 years. She has hypertension, diabetes, and arthritis, and is mildly obese. She comes to you today for a routine visit. She tells you that she is doing well but her memory is failing because she is getting old.

She said that she would go to the market and come back with only two of the three things that she had intended to get. She has misplaced things and has forgotten conversations that she may have had with her son. She never had these problems before. She was always proud of her math skills (she was an accountant and was the first in her family to finish college) and of her ability to remember her activities for the day without a planner. Although she is still writing her own checks and paying her bills, she noticed that it is taking her a lot longer to balance her checkbook. Her son is worried that his mother has Alzheimer's disease. He thinks that these problems may have gotten worse after he moved out of his mother's building. Eight months ago while in the planning phase of moving, Mrs. W. had expressed concerns about her ability to live by herself in the building. Her son had invited her to come live with him but she refused. She did not want to leave the apartment that she has lived in for 50 years.

On your exam, you noted that although Mrs. W. was cooperative and would smile intermittently, she was definitely not her outspoken self. You asked her if she was sad or depressed and she said no. She drew a clock for you and it was correct. She scored a 30/30 on the Mini–Mental State Examination (MMSE) and a 4/15 on the Geriatric Depression Scale (GDS).

Screening for Depression and Dementia

Depression is a common and treatable condition in older individuals. Early diagnosis and appropriate treatment with medication or psychotherapy are critical to management; unfortunately, however, it is both underdiagnosed and undertreated in the elderly population. The U.S. Preventive Services

Task Force recommends that physicians maintain a high index of suspicion for elderly patients, especially those with a family or personal history of depression, chronically ill or home-bound elders, and those with recent personal loss, sleep disorders, and memory impairment.

A "yes" response to the question "Do you often feel sad or depressed?" has a sensitivity of 83% and specificity of 79% (95), and should provoke a more thorough assessment. The Geriatric Depression Scale (GDS-15 or -30) is even more sensitive. The GDS-15 cutoff score of 5 had 100% sensitivity and 72% specificity in detecting cases of depression, more than three quarters of which had been undiscovered by the primary care physicians at least as long as the year prior to the clinical interview (96). The GDS, however, is a screening instrument and does not make the diagnosis.

Dementia, particularly Alzheimer's disease, increases in prevalence as the population ages. It is a chronic, progressive disease whose etiology is not yet known and for which there is currently no effective curative treatment. A systematic review of studies by the American Academy of Neurology indicates that individuals classified as having mild cognitive impairment (but not meeting clinical criteria for dementia) have a high risk of progressing to dementia or Alzheimer's disease (estimated rate between 6% and 25% per year, compared to an incidence of dementia in the overall population of older persons of 0.2% in the 65 to 69 age range to 3.9% in the 85 to 89 age range) (97). For the purposes of the systematic review, the criteria for mild cognitive impairment included objective memory impairment as well as patient memory complaint, preferably corroborated by an informant, but normal general cognitive function and activities of daily living.

Early diagnosis (case finding) is increasingly important as potentially helpful palliative treatments are available, but as yet there is insufficient evidence to screen elderly adults in whom there is no suspicion of cognitive impairment. For patients (or family informants) reporting memory difficulties, the U.S. Preventive Task Force advises screening; recommended instruments include the Mini–Mental Status Examination (MMSE), the Short Portable Mental Status Questionnaire, and the clock-drawing test. A very simple three-item recall test has a sensitivity of 90% for patients unable to remember all three items after 1 minute (98). In general, mild-to-moderate cognitive impairment is indicated by scores between 18 and 24 on the MMSE. The MMSE must be adjusted for high education or intelligence levels. The clock-drawing test, despite multiple scoring systems, has a mean sensitivity and specificity of 85% and a likelihood ratio of >10 (99). Abnormal entries in the fourth quadrant of the clock alone are almost diagnostic of dementia (100). It is important to note that depression, language differences, hearing impairment, and aphasia can affect the accuracy of cognitive screening tests. In addition, because dementia cannot reliably be screened in the presence of delirium, differentiating between the two must be a priority and the Confusion Assessment Method (CAM) has a high specificity for detecting delirium (101,102) (see Chapter 13: Depression, Dementia, Delirium, page 216).

Case I

Mr. M., an 82-year-old man with coronary artery disease, with two prior myocardial infarctions, is brought to your office by his daughter because she thinks that he is depressed. He no longer does his usual activities. He used to enjoy listening to the radio, reading the newspaper, and watching television. In the last 2 years, he gradually withdrew himself from these activities and now he stays in his room all day except for meals. She is very concerned and asks you for help.

When you ask Mr. M. why he's not leaving his room and why he is no longer enjoying his favorite activities, he replied in a loud defensive voice, "What is the point, I can't understand what they are saying anyway. Besides, the newspaper print is just getting smaller each year. It looks like ants. Who can read that thing?"

Screening for Visual Acuity and Glaucoma

Routine vision screening utilizing Snellen acuity testing to detect diminished visual acuity is recommended for older individuals, although there have not been any trials in older individuals that primarily assessed vision per se (103,104). Analysis of multiphasic assessment trials where visual acuity testing was included has not revealed a benefit. Despite a lack of evidence supporting routine screening for glaucoma, screening older persons can be justified but is best done by eye specialists, not primary care physicians (105) (see Chapter 9: Vision and Hearing Impairments, page 143.)

Screening for Hearing Impairment

A very common problem in older adults, hearing impairment is most easily and reliably screened for by periodically asking patients whether they are experiencing any problems with their hearing (106). If yes, referral for formal hearing evaluation is indicated. Even those already wearing hearing aids can benefit from routine screening: in one study, 10 out of 11 older hearing aid users were discovered upon testing in a screening clinic to require major readjustment or complete replacement of the device (107). Hearing aids are often helpful in appropriate persons and are smaller and cosmetically more appealing than in the past (see Chapter 9: Vision and Hearing Impairments, page 152).

Case J

Mrs. N. is a 72-year-old white female with recently diagnosed hypertension who presents for follow-up. Her blood pressure today is 160/85. You ask her if she took her diuretic this morning and she tells you that she has stopped taking it because she was "wetting" herself. She said this problem has been going on for 2 to 3 years. She was too embarrassed to tell you. She would feel the urge and before she can get to the bathroom, she would have "wet myself." This would happen about 8 to 10 times a day. The diuretic was making it worse. Her adult diapers, which were initially sufficient, would overflow when she was on the diuretic, making her fearful of leaving the house.

Incontinence

Patients are often reluctant to mention or seek help for urinary or fecal incontinence, yet both are common problems with aging, affecting independence and quality of life. In addition to the significant social and emotional toll, incontinence may be both a marker for and a contributing cause of frailty in elderly patients. Frequent urinary incontinence (weekly or more often) is associated with an increased risk of falls and non-spine fractures in older women (108).

Screening is simple. All older patients should be asked, "Do you ever lose your urine and get wet?" Affirmative answers should be followed up with the question, "Have you lost urine on at least 6 separate days?" Fecal incontinence can be screened for in a similar manner. Few trials have evaluated the outcomes of screening for either condition on function or quality of life, but incontinence is a common and potentially avoidable cause for nursing home admissions. (See Chapter 29: Urinary Incontinence, page 512.)

Case K

Mrs. E. is an active 82-year-old with hypertension, osteoporosis, and osteoarthritis, who is interested in starting an exercise program. She plans to sign up for membership at her local gym with her friend and was wondering what kind of activities she should participate in. You tell her that it is a great idea and that any physical activity will improve her hypertension and physical well-being. For her osteoporosis, you recommend weight-bearing exercises. For her arthritis, water exercises are the best. You tell her that the water buoyancy takes the pressure off the joints, enabling muscle strengthening and cardiopulmonary exercise without the pain; however, because the bones are not stressed with water exercises, it is not effective in osteoporosis prevention.

Exercise

Regular physical activity has been shown in numerous studies to be an extremely important preventive intervention for older adults. Exercise promotes health and stimulates a sense of well-being. Included among the many benefits of regular exercise for older people are the following: an increase in lean body mass and strength; a reduction in risk for coronary artery disease, hypertension, and diabetes; a diminished risk for falling; a delay in overall functional decline; a decrease in depression; a reduction in pain from arthritis; and improved longevity (109,110). Of all the benefits, perhaps the most important are those gleaned from preventing age-associated functional decline and the reversal of effects of adverse health episodes (111–119).

Exercise, if approached properly, is safe even into advanced age (120). Both resistance training and aerobic exercise are important and efficacious. Resistance training is most helpful for improving balance and muscular strength. Aerobic exercise is most helpful for improvement in cardiopulmonary fitness and stamina (121).

Giving permission to older patients and encouraging regular physical activity are more important than the exact exercise program undertaken. Regular activity, taking into account the older individual's preferences, and compliance are key factors for success. Appropriate exercise can include regimens easily integrated into a routine day such as walking, climbing and descending stairs, swimming, gardening, and bicycling (mobile or stationary). For individuals unable to ambulate or transfer independently, exercises can be done in bed or in a chair. Regular exercise is therefore appropriate for people at any age and almost all stages of functional status (see Chapter 10: Exercise and Rehabilitation, page 164.)

Conclusion

As the quantity of prevention-related information increases and dissemination becomes quicker and more widespread, shared decision making between clinician and patient will become increasingly important. Availability of sites beyond the physician's office—the Internet, the workplace, senior centers, and schools, for example—will facilitate broader access to disease prevention and health promotion measures. As more individuals live longer with more active lives, attention to lifestyle habits, quality of life issues, risk factors for diseases, and genuine health promotion activities will demand more attention in the disease prevention/health promotion arena. Table 8.2 provides likelihood ratios and sensitivities for several common in-office geriatric screening instruments. Tables 8.3 through 8.5 summarize evidence-based recommendations for inclusion or exclusion of preventive measures in the older adult population. How often to perform

TABLE 8.2. Sensitivity and specificity of common screening instruments by blinded assessment (%) (99)

Condition	Description of screening test	Sensitivity (±95% CI)	Specificity (±95% CI)	Likelihood ratio
Nutrition	• Ask: "Have you lost 10lb over the past 6 months without trying to do so?" • Weigh the patient.	0.65 (0.56, 0.74)	0.87 (0.81, 0.93)	5.0
Vision	• Ask: "Do you have difficulty driving, watching TV, or reading, or doing any your daily activities because of your eyesight?" • If yes, test each eye with Snellen chart while patient wears corrective lenses (if applicable).	0.67 (0.58, 0.76)	0.86 (0.79, 0.93)	4.8
Hearing	• Set audioscope to 40dB. • Test hearing using 1000 and 2000Hz.	0.93 (0.88, 0.98)	0.60 (0.51, 0.69)	2.3
Cognition/memory	• Three-item recall test	0.90 (0.84, 0.96)	0.64 (0.55, 0.73)	2.5
Incontinence	• Ask: "In the last year, have you ever lost your urine and gotten wet?" • If yes, ask: "Have you lost your urine on at least 6 separate days?"	0.89 (0.83, 0.95)	0.95 (0.91, 0.99)	17.8
Depression	• Ask: "Do you often feel sad or depressed?"	0.83 (0.76, 0.90)	0.79 (0.71, 0.87)	4.0
Physical disability	Ask 6 questions: "Are you able to . . . • do strenuous activities like fast walking or bicycling?" • do heavy work around the house like washing windows, walls, or floors?" • go shopping for groceries or clothes?" • get to places out of walking distance?" • bathe, either a sponge bath, tub bath, or shower?" • dress, like putting on a shirt, buttoning and zipping, or putting on shoes?"	0.91 (0.86, 0.96)	0.50 (0.41, 0.59)	1.8

Source: Adapted from Moore AA, Siu AL. Screening for common problems in ambulatory elderly: clinical confirmation of a screening instrument. Am J Med 1996;100(4):438–443, with permission from Elsevier. Reprinted as appears in Bloom HG. Prevention. In: Cassel CK, Leipzig RM, Cohen HJ, et al., eds. Geriatric Medicine, 4th ed. New York: Springer, 2003.

TABLE 8.3. Common screening measures recommended on good evidence for the geriatric patient

Screening or counseling	USPSTF	CTF	AAFP	ACP	AMA	Specialist organizations	High-risk elderly patients
Screening for hearing impairment	Y	Y					
Screening for visual impairment	Y	Y	Y			American Academy of Ophthalmologists, American Optometric Association	African-Americans and Caucasians; diabetics; family history of ocular disease
Counseling on well-balanced diet/ use of BMI tables	Y	Y	Y			Institute of Medicine, American Academy of Clinical Endocrinologists	
Counseling on physical activity	Y	Y					
Counseling on falls/injury prevention	Y	I					
Screening for elder abuse	Y*	I				Lachs; Moore & Siu (see references)	Injured older patients
Screening for IADL/ADL limitations							
Screening for substance abuse	Y	Y				Substance Abuse and Mental Health Administration	Personal history of substance abuse; patients with major life changes
Screening for hypertension (BP)	Y	Y	Y	Y		American Heart Association	
Screening for lipid disorders	Y			I		National Cholesterol Education Program's Adult Treatment Panel II, National Institutes of Health, American Heart Association	
Screening for oral health	Y	I				National Cancer Institute, American Cancer Society	Tobacco or alcohol users; patients with suspicious lesions
Annual influenza vaccination	Y	Y			Y	American College of Preventive Medicine, CDC	Patients with chronic pulmonary, cardiovascular, or metabolic

Preventive service			Recommending organizations	High-risk groups/comments
Pneumococcal vaccination	Y	I*	Y	Advisory Committee on Immunization Practices; American College of Preventive Medicine, CDC Advisory Committee on Immunization Practices	disorders; institutionalized patients Patients with chronic pulmonary, cardiovascular, or metabolic disorders; institutionalized immunocompetent elderly patients
Tetanus-diphtheria vaccination	Y	Y	Y	CDC Advisory Committee on Immunization Practices	
Screening for breast cancer, ages 50–69 (mammography)	Y	Y	Y	American College of Preventive Medicine; NIH consensus conference, National Cancer Institute, American Cancer Society, American College of Radiologists, American College of Obstetricians & Gynecologists, American Geriatric Society	
Screening for breast cancer, ages 50–69 (clinical breast exam)	Y	Y	Y	National Cancer Institute; American College of Obstetrics and Gynecology; American Cancer Society; American College of Radiology; American Society of Clinical Oncology	
Screening for breast cancer (breast self-exam)	I			American College of Radiology, American Society of Clinical Oncology	

(Continued)

TABLE 8.3. *Continued*

Screening or counseling	USPSTF	CTF	AAFP	ACP	AMA	Specialist organizations	High-risk elderly patients
Screening for cervical cancer (Pap smear, up to age 69)	Y*	Y	Y	Y		American College of Preventive Medicine; National Cancer Institute	Previous irregular tests; immigrants from developing nations who have never been screened
Screening for colorectal cancer (annual FOBT)	Y	I		Y		American Cancer Society, American Gastroenterology Association	Familial polyposis; family history of colorectal cancer in a first-degree relative; inflammatory bowel disease
Screening for colorectal cancer (sigmoidoscopy)	Y	I		Y		American Cancer Society	Same as above
Screening for colorectal cancer (colonoscopy)	I	I*		Y*		American Cancer Society	Same as above

USPSTF, U.S. Preventive Services Task Force; CTF, Canadian Task Force on the Periodic Health Examination; AAFP, American Academy of Family Physicians; ACP, American College of Physicians; AMA, American Medical Association; Y, yes; N, no; I, insufficient evidence; * screen high-risk patients; ADL, activities of daily living; FOBT, fecal occult blood test; IADL, instrumental activities of daily living.
Source: Bloom HG. Prevention. In: Cassel CK, Leipzig RM, Cohen HJ, et al, eds. Geriatric Medicine, 4th ed. New York: Springer, 2003.

TABLE 8.4. Common screening measures to consider recommending, despite lack of conclusive evidence

Screening measure:	USPSTF	CTF	AAFP	ACP	AMA	American College of Preventive Medicine	Specialty organizations	High-risk patients
Screening for cognitive impairment (MMSE, SPMSQ, or clock-drawing test)	I*	I*						Difficulties in daily activities, self-reported (or reported by reliable informant)
Screening for depression (GHQ or Zung self-rating scale)	I*	N						Family/personal history of depression; patients with chronic illness, pain, sleep disorders, or multiple unexplained somatic complaints
Screening for gait/ mobility problems		Y						Over age 75; using ≥4 prescription medications, especially psychoactive or antihypertensive drugs
Screening for diabetes mellitus (plasma glucose measurement)	I*	N*	N*	N*			American Diabetes Association	Obese patients; family history of disease; Native Americans, Hispanics, African Americans
Screening for thyroid disease (thyroid function tests)	I	I	Y	Y*			American Thyroid Association, American Academy of Clinical Endocrinologists	Post-menopausal women with vague complaints; patients with possible symptoms
Screening for thyroid disease (neck palpation)	N*	N	N*				American Cancer Society	Patients with history of head/neck irradiation
Screening for prostate cancer (DRE)	N	I		N		N	American Cancer Society, American Urologic Society, American College of Radiology	

(Continued)

TABLE 8.4. *Continued*

Screening measure:	USPSTF	CTF	AAFP	ACP	AMA	American College of Preventive Medicine	Specialty organizations	High-risk patients
Screening for prostate cancer (PSA)	N	N		N		N	American Cancer Society, American Urologic Society, American College of Radiology	
Screening for prostate cancer (TRUS)	N	N						
Screening for skin cancer (clinical skin exam)	I*	N*	N*		N	N	American Cancer Society, National Institutes of Health, National Cancer Inst., American Academy of Dermatology, American College of Preventive Medicine*	Fair-skinned men and women aged >65, patients with atypical moles, and those with >50 moles
Screening for ovarian cancer	N	N	Y	N*	Y		National Institutes of Health, American Cancer Society, National Cancer Institute, American Medical Women's Association	Family history of ovarian cancer

USPSTF, U.S. Preventive Services Task Force; CTF, Canadian Task Force on the Periodic Health Examination; AAFP, American Academy of Family Physicians; ACP, American College of Physicians; AMA, American Medical Association; CDC, Center for Disease Prevention and Control; MMSE, Mini–Mental State Examination; DRE, digital rectal examination; GHQ, general health questionnaire; PSA, prostate-specific antigen; SPMSQ, short portable mental status questionnaire; TRUS, transrectal ultrasound; Y, yes; N, no; I, insufficient evidence; *screen high-risk patients.
Source: Bloom HG. Prevention. In: Cassel CK, Leipzig RM, Cohen HJ, et al., eds. Geriatric Medicine, 4th ed. New York: Springer, 2003.

TABLE 8.5 Screening measures for which evidence does *not* support recommending

Screening measure	Does NOT recommend:				Recommends	Screen high-risk individuals
	USPSTF	CTF	AAFP	ACP		
Annual electrocardiogram	I	N		N	American College of Cardiologists/American Heart Association, American College of Sports Medicine	
Screening for osteoporosis (bone densitometry)	I*	N*			National Osteoporosis Foundation, American Academy of Clinical Endocrinologists*	Women with history of fractures; loss of height with back pain; advanced age; Caucasian race; low body weight; bilateral oophorectomy before menopause; women considering estrogen prophylaxis
Screening for lung cancer	N	N	N	N		
Screening for pancreatic cancer	N	N	N			
Screening for bladder cancer	N*	N	N*	N		Smokers; patients who worked in rubber or dye professions
Screening for asymptomatic carotid disease	I	N	N*	N		Patients with risk factors for cardio- or cerebrovascular disease
Screening for peripheral artery disease	N*		N		American Heart Association*	Diabetics
Screening for abdominal aortic aneurysm (AAA)	I*	I*				Men over 60 who are smokers, hypertensives, claudicants, or have family history of AAA

(*Continued*)

TABLE 8.5 *Continued*

Screening measure	Does NOT recommend:				Recommends	Screen high-risk individuals
	USPSTF	CTF	AAFP	ACP		
Screening for asymptomatic bacteriuria	I	I				
Screening for iron-deficiency anemia	N	N	N*			Recent immigrants from developing nations
Screening for tuberculosis	N*	N*	N*	N*		Recent immigrants from developing nations; patients from underserved, low-income populations, patients with diabetes, renal failure, HIV; substance abusers; nursing home residents

USPSTF, U.S. Preventive Services Task Force; CTF, Canadian Task Force on the Periodic Health Examination; AAFP, American Academy of Family Physicians; ACP, American College of Physicians; AMA: American Medical Association; Y, yes; N, no; I, insufficient evidence; *screen high-risk patients.

Source: Bloom HG. Prevention. In: Cassel CK, Leipzig RM, Cohen HJ, et al., eds. Geriatric Medicine, 4th ed. New York: Springer, 2003.

various preventive measures and what age (chronologic or physiologic) to stop certain interventions, with few exceptions (e.g., influenza vaccine yearly) has not been well studied. Until better evidence is available, common sense should prevail.

General Principles

* Primary prevention is the avoidance of a disease before it can begin. Physicians can intervene by identifying and eliminating risk factors with effective counseling.
* Secondary prevention, or screening for occult disease, is looking for early markers of a disease before it becomes symptomatic and then intervening early enough to positively affect outcomes. Breast exams, mammograms, Pap smears, fecal occult blood tests, and sigmoidoscopy, which are used to identify malignancies, fall into this category.
* Screening measures specific to the older adult assess osteoporosis, malnutrition, depression, dementia, visual acuity and hearing impairment, incontinence, functional decline, and frailty.
* The goal of all preventive measure is to decrease suffering, to reduce morbidity and mortality, and to improve quality of life.
* Although there are general prevention guidelines to help the physician, all decisions must be a joint effort with preference given to patient's lifestyle and values.

Suggested Readings

Bloom HG. Prevention. In: Cassel CK, Leipzig RM, Cohen HJ, et al., eds. Geriatric Medicine, 4th ed. New York: Springer, 2003:169–184.

Petersen RC, Stevens JC, Ganguli M, et al. Practice parameter: early detection of dementia: mild cognitive impairment (an evidence-based review). Report of the Quality Standards Subcommittee of the American Academy of Neurology. Neurology 2001;56(9):1133–1142. *An excellent review of studies on the sensitivity and specificity of the various instruments in the detection of dementia.*

References

1. U.S. Department of Health and Human Services. Healthy People 2000: National Health Promotion and Disease Prevention Objectives. DHHS publication no. PHS 91–50213. Washington, DC: Government Printing Office, 1991.
2. Fries JF, Koop CE, Beadle CE, et al. Reducing health care costs by reducing the need and demand for medical services. N Engl J Med 1993;329: 321–325.

3. Patterson C, Chambers LW. Preventive health care. Lancet 1995;345:1611–1615.
4. Centers for Disease Control and Prevention. CDC Surveillance Summaries, Dec. 17, 1999. MMWR 1999;48 (No. SS-8).
5. Centers for Disease Control and Prevention. Prevention and Control of Influenza: Recommendations of the Advisory Committee on Immunization Practices (ACIP). MMMW 2000;49:1–38.
6. Patriarca PA, Weber JA, Parker RA, et al. Efficacy of influenza vaccine in nursing homes. Reduction in illness and complications during an influenza A (H3N2) epidemic. JAMA 1985;253:1136–1139.
7. Gross PA, Hermogenes AW, Sacks HS, Lau J, Levandowski RA. The efficacy of influenza vaccine in elderly persons. A meta-analysis and review of the literature. Ann Intern Med 1995;123:518–527.
8. Couch RB. Drug Therapy: Prevention and treatment of influenza. N Engl J Med 2000;343:1778–1787.
9. Govaert TM, Thijs CT, Masurel N, et al. The efficacy of influenza vaccination in elderly individuals. A randomized double-blind placebo-controlled trial. JAMA 1994;272(21):1661–1665.
10. Couch RB. Drug therapy: prevention and treatment of influenza. N Engl J Med 2000;343:1778–1787.
11. Carman WF, Elder AG, Wallace LA, et al. Effects of influenza vaccination of health-care workers on mortality of elderly people in long-term care: a randomised controlled trial. Lancet 2000;355(9198):93–97.
12. Potter J, Stott DJ, Roberts MA, et al. Influenza vaccination of health care workers in long-term-care hospitals reduces the mortality of elderly patients. J Infect Dis 1997;175(1):1–6.
13. Mast EE, Harmon MW, Gravenstein S, et al. Emergence and possible transmission of amantadine-resistant viruses during nursing home outbreaks of influenza A (H3N2). Am J Epidemiol 1991;134(9):988–997.
14. Libow LS, Neufeld RR, Olson E, Breuer B, Starer P. Sequential outbreak of influenza A and B in a nursing home: efficacy of vaccine and amantadine. J Am Geriatr Soc 1996;44(10):1153–1157.
15. Schilling M, Povinelli L, Krause P, et al. Efficacy of zanamivir for chemoprophylaxis of nursing home influenza outbreaks. Vaccine 1998;16(18): 1771–1774.
16. Drinka PJ, Gravenstein S, Schilling M, Krause P, Miller BA, Shult P. Duration of antiviral prophylaxis during nursing home outbreaks of influenza A: a comparison of 2 protocols. Arch Intern Med 1998;158(19):2155–2159.
17. Sims RV, Steinmann WC, McConville JH, King LR, Zwick WC, Schwartz JS. The clinical effectiveness of pneumococcal vaccine in the elderly (published erratum appears in Ann Intern Med 1988;109(9):762–763). Ann Intern Med 1988;108:653–657.
18. Shapiro ED, Berg AT, Austrian R, et al. The protective efficacy of polyvalent pneumococcal polysaccharide vaccine. N Engl J Med 1991;325:1453–1460.
19. Butler JC, Breiman RF, Campbell JF, Lipman HB, Broome CV, Facklam R. Pneumococcal polysaccharide vaccine efficacy. An evaluation of current recommendations. JAMA 1993;270:1826–1831.
20. Farr BM, Johnston BL, Cobb DK, et al. Preventing pneumococcal bacteremia in patients at risk. Results of a matched case-control study. Arch Intern Med 1995;155:2336–2340.

21. Shapiro ED, Berg AT, Austrian R, et al. The protective efficacy of polyvalent pneumococcal polysaccharide vaccine. N Engl J Med 1991;325(21):1453–1460.

22. Butler JC, Breiman RF, Campbell JF, Lipman HB, Broome CV, Facklam R. Pneumococcal polysaccharide vaccine efficacy. An evaluation of current recommendations. JAMA 1993;270:1826–1831.

23. Shapiro ED, Berg AT, Austrian R, et al. The protective efficacy of polyvalent pneumococcal polysaccharide vaccine. N Engl J Med 1991;325(21):1453–1460.

24. Butler JC, Breiman RF, Campbell JF, Lipman HB, Broome CV, Facklam R. Pneumococcal polysaccharide vaccine efficacy. An evaluation of current recommendations. JAMA 1993;270:1826–1831.

25. Centers for Disease Control. Tetanus surveillance-United States 1989–1990. MMWR 1992:1–9.

26. Sutter RW, Cochi SL, Brink EW, Sirotkin BI. Assessment of vital statistics and surveillance data for monitoring tetanus mortality, United States, 1979–1984. Am J Epidemiol 1990;131:132–142.

27. U.S. Preventive Services Task Force. Adult Immunizations. Guide to CLINICAL PREVENTIVE SERVICES. Baltimore: Williams & Wilkins, 1996: 791–814.

28. Smith RA, von Eschenbach AC, Wender R, et al. American Cancer Society guidelines on screening and surveillance for the early detection of adenomatous polyps and cancer: update 2001. In: American Cancer Society Guidelines for the Early Detection of Cancer. Update of Early Detection Guidelines for Prostate, Colorectal, and Endometrial Cancers and Update 2001: Testing for Early Lung Cancer Detection. CA Cancer J Clin 2001;51(1):38–75.

29. Mandel JS, Church TR, Ederer F, Bond JH. Colorectal cancer mortality: effectiveness of biennial screening for fecal occult blood. J Natl Cancer Inst 1999;91:434–437.

30. Hardcastle JD, Chamberlain JO, Robinson MH, et al. Randomised controlled trial of faecal-occult-blood screening for colorectal cancer. Lancet 1996;348:1472–1477.

31. Kronborg O, Fenger C, Olsen J, Jorgensen OD, Sondergaard O. Randomised study of screening for colorectal cancer with faecal-occult-blood test [see comments]. Lancet 1996;348:1467–1471.

32. Mandel JS, Church TR, Bond JH, et al. The effect of fecal occult-blood screening on the incidence of colorectal cancer. N Engl J Med 2000;343: 1603–1607.

33. Imperiale TF, Wagner DR, Lin CY, Larkin GN, Rogge JD, Ransohoff DF. Risk of advanced proximal neoplasms in asymptomatic adults according to the distal colorectal findings. N Engl J Med. 2000;343(3):169–174.

34. Lieberman DA, Weiss DG, Bond JH, Ahnen DJ, Garewal H, Chejfec G. Use of colonoscopy to screen asymptomatic adults for colorectal cancer. Veterans Affairs Cooperative Study Group 380. N Engl J Med 2000 Jul 20;343(3): 162–168.

35. Tinetti ME, Stone L, Cooney L, Kapp MC. Inadequate barium enemas in hospitalized elderly patients. Incidence and risk factors. Arch Intern Med 1989;149(9):2014–2016.

36. Gurwitz JH, Noonan JP, Sanchez M, Prather W. Barium enemas in the frail elderly. Am J Med 1992;92(1):41–44.

37. Woolf SH. The best screening test for colorectal cancer. N Engl J Med 2000;343:1641–1643.
38. Winawer SJ, Zauber AG, Ho MN, et al. Prevention of colorectal cancer by colonoscopic polypectomy. The National Polyp Study Workgroup. N Engl J Med 1993;329:1977–1981.
39. Rex DK, Johnson DA, Lieberman DA, Burt R, Sonnenberg A. Colorectal cancer prevention 2000: screening recommendations of the American College of Gastroenterology. American College of Gastroenterology. Am J Gastroenterol 2000;95:868–877.
40. Bond JH. Virtual colonoscopy—promising, but not ready for widespread use. N Engl J Med 1999;341:1540–1542.
41. Jansen MC, Bueno-de-Mesquita HB, Buzina R, et al. Dietary fiber and plant foods in relation to colorectal cancer mortality: the Seven Countries Study. Int J Cancer 1999;81(2):174–179.
42. Fuchs C, Giovannucci E, Colditz G, et al. Dietary fiber and the risk of colorectal cancer and adenoma in women. N Engl J Med 1999;340:169–176.
43. Byers T. Diet, colorectal adenomas, and colorectal cancer. N Engl J Med 2000;342:1206–1207.
44. Schatzkin A, Lanza E, Corle D, et al. Lack of effect of a low-fat, high-fiber diet on the recurrence of colorectal adenomas. Polyp Prevention Trial Study Group. N Engl J Med 2000;342(16):1149–1155.
45. Alberts DS, Martinez ME, Roe DJ, et al. Lack of effect of a high-fiber cereal supplement on the recurrence of colorectal adenomas. Phoenix Colon Cancer Prevention Physicians' Network. N Engl J Med 2000;342(16):1156–1162.
46. Janne PA, Mayer RJ. Chemoprevention of colorectal cancer. N Engl J Med 2000;342(26):1960–1968.
47. Minton SE. Chemoprevention of breast cancer in the older patient. Hematol Oncol Clin North Am 2000;14:113–130.
48. Smith-Bindman R, Kerlikowske K, Gebretsadik T, Newman J. Is screening mammography effective in elderly women? Am J Med 2000;108:112–119.
49. Chu KC, Tarone RE, Kessler LG, et al. Recent trends in U.S. breast cancer incidence, survival, and mortality rates. J Natl Cancer Inst 1996;88:1571–1579.
50. Kerlikowske K, Barclay J. Outcomes of modern screening mammography. J Natl Cancer Inst Monogr 1997;63:105–111.
51. Olsen O, Gotzsche PC. Screening for breast cancer with mammography (Cochrane Review). Cochrane Database Syst Rev 2001;4:CD001877.
52. Smith-Bindman R, Kerlikowske K, Gebretsadik T, Newman J. Is screening mammography effective in elderly women? Am J Med 2000;108:112–119.
53. Leitch M, Dodd GD, et al. Breast cancer screening in older women. AGS Clinical Practice Committee. J Am Geriatr Soc 2000;48:842–844.
54. U.S. Preventive Services Task Force. Screening for Breast Cancer. In: DiGuiseppi C, ed. Guide to Clinical Preventive Services. Baltimore: Williams & Wilkins, 1996:73–87.
55. Minton SE. Chemoprevention of breast cancer in the older patient. Hematol Oncol Clin North Am 2000;14:113–130.
56. Gail MH, Brinton LA, Byar DP, et al. Projecting individualized probabilities of developing breast cancer for white females who are being examined annually. J Natl Cancer Inst 1989;81(24):1879–1886.

57. Siegler EE. Cervical carcinoma in the aged. Am J Obstet Gynecol 1969; 103:1093–1097.
58. Mandelblatt JS, DB H. Primary care of elderly women: is Pap smear screening necessary? Mt Sinai J Med 1985;52:284–290.
59. U.S. Preventive Services Task Force. Guidelines from Guide to Clinical Preventive Services, 2nd ed. 1995; Williams & Wilkins: Baltimore.
60. Cervical cancer. NIH Consensus Dev. Conference Statement on Cervical Cancer. 1996;14(1):1–3.
61. Flood AB, Wennberg JE, Nease RF, Fowler FJ, Ding J, Hynes LM. The importance of patient preference in the decision to screen for prostate cancer. Prostate Patient Outcomes Research Team. J Gen Intern Med 1996;11:342–349.
62. Friedrich MJ. Issues in prostate cancer screening. JAMA 1999;281: 1573–1575.
63. U.S. Preventive Services Task Force. Guide to Clinical Preventive Services. Baltimore: Williams & Wilkins, 1996.
64. Martinez de Hurtado J, Chechile Toniolo G, Villavicencio Mavrich H. The digital rectal exam, prostate-specific antigen and transrectal echography in the diagnosis of prostatic cancer. Arch Esp Urol 1995;48(3):247–259.
65. De Parle N. From the Health Care Financing Administration. JAMA 2000;283(12):1558.
66. U.S. Preventive Services Task Force. Screening for Hypertension. Guide to Clinical Preventive Services. Baltimore: Williams & Wilkins, 1996: 39–51.
67. Gorelick PB, Sacco RL, Smith DB, et al. Prevention of a first stroke: a review of guidelines and a multidisciplinary consensus statement from the National Stroke Association. JAMA 1999;281:1112–1120.
68. Mulrow CD, Cornell JA, Herrera CR, Kadri A, Farnett L, Aguilar C. Hypertension in the elderly. Implications and generalizability of randomized trials. JAMA 1994;272:1932–1938.
69. U.S. Preventive Services Task Force. Screening for Hypertension. Guide to Clinical Preventive Services. Baltimore: Williams & Wilkins, 1996:39–51.
70. SHEP Cooperative Research Group. Prevention of stroke by antihypertensive drug treatment in older persons with isolated systolic hypertension. Final results of the Systolic Hypertension in the Elderly Program. JAMA 1991; 265(24):3255–3264.
71. The Sixth Report of the Joint National Committee on Prevention, Detection, Evaluation, and Treatment of High Blood Pressure. The National Heart, Lung, and Blood Institute (NHLBI), National Institutes of Health, November, 1997 Bethesda, MD.
72. Joint National Committee on Detection E, and Treatment of High Blood Pressure. The fifth report of the Joint National Committee on Detection. Evaluation, and Treatment of High Blood Pressure. NIH Publication 1993: 93–1088. Bethesda, MD: NIH, 1993.
73. Corti MC, Guralnik JM, Salive ME, et al. Clarifying the direct relation between total cholesterol levels and death from coronary heart disease in older persons. Ann Intern Med 1997;126:753–760.
74. U.S. Preventive Services Task Force. Screening for Lipid Disorders: Recommendations and Rationale. Am J Prev Med 2001;20(3S):73–76.

75. Guidelines for using serum cholesterol, high-density lipoprotein cholesterol, and triglyceride levels as screening tests for preventing coronary heart disease in adults. American College of Physicians. Part 1. Ann Intern Med 1996; 124(5):515–517.

76. Garber AM, Browner WS, Hulley SB. Cholesterol screening in asymptomatic adults, revisited. Part 2. Ann Intern Med 1996;124(5):518–531.

77. Leaf DA. Lipid disorders: applying new guidelines to your older patients. Geriatrics 1994;49(5):35–41.

78. Ginsberg HN, Goldberg IJ. In: Harrison's Principles of Internal Medicine, 14th ed. New York: McGraw-Hill, 1998:2138–2149.

79. Executive Summary of the Third Report of The National Cholesterol Education Program (NCEP) Expert Panel on Detection, Evaluation, and Treatment of High Blood Cholesterol in Adults (Adult Treatment Panel III). JAMA 2001;285(19):2486–2497.

80. Goldberg TH, Chavin SI. Preventive medicine and screening in older adults. J Am Geriatr Soc 1997;45:344–354.

81. Butler RN, Rubenstein AH, Gracia AM, Zweig SC. Type 2 diabetes: causes, complications, and new screening recommendations. I. Geriatrics. 1998; 53(3):47–50, 53–54.

82. Goldberg TH, Chavin SI. Preventive medicine and screening in older adults. J Am Geriatr Soc 1997;45:344–354.

83. Goldberg TH. Update: Preventive medicine and screening in older adults. J Am Geriatr Soc 1999;47:122–123.

84. Association AD. Report of Expert Committee on the Diagnosis and Classification of Diabetes Mellitus. Diabetes Care 1997;20:1183–1197.

85. Siris ES, Miller PD, Barrett-Connor E, et al. Identification and fracture outcomes of undiagnosed low bone mineral density in postmenopausal women: results from the National Osteoporosis Risk Assessment. JAMA 2001;286(22):2815–2822.

86. U.S. Preventive Services Task Force, Guidelines from Guide to Clinical Preventive Services, 2nd ed. 1995 Section I. Screening Part H. Musculoskeletal Disorders and Section III, Immunizations and Chemoprophylaxis. Williams & Wilkins: Baltimore.

87. Writing Group for the Women's Health Initiative Investigators. Risks and benefits of estrogen plus progestin in healthy postmenopausal women. JAMA 2002;288:321–333.

88. Grady D, Herrington D, Bittner V, et al. Cardiovascular disease outcomes during 6.8 years of hormone therapy. Heart and estrogen/progestin replacement study follow-up (HERS II). JAMA 2002;288:49–57.

89. NIH Consensus Development Panel on Osteoporsis, Prevention, Diagnosis, and Therapy. JAMA 2001;285:785–795.

90. Hough S. Osteoporosis Clinical Guideline. South African Medical Association Osteoporosis Working Group. S Afr Med J 2000;90(9 pt 2):907–944.

91. Goldberg TH. Update: preventive medicine and screening in older adults. J Am Geriatr Soc 1999;47:122–123.

92. Reuben DB. Greendale GA, Harrison GG. Nutrition screening in older persons. J Am Geriatr Soc 1995;43(4):415–425.

93. Goodwin JS. Social, psychological, and physical factors affecting the nutritional status of elderly subjects: separating cause and effect. Am J Clin Nutr 1989;50:1201–1209.

94. Posner BM, Jette AM, Smith KW, et al. Nutrition and health risks in the elderly: the Nutrition Screening Initiative. Am J Public Health 1993;83: 972–978.

95. Moore AA, Siu AL. Screening for common problems in ambulatory elderly: clinical confirmation of a screening instrument. Am J Med 1996;100(4): 438–443.

96. Arthur A, Jagger C, Lindesay J, Graham C, Clarke M. Using an annual over-75 health check to screen for depression: validation of the short geriatric depression scale (GDS15) within general practice. Int J Geriatr Psychiatry 1999;14:431–439.

97. Petersen RC, et al. Practice parameter: early detection of dementia: mild cognitive impairment (an evidence-based review). Report of the Quality Standards Subcommittee of the American Academy of Neurology. Neurology 2001;56(9):1133–1142.

98. Moore AA, Siu AL. Screening for common problems in ambulatory elderly: clinical confirmation of a screening instrument. Am J Med 1996;100(4): 438–443.

99. Shulman KI. Clock-drawing: is it the ideal cognitive screening test? Int Geriatr Psychiatry 2000;15:548–561.

100. Sherman FT. Functional assessment. Easy-to-use screening tools speed initial office work-up. Geriatrics 2001;56(8):36–40.

101. Agency for Health Care Policy and Research. Clinical Practice Guideline. Recognition and Initial Assessment of Alzheimer's Disease and Related Dementias. AHCPR Publication No. 97–R123, September 1996.

102. Inouye SK, et al. Clarifying confusion: the confusion assessment method. A new method for detection of delirium. Ann Intern Med 1990;113:941–948.

103. U.S. Preventive Services Task Force. Screening for Visual Impairment. Guided to Clinical Preventive Services. Baltimore: Williams & Wilkins, 1996:373–382.

104. Smeeth L, Iliffe S. Effectiveness of screening older people for impaired vision in community setting: systematic review of evidence from randomised controlled trials. BMJ 1998;316:660–663.

105. U.S. Preventive Services Task Force. Screening for glaucoma. In: Guide to Clinical Preventive Services. Baltimore: Williams & Wilkins, 1996: 383–391.

106. U.S. Preventive Services Task Force. Screening for Hearing Impairment. Guide to Clinical Preventive Services. Baltimore: Williams & Wilkins, 1996:393–405.

107. Sangster JF, Gerace TM, Seewald RC. Hearing loss in elderly patients in a family practice. Can Med Assoc J 1991;144(8):981–984.

108. Brown JS, Vittinghoff E, Wyman JF, et al. Urinary incontinence: does it increase risk for falls and fractures? Study of Osteoporotic Fractures Research Group. J Am Geriatr Soc 2000;48(7):721–725.

109. Christmas C, Andersen RA. Exercise and older patients: guidelines for the clinician. J Am Geriatr Soc 2000;48:318–324.

110. Singh NA, Clements KM, Singh MA. The efficacy of exercise as a long-term antidepressant in elderly subjects: a randomized, controlled trial. J Gerontol [A] Biol Sci Med Sci 2001;56(8):M497–M504.

111. Evans WJ. Exercise training guidelines for the elderly. Med Sci Sports Exerc 1999;31:12–17.

112. Ettinger WH, Afable RF. Physical disability from knee osteoarthritis: the role of exercise as an intervention. Med Sci Sports Exerc 1994;26: 1435–1440.
113. Ettinger WH. Physical activity, arthritis, and disability in older people. Clin Geriatr Med 1998;14:633–640.
114. Judge JO, Schechtman K, Cress E. The relationship between physical performance measures and independence in instrumental activities of daily living. The FICSIT Group. Frailty and Injury: Cooperative Studies of Intervention Trials. J Am Geriatr Soc 1996;44:1332–1341.
115. O'Connor PJ, Aenchbacher LE, Dishman RK. Physical activity and depression in the elderly. J Aging Physiol Activ 1993;1:34–58.
116. Camacho TC, Roberts RE, Lazarus NB, Kaplan GA, Cohen RD. Physical activity and depression: evidence from the Alameda County Study. Am J Epidemiol 1991;134:220–231.
117. Davis MA, Ettinger WH, Neuhaus JM, Mallon KP. Knee osteoarthritis and physical functioning: evidence from the NHANES I Epidemiologic Followup Study. J Rheumatol 1991;18:591–598.
118. Ettinger WH, Burns R, Messier SP, et al. A randomized trial comparing aerobic exercise and resistance exercise with a health education program in older adults with knee osteoarthritis. The Fitness Arthritis and Seniors Trial (FAST). JAMA 1997;277:25–31.
119. Blair SN, Kampert JB, Kohl HW, et al. Influences of cardiorespiratory fitness and other precursors on cardiovascular disease and all-cause mortality in men and women. JAMA 1996;276:205–210.
120. Stewart AL, et al. Physical activity outcomes of CHAMPS II: a physical activity promotion program for older adults. J Gerontol A Biol Sci Med Sci 2001;56(8):M465–M470.
121. Christmas C, Andersen RA. Exercise and older patients: guidelines for the clinician. J Am Geriatr Soc 2000;48:318–324.

9
Vision and Hearing Impairments

HELEN M. FERNANDEZ

Learning Objectives

Upon completion of the chapter, the student will be able to:

1. Recognize the changes in vision and hearing that are considered to be part of normal aging and those secondary from disease.
2. Identify the most common age-associated disease changes in vision and hearing.
3. Describe the management considerations in visual and hearing impairment among older adults.

Vision Impairment

Case A

Ms. A. Brown is a 78-year-old woman with a history of osteoporosis and hypertension. She presents to your practice for a routine checkup. She has no presenting complaints and no recent illnesses. Her only concern is that as a mentor for a high school after-school program, she needs to drive to the school after 5 p.m. This past winter she noticed that she has had more difficulty driving in the dark and hit a trash bin on two occasions. She thinks she may be having some trouble with her eyes. In the summer months, she has never had an accident and has always been a careful driver. She denies any alcohol or drug use.

Material in this chapter is based on the following chapters in Cassel CK, Leipzig RM, Cohen HJ, Larson EB, Meier DE, eds. Geriatric Medicine: An Evidence-Based Approach, 4th ed. New York: Springer, 2003: Rosenthal BP. Changes and Diseases of the Aging Eye, pp. 883–891. Gates GA, Rees TS. Otologic Changes and Disorders, pp. 893–900. Selections edited by Helen M. Fernandez.

General Considerations

The eye is a complex dynamic structure that undergoes physiologic, functional, and significant pathologic changes with age. In addition, vision may be affected by systemic conditions that are more prevalent after the age of 50, such as hypertension and diabetes.

Definitions related to vision loss are important in a discussion on the demographics and epidemiology of the aging eye. *Vision impairment* is a condition that encompasses the continuum from near-normal vision with a slight deficit in the visual acuity or visual field to low vision with significantly reduced vision to profound vision loss and blindness (no light perception) (1,2). *Blindness* is defined as no usable vision with the exception of light perception. *Legal blindness* is defined as a visual acuity of 20/200 or less in the better eye or a visual field of 20 degrees or less in the better eye in the widest meridian (3).

Age-Related Changes to the Ocular Structures and Vision

Visual performance is not just limited to changes in the eye itself, but may also be affected by changes to the surrounding structures, such as the eyelids, orbit, internal and external muscles, as well as the visual pathways (4–10). There are other common functional and physiologic changes that take place in the aging visual system, including a decrease in visual acuity, accommodation, visual field, contrast sensitivity function, color vision, and recovery from a glare source. Functional losses may ultimately affect the most basic of activities of daily living, including reading, driving performance, and the ability to recognize faces (10). For the age-associated changes in the ocular anatomy and vision, see Table 9.1.

Epidemiology and Risk Factors

The Lighthouse National Survey on Vision Loss (11) found that the prevalence of vision impairment substantially increases with age. In fact, 17% of Americans of ages 65 to 74 years (representing 3.1 million persons) and 26% of Americans (3.5 million persons) of ages 75 years and older self-report some form of vision impairment.

Moderate and significant vision impairment can result in an inability to continue to perform activities of daily living (ADLs), such as reading, driving, watching television, or writing a check (12,13). It could result in a loss of independence and social integration, as well as result in depression (14,15).

Case B

Mrs. F. Gordon is a 69-year-old African-American woman who recently went to a department store eyeglass dispensary. She was told that her "eye pressures were high" and that she should see her primary care physician as soon as possible. She remembered that her mother also had a vision problem and eventually went blind in her later years.

TABLE 9.1. Age-associated changes in ocular anatomy and vision

Ocular site	Anatomic function	Age-associated changes
Eyelids	Help spread the tear film Prevent desiccation of the cornea	Thin out with age The dermis becomes dehydrated and loses it vascularity The loss in tonicity results in a lid droop (ptosis) that may obscure the pupil
Tear layer	Protects the cornea, inner surface of the lids	Tear production begins to decrease markedly after age 40; by age 50 an individual produces half the tears produced at age 20 and by age 80 one quarter in males and females May cause erosion of the cornea, dry spots, neovascularization and scarring
Conjunctiva	Protects the eye from infection and injury	Subject to infectious, allergic, metabolic, degenerative, vascular, and neoplastic changes in the elderly
Cornea	One of the two major refracting structures of the eye (the other being the lens) that enable light to reach the retina	Affected by pathologic and degenerative changes, becomes yellower with age, loses some of transparency, and becomes more astigmatic in shape Corneal disease in the elderly may be the result of infections, metabolic changes, viruses, fungi, a decrease in the tear film, trigeminal nerve involvement, degenerations, and neoplasms
Aqueous fluid/canal of Schlemm	Helps to maintain the intraocular pressure of the eye eventually drained through a structure known as Schlemm's canal and onto the venous system	Any change in the outflow of aqueous through Schlemm's canal can result in an elevation of the intraocular eye pressure This elevation in pressure, known as glaucoma, in turn can result in damage to the optic nerve as well as the retina

(Continued)

TABLE 9.1. *Continued*

Ocular site	Anatomic function	Age-associated changes
Lens	Commonly known as the crystalline lens, because of its impressive regularity, precise organization, and clarity in the early years of life	Weale (57) found that aging changes affect the transmission of light through the lens in the visible and the ultraviolet regions of the spectrum Yellowing of the crystalline lens due to the slow growth of the lens throughout life These factors result in a significant decrease of light reaching the retina with advancing age
Vitreous	Occupies the central cavity of the eye and helps to maintain its shape	Generally transparent throughout life but may contract, liquefy, shrink, and possibly detach in the aging eyes
Retina	Contains rods and cones The cones tightly packed into the central area of the eye, known as the macula The rods, which occupy the majority of the peripheral retina, respond to black and white, low levels of illumination and are important in mobility	The central as well as the peripheral retina may be significantly affected by pathologic changes later in life by conditions such as macular degeneration, diabetic retinopathy, retinal detachment, central and branch artery and vein occlusions, and hemorrhagic disease
Optic nerve	Transmits the images falling on the retina to the visual pathway and eventually the visual cortex; it is also synonymous with the blind spot of the eye and contains no light sensitive receptors where it exits the eye	The optic nerve may be affected by a number of disease processes including glaucoma, multiple sclerosis, and brain tumors
Pupil	It dilates under conditions of dim illumination and constricts when the illumination is increased	Lowenfeld (58) found that the pupillary aperture decreases by about 2.5 mm between the ages of 20 and 80 due to the loss in muscle tonus; this resultant decrease in the ambient light reaching the photosensitive layer, the retina, in turn may affect mobility as well as reading performance Morgan (59) found that the pupillary response to ambient light diminishes with age and results in a smaller pupillary diameter

Source: Adapted from Rosenthal BP. Changes and Diseases of the Aging Eye. In: Cassel CK, Leipzig RM, Cohen HJ, et al., eds, Geriatric Medicine, 4th ed. New York: Springer, 2003.

Glaucoma

Glaucoma is a group of diseases rather than a single disease. It is generally classified into open- and closed-angle types. It is estimated that 2 million to 4 million people of ages 40 and over have glaucoma (16,17). A change in resistance to outflow appears to be a primary causative agent in glaucoma that is associated with the normal aging changes. The aging changes include a loss of cells, an increase in pigment in the endothelial cells of the trabecular meshwork, an increase in thickening of the meshwork, and a deposition of plaque in key areas (18).

The diagnosis of glaucoma is generally made on the basis of elevated intraocular pressure, changes in the visual field, changes in the appearance of the optic nerve and optic disk, changes in the nerve fiber layer, and family history (19). The symptoms of glaucoma may include halos around lights, difficulty with mobility, difficulty in seeing under low levels of illumination, and difficulty with contrast. Glaucoma, if left untreated, results in significant changes in the ganglion cell layer of the retina, optic nerve, and visual field.

Tonometry is the measurement of eye pressure and has traditionally been one of the tests to diagnose as well as manage glaucoma. However, damage may take place in the optic nerve, even with "normal" eye pressures for that individual. Visual field testing (perimetry) is another measure used to determine the extent of vision loss in glaucoma. The newer types of automated perimeters help to precisely measure the damage to the visual field in decibels and is very analogous to a hearing test. This enables the examiner to measure the effect of the various treatments used to preserve the remaining visual field.

Traditional treatment for glaucoma has included the instillation of eyedrops as well as surgery. However, there are numerous new medications that work on different mechanisms in the eye to reduce the eye pressure. Some beta-blockers are used to inhibit aqueous production by blocking beta-receptors in the ciliary body. There are also carbonic anhydrase inhibitors that similarly reduce the production of aqueous, whereas epinephrine reduces aqueous production and to a lesser extent increases the outflow of the fluid. In addition, there are adrenergic agonists, pilocarpine, and prostaglandin analogues that also increase aqueous outflow. Unfortunately, laser surgery or other filtering procedures may be indicated if damage continues.

Case C (Part 1)

Mr. F. Thompson is a 58-year-old business executive who used to be a copy editor for a city newspaper before moving on to the business aspect of journalism. He prided himself of his editing skills even before the advent of mainstream word processing. He now presents to your practice because he is having trouble reading the *Wall Street Journal.* He describes problems with focusing that requires him to hold the newspaper at arm's length. He asks you if this is just part of growing old or may be related to something else?

Presbyopia

Presbyopia, the most common of the normal aging changes, begins in the fourth decade. It is a natural age-related condition that is the result of a gradual decrease in accommodative amplitude, from about 15 diopters (D) in early childhood to 1 D before the age of 60 years (20–23). Clinically, it is the inability to focus clearly on close objects or to see print clearly. The lens, which is a flexible structure that can change its shape into a more or less convex structure, begins to lose its elasticity in the third and fourth decade. But reading is not generally affected until the early or mid-40s.

Major risk factors for presbyopia are age, short stature, occurrence of certain systemic diseases, such as diabetes, cardiovascular disease, medications, trauma, hyperopia (farsightedness), and side effects of drugs (24–26). However, there are still major unanswered questions on the influence of genetics, caloric intake, hypertension, ethnic and racial factors, and environmental influences.

Presbyopia was traditionally treated with reading lenses, contact lenses, bifocals, or trifocals. The latest optical designs include bifocal contact lenses as well as optical systems that allow the viewer to see simultaneously at distance and near. One of the more recent changes in the treatment of presbyopia, known as *monovision*, involves correction of the dominant eye for distance vision. Patients may either wear a contact lens or, more recently, have corrective surgery on the cornea to correct for near vision. This is done by inserting an intraocular lens to correct for close vision. One of the newest surgical advances includes a foldable silicone multifocal intraocular lens that allows the viewer to see clearer at different distances.

Cataracts

The prevalence of cataract is said to be 18% of persons aged 65 to 74, and 46% of persons aged 75 to 85 (27–29). There is a steady increase in cataracts with age (30). Some of the risk factors for cataract development include excessive exposure to sunlight (ultraviolet B), age, cigarette smoking (31), high cholesterol and triglycerides, diabetes mellitus, cortisone medication, and eye injury (32).

Surgical treatments for cataracts have dramatically shifted to a procedure known as *extracapsular cataract extraction* (33). Ophthalmic treatment for cataract has also evolved rapidly over the last 25 years from the prescription of thick heavy glass and plastic lenses to contact lenses to the posterior chamber–placed intraocular lens (IOL) implant (34). The IOL implant is the treatment of choice for more than 95% of persons undergoing cataract surgery in the developed world.

Vitreous Hemorrhage

The vitreous is generally transparent throughout life but may contract, liquefy, shrink, and possibly detach in the aging eyes. Vitreous hemorrhage is often a complication of proliferative diabetic retinopathy and results in a clouding of the vitreous. (For further details on this condition, see Chapter 59: Changes and Diseases of the Aging Eye. In: Cassel CK, et al., eds; Geriatric Medicine, 4th ed., page 887.)

Case C (Part 2)

You diagnosed Mr. Thompson as having presbyopia, and you prescribed corrective lenses for him. Now at age 68, Mr. Thompson complains that his vision is getting more blurry. He has trouble distinguishing faces and has stopped reading the newspaper because at times he cannot make out the words.

Macular Degeneration

There are over 13.2 million Americans (15%) who have signs of age-related macular degeneration. That number climbs to one in three over the age of 75 (35). It is estimated that as the population ages, more people will become legally blind from macular degeneration than from glaucoma and diabetic retinopathy combined (36).

Age-related macular degeneration (AMD), formerly known as senile macular degeneration, is primarily found in the Caucasian population. Known risk factors include smoking, light-colored irises, women over 60, familial history, postmenopausal women who have not undergone hormonal replacement therapy, individuals taking antihypertensive drug therapy, and individuals having a high serum cholesterol level (37). Visual function may be dramatically affected in macular degeneration. Age-related macular degeneration might also be manifested by blurred vision; difficulty in seeing words, letters, faces, or street signs, as well as difficulty in differentiating colors.

There are primarily two types of age-related macular degeneration. The *dry (atrophic) type*, for which there is no treatment at this time, accounts for 90% of the new cases diagnosed. The *wet type*, also known as choroidal neovascularization or exudative maculopathy, accounts for the remaining

10% of the cases. The wet AMD is generally characterized by a more profound loss of visual function.

Remediation includes traditional "thermal" laser as well as nonthermal photodynamic therapy for the wet AMD. The latter treatment may arrest the progressive loss of vision but never results in complete restoration of visual function. Additional research on AMD is being done with low-dose radiation, submacular surgery, cell transplantation, macular translocation, blood filtration, and vasogenic factors that stimulate the growth of new blood vessels.

Diabetic Retinopathy

Diabetic retinopathy is a microvascular complication of chronic diabetes mellitus (38). Of the estimated 12.7 million people in the United States who are over the age of 40 and have diabetes, 4.8 million (38%) have diabetic retinopathy, the majority having the more common background diabetic retinopathy. However, there are 700,000 people who have the proliferative, more destructive type of the disease. It is also estimated that 12,000 to 24,000 lose their sight from diabetic retinopathy (39).

In addition to the ongoing medical care, the diabetic may need laser photocoagulation and cataract extraction as the disease progresses. Vision rehabilitation is often indicated for the diabetic, especially those with advanced vision loss (see Chapter 24: Diabetes Mellitus, page 437).

Visual Field Loss

The etiology of visual field loss is generally glaucoma, stroke, or brain tumor. Approximately 92% of all strokes occur in patients aged 50 and older (40). The incidence doubles with each successive decade (41). The ocular consequences of stroke are often serious and may include transient vision loss as well as the loss of the right or the left side of vision (hemianopia) in both eyes or partial field loss. Hemianopia can also be the result of brain tumors that affect the individual between 50 and 70 years of age (49). Depending on the location of the visual field loss, reading and mobility may be affected. Individuals with hemianopia often read the entire eye chart to the 20/20 line because of macular sparing. However, there may still be an absolute or relative loss in the visual field. Many people are unaware that the vision is actually lost and can injure themselves unless instructed on the management of using the residual vision.

Stroke rehabilitation often requires a team approach and usually includes a variety of professionals for reeducation in the areas of vision, mobility, speech, and cognitive functioning. The low-vision specialist may recommend techniques, optical and nonoptical devices, as well as special lens systems to enhance visual performance.

Case C (Part 3)

Mr. Thompson is diagnosed with dry-type macular degeneration. He tells you that he has heard of this condition before and knows that there are no effective treatments. Yet he wants to explore other modalities such as visual aids to help with his daily performance of his ADLs.

Low Vision and Vision Rehabilitation

Vision rehabilitation may be an essential component in the management of the person with a visual impairment from macular degeneration, inoperable cataracts, glaucoma, diabetic retinopathy, and visual field loss from a stroke or tumor. Vision rehabilitation may involve many other professionals, including the eye care professionals specializing in low vision, the optometrist (OD) or ophthalmologist (MD), as well as vision rehabilitation teachers, orientation and mobility instructor, social workers, and occupational therapists. The low-vision specialist will prescribe specialized optical, nonoptical, and electronic low-vision devices for distance and near tasks. A rehabilitation teacher may be called on to teach how to safely manage the kitchen and personal affairs, and an orientation or mobility instructor may be involved to teach safe independent cane travel.

A low-vision evaluation is an eye examination that may be ordered when the vision is not corrected with ordinary glasses, contact lenses, or medical treatment including surgery. The examiner uses specialized eye charts to test visual acuity function at distance and near, which are used to determine the visual potential. Various researchers have outlined specialized tests of visual function, including a contrast sensitivity test, evaluation of the macular function with the Amsler grid, visual field tests, color vision analysis, and photostress tests that may be indicated (42–45).

There is value in the prescription of specialized low-vision devices for persons with a visual impairment. These devices would be especially valuable for persons having a visual acuity ranging from 20/40 to 20/800 as well as for those with visual field and loss in contrast sensitivity function (46). These specialized low-vision devices include high-powered reading lenses (microscopic lenses), hand and stand magnifiers, handheld and head-borne telescopic systems, absorptive and tinted lenses, closed-circuit televisions, and systems for persons with visual field defects. In addition, there are numerous nonoptical devices, including lighting and illumination systems, reading stands, talking devices, and high-contrast devices, that will help to improve visual performance.

Hearing Impairment

Case D (Part 1)

Mr. E. Day is a 74-year-old Caucasian man who presents to your office. His wife, Joyce, accompanies him. She complains that Mr. Day is withdrawn and does not participate in conversations with their friends. She tells you that he had always been a very sociable kind of guy. Also, their neighbors have complained about how loud the television volume is whenever Mr. Day is watching.

General Considerations

Age-related hearing loss is one of the most frequent health problems encountered in geriatric medicine. It is the third most prevalent major chronic disability in the over 65-year-old age group. Unfortunately, hearing loss is a disorder that is frequently unrecognized, frequently misunderstood, and all too frequently neglected, by the affected themselves as well as by health care providers.

Age-Related Changes to Auditory Structures and Hearing

The aging process has three distinct components: physiologic degeneration, extrinsic insults, and intrinsic insults. In the auditory system, the extrinsic component (*nosocusis*) includes hearing loss due to otologic disease, hazardous noise exposure, acoustic trauma, and ototoxic agents. The intrinsic component (*sociocusis*) indicates the wear-and-tear effects of exposure to the everyday sounds of normal living (47). People who live in nonindustrialized regions avoid both nosocusis and sociocusis and demonstrate excellent hearing into old age (48).

In our industrialized society, it is difficult to escape from noise pollution. It is likely that much of the variance in levels of presbycusis is due to unmeasured effects of noise damage, which is the most common form of ototoxicity. The effects of systemic disease on hearing are still incompletely understood, but may contribute as well.

Presbycusis

Presbycusis, literally meaning "elder hearing," is the generic term applied to age-related hearing loss and is used to signify the sum of all the processes that affect hearing with the passage of time. The prevalence of self-reported hearing problems among the elderly is 30% (49). The prevalence increases substantially with age, with 24% between the ages of 65 and 74, and up to 39% of those over the age of 75 years. It is estimated that by the year 2030, older adults will comprise 32% of the population, and it is predicted that as many as 60% to 75% of the elderly will suffer hearing loss, approximately 21 million persons.

Age-related hearing loss is manifested by deterioration in each of the two critical dimensions of hearing: reduction in threshold sensitivity and reduction in the ability to understand speech. The loss in threshold sensitivity is insidious in onset, beginning in the highest frequencies (8000 Hz) and slowly progressing to involve those frequencies important in speech understanding (1000- to 3000-Hz range). The most common complaint of presbycusic patients is not "I can't hear" but rather "I can't understand." The high-frequency hearing impairment causes the voiceless consonants (t, p, k, f, s, and _ch_) to be rendered unintelligible. For example, people confuse "mash," "math," "map," and "mat," or "Sunday" with "someday." Seniors often complain that others mumble and they cannot participate in conversations because bits and pieces of speech are missing. As the hearing loss worsens and affects the lower frequencies with advancing years, the older person requires greater volume for speech detection and often needs repetition or confuses what is said. Everyday sounds, such as beepers, turn signals, and escaping steam are not heard, which places the hearing impaired at greater risk of injury and makes them more isolated from the everyday world.

Types of Hearing Loss

Hearing loss is traditionally classified as conductive, sensorineural, and central. These types are based on the site of structural damage or blockage in the auditory system.

Conductive Hearing Loss

Conductive hearing loss arises from obstruction of sound transfer through the external or middle ear space. Cerumen impaction represents the most common external ear cause of conductive hearing loss and is a frequently overlooked problem in elderly people whose ear canals often "collapse" with age. Cerumen impaction is commonly the result of misguided attempts by people to clean their ear canals with cotton-tipped ear buds. Other types of conductive loss, such as otitis media and otosclerosis, seldom arise primarily in the senior years. Unilateral middle ear effusion can be a sign of nasopharyngeal cancer, but is more commonly the result of an ear infection.

Sensorineural Hearing Loss

A sensorineural hearing loss involves damage to the cochlea and/or fibers of the eighth cranial nerve. "Nerve deafness" and "perceptive deafness" are obsolete terms for sensorineural hearing loss but are occasionally encountered. Sensorineural hearing loss may be sensory only (cochlear hair cell loss), may involve the auditory nerve or brainstem (neural), or both. Newer diagnostic methods permit finer distinctions between sensory and neural losses. Sensorineural hearing loss due to presbycusis affects both ears equally and generally begins in the higher frequencies. Unilateral sensorineural hearing loss may be caused by a neoplasm (acoustic neuroma), acoustic trauma (blast injury), or a viral infection or vascular event (sudden sensorineural hearing loss). Sudden sensorineural hearing loss may be accompanied by vestibular symptoms of vertigo, dizziness, and nystagmus. Idiopathic sudden sensorineural hearing loss often recovers with prompt corticosteroid therapy. Therefore, immediate otologic referral is indicated for evaluation and treatment. Metabolic causes of hearing impairment are seen in endocrine diseases: thyroid, pancreatic, and adrenal, renal disease, diabetes mellitus, and hypertension.

Central Hearing Loss

Central auditory dysfunction is far less common and is seen in conditions such as stroke and Alzheimer's disease, neoplasm, multiple sclerosis, and degenerative disorders (49).

Diagnostic Evaluation

Signs and Symptoms

The otologic examination is preceded by a carefully taken patient history. In the case of hearing loss, the time of onset, whether the loss was gradual or sudden, and the presence or absence of associated symptoms, especially vertigo, tinnitus, discharge, or pain, should be noted. Family history, noise exposure history, previous ear or head trauma, and use of ototoxic drugs should also be included. People with substantial exposure to workplace noise, recreational noise, and firearm use are more likely to have irreversible high-frequency hearing loss. Medication history should be explored to determine possible ototoxicity. Aminoglycoside antimicrobials, cisplatinum, loop diuretics, and antiinflammatory agents may contribute to hearing loss. Metabolic evaluation is indicated if the patient has not had a recent health examination. Diabetes, hypertension, and hyperlipidemia should be excluded as cofactors. Patients receiving renal dialysis often have poorer hearing than would be expected from age alone. Hearing loss does cluster in families, particularly the trial form of presbycusis.

The physical examination of the ear canal and tympanic membrane is typically normal in most older adults, with the exception of cerumen accumulation in some. Cerumen removal with either ear canal irrigation, often preceded by use of cerumen-dissolving drops (10% sodium bicarbonate is the most effective), or manual (instrumental) removal is necessary. While the removal of occluding cerumen for some individuals can result in hearing improvement, most often the locus of the hearing loss is in the sensorineural system. Itching and dryness of the external canal is a common complaint among older adults. Although the itching is often temporarily relieved by use of cotton-tipped ear buds, this inevitably worsens the dryness and itching due to trauma to the canal. Aging causes atrophy of the canal epithelium and underlying sebaceous and cerumen glands, which results in decreased hydration of the canal skin and increased susceptibility to abrasion from cotton-tipped ear buds. Patients should avoid putting anything in their canals. Canal itching can be controlled with steroid-based creams as needed.

Examination of the tympanic membrane should be accompanied by pneumatic otoscopy to assess tympanic membrane mobility. In people with middle ear effusion, the drum does not move or moves very little. Relying on the "color" of the tympanic membrane to diagnose effusion may be misleading. Commonly seen is opacification of the normally translucent tympanic membrane (tympanosclerosis). This has no effect on conduction of sound energy into the inner ear and is simply a manifestation of age. There are several "warning signs" associated with the history and physical examination that should prompt referral to an otolaryngologist for complete evaluation and treatment. These include acute or chonic dizziness, pain or discomfort in the ear and any unilateral hearing loss.

Ancillary Tests

Imaging studies are not indicated except where the loss is unilateral or significantly asymmetric, or where tinnitus is unexplained by the audiogram. Screening magnetic resonance imaging (MRI) scans using the T2 fast spin echo technique provide superb visualization of the 8th nerve and brainstem and can detect tumors in the millimeter range, even before hearing is affected (50).

TABLE 9.2. Guidelines for communicating with the hearing-impaired

Get listener's attention before speaking.
Face listener directly to give visual cues.
Do not cover mouth while talking or turn away.
Try to reduce background noise; turn down TV, radio, etc.
Use facial expressions and gestures.
Speak slowly and clearly with more pauses than usual.
Speak only slightly louder than normal; do not shout.
Rephrase if listener does not understand rather than repeating word for word.
Alert listener to changes in topic before proceeding.
Do not turn and walk away while talking.
Use written notes if necessary.

Source: Gates GA, Rees TS. Otologic changes and disorders. In: Cassel CK, Leipzig RM, Cohen HJ, et al., eds. Geriatric Medicine, 4th ed. New York: Springer, 2003.

Screening Audiometry

Although it would seem prudent for health care providers to screen for one of the most prevalent chronic conditions affecting the elderly, this is unfortunately not the practice with hearing loss identification (51). Moreover, even when elderly patients have discussed their hearing difficulties with their primary care providers, they are often told that their hearing loss is minor or that it cannot be improved with a hearing aid (52). When one considers the adverse effects of hearing loss on quality of life and that such effects are reversible with hearing aids, it is surprising that in-office hearing loss screening is not common practice.

The use of screening audiometry is the tool of choice in the identification of hearing loss. Screening audiometry can be quickly and easily administered by a trained office nurse or medical assistant. The equipment needed for screening audiometry is lightweight and low cost. There are portable, battery-operated audiometers and even specially developed otoscopes with audiometric capabilities available for the practitioner (53). A portable audiometer can be used to screen hearing at 1000, 2000, and 3000 Hz at intensity levels of 25 dB (normal), 40 dB (borderline), and 60 dB hearing loss (HL). Failure at any one frequency at 25 dB for younger adults or 40 dB for older adults suggests the need for referral for a complete audiologic evaluation (54).

Case D (Part 2)

You ask Mr. Day if he thinks he has a hearing problem. He states that perhaps he does but that he suspects it is part of growing older.

Self-Assessment Screening Methods

The simplest self-assessment screening method is to ask patients if they think they have a hearing problem. This single question is more sensitive than multiitem questionnaires, which are more specific. A number of self-assessment inventories have been developed as a means of evaluating hearing handicap. These scales quantify hearing handicap by including questions about the self-perceived situational and psychosocial effects of decreased hearing on various aspects of daily function. One of these scales, the Hearing Handicap Inventory for the Elderly–Screening Version (HHIE-S), is specifically designed for use with noninstitutionalized elderly (55,56). For details on the scoring of the HHIE-S, see Chapter 60: Otologic Changes and Disorders. In: Cassel CK et al., eds; Geriatric Medicine, 4th ed., page 896.

Patients who fail audiometric screening tests, or have a high self-perceived hearing handicap, should be referred for formal audiologic and otologic assessment. This evaluation delineates the pattern and degree of loss, indicates the likely site of loss, and predicts the suitability of otologic treatment or amplification for rehabilitation. Central auditory tests are widely available and should be considered when the possibility of early dementia exists.

Management Considerations

Medical-Surgical Treatment

Hearing loss due to conductive deficits (e.g., otosclerosis, otitis media, eardrum perforations, etc.) can most often be successfully treated with medical or surgical intervention by an otolaryngologist. Eardrum perforations can be surgically repaired (myringoplasty), middle ear fluid can be removed and the middle ear aerated (myringotomy with placement of a pressure-equalization tube), a nonmobile stapes can be removed and replaced with a prosthesis (stapedectomy), and an absent or disarticulated ossicle can be replaced with a prosthesis (ossicular chain reconstruction). These procedures generally can eliminate the conductive hearing loss and return hearing to normal or near-normal levels.

Case D (Part 3)

After completing a thorough history and physical examination, screening assessments and audiometry, Mr. Day is diagnosed with bilateral sensorineural hearing loss due to presbycusis. He agrees to consider hearing aids but he desires aids that are not "so obvious."

Hearing Aid Amplification

The most common site of age-related hearing loss is dysfunction in the cochlea or associated neural structures. Of all patients with sensorineural hearing loss, less than 5% can be helped medically. Consequently, hearing aid amplification is the principal resource for improving communication and reducing hearing handicaps in persons with sensorineural hearing loss. Unfortunately, only 10% of people who might benefit from an aid actually own one, which indicates a substantial underservice. Current hearing aids include devices that fit behind the ear, in the ear, in the canal, and, most recently, completely in the canal. Those older adults with dexterity problems or vision impairments are often unable to insert and adjust the smaller aids properly and are better served with larger hearing aids. The audiologist reviews such issues with the hearing-impaired individual during the prefitting session.

Conventional hearing aids typically use omnidirectional microphones, which pick up sounds from all directions. While these microphones are helpful in quiet situations, persons often complain of amplification of background noise in restaurants and groups. Directional and dual microphones are now available in hearing aids, which attenuate sounds from the back or side and focus on sounds from the front of the listener. The hearing aid user can choose either the directional microphone or omnidirectional microphone to suit the listening situation.

The most recent introduction in hearing aid technology is the fully digital instrument. These aids offer complex sound processing, fitting flexibility, precision in signal manipulation, multiple memories, multiple channels, and automatic feedback reduction capabilities, which are not available in conventional devices. While digital aids are considerably more expensive than conventional aids, the benefits may by justified by many hearing-impaired persons. One must consider the acoustic and communicative needs of an individual patient and determine the appropriate level of hearing aid technology. If the patient does not participate in social activities and has few demands placed on his/her hearing, a digital hearing aid is inappropriate. If, on the other hand, the patient is socially active and encounters a variety of listening environments and high hearing demands, digital hearing aids with multiple memories and dual-microphone technology are highly beneficial and worth the added cost.

The industry standard of practice is to provide the user with at least a 30-day trial period with amplification and to refund the cost of the hearing aid if it is returned. The new amplification systems are considerably more expensive than conventional hearing aids. Currently, digital in-the-canal aids cost approximately $2500 per aid, and binaural aids are typically most beneficial. Neither Medicare nor most insurance carriers provide financial coverage for hearing aids. The specific hearing needs, lifestyle, and adaptability of the hearing aid wearer must be taken into account during the prefitting process.

Assistive Listening Devices

Assistive listening devices (ALDs) comprise a growing number of situation-specific amplification systems designed for use in difficult listening environments. They commonly use a microphone placed close to the desired sound source (e.g., a television, theater stage, or speaker's podium), and sound is directly transmitted to the listener. Several transmission methods include infrared, audio loop, FM radio, or direct audio input. Desired sounds are enhanced while competing extraneous noises are decreased, thus permitting improved understanding. These ALDs are becoming more available in churches, theaters, and classrooms, enabling hearing-impaired seniors to avoid the isolation imposed by the inability to hear a sermon, play, or public address.

Other assistive listening devices, such as small portable pocket amplifiers, are very helpful in medical situations. These amplifiers are particularly well suited for health care professionals' communication with the hearing-impaired elderly. Often it is in the setting of acute health care delivery that older patients have misplaced or forgotten their own hearing aids. Portable amplifiers can save the voice and patience of the health care provider and allow respectful and private interactions to take place.

For further details on assistive listening devices, implantable hearing aids and cochlear implants, see Chapter 60: Otologic Changes and Disorders. In: Cassel CK et al., eds; Geriatric Medicine, 4th ed., page 898.

Audiologic Rehabilitation

Audiologic rehabilitation can include speech reading (lip-reading) training, auditory training, and hearing loss counseling. Speech reading training teaches the use of visual cues to help in understanding speech. Cues include the use of lip movement, facial expression, body gestures, and context. Auditory training teaches strategies to improve listening skills and encourages the acceptance of amplified sound. For further details on audiologic rehabilitation, see Chapter 60: Otologic Changes and Disorders. In: Cassel CK et al., eds; Geriatric Medicine, 4th ed., page 898.

Case D (Part 4)

Mrs. Day asks what she and her family and friends can do to make conversations easier for her husband.

Effective Communication with the Hearing-Impaired

Table 9.2 lists several ways to enhance communication with hearing-impaired persons. These "guidelines" can be very helpful for improved communication in the practitioner-patient relationship.

General Principles

- Visual performance is not just limited to changes in the eye itself but may also be affected by changes to the surrounding structures, such as the eyelids, orbit, internal and external muscles, as well as the visual pathways.
- The functional losses may ultimately affect the most basic of activities of daily living, including reading, driving, and recognizing faces.

- Age-related hearing loss is the third most prevalent major chronic disability in the over-65 age group.
- Hearing loss is a normal accompaniment of old age. The health care provider should be alert to the signs of hearing impairment and assist the patient in obtaining and using appropriate rehabilitation.
- Unfortunately, hearing loss is frequently unrecognized, frequently misunderstood, and all too frequently neglected, both by the affected themselves and by health care providers.

Suggested Readings

Gates GA, Rees TS. Otologic changes and disorders. In: Cassel CK, Leipzig RM, Cohen HJ, et al., eds. Geriatric Medicine, 4th ed. New York: Springer, 2003: 893–900.

Rosenthal BP. Changes and diseases of the aging eye. In: Cassel CK, Leipzig RM, Cohen HJ, et al., eds. Geriatric Medicine, 4th ed. New York: Springer, 2003: 883–892.

References

1. Colenbrander A. Dimensions of visual performance. Trans Am Acad Ophthalmol Otolaryngol 1977;83;322.
2. Bailey IL. Measurement of visual acuity—towards standardization. In: Vision Science Symposium. Bloomington, IN: Indiana University, 1988:215–230.
3. Silverstone B, Lang MA, Rosenthal BP, Faye EE. The Lighthouse Handbook on Vision Impairment and Vision Rehabilitation, vol 1, Vision Impairment. New York: Oxford University Press, 2000.
4. Dutton JJ. Gliomas of the anterior visual pathway. Surv Ophthalmol 1992;38:427–452.
5. Sadun AA, Rubin R. Sensory neuro-ophthalmology and vision impairment. In: Silverstone B, Lang MA, Rosenthal BP, Faye EE, eds. The Lighthouse Handbook on Vision Impairment and Vision Rehabilitation. New York: Oxford University Press, 2000.
6. Arnold AC, Hepler RS. Natural history of nonarteritic anterior ischemic optic neuropathy. J Neuro-Ophthalmol 1994;14:66–69.
7. Gentile M. Functional Visual Behavior: A Therapist's Guide to Evaluation and Treatment Options. American Occupational Therapy Association, 1997.
8. Beard C. Ptosis. St. Louis: CV Mosby, 1976.
9. Mahoney BP. Sjogren syndrome. In: Mark ES et al., eds. Primary Eyecare in Systemic Disease. Norwalk, CT: Appleton and Lange, 1995.
10. Bullimore MA, Bailey IL, Wacker RT. Face recognition in age-related maculopathy. Invest Ophthalmol Vis Sci 1991;1:776–783.
11. The Lighthouse Inc. The Lighthouse National Survey on Vision Loss: The Experience, Attitudes, and Knowledge of Middle-Aged and Older Americans. New York: The Lighthouse, 1995.

12. Kircher C. Economic aspects of blindness and low vision: a new perspective. J Vis Impair Blindness 1995;89:506–513.
13. Horowitz A. Vision impairment and functional disability among nursing home residents. Gerontologist 1994;34(3):316–323.
14. Horowitz A, Reinhardt JP. Mental health issues in vision impairment. In: Silverstone B, Lang MA, Rosenthal BP, Faye EE, eds. The Lighthouse Handbook on Vision Impairment and Vision Rehabilitation. New York: Oxford University Press, 2000.
15. Kleinschmidt JJ, Trunnell EP, Reading JC, White GL, Richardson GE, Edwards ME. The role of control in depression, anxiety, and life satisfaction among the visually impaired older adult. J Health Educ 1995;26:26–36.
16. Prevent Blindness America. Vision Problems in the U.S., 1994.
17. Glaucoma Foundation, Inc. http://www.glaucomafoundation.org, 2000.
18. Lewis T, Fingeret M. Primary Care of the Glaucomas. New York: McGraw-Hill, Medical Publishing Division, 2000.
19. Yablonski ME, Zimmerman TJ, Kass MA, Becker B. Prognostic significance of optic disc cupping in ocular hypertensive patients. Am J Ophthalmol 1980;89:585–590.
20. Beers APA, van der Hiejde GI. Age-related changes in the accommodative mechanism. Optom Vis Sci 1996;73:235–242.
21. Hamasaki D, Ong J, Marg E. The amplitude of accommodation in presbyopia. Am J Optom 1956;33:3–14.
22. Ramsdale C, Charman WN. A longitudinal study of the changes in the state accommodative response. Ophthalmic Physiol Opt 1989;9:255–263.
23. Wagstaff DF. The objective measurement of the amplitude of accommodation. Part VII. Optician 1966;151:431–436.
24. Pointer JS. Broken down by age and sex. The optical correction of presbyopia revisited. Ophthalmic Physiol Opt 1995;15(5):439–443.
25. Patorgis CJ. Presbyopia. In: Amos JF, ed. Diagnosis and Management in Vision Care. Boston: Butterworths, 1987:203–238.
26. Jain IS, Ram J, Bupta A. Early onset of presbyopia. Am J Optom Physiol Opt 1982;59:1002–1004.
27. Leske MC, Sperduto RD. The epidemiology of senile cataract: a review. Am J Epidemiol 1983;118(2):152–165.
28. Taylor HR, West SK, Rosenthal FS, et al. Effect of ultraviolet radiation on cataract formation. N Engl J Med 1988;319(22):1429–1433.
29. Klein BEK, Klein RK, Linton KLP. Prevalence of age-related lens opacities in a population. The Beaver Dam Eye Study. Ophthalmology 1992;99:546–552.
30. Kahn HA, Leibowitz HM, Ganley JP, et al. The Framingham Eye Study: I. Outline and major prevalence findings. Am J Epidemiol 1977;106:17–32.
31. Rouhianen P, Rouhianen H, Salonen JT. Association between low plasma vitamin E concentration and progression of early cortical lens opacities. Am J Epidemiol 1996;144:496–500.
32. Faye EE, Rosenthal BP, Sussman-Skalka CJ. Cataract and the Aging Eye. Lighthouse International, Center for Vision and Aging; New York, 1995.
33. Jaffe NS, Jaffe MS, Jaffe GF. Cataract Surgery and Its Complications, 5th ed. St. Louis: Mosby Yearbook, 1990:34.

34. Lindquist TD, Lindstrom RL. Ophthalmic Surgery: Looseleaf and Update Service. St. Louis: Mosby-Yearbook, 1994:I-F-1.
35. Prevent Blindness America. Vision Problems in the U.S.; Chicago, IL 1994.
36. National Advisory Eye Council. Vision research—a national plan: 1994–1998. NIH publication No. 95–3186. Bethesda, MD: National Institutes of Health, 1993.
37. Rosenthal BP. Living Well with Macular Degeneration. New York: NAL Penguin/Putnam Books, 2001.
38. Leonard B, Charles S. Diabetic retinopathy. In: Silverstone B, Lang MA, Rosenthal BP, Faye EE, eds. The Lighthouse Handbook on Vision Impairment and Vision Rehabilitation. New York: Oxford University Press, 2000.
39. Will JC, Geiss LS, Wetterhall SF. Diabetic retinopathy (letter to the editor). N Engl J Med 1990;323:613.
40. Cockburn DM. Ocular implications of systemic disease in the elderly. In: Rosenbloom A, Morgan M, eds. Vision and Aging. Boston: Butterworth-Heinemann, 1993.
41. Blaustein BH. Cerebrovascular disease. In: Thomann KH, Marks ES, Adamczyk DT, and Marks E. Norwalk CT: Appleton & Lange, 1995, page 55. Primary Eyecare in Systemic Disease.
42. Rosenthal BP, Fischer ML. Optometric assessment of low vision. In: Gentile M, ed. Functional Visual Behavior: A Therapist's Guide to Evaluation and Treatment Options. Bethesda, MD: American Occupational Therapy Association, 1997:345–373.
43. Cole RG, Rosenthal BP. Remediation and Management of Low Vision. St. Louis: Mosby, 1997.
44. Rosenthal BP, Cole RG. Functional Assessment of Low Vision. St. Louis: Mosby, 1996.
45. Faye EE. Clinical low vision, 2nd ed. Boston: Little, Brown, 1984.
46. Rosenthal BP, Williams DR. Devices primarily for people with low vision. In: Silverstone B, Lang MA, Rosenthal BP, Faye EE, eds. The Lighthouse Handbook on Vision Impairment and Vision Rehabilitation, vol 1, Vision Impairment. New York: Oxford University Press, 2000.
47. Gates GA, Cooper JC. Incidence of hearing decline in the elderly. Acta Otolaryngol 1991;111:240–248.
48. Gates GA, Cobb JL, D'Agostino RB, et al. The relation of hearing in the elderly to the presence of cardiovascular disease and cardiovascular risk factors. Arch Otol Head Neck Surg 1993;119:156–161.
49. Lavizzo-Mourey RJ, Siegler EL. Hearing impairment in the elderly. J Gen Intern Med 1992;7:191–198.
50. Frank T, Petersen DR. Accuracy of a 40 dB HL Audioscope and audiometer screening for adults. Ear Hear 1987;8:180–183.
51. Mulrow CD, Aguilar C, Endicott JE, et al. Quality-of-life changes and hearing impairment: a randomized trial. Ann Intern Med 1990;113(3):188–194.
52. ASHA Ad Hoc Committee on Hearing Screening in Adults. Considerations in screening adults/older persons for handicapping hearing impairments. ASHA 1992;8:81–87.
53. Ventry IM, Weinstein BE. The Hearing Handicap Inventory for the Elderly: a new tool. Ear Hear 1982;3:128–134.

54. Weinstein BE. Age-related hearing loss: how to screen for it, and when to intervene. Geriatrics 1994;49:40–45.

55. Gates GA, Karzon RK, Garcia P, et al. Auditory dysfunction in aging and senile dementia of the Alzheimer's type. Arch Neurol 1995;52:626–634.

56. Malinoff RL, Weinstein BE. Changes in self-assessment of hearing handicap over the first year of hearing aid use by older adults. J Am Acad Rehabil Audiol 1989;22:54–60.

57. Weale RA. Age and the transmittance of the human crystalline lens. J Physiol 1988;395:577–587.

58. Lowenfeld IE. Pupillary changes related to age. In: Thompson HS, Daroff R, Frisen L, et al., eds. Topics in Neuro-Ophthalmology. Baltimore: Williams and Wilkins, 1979:124–150.

59. Morgan MW. Changes in visual function in the aging eye. In: Rosenbloom AA, Morgan MW, eds. Vision and Aging. New York: Fairchild, 1986:121–134.

10
Exercise and Rehabilitation

Sandra E. Sanchez-Reilly

Learning Objectives

Upon completion of the chapter, the student will be able to:

1. Outline the importance of exercise and its implications in the well-being of older adults.
2. Identify the different components of an exercise program for the elderly.
3. Differentiate among several types of disability and its effects in activities of daily living in geriatric patients.
4. Define rehabilitation and recognize the importance of an interdisciplinary team in the process of function restoration in the elderly.

Exercise

Case A (Part 1)

Mr. M. is a 76-year-old man who lives at home. He has a history of controlled hypertension and diet-controlled diabetes. He is also slightly overweight. Mr. M. has been coming regularly for checkups for a couple of years, and now his wife wants him involved in an exercise program to lose weight and control his blood pressure. During his checkup visit, Mr. M. asks questions about exercise for the elderly. He has never followed any exercise program. "I drive everywhere," he states.

Material in this chapter is based on the following chapters in Cassel CK, Leipzig RM, Cohen HJ, Larson EB, Meier DE, eds. Geriatric Medicine: An Evidence-Based Approach, 4th ed. New York: Springer, 2003: Brummel-Smith K. Rehabilitation, pp. 259–277. Larson EB, Bruce RA. Exercise, pp. 1023–1029. Selections edited by Sandra E. Sanchez-Reilly.

General Considerations

The health benefits of exercise, particularly in a sedentary society, have gained an increasingly compelling evidence base in the past decade. For earlier generations of seniors, exercise was a regular feature of everyday life. Beginning sometime after the Industrial Revolution and culminating in today's most advanced societies, there is a seemingly inevitable trend of everyday life requiring progressively less energy expenditure through exercise.

Aging and Exercise

The health benefits of exercise may be even greater for older persons than for younger persons. Younger adults have considerably more physiologic reserve—both muscular strength and cardiovascular capacity. Older individuals, in contrast, experience a progressive decline in many physiologic functions, including muscular strength and cardiovascular capacity (1,2). Habitual exercise, by improving strength and maximum aerobic capacity (VO_2 max) as a result of conditioning effects, can slow development of disability and thereby prolong active life expectancy (3,4).

In addition to habitual exercise for conditioning, there is increasing evidence that resistance exercise to improve muscle strength, along with more tailored exercise therapies, including those designed to improve balance and rehabilitate persons with various chronic disease and acute ailments, may be of particular value for older patients (5–7). Thus, exercise should be considered an important part of general care of healthy aging persons as well as persons with age-related illnesses (8). For further details on the changes with aging that relate to exercise, see Chapter 69: Exercise. In: Cassel CK, et al., eds; Geriatric Medicine, 4th ed., page 1023.

Case A (Part 2)

Mr. M. is highly motivated, but slightly scared about starting an exercise program. "I can fall; I may have a sudden heart attack," he says. Mr. M.'s physician reassures him, explaining to the patient the process to follow: It should be a program designed to increase conditioning, to improve muscle strength, with minimal risk of injury, and, most importantly, it should be fun!

Exercise Programs for Older Persons

It is tempting (and probably justified) to simply prescribe exercise as a general tonic for all older persons. However, there are special benefits for older persons with chronic disease and disabilities for whom more focused prescriptions should be provided. Current evidence supports exercise programs for persons with ischemic heart disease, including those with congestive heart failure, osteoporosis, osteoarthritis, spinal stenosis, degenerative central nervous system diseases like Parkinson's disease, diabetes mellitus, hypertension, peripheral vascular disease, and possibly psychiatric illnesses, like depression and anxiety disorders (9–14).

Hazards of Exercise

The most important concern with regard to the overall health benefits of exercise in older persons is the risk of exercise (15). Except for the risks, exercise is essentially a low-cost intervention and may require relatively little in the way of health care resources. Thus, the key element to the question of efficacy in older persons is risk and injuries.

The hazards of exercise are related to extremes of intensity and duration. When exercise is excessively intense and/or prolonged, extreme fatigue, exhaustion, or delayed recovery is experienced. In addition, more prolonged or intense exercise is associated with increased risk of injury (16). Injuries and sudden death are the most important complication for elderly persons.

The risk of sudden death and nonfatal myocardial infarction is quite small, but detectable, during unsupervised activity (17). Risk factors for sudden death among those participating in exercise programs include attaining a heart rate in excess of 85% of that individual's maximum; marked ST depression with exercise despite the absence of chest pain; poor adherence to limiting heart rate; and attainment of above average VO_2 max for gender and age due to peripheral mechanisms. Overall, however, the risk of primary cardiac arrest in more active individuals is less. The incidence of primary cardiac arrest attributable to lack of exercise was greatest in older, hypertensive, or obese males (18). Bouts of heavy exertion in sedentary people appear to pose a threat.

Thus, any general exercise program should be moderate in intensity and duration and should minimize risk of injury, cardiac arrest, and nonfatal myocardial infarction, as well as excessive fatigue. It may also be important to maintain adequate hydration to counteract fluid losses of sweating.

Goals of an Exercise Program

Four goals should be a part of an exercise program established for older individuals. First, the program should increase conditioning, especially endurance. Second, the intervention should improve muscle strength, especially lower extremity strength, given the importance of walking to independent functioning. Both of these goals are likely to improve a person's ability to perform activities of daily living, decrease fatigue associated with the day's activity, improve a sense of well-being, and perhaps forestall such adverse events as falls by improving muscle strength. Third, the program should minimize risk of injury due to exercise. Fourth, the program should promote enjoyment without causing excessive fatigue.

The components of the exercise program include two essentials: The first is dynamic aerobic exercise in the form of walking, swimming, cycling, jogging, and other similar activities. The second is lower extremity strengthening. Also desirable are a period to warm up and cool down and muscle and tendon stretching.

The exercise program should be tailored, especially so for older individuals. The program should take account of an individual's physical capacities and coexistent disabilities as well as mitigating social, psychological, and economic factors. Among all forms of exercise available to the elderly, brisk walking is one of the most ideal, and it has been recommended by a number of groups (19–21).

Normal Response to Exercise and Warning Signs

Physicians and other health professionals should be prepared to give appropriate guidelines for exercise. In particular, habitually sedentary persons may need to be advised of the normal responses to exercise, which include increased heart rate and breathing; mild perspiration; an increased awareness of one's heartbeat; and, at least initially, mild muscle aches. Such responses are normal and do not indicate that a person should stop exercising. The warning signs of excessive exercise include severe dyspnea, wheezing, and coughing; any form of chest discomfort; excessive perspiration; syncope or near syncope; prolonged fatigue and exhaustion lasting at least half an hour after exercise; and local muscle or joint discomfort. Heart rate guidelines are most appropriate for persons with coexistent cardiac disease. An exercise tolerance test facilitates calculating the desired heart rate based on the observed or extrapolated maximal heart rate. The typical target heart rate for achieving a conditioning effect is 70% to 80% of maximal heart rate. There also are tables listing average exercise heart rates for various age groups; however, such tables may be less useful given the wide variation in baseline and maximal aerobic capacity seen in the elderly.

Pacing

It is perhaps more useful to teach individual guidelines for pacing. One guideline is the so-called *talk test*, in which persons know they are not exercising excessively when they can carry on a normal conversation while exercising. For many elderly persons, a reliable heart rate guide is to aim for an exercise heart rate 15 to 20 beats per minute over their resting heart rate. Most persons who have not exercised excessively will also find that their pulse returns to resting levels or nearly so within 20 minutes after stopping exercise. Perhaps the most important pacing guide is to emphasize starting a program slowly and increasing activity by small increments.

Many older persons abandon exercise programs because they expect too much too fast, become discouraged, and thereby give up their programs before benefits are achieved.

Duration

The duration to be prescribed is driven by the amount of time required to produce the conditioning effect. In general, a minimum of 20 to 30 minutes of aerobic exercise three times per week at 70% to 80% of maximum heart rate is required to achieve a conditioning effect, which will begin approximately 2 weeks after commencing the exercise program. Moderate exercise (like brisk walking) is more likely to produce a conditioning effect at levels of 30 to 40 minutes 5 days per week, which is the level recommended by the U.S. Prevention Services Task Force.

Compliance

Lack of compliance, along with insufficient physician counseling, is the major barrier to successful exercise programs in the elderly (22). This is a common issue for many health promotion activities. A related issue is the relative lack of social and community resources for habitual activity. Much of the advancing technology consists of labor-saving devices. Especially in large, northern cities, there may be few opportunities and almost no facilities for older persons to get habitual exercise.

Rehabilitation

Case B (Part 1)

Mrs. F. is an 83-year-old woman who has poorly controlled diabetes and hypertension. She has been somewhat noncompliant with her medications. She is currently in the hospital after developing right-sided weakness and expressive aphasia. She was diagnosed with a stroke and treated accordingly. She has slightly regained motor function and speech, and she is medically stable. However, she is not yet ready to go back home. Mrs. F. is saddened about her medical condition, but she wants to do her best so she can be who she was before: a very independent woman.

General Considerations

Rehabilitation is a process of care directed at restoring or maintaining a person's ability to live independently. Interventions are directed at helping the patient to recover from and adapt to the loss of physical, psychological, or social skills that occurred as a result of illness or trauma.

Disability is a common problem among older Americans (Table 10.1). Kunkel and Applebaum (23) estimate that by the year 2020, between 9.7 and 13.6 million older people will have moderate to severe disability—an 85% to 167% increase over current levels. Clinical geriatrics emphasizes the functional approach in the care of the patient. By enhancing the person's functional abilities, the impact of a disability can be lessened. Rehabilitation is a basic foundation of geriatric care. All health care providers should promote a rehabilitation orientation when caring for older persons (24).

Demographics of Disability

A large percentage of persons with a disability are elderly. Conditions for which rehabilitation interventions are beneficial disproportionately affect the elderly population. Arthritis is the most common condition affecting older persons and the most common cause of disability (25). The incidence of stroke peaks in the seventh and eighth decades (26). The average 80-year-old white woman has a 1% to 2% risk of hip fracture per year (27). Most amputations are performed in the geriatric age group (28). Even without such catastrophic diagnoses, the prevalence of limited activities due to chronic conditions is very high, particularly in those over age 75.

Components of Rehabilitation

Rehabilitation comprises a number of components of care. These are summarized in Table 10.2. Each of these components requires special attention in geriatric patients. The foundation of rehabilitation is the restoration of lost functional abilities. By using directed exercises, with the assistance of physical, occupational, and often communication therapists, the patient can relearn how to carry out daily activities. Various adaptive equipment, such as rocker knives, sock-donners, and dressing sticks have been shown in randomized trials to enable a person to function independently and reduce health care costs (Table 10.3) (29).

Case B (Part 2)

Mrs. F. is transferred from the hospital to an acute rehabilitation facility. She is very motivated to do everything she can to improve her functional status. An interdisciplinary team, composed by her physician, the speech pathologist, occupational therapists, physical therapists, recreation therapists, and a rehabilitation nurse, evaluates Mrs. F. She improves remarkably.

TABLE 10.1. The World Health Organization's definitions of disability

Disease	"An intrinsic pathology or disorder . . . [which] may or not make [itself] evident clinically"
Impairment	"A loss or abnormality of psychological, physiological, or anatomical structure or function at organ level"
Disability	"A restriction or lack of ability to perform an activity in normal manner, a disturbance in the performance of daily tasks"
Handicap	"A disadvantage due to impairment or disability that limits or prevents fulfillment of a role that is normal (depends on age, sex, socio-cultural factors for the person)"

Source: Adapted from World Health Organization. International Classification of Impairments, Disabilities, and Handicaps. Geneva: WHO, 1980. Table reprinted as appears in Brummel-Smith K. Rehabilitation. In: Cassel CK, Leipzig RM, Cohen HJ, et al., eds. Geriatric Medicine, 4th ed. New York: Springer, 2003.

Rehabilitation Teams

Both multidisciplinary and interdisciplinary teams are used in rehabilitation (Table 10.4). Geriatric providers and physiatrists (specialists in physical medicine and rehabilitation) are often involved in interdisciplinary teams, whereas most primary care physicians function in a multidisciplinary setting. A *multidisciplinary* team works in a consulting relationship, each person seeing the patient individually and communicating with other team members by written notes or telephone calls. The decision to involve other team members usually is made by the physician. An *interdisciplinary* team functions in a setting where all team members can meet periodically to discuss the patient's problems and progress. Although each team member has a specific area of expertise, often there is considerable overlap in roles. With more complex cases, such as those seen in inpatient or long-term-care rehabilitation, an interdisciplinary team is usually required.

Ideally, team members should meet periodically to discuss their assessments, establish goals, provide updates on progress toward those goals, and estimate the duration of the program needed to meet the goals. A written summary of the meeting is placed in the patient's record. Some teams also provide a copy to the patient and the family.

TABLE 10.2. Components of rehabilitation

Stabilize the primary disorder
Prevent secondary complications
Treat functional deficits
Promote adaptation
Adaptation of the person to his/her disability
  Adaptation of the environment to the person
  Adaptation of the family to the person

Source: Brummel-Smith K. Rehabilitation. In: Cassel CK, Leipzig RM, Cohen HJ, et al., eds. Geriatric Medicine, 4th ed. New York: Springer, 2003.

TABLE 10.3. Tools for activities of daily living

Bathing: handheld shower hoses, bath seats, benches, long handled scrubbers, grab bars
Ambulation: canes, walkers, special shoes, wheelchairs
Toileting: raised toilet seats, arm attachments, grab bars
Transfers: side rails, sliding boards, trapeze bars
Eating: large handle utensils, rocker knives, plate guards, plate holders, hand braces
Dressing: button hooks, Velcro closures, sock-donners, clothes hooks

Source: Brummel-Smith K. Rehabilitation. In: Cassel CK, Leipzig RM, Cohen HJ, et al., eds. Geriatric Medicine, 4th ed. New York: Springer, 2003.

The role of the physician on the team is to provide medical expertise and often to serve as facilitator of the team process. Physicians must be extremely careful in this dual role as both the expert and the facilitator. Hierarchical relationships are common in medical settings, and the physician-expert may inhibit the functioning of other team members. If that happens, the flow of information necessary to make critical decisions may be impeded. Although the final responsibility of the clinical decision rests with physicians, they must always promote the reasoned deliberation of other team members. Group communication skills and knowledge of team dynamics, attributes often ignored in medical school training, are important for efficient and mutually satisfying teamwork.

Rehabilitation in Different Care Sites

Rehabilitation interventions can be provided in a variety of continuing care sites (Table 10.5). Medicare covers most of these services, but Medicaid's

TABLE 10.4. Roles of selected team members

Physiatrist: provides consultation regarding complex functional limitations and interventions to improve function; conducts diagnostic tests such as nerve conduction studies and may perform invasive interventions such as nerve blocks
Physical therapist: deals with problems in mobility and transfers, gait training, use of braces for mobility; involved in training in the use of canes, walkers, and wheelchairs
Occupational therapist: works with patient to improve skills in activities of daily living (ADL), uses a variety of interventions and teaches the patient how to use assistive devices for ADL; may also produce or train in the use of splints
Recreation therapist: helps the patient to recover or learn new skills in vocational activities
Speech and language pathologist: helps the patient to improve communication skills; trains patient to use alternative forms of communication if needed; may be involved in swallowing programs
Orthotist: fashions braces and splints
Rehabilitation nurse: in addition to providing nursing care, assists the patient in utilizing new techniques learned from the above-mentioned therapists; involved in family training

Source: Brummel-Smith K. Rehabilitation. In: Cassel CK, Leipzig RM, Cohen HJ, et al., eds. Geriatric Medicine, 4th ed. New York: Springer, 2003.

TABLE 10.5. Sites for rehabilitation

Home: requires a committed in-home caregiver, reasonably accessible (or modifiable) environment, and access to home health services

Outpatient facility: requires a dependable means of transportation, enough medical stability to tolerate outings into the community, reasonable cognition to retain between visits newly learned information

Nursing home: best if a rehabilitation-oriented facility, needs dependable access to therapists, burden of documentation by physicians and therapy staff is high

Acute hospital: limited time available for providing rehabilitation; even small amounts of therapy may be beneficial; attention should be paid to limiting functional decline

Rehabilitation hospital: intensive services (minimum 3 hours per day) may limit ability of frail elders to participate; evidence that greatest gains in stroke rehabilitation happen in this setting

Source: Brummel-Smith K. Rehabilitation. In: Cassel CK, Leipzig RM, Cohen HJ, et al., eds. Geriatric Medicine, 4th ed. New York: Springer, 2003.

reimbursement policies vary from state to state (see Chapter 5: Medicare and Medicaid, page 73). Medicare and most third-party reimbursement require that there be documentation that the patient is progressing toward the goals and that therapy must not be used for maintenance of function only. Algorithms have been developed for determining the proper site of rehabilitation for older persons with functional decline, and for stroke (see Chapter 15: Transient Ischemic Attacks and Stroke, page 267) (30).

Assessment for Rehabilitation Potential

The first step in the assessment for rehabilitation potential is awareness that rehabilitation interventions may be of benefit. Once that idea is entertained, a number of features must be considered. Factors associated with a better prognosis include recent health changes, less severe deficits, an assertive personality, a supportive family system, and adequate financial resources. A poorer prognosis exists for patients with low motivation, more severe health problems (especially if associated with cognitive impairments), and inadequate financial resources or support systems. However, because of the great variability seen in older persons, no single factor should automatically exclude a person from a trial of rehabilitation interventions.

When there is doubt, the patient should undergo a comprehensive assessment before a final determination is made. The assessment should identify what demands the patient will encounter in the expected living environment and whether he or she has the ability to meet those demands. A complete assessment includes evaluation of the patient's physical impairments, cognitive and psychological functioning, the social environment, and economic resources. The patient's prior levels of functioning and present capabilities should both be determined.

Two scales have been widely used to measure progress in rehabilitation. The oldest is the Barthel Index. Using this 100-point scale, some investigators have shown that discharge to home is unlikely with scores below 29 and very likely with scores above 60. The most widely used scale in rehabilitation currently is the Functional Independence Measure (FIM) (31). For further details on the Barthel Index and the FIM, see Chapter 23: Rehabilitation. In: Cassel CK, et al., eds; Geriatric Medicine, 4th ed., page 264.

There are specific approaches to rehabilitation of older persons with various common conditions. For further details, see Chapter 15: Transient Ischemic Attacks and Stroke, page 279; Chapter 16: Parkinson's Disease and Related Disorders, page 298; and Chapter 18: Osteoarthritis, page 322.

General Principles

- There is now growing evidence that exercise programs offer measurable health benefits for older persons, ranging from increased life expectancy to mitigation of adverse sequelae of aging and of many chronic diseases.
- Active elderly adults may have improved ability to withstand the stress of illness, more rapid recovery from illness or injury, and greater likelihood to have the ability to perform ADLs during the course of an acute illness or during exacerbations of chronic illnesses.
- Four goals of an exercise program for older individuals: increase conditioning, improve muscle strength, minimize risk of injury due to exercise, and promote enjoyment without causing excessive fatigue.
- The two essential components of the exercise program: *dynamic aerobic* exercise (walking, swimming, cycling, jogging) and *lower extremity strengthening*. Also desirable are a period to warm up and cool down and muscle and tendon stretching.
- *Rehabilitation* is a process of care directed at restoring or maintaining a person's ability to live independently and should be considered for all geriatric patients with functional losses.
- Factors associated with a better prognosis include recent health changes, less severe deficits, an assertive personality, a supportive family system, and adequate economic resources.
- An *interdisciplinary team approach* to rehabilitation is required due to the complex nature of the various interventions. Patients and their families must be involved in decisions regarding rehabilitation treatment.

Suggested Readings

Brummel-Smith K. Rehabilitation. In: Cassel CK, Leipzig RM, Cohen HJ, et al., eds. Geriatric Medicine, 4th ed. New York: Springer, 2003:259–277.

Larson EB, Bruce RA. Exercise. In: Cassel CK, Leipzig RM, Cohen HJ, et al., eds. Geriatric Medicine, 4th ed. New York: Springer, 2003:1023–1030.

Mulrow CD, Gerety MD, Kanton D, et al. A randomized trial of physical rehabilitation for very frail nursing home residents. JAMA 1994;271:519–524. *This article addresses the different efforts made to improve functional status of fragile older adults.*

Tinetti ME, Baker DI, McAvay MS, et al. A multifactorial intervention to reduce the risk of falling among elderly people living in the community. N Engl J Med 1994;331:821–827. *An excellent review on how to approach the elderly patient from an interdisciplinary point of view.*

Wee CC, McCarthy EP, Davis RB, Phillips RS. Physician counseling about exercise. JAMA 1999;282:1583–1588. *This article summarizes the recommendations given to all patients, particularly older adults to start and maintain an exercise program that is adequate to their needs.*

References

1. Astrand PO. Physical performance as a function of age. JAMA 1968;205: 729–733.
2. Larson EB, Bruce RA. Exercise and aging. Ann Intern Med 1986;105: 793–785.
3. Fries JF, Singh G, Morfeld D, Hubert HB, Lane WE, Brown BW. Running and the development of disability with age. Ann Intern Med 1994;121: 502–509.
4. Katz S, Branch LG, Branson MH, Papsidero JA, Beck JC, Greer DS. Active life expectancy. N Engl J Med 1983;309:1218–1224.
5. Fiatarone MA, Marks EC, Ryan ND, et al. High intensity strength training in nonagenarians. JAMA 1990;263:3029–3034.
6. Buchner DM, Cross ME, de Lateur BJ, et al. The effect of strength and endurance training on gait, balance, fall risk and health services use in community-living older adults. J Gerontol Med Sci 1997;52A:M218–224.
7. Wolff J, van Croonenborg JJ, Kemper HC, Kostense PJ, Twisk JW. The effect of exercise training on bone mass: A meta-analysis of published clinical trials in pre- and postmenopausal women. Osteoporos Int 1999;9:1–12.
8. Girolami B, Bernardi E, Prinz MH, et al. Treatment of intermittent claudication with physical training, snacking cessation, pentoxifylline, or nafronyl: a meta-analysis. Arch Intern Med 1999;159:337–345.
9. Hambrecht R, Wolf A, Grelen S, et al. Effect of exercise on coronary endothelial function in patients with coronary artery disease. N Engl J Med 2000;342:454–460.
10. Kasch FW, Boyer JL, Schmidt DK, et al. Aging of the cardiovascular system during 33 years of aerobic exercise. Aging 1999;28:531–536.
11. Paluska SA, Schwenk TL. Physical activity and mental health: current concepts. Sports Med 2000;29:167–180.

12. Singh NA, Clements KM, Fiatarone MA. A randomized trial of progressive resistance training in depressed elders. J Gerontol [A] Biol Sci Med 1997;52: 27–35.
13. Wei M, Gibbons LW, Kampert JB, Nichamon MZ, Blair SW. Low cardiorespiratory fitness and physical inactivity as predictors of mortality in men with Type 2 diabetes. Ann Intern Med 2000;132:605–611.
14. Walker RD, Nawaz S, Wilkinson CH, Saxton JM, Pockley AG, Wood RF. Influence of upper and lower-limb exercise program on cardiovascular function and walking distances in patients with intermittent claudication. J Vasc Surg 2000;31:662–669.
15. Koplan JP, Siscovick DS, Goldbaum GM. Risks of exercise: Public health view of injuries and hazards. Public Health Reports 1985;100:189–194.
16. Koplan JP, Powell KE, Sikes RK, Shirley RW, Campbell OC. An epidemiologic study of the benefits and risks of running. JAMA 1982;248: 3118–3121.
17. Siscovick DS, Weiss NS, Fletcher RH, et al. The incidence of primary cardiac arrest during vigorous exercise. N Engl J Med 1984;311:874–877.
18. Siscovick DS, Weiss NS, Fletcher RH, Schoenbach VJ, Wagner EH. Habitual vigorous exercise and primary cardiac arrest: effect of other risk factors on the relationship. J Chron Dis 1984;37:625–631.
19. American Association of Retired Persons. Pep Up Your Life—A Fitness Book for Midlife and Older Person. Washington, DC: AARP (1909 K Street), 1991.
20. U.S. Department of Health and Human Services, Public Health Services, National Institutes of Health. Exercise and Your Heart. Bethesda, MD: DHHS, 1981.
21. Mielchen SD, Larson EB, Wagner E, et al. Getting Started: A Guide to Physical Activity for Seniors. Seattle: Center for Health Promotion, Group Health Cooperative, 1987.
22. Wee CC, McCarthy EP, Davis RB, Phillips RS. Physician counseling about exercise. JAMA 1999;282:1583–1588.
23. Kunkel SR, Applebaum RA. Estimating the prevalence of long-term disability for an aging society. J Gerontol 1992;47:S253–260.
24. Frieden RA. Geriatrics and rehabilitation medicine: common interests, common goals. Mt Sinai J Med 1999;66:145–151.
25. Boult C, Kane RL, Louis TA, et al. Chronic conditions that lead to functional limitation in the elderly. J Gerontol 1994;49:M28–36.
26. Lorish TR. Stroke rehabilitation. Clin Geriatr Med 1993;4:705–716.
27. Ackerman RJ. Medical consultation for the elderly patient with hip fracture. J Am Board Fam Pract 1998;11:366–377.
28. Esquenazi A, Vachranukunkeit T, Torres M, et al. Characteristics of a current lower extremity amputee population: review of 918 cases. Arch Phys Med Rehabil 1984;65:623.
29. Mann WC, Ottenbacher KJ, Fraas L, Tomita M, Granger CV. Effectiveness of assistive technology and environmental interventions in maintaining independence and reducing home care costs for the frail elderly. A randomized controlled trial. Arch Fam Med 1999;8:210–217.
30. Gresham GE, Duncan PW, Stason WB, et al. Post-Stroke Rehabilitation: Assessment, Referral, and Patient Management. Clinical Practice Guideline: Quick Reference Guide for Clinicians, No. 16. AHCPR publication No.

95-0663. Rockville, MD: U.S. Department of Health and Human Services, Public Health Service, Agency for Health Care Policy and Research, May 1995.

31. Mahoney F, Barthel D. Functional evaluation: Barthel Index. Maryland State Med J 1965;14:61–65.

32. World Health Organization. International Classification of Impairments, Disabilities, and Handicaps. Geneva: WHO, 1980.

11
Nutrition

Sandra E. Sanchez-Reilly

Learning Objectives

Upon completion of the chapter, the student will be able to:

1. Assess the nutritional status and needs of an elderly patient.
2. Identify nutritional deficiencies and their consequences in older adults.
3. Outline differences between younger and older adults from a nutritional point of view.

Case (Part 1)

Mrs. Smith is a 79-year-old woman who comes to her physician for her regular checkup. Her daughter, who comes with her, is very concerned about Mrs. Smith's dietary intake. "She is not eating what she used to," she says. Mrs. Smith has a past medical history of stable angina, hypertension, and osteoarthritis that limits her daily activities due to pain.

General Considerations

Management of nutritional problems in the elderly constitutes an important challenge. Few health care professionals pay much attention to the nutritional status of their patients, which may have adverse effects on morbidity, mortality, and quality of life. Although overnutrition is a common

---

Material in this chapter is based on the following chapter in Cassel CK, Leipzig RM, Cohen HJ, Larson EB, Meier DE, eds. Geriatric Medicine: An Evidence-Based Approach, 4th ed. New York: Springer, 2003: Lipschitz DA. Nutrition, pp. 1009–1021. Selections edited by Sandra E. Sanchez-Reilly.

problem in younger persons, aging is associated with increases in the incidence of weight loss, being underweight, and having protein-energy malnutrition. Identifying and appropriately treating the underlying cause is a critical component of nutritional rehabilitation (1).

Energy Requirements

Aging results in a significant decrease in energy needs (2) (Table 11.1). The major mechanism is a decrease in resting energy expenditure as a consequence of declines in muscle mass. Diminished energy needs also result from age-related declines in physical activity. Decreased activity is the result primarily of coexisting diseases, such as bone and joint disorders, loss of postural stability, and chronic diseases that may limit activity, such as angina pectoris and intermittent claudication.

Total caloric (food) intake is determined primarily by energy needs. Thus, a 30% reduction in energy need will be accompanied by a 30% reduction of food intake. Compared with younger subjects, individuals over the age of 70 consume a third fewer calories. The importance of this effect relates to the fact that the average intake of all nutrients is reduced in parallel, yet the requirements for virtually every other nutrient, with the exception of carbohydrates, do not decline significantly with age. As a consequence, epidemiologic studies of dietary intakes of healthy elderly individuals reveal deficient intakes. In the presence of disease with increased nutritional requirements or because of declining intake caused by anorexia, severe nutritional deficiencies are very common in hospitalized or institutionalized elderly individuals with acute or chronic diseases.

Case (Part 2)

During Mrs. Smith's doctor's visit, her physician decides to ask the patient and her daughter about specific dietary intake products. Mrs. Smith lives alone, and usually prepares her meals. Many of her dietary intakes come from canned containers that she buys at the supermarket, "easy to make because of my arthritis.".

TABLE 11.1 Energy and protein requirements: changes in the elderly

Energy requirements	Protein requirements
Decrease in energy needs (30%)	Increased protein requirements
Decrease in muscle mass	Requirements even more increased in acute disease
Decrease in physical activity	Very important in wound healing
Coexisting diseases	No significant reductions on albumin

Source: Adapted from Lipschitz DA. Nutrition. In: Cassel CK, Leipzig RM, Cohen HJ, et al., eds. Geriatric Medicine, 4th ed. New York: Springer, 2003:1009–1021.

Protein Requirements

On first principles it seems likely that, because of declines in muscle mass, aging should result in decreased protein needs (Table 11.1). Although aging results in significant declines in muscle mass, protein synthetic and degradation rates are only minimally compromised. Visceral protein stores and turnover are generally unchanged with aging so that no significant reductions are noted in serum albumin, retinol binding protein, or prealbumin.

At the current time a protein intake of 1 g/kg body weight is recommended for healthy elderly. Most importantly, the presence of acute or chronic diseases further increases protein requirements. In this circumstance, protein intake in the older patient is frequently grossly inadequate. This is particularly important in wound healing and in pressure ulcer, where inadequate protein intake adversely affects outcome.

Case (Part 3)

Mrs. Smith thinks her diet is well balanced, although she admits to skipping some meals. She is concerned about her angina, and she has heard from friends that she should be very careful with her diet because "cholesterol and fat can cause heart attacks and strokes. She is also concerned because she does not look the same as she did before. She says she looks bigger."

Fat Requirements

Aging does not alter any of the specific requirements for any of the essential lipids (4). Advancing age is generally associated with an increase in the proportion of body weight as fat, which is the result of decreases in muscle mass accompanied by an increase in fat mass. Body fat stores increase until the seventh decade, after which reductions in total weight and fat stores are frequently noted. Although obesity is not as common a problem in the elderly as it is in younger individuals, approximately 20% of subjects over the age of 65 are significantly overweight. There is evidence that the risks of atherosclerotic heart disease and stroke in the elderly can be reduced by consuming a diet low in saturated fats and cholesterol.

These facts make dietary recommendations in the elderly difficult. For older individuals, a palatable acceptable diet is very important.

Recommending drastic changes in dietary intake, therefore, should be undertaken with caution and with careful clinical judgment. For individuals in their late sixties and early seventies who are very healthy and ambulatory but significantly overweight, hypercholesterolemic, and perhaps hypertensive, an effort to reduce calories, fat, and sodium intake is warranted. In many circumstances, drastic reductions in diet may not be beneficial; this particularly applies to institutionalized elderly, for whom medically prescribed diets are frequently not palatable, are not adequately consumed, and may result in weight loss. It must be noted that the value of serum or high-density lipoprotein (HDL) cholesterol in the prediction of coronary artery disease is less for the elderly than it is for younger patients (3). For this reason, the efficacy of aggressive dietary or pharmacologic attempts to lower cholesterol in subjects over the age of 70 is far from clear.

Water Requirements

In the elderly, fluid balance is extremely important because of the propensity of the elderly to develop dehydration and the ease at which overhydration can occur in elderly individuals with compromised renal function or other disorders associated with fluid retention. As a general rule, water intake should be 1 mL/kcal or 30 mL/kg body weight. Dehydration is extremely prevalent in hospitalized elderly and is the single most common cause of an acute confusional state in the elderly; this is primarily related to the well-described age-related decline in thirst drive. Studies have demonstrated a decreased ability of the elderly to respond to fluid deprivation, which becomes a particularly serious problem in frail elderly who develop a minor pathologic insult, such as a respiratory or urinary tract infection, resulting in fever, increased metabolism, and fluid loss. If fluid intake does not readily replace fluid lost, dehydration rapidly develops.

Mineral Requirements

Numerous studies indicate that, for a wide variety of minerals and vitamins, intake is significantly lower than the recommended daily allowance (RDA) for a large proportion of ambulatory elderly (Table 11.2) (4).

Vitamin Requirements

Studies have shown that dietary intake of many vitamins is inadequate in the elderly, including an intake of 50% or less for folic acid, thiamine, vitamin D, and vitamin E. In other studies intakes were shown to be less

TABLE 11.2. Mineral intake considerations in the elderly

	Calcium	Zinc	Iron	Selenium	Copper	Chromium
ROLE	Major role in bone metabolism Calcium intake in the elderly should be 1–1.5 g/day	Major role in wound healing May help to improve immune function and slows the rate of development of macular degeneration in the elderly	Aging is associated with a gradual increase in iron stores in both men and women (different from younger adults) Iron deficiency is rare in the elderly, and, if present, it is caused by a pathologic blood loss	May minimize free radical accumulation There is suggestive evidence that selenium deficiency may contribute to age-related declines in cellular function	Aging is associated with increase in serum copper concentrations; the significance of this is unknown	Plays an important role in carbohydrate metabolism Tissue chromium levels decline with age
DEFICIENCY	Lifelong inadequate intakes of calcium contribute to the high prevalence of osteoporosis in the elderly	Modest deficiency contributes to anorexia in debilitated patients	There is a correlation between iron stores and risks of neoplasia and coronary artery disease, so, unless needed, supplemented iron may not be desirable in older adults	Its deficiency is frequent in the elderly Selenium deficiency syndromes are rare; when they occur they may produce cardiomyopathy, nail abnormalities and myopathies; also decline in immune function	Copper deficiency is rare and only reported in parenteral nutrition	It may contribute to glucose intolerance in the elderly (although replacement is still controversial)

Source: Adapted from Lipschitz DA. Nutrition. In: Cassel CK, Leipzig RM, Cohen HJ, et al., eds. Geriatric Medicine, 4th ed. New York: Springer, 2003:1009–1021.

than 66% of the RDA for most vitamins. It must be emphasized that deficiencies identified on the basis of inadequate intake are invariably significantly higher than the prevalence of biochemical deficiency of most vitamins (Tables 11.3 and 11.4).

TABLE 11.3. Water-soluble vitamin intake considerations in the elderly

Water-soluble vitamins	Vitamin C	Studies have indicated inadequate dietary vitamin C in the elderly. In debilitated elderly patients, there is some evidence that vitamin C supplementation improves the rate of wound and pressure ulcer healing (5). Other studies have shown a high prevalence of vitamin C supplementation in the elderly. There is little evidence that megadoses of vitamin C have any relevant side effects, although falsely negative occult bloods have been reported, as have inaccuracies in serum and urine glucose determinations.
	Thiamine	Clinically relevant deficiencies of the B vitamins are very rare in the elderly. Thiamine deficiency, however, is common in elderly alcoholics and can be an important contributing factor in the development of disordered cognition, neuropathies, and perhaps cardiomyopathies. Relevant deficiencies of this vitamin are relatively common in institutionalized elderly.
	Folic acid	Like thiamine, folate deficiency in the elderly is predominantly found in alcoholics. It is also common in elderly subjects who are taking drugs that interfere with folate metabolism (trimethoprim, methotrexate, and phenytoin) or in disorders associated with increased folate needs (hemolytic anemia and ineffective erythropoiesis). Folate deficiency may result in cognitive loss or significant depression and should always be evaluated in the workup of elderly subjects with a memory disorder.
	Vitamin B_{12}	Low serum vitamin B_{12} concentrations have been shown to occur in as many as 10% of otherwise healthy elderly subjects. Many comprehensive workups indicate early pernicious anemia, the commonest cause of vitamin B_{12} deficiency, whereas in others no obvious cause can be identified. B_{12} deficiency classically causes a severe megaloblastic anemia. Not uncommonly, the nonhematologic manifestations of B_{12} deficiency can occur in the absence of anemia; these include gait disorders, sensory and motor neurologic deficits, and highly significant memory loss. This vitamin should be measured routinely in the workup of any elderly patient with disordered cognition or depression, and replacement therapy should be given to any patients in whom low serum levels are found. The lower limit of normal varies in different laboratories, but a value below 150 pg/mL is highly suspect and should always result in the commencement of replacement therapy.

Source: Adapted from Lipschitz DA. Nutrition. In: Cassel CK, Leipzig RM, Cohen HJ, et al., eds. Geriatric Medicine, 4th ed. New York: Springer, 2003:1009–1021.

TABLE 11.4. Fat-soluble vitamin intake considerations in the elderly

Fat-soluble vitamins	Vitamin A	Vitamin A is one of the only nutrients in which requirements decrease with advancing age. Studies have shown that aging is associated with an increase in absorption of vitamin A from the gastrointestinal tract, accompanied by a reduction of hepatic uptake. These effects make the elderly susceptible to toxicity if excessive amounts of the vitamin are consumed as a supplement. Side effects of daily intakes in excess of 50,000 IU include headaches, lassitude, reduction in white cell counts, impaired hepatic function, and bone pain. The vitamin plays an important role in visual acuity. However, there is no evidence that vitamin A supplements improve age-related declines in eyesight. Vitamin A and its precursor beta-carotene have been suggested as exerting a protective effect against an array of neoplasms. Recent large-scale controlled trials, however, have failed to definitively prove a beneficial effect of beta-carotene in the development of skin cancers.
	Vitamin D	Recent studies suggest that vitamin D deficiency may be a serious concern in the elderly. In addition to the vitamin's known role in bone metabolism, it also affects macrophage function in general and pulmonary macrophages in particular. Vitamin D deficiency increases susceptibility to the development of pulmonary tuberculosis by compromising macrophage function. This has been suggested as contributing to the high prevalence of tuberculosis in nursing home patients in whom deficiencies are common and aggravated by diminished exposure to sunlight. In any patient with severe osteoporosis, fracture, or bone pain, vitamin D—induced osteomalacia must be excluded.
	Vitamin E	Vitamin E (α-tocopherol) is abundant in the diet and deficiencies of the vitamin virtually never occur. It is involved in the function of the enzyme glutathione peroxidase, which is involved in free radical generation. The vitamin also affects the biophysical properties of the cell membrane, reducing the age-related increase in membrane microviscosity. It also influences immune function, and recent evidence indicates that administration of the vitamin enhances immune function in the elderly and may minimize infectious risk. Vitamin E has also been used for the treatment and prevention of Alzheimer's disease.
	Vitamin K	Vitamin K is essential for the production of a number of factors involved in both the intrinsic and extrinsic clotting cascade. There is evidence that vitamin K administration is beneficial in elderly people who have an unexplained prolongation of their prothrombin time. Although dietary intake is adequate, deficiencies can result from the administration of drugs (such as antibiotics) that interfere with the vitamin's absorption or interfere with bacterial flora.

Source: Adapted from Lipschitz DA. Nutrition. In: Cassel CK, Leipzig RM, Cohen HJ, et al., eds. Geriatric Medicine, 4th ed. New York: Springer, 2003:1009–1021.

Diagnostic Evaluation

A high index of suspicion for nutritional problems is very important in patients who have a primary diagnosis associated with malnutrition, such as chronic alcoholism; disorders of cognition; chronic myocardial, renal, or pulmonary insufficiency; malabsorption syndromes; and multiple medication use (5). In addition, particular attention should focus in the history on evidence of anorexia, early satiety, nausea, change in bowel habits, fatigue, apathy, or memory loss. Physical findings that may also provide clues to the presence of nutritional deficits include poor dentition, cheilosis, angular stomatitis, and glossitis, which is common in a number of vitamin deficiencies. Pressure ulcers or poorly healing wounds, edema, dehydration, and poor dental status are common physical findings in severely malnourished patients (6).

Clinically, a number of important questions must be addressed in the nutritional assessment. Increased risk of malnutrition can usually be identified from the history and physical examination. Commonly recognized risk factors are listed in Table 11.5.

Case (Part 4)

Mrs. Smith's physical exam reveals a 7-lb weight loss from her previous visit 1 year ago, although she states she did not notice any. She also looks pale, and slightly distracted. Her vital signs are stable. Her Mini–Mental State Examination shows a score of 26/30 (mild cognitive disorder), diminished from the last visit. The rest of her physical exam is unremarkable, except for decreased patellar reflexes and decreased sensation in the lower limbs.

Has the Patient Lost Weight?

Weight loss is perhaps the most important finding indicating the presence of malnutrition. Recent studies have clearly indicated that this finding in patients with serious disease is a very poor prognostic sign and is associated with increased morbidity and mortality (7). To be significant, weight loss must be involuntary, and must have exceeded 10% or more of body weight in 6 months, 7.5% or more in 3 months, or 5% or more in 1 month. In older persons, any weight loss that clearly cannot be ascribed to alterations in fluid balance should be taken seriously. Any significant weight loss that is involuntary indicates that nutritional intake is inadequate and that the patient's needs are not being met.

TABLE 11.5. Causes of weight loss in the elderly

Anorexia
Depression
Medications
   Digoxin
   Serotonin reuptake inhibitors
Diseases
   Cancer
   Chronic organ failure (cardiac, renal, pulmonary)
Chronic infections
   Tuberculosis
Polymyalgia rheumatica and other collagen vascular
diseases
Single-nutrient deficiencies that affect taste and appetite
   Vitamin A
   Zinc
Malabsorption
   Intestinal ischemia
   Celiac disease
Swallowing disorders
   Neurologic
   Esophageal candidiasis
   Web stricture
   Dental disease
Metabolic
   Thyroid disease
   Diabetes
   Liver disease
Social
   Isolation
   Poverty
   Caregiver fatigue
   Neglect
   Abuse
      Physical
      Alcohol
   Food preference not met
   Inappropriate food choices
Physical
   Inability to purchase or cook food
   Decreased activity
No cause identified

Source: Lipschitz DA. Nutrition. In: Cassel CK, Leipzig RM, Cohen HJ, et al., eds. Geriatric Medicine, 4th ed. New York: Springer, 2003.

Is the Patient Underweight?

To determine if the patient is underweight or has lost weight requires an evaluation of body composition (8). In this regard, virtually every anthropometric measure of body composition employs height as the reference point. In both men and women, height decreases by approximately 1 cm per decade after the age of 20. This is caused by vertebral bony loss, increased laxity of vertebral supportive ligaments, reductions in disk spaces, and alterations in posture. Historical estimations of height are also frequently inaccurate in the elderly, and its measurement is difficult in bedridden patients or in those with significant postural abnormalities. For this reason, it has been suggested that alternatives to height should be used in the development of standards for body composition for the elderly. Options suggested include arm length and knee-height measurements.

In general, a gradual increase in weight occurs with advancing age, peaking in the early forties in men and a decade later in women. After age 70, reductions in weight are not uncommon. Lean body mass decreases by approximately 6.0% per decade after the age of 25. By the age of 70, lean body mass has decreased an average of 5 kg for women and 12 kg for men. Thus, in the elderly, fat constitutes a far greater percentage of total weight than it does in younger patients.

Fat distribution also alters with aging. Truncal and intraabdominal fat content increase whereas limb fat diminishes. Skinfold measurements are often employed to estimate fat and muscle stores. In the elderly, subscapular and suprailiac skinfolds are the best predictors of fat stores in men, whereas the triceps skinfold and thigh measurements are of greater value in women. Evaluating ideal body weight for height can be employed to determine if a patient is underweight, defined as being 15% below the ideal weight for that individual patient.

A more accurate assessment is the determination of the body mass index (BMI), which is the ratio of weight to height squared. It is generally recommended that persons over the age of 65 have a BMI between 24 and 29. As a general rule, a BMI below 22 is a cause for concern and indicates that the patient is significantly underweight, whereas a value above 29 indicates obesity.

Case (Part 5)

Mrs. Smith is sent by her physician for blood testing. Among other tests, her albumin level is 3.1 mg/dL.

Does the Patient Have Protein-Energy Malnutrition?

This condition is best described as a metabolic response to stress that is associated with increased requirement for energy and protein. The metabolic response to a stress such as injury or infection is characterized by hormonal changes and the release of cytokines that lead to the development of anorexia, despite the presence of increased nutrient needs. In older persons, the negative sequelae of this response can develop quickly. *Protein-energy malnutrition* (PEM) is associated with marked depletion of visceral protein stores characterized by the presence of hypoalbuminemia. Inadequate supply of protein leads to liver dysfunction, which contributes to the low serum albumin. Decreased clearance of drugs and toxins also occurs, increasing the risk of toxicities and adverse drug reactions. Inadequate supply of protein primarily affects organ systems with the highest turnover of cells, which are the skin, immunohematopoietic system, and gastrointestinal tract. Thus, PEM is characterized by a dry skin and "flaky paint" dermatitis. Impaired immune responses lead to compromised host defenses, increasing the risk of life-threatening infections. Malabsorption also develops as a result of impaired jejunal and ileal mucosal cell proliferation, creating a vicious cycle of malnutrition causing malabsorption and worsening malnutrition. As a result of disease and deficiencies of taste-related nutrients, anorexia is usually present. The disorder is also referred to as hypoalbuminemia malnutrition and is usually diagnosed by the presence of a serum albumin level of less than 3.0 g/dL.

This disorder leads to the development of confusion, hypotension, and a vicious cycle in which the patient's overall condition can deteriorate very rapidly (9). If nutritional needs are not met within 2 to 3 days of the onset of the acute illness, the declines in immune, hepatic, and gastrointestinal function appear to contribute significantly to increased morbidity, mortality, and prolonged hospital stays.

Case (Part 6)

Mrs. Smith is also diagnosed with vitamin B_{12} deficiency. After a long discussion with her physician and her family, specific dietary recommendations are given, and B_{12} supplementation is started.

Does the Patient Have Isolated Nutrient Deficiencies?

These deficiencies are quite rare in older persons but should be considered in special circumstances. Zinc deficiency has been reported to be increased in patients with pressure ulcers and may contribute to decreased rates of healing. For this reason, zinc supplementation is frequently prescribed for patients with pressure ulcers. Vitamin D deficiency is relatively common in homebound and institutionalized older persons and may contribute to declines in host defense mechanisms in the elderly. Frank osteomalacia has also been reported. Folate deficiency is limited to patients with malabsorption and to older alcoholics. Vitamin B_{12} deficiency has been reported to be frequent in older persons. Its level should be measured in any patient being evaluated for memory loss and if levels are low, it warrants replacement.

Management Considerations

Weight Loss and Being Underweight

The initial approach to management should be a careful attempt to identify the cause of the weight loss and, if found, to aggressively attempt correction. Table 11.5 lists the common causes of weight loss in older persons, highlighting potentially correctable causes. Identifying a potentially treatable cause such as drug use (digoxin, fluoxetine), thyrotoxicosis, and depression can usually result in weight gain if the underlying condition is corrected with appropriate medical interventions. Other conditions that may well contribute to weight loss that are potentially improvable include social or economic isolation, difficulties with cooking or feeding as a consequence of physical disability, dental or swallowing problems, and not having palatable or preferred foods.

Older persons who have experienced weight loss are consuming inadequate calories to meet their needs. Thus nutritionally the aim must be to increase caloric intake. This can be achieved by assuring the use of palatable meals, often recommending diets high in both protein and fats. Patients who fail to respond to treatment of their underlying medical condition and fail to gain weight despite nutritional and physical rehabilitation carry a very poor prognosis.

Protein Energy Malnutrition

In the acutely ill patient, attention should first be directed at correcting the major medical abnormalities. Thus, management of infections, control of blood pressure, and the restoration of metabolic, electrolyte, and fluid homeostasis must assume priority. During this period, fluid and nutrient intake should be recorded so that an assessment of future needs can be made. Once the acute process has stabilized, daily calorie counts should be performed and the patients should be encouraged by the staff to voluntarily consume as much of their food as possible. The aim is to obtain a caloric intake of approximately 35 kcal/kg, based on an ideal rather than the actual body weight.

In clinical practice, only 10% of elderly subjects with PEM can consume sufficient food voluntarily to correct their nutritional deficiency. Thus, most subjects require a more aggressive form of nutritional intervention. As a general rule, more aggressive attempts to ensure adequate nutrient intake must commence within 48 hours of admission. For those patients requiring short-term support (fewer than 10 days), peripheral hyperalimentation is the method of choice. Using this approach it is possible, through a peripheral vein, to provide adequate calories and protein to meet the patient's needs using amino acid solutions, 10% dextrose, and intralipid.

Enteral Hyperalimentation

Nasogastric feeding should be avoided in any confused older patient because of the risk of aspiration and the need for restraints to prevent the patient from pulling out the uncomfortable and irritating tubes. For those who are not confused and who have a normal gastrointestinal tract, enteral hyperalimentation through a small-bore nasogastric polyethylene catheter should be considered. These tubes are nonirritating and do not interfere with patient mobility or the ability to swallow food. It is extremely important that after the tube is passed, placement in the stomach be confirmed before commencing nutritional feedings. For patients likely to require nutritional support for periods of 6 weeks or longer, a feeding gastrostomy or jejunostomy is recommended. For both nasogastric feeding gastrostomies, infusions should begin with an undiluted, commercially available polymeric dietary supplement at a continuous rate of 25 mL/h. The supplement should contain no more than 1 kcal/mL, as caloric-dense fluids are too viscous to pass through the tube with ease. The rate can gradually be increased so that after 48 hours the total daily protein and calorie requirements of the patient are met by this route.

One of the most commonly encountered side effects is excessive fluid retention. When nutritional support begins, weight gain is invariably noted within the first 2 to 3 days. This almost certainly reflects fluid retention, as the weight gain is associated with significant reductions in the serum albumin and hemoglobin levels. The average increase in weight during this time is 1.3 kg, whereas the level of the serum albumin falls from a mean of 2.8 g/dL to 2.3 g/dL at day 3. In elderly subjects with inadequate renal function, excessive retention of fluid can occasionally result in peripheral edema or even heart failure. When this occurs, diuretic therapy can correct the underlying problem, or the use of calorie-dense supplements should be considered. Hyponatremia and hypocalcemia occur frequently. In addition, hypophosphatemia and decreased magnesium levels can occur, resulting in worsening confusion and delirium. Hyperglycemia and glycosuria are occasionally noted, and frank diabetic coma can develop. An additional problem seen occasionally is severe diarrhea. The risk of diarrhea can be minimized if supplements are given by slow infusion. Bolus administration of dietary supplements through a nasogastric tube increases the risk of diarrhea and enhances the possibility of vomiting and aspiration pneumonia. Because a major goal of any geriatric rehabilitation is to improve functional independence and improve strength, strategies aimed at improving muscle mass are particularly important. Aggressive nutritional intervention is only a part of a complete strategy aimed at restoring, in the appropriate patient, functional independence.

General Principles

- Although overnutrition is a common problem in younger persons, aging is associated with increases in the incidence of weight loss, being underweight, and having protein-energy malnutrition. Identifying and appropriately treating the underlying cause is a critical component of nutritional rehabilitation.
- However, it is important to simultaneously ensure that the patient's energy and protein needs are met, which can be done by dietary manipulation and by the use of dietary supplements.
- The diagnostic evaluation of weight loss includes asking the following questions:
  - Has the patient lost weight?
  - Is the patient underweight?
  - Does the patient have protein energy malnutrition?
  - Does the patient have isolated nutrient deficiencies?

Suggested Readings

Chernoff R. Effects of age on nutrient requirements. Clin Geriatr Med 1995;11(4):641–651. *A summary of nutritional needs of the elderly and the most common nutritional deficiencies and their clinical manifestations.*

Gersovitz M, Motil K, Munro H, et al. Human protein requirements: assessment of the adequacy of the current recommended dietary allowance for dietary protein in elderly men and women. Am J Clin Nutr 1982;35:6–14. *Illustrates the specific nutritional requirements for the elderly.*

Lipschitz DA. Nutrition. In: Cassel CK, Leipzig RM, Cohen HJ, et al., eds. Geriatric Medicine, 4th ed. New York: Springer, 2003:1009–1022.

References

1. McCarter RJM. Role of caloric restriction in prolongation of life. Clin Geriatr Med 1995;11:553–565.
2. Shock NW, Gruelich RC, Andres R, et al., eds. Normal Human Aging: The Longitudinal Study of Aging. NIH publication No. 84–2450. Washington, DC: National Institutes of Health, 1984.
3. Gersovitz M, Motil K, Munro H, et al. Human protein requirements: assessment of the adequacy of the current recommended dietary allowance for dietary protein in elderly men and women. Am J Clin Nutr 1982;35:6–14.
4. Chernoff R. Effects of age on nutrient requirements. Clin Geriatr Med 1995;11(4):641–651.
5. Ham RJ. The signs and symptoms of poor nutritional status. Prim Care 1994;21:33–67.

6. Allman R. Pressure sores among the elderly. N Engl J Med 1989;320: 850–853.
7. Sullivan DH, Walls RC. Impact of nutritional status on morbidity in a population of geriatric rehabilitation patients. J Am Geriatr Soc 1994;42:471–477.
8. The Nutrition Screening Initiative. Incorporating Nutrition Screening and Interventions into Medical Practice: A Monograph for Physicians. Washington, DC: Nutrition Screening Initiative, 1994.
9. Silver AJ, Morley JE. Role of the opioid system in the hypodypsia associated with aging. J Am Geriatr Soc 1992;40:556–560.

12
The Older Surgical Patient

Hannah I. Lipman

Learning Objectives

Upon completion of the chapter, the student will be able to:

1. Identify risk factors for perioperative complications in elderly surgical patients and recommend strategies to decrease this risk.
2. Understand the considerations specific to elderly patients regarding the use of anesthetic agents.
3. Identify the indications for perioperative noninvasive and invasive monitoring.
4. Understand the impact of the presence of common comorbid conditions on the management of the elderly surgical patient.
5. Assess nutritional status in the elderly surgical patient and recommend strategies to improve nutritional reserve.
6. Understand the risk for postoperative delirium and identify strategies to reduce its severity.

Case (Part 1)

Mrs. Marlowe is a 90-year-old woman with recently diagnosed colon cancer who lives independently. She has a medical history of diabetes mellitus, hypertension, hyperlipidemia, hypothyroidism, and a remote history of myocardial infarction. She has decided to undergo colon resection. Her daughter tells you she believes her mother is too old to undergo the surgery and asks you to explain the risks.

What is Mrs. Marlowe's risk? What further information is needed to assess her risk?

Material in this chapter is based on the following chapters in Cassel CK, Leipzig RM, Cohen HJ, Larson EB, Meier DE, eds. Geriatric Medicine: An Evidence-Based Approach, 4th ed. New York: Springer, 2003: Pompei P. Preoperative Assessment and Perioperative Care, pp. 213–227. Silverstein JH. Anesthesia for the Geriatric Patient, pp. 229–238. Rosenthal RA. Surgical Approaches to the Geriatric Patient, pp. 239–257. Selections edited by Hannah I. Lipman.

General Considerations

The increasing number of older persons undergoing surgery is due both to our aging population and to important recent advances in surgical and anesthetic techniques. Currently, about one third of all operations in the United States are done on persons 65 years of age and older compared to about 20% in 1980 (1). Over the next three decades, the number of patients over age 65 who undergo noncardiac surgery is projected to increase from 7 million to 14 million (2).

The types of surgical procedures commonly performed on older persons reflect the prevalence of chronic diseases in this population: intraocular lens implants for cataracts, prostate gland resections for hyperplasia, colorectal procedures for cancer, orthopedic procedures for osteoarthritis and fractures, and arterial reconstruction for vascular disease. The introduction of neuroleptic anesthesia, sophisticated perioperative monitoring technology, and effective prophylaxis against deep venous thrombosis have contributed to lower surgical mortality for older adults (3). Endoscopic and other minimal access techniques have added to the ease and safety of operative therapy and have led to reduced mortality, increased ambulatory surgery, and shorter hospital stays (4,5).

Returning patients quickly to their usual environment and functional status reduces complications related to medications and immobilization associated with hospitalization. Current estimates of 30-day perioperative mortality for properly prepared surgical patients over age 65 are 5% to 10% (6–8).

It has been shown that mortality for many types of surgical procedures is associated with increasing comorbidity with age, rather than chronological age alone (9). The American Society of Anesthesiologist (ASA) Physical Status Classification is a reliable and accurate predictor of surgical mortality. It stratifies patients based on comorbid conditions and functional status into five classes (Table 12.1) (10). Curves for mortality versus ASA class in older patients are nearly superimposable on those of younger patients (11). Even in patients over age 80, ASA classification has been shown to accurately predict postoperative mortality (12).

TABLE 12.1. The American Society of Anesthesiologists (ASA) Physical Status Classification System (10)

Class I	A normal healthy patient for elective operation
Class II	A patient with mild systemic disease
Class III	A patient with severe systemic disease that limits activity but is not incapacitating
Class IV	A patient with incapacitating systemic disease that is a constant threat to life
Class V	A moribund patient not expected to survive 24 hours with or without operation

Source: Reprinted from American Society of Anesthesiologists. New classification of physical status. Anesthesiology 1963;24:111, with permission from Lippincott, Williams, & Wilkins.

Surgery, as a therapeutic alternative, has an essential role in the medical care of the geriatric patient. Certain types of cancer, coronary artery disease, and arthritis, common diseases that accompany aging, can be effectively treated and often cured by operation.

Assessing Individual Risk

With the increasing rate of operative therapy among older patients, there is an increasing demand by surgeons for medical consultation in the perioperative period. Though the request is often for preoperative clearance, both the unstated expectations of the requesting physician and the responsibilities of the consultant are much more specific. The purpose of a preoperative assessment is (1) to identify factors associated with increased risks of specific complications related to the anticipated procedure and (2) to recommend a management plan that would minimize these risks. The consultant must give careful attention to the extent and severity of comorbid conditions, the current and anticipated pharmacologic therapy, and the functional and psychological state of the patient. These patient-specific risk factors are only part of the required assessment; the type and technical difficulty of the procedure, the skill of the surgeon, and the anesthetic management all contribute to the risks of complications (3). The most common postoperative medical complications include respiratory problems, congestive heart failure, delirium, and thromboembolism (13).

Identification of Persons at Risk

Assessing an individual patient's risk for postoperative complications is an important aspect of preoperative evaluation. This process allows physicians to focus treatments on modifiable factors, anticipate specific problems, and provide patients and families with more precise, individual-specific, prognostic information.

The ASA classification has been introduced as one measure used to predict operative mortality. Other standard measures of functional status have also proven to be predictive of postoperative outcome. Such measures associated with *poorer* surgical outcome include activities of daily living (ADL) impairment (14), limited preoperative physical activity level (14), inability to increase O_2 delivery to three times the basal level (measured by cardiopulmonary O_2 consumption exercise testing) (15,16), lower Charlson comorbidity index score (17–19), and hypoalbuminemia (20).

Cardiac complications are among the most common and most serious postoperative problems. These included recent myocardial infarction, uncompensated congestive heart failure, electrocardiographic evidence of a rhythm other than sinus or premature atrial contractions, and more than five premature ventricular contractions per minute. The usefulness of the multifactorial index of cardiac risk that was developed has been repeatedly confirmed (19–25). Most recently, Goldman (25) and others have revised and validated a simple index for predicting cardiac risk of noncardiac surgery (26). Stable patients undergoing nonurgent, major, noncardiac surgery were assessed for the presence or absence of the following six factors: high-risk type of surgery, history of ischemic heart disease, history of congestive heart failure, history of cerebrovascular disease, preoperative treatment with insulin, and preoperative serum creatinine of greater than 2.0 mg/dL. The rates of major cardiac complications among patients with 0, 1, 2, and 3 or more of these factors were 0.5%, 1.3%, 4%, and 9%, respectively. This index performed better than the original Goldman index and several other risk-prediction indices.

Management Plan for Minimizing Risks

Beyond the identification of groups of patients at increased risk for developing cardiac complications are management algorithms that can guide the physician beyond the assessment phase (27,28). The guideline for assessing and managing the risk of perioperative cardiac complications in noncardiac surgery from the American College of Physicians starts with an assessment of the patient's risk for cardiac complications using the Modified Cardiac Risk Index. Patients in the low-risk category can proceed to surgery without additional evaluation or treatment. Patients in the intermediate-risk category not undergoing a vascular procedure can also proceed to surgery. Patients in the intermediate-risk category undergoing vascular surgery are advised to have a cardiac stress test. If negative, they can proceed to surgery; if positive, they are treated like patients who fall into the high-risk category based on the Modified Cardiac Risk Index. Patients in the high-risk category and those in the intermediate-risk category with an abnormal cardiac stress test should have a further evaluation of the nature of their risk. If the risk is due to ischemic heart disease, eligibility for coronary revascularization should be considered before proceeding with elective noncardiac surgery. If the risk is due to congestive heart failure, dysrhythmias, or other modifiable factors, these should be optimally managed before proceeding to surgery. If the risks are nonmodifiable, consideration should be given to canceling or altering the anticipated surgery. The stepwise approach of this guideline provides the clinician with an organized, systematic approach to assessment and management. (For the algorithm, see Chapter 20: Preoperative Assessment and Perioperative Care. In: Cassel CK, et al., eds. Geriatric Medicine, 4th ed. New York: Springer, 2003, page 215.)

Case (Part 2)

How would your recommendations change if Mrs. Marlowe had chronic stable angina? Aortic stenosis? Elevated jugular venous pressure (JVP) and rales? A significant smoking history? If she had a hip fracture and required open reduction and internal fixation (ORIF)? If she required repair of an abdominal aortic aneurysm?

What special considerations must be given to the intraoperative management of Mrs. Marlowe?

Anesthetic Technique

General Anesthesia

Anesthesia generally consists of analgesia, control of the physiologic responses to surgical stimuli, hypnosis or amnesia, and maintenance of adequate operating conditions, primarily muscle relaxation. Agents are chosen to produce the desired effect and minimize side effects. The guiding principle for anesthesia use in the elderly surgical patient is that less of the drug is usually required.

The volatile anesthetic agents isoflurane, ethrane, sevoflurane, and desflurane are administered by inhalation as part of the gas mixture used to ventilate patients under general anesthesia. Induction of anesthesia is most commonly undertaken with intravenous hypnotic agents. They have the principal advantage of a rapid induction of unconsciousness. The principal agents used are the barbiturates thiopental (Pentothal), thiamylal (Surital), and methohexital (Brevital) and an agent of a unique class called propofol (Diprivan). (For further details on the other anesthetic agents used in general anesthesia, see Chapter 21: Anesthesia for the Geriatric Patient. In: Cassel CK, et al., eds. Geriatric Medicine, 4th ed., page 229.)

Regional Anesthesia

Regional anesthesia is frequently advocated for the elderly patient because of the presumed advantage of reduced stress and less mental confusion in the perioperative period. Unfortunately, no large study has been able to confirm this perception (29). For many years, the prevailing dogma was that minimal alterations in the pharmacokinetics or pharmacodynamics of local anesthetics occurred with aging. In recent years, increasing knowledge has refined our understanding of the effects of age on local anesthetic agents. The effects are not as prominent as for many of the general anesthetic agents.

Neuraxial Anesthesia

Neuraxial anesthesia involves blockade of nerves within the spinal cord. This may be accomplished by injecting agents into the cerebrospinal fluid that surrounds the spinal nerves in the subarachnoid space. This technique is referred to as *spinal* or *subarachnoid anesthesia*. *Epidural anesthesia* involves the placement of drug in the epidural space, which is the area outside the dural sac but inside the vertebral canal. Spinal anesthesia is frequently selected for elderly patients. However, the high incidence of osteoarthritis in the spinal column frequently diminishes flexion and impairs positioning of the patient that is necessary to institute spinal anesthesia. Alterations of the technique are available to facilitate placement of the needle into the subarachnoid space (30). Spinal anesthesia is frequently associated with profound decreases in cardiac output and blood pressure, and patients over 60 years of age frequently manifest 30 to 40 mmHg decrease in blood pressure with anesthetic levels up to the T5 dermatome (31,32). Another important complication of spinal anesthesia is the development of a postspinal headache, but this is principally a complication of younger patients and is relatively rare in the elderly.

Sedation (Conscious Sedation)

Sedation and analgesia describe a state that allows patients to tolerate unpleasant procedures while maintaining adequate cardiorespiratory function and the ability to respond purposefully to verbal command and tactile stimulation (33). *Sedation/analgesia* is preferred to the more common term *conscious sedation*, which is difficult to define.

Patients undergoing sedation/analgesia should be thoroughly evaluated and prepared prior to the procedure. They should be fasting. Vital signs, including pulse oximetry, respiratory activity, and level of consciousness, which may be assessed using spoken responses, should be monitored and recorded. Patients whose only response is reflex withdrawal from painful stimuli may be approaching a state of general anesthesia. Elderly patients or those with severe cardiac, pulmonary, hepatic, or renal disease are at increased risk for developing complications related to sedation/analgesia. However, no specific recommendations were advanced by the American Society of Anesthesiologists Task Force on Sedation and Analgesia to address sedation/analgesia in the elderly.

Intraoperative Monitoring for all Procedures

Blood pressure, electrocardiogram (ECG), and oxygen saturation should be monitored in all elderly patients undergoing any procedure. However, for larger or prolonged surgeries, invasive monitoring should be considered. Placement of a central venous catheter intraoperatively is indicated if a patient shows signs of hemodynamic instability, hypovolemia, unresponsive to fluid repletion. In addition, a central catheter may be indicated for venous access if irritating medications need to be administered or if the patient has difficulty maintaining a peripheral intravenous line for multiple days. (For further details on intraoperative monitoring, see Chapter 21: Anesthesia for the Geriatric Patient. In: Cassel CK, et al., eds. Geriatric Medicine, 4th ed., page 236.)

Case (Part 3)

Mrs. Marlowe is now in the recovery room, but she has severe pain. She is confused and is unable to localize her pain. Her blood pressure is 200/100 mmHg. What should be done?

Management of Selected Problems

Hypertension

Uncontrolled hypertension is a well-established risk factor for stroke, myocardial infarction, and renal dysfunction. In the preoperative period, when the blood pressure is 180/110 mmHg or greater, elective operations should be postponed until better control of the hypertension is achieved (27). An increased incidence of myocardial ischemia is seen not only among patients with preoperative hypertension, but also in those patients who have major fluctuations in blood pressure during a surgical procedure. This variability is more common in patients with established hypertension (34).

Patients with chronic hypertension undergoing elective operations are probably at no increased risk for cardiac complications as long as the preoperative diastolic pressure is stable and less than 110 mmHg and large fluctuations in the mean arterial pressure can be avoided intraoperatively (34). For this reason, and because of the potential for untoward responses to newly introduced antihypertensive agents, it is generally not advisable to begin a new drug regimen for blood pressure control in the few days before surgery. When therapy needs to be initiated or adjusted, it is preferable to postpone the procedure until the patient's response to a new regimen can be observed and a steady state achieved. Oral medications used to control hypertension preoperatively should be given on the day of surgery with a sip of water and restarted as soon as possible postoperatively (29). The risks of severe hypertension from withholding antihypertensive medications far outweigh the potential adverse effects of giving these medications preoperatively. Clinicians must be alert to the negative chronotropic and inotropic effects of some β-adrenergic blockers and calcium channel antagonists that may exacerbate similar pharmacologic effects of inhalation anesthetics.

In the postoperative period, patients with significant elevations in blood pressure should be fully evaluated. Occasionally, uncontrolled pain or a distended bladder is the cause of the hypertension, and treatment is directed at these precipitating factors. If secondary causes of hypertension are excluded, antihypertensive drug treatment is indicated. Parenteral or oral calcium channel antagonists, beta-blockers, and drugs that block both α- and β-adrenergic receptors have been very useful in controlling postoperative hypertension in older patients.

The ability to quickly titrate the dose of parenterally administered medications to blood pressure response is a significant advantage. Beta-blockers must be used cautiously in patients predisposed to congestive heart failure because of negative inotropic effects. The negative chronotropic effects of this class of drugs can blunt the normal compensatory response of increased heart rate to a sudden loss of intravascular volume, such as a major postoperative bleeding episode. Other relative contraindications to beta-blockers include a history of bronchospasm, claudication, and diabetes mellitus. Potent vasodilators, such as hydralazine, can be hazardous in the subset of patients with hypertensive, hypertrophic cardiomyopathy who have a small left ventricular chamber and good contractile function; these patients depend heavily on adequate diastolic filling that can be compromised by rapid vasodilation and reflex tachycardia. Nitroprusside can effectively control significant hypertension, but its use requires careful monitoring of the patient, usually in an intensive care unit with an intra-arterial catheter to continuously measure the blood pressure response.

Atherosclerotic Disease

Many older surgical patients can be expected to have atherosclerosis. The identification and management of occlusive coronary disease in the surgical patient is especially important, because the mortality of perioperative myocardial infarction has been estimated to be about 40% (31). Useful guidelines for the assessment and management of patients with coronary artery disease have been developed (27,28,32). Management of patients with known or suspected coronary artery disease should include the perioperative use of beta-blockers, if there is no contraindication. The use of these medications has been shown to significantly reduce the risk of postoperative cardiac complications among patients undergoing noncardiac surgery including vascular procedures (33–35). In individuals with significant risk, especially if their ability to communicate their symptoms is impaired, it is reasonable to assess a postoperative ECG.

Carotid occlusions and peripheral vascular disease are also prevalent among older persons. The presence of a carotid bruit has been judged to be supportive evidence of atherosclerosis, but has not been shown to increase the risk of postoperative stroke (36). Clinical factors that have been shown to increase the incidence of perioperative stroke include cerebrovascular disease, chronic obstructive pulmonary disease, and peripheral vascular disease (37). Patients experiencing transient ischemic attacks, for whom carotid endarterectomy is recommended, should have this procedure done prior to elective noncardiac surgery.

Peripheral vascular disease very commonly coexists with significant atherosclerotic coronary artery disease. If the peripheral vascular disease is serious enough to limit the patient's activity, exertional angina may be masked. Symptoms or signs of arterial disease should prompt the consultant to evaluate the patient for the presence of ischemic heart disease.

Congestive Heart Failure

In the original Goldman index of cardiac risk factors in noncardiac surgery, the preoperative conditions associated with the most points predictive of an adverse outcome are the presence of an S_3 gallop and jugular venous distention, two of the classic signs of uncompensated congestive heart failure.

In the management of surgical patients with congestive heart failure, it is important to optimize their medication regimen and to monitor carefully their volume status and cardiac output. The standard treatment of systolic cardiac dysfunction includes the use of diuretics and medications to reduce afterload. Positive inotropic agents may be required. Heart rate and rhythm contribute significantly to cardiac output and may require monitoring and special interventions. This is especially true in patients with diastolic dysfunction, often due to hypertensive cardiomyopathy, in which the left ventricular end-diastolic volume is dependent on atrial contraction and adequate filling time. Also, invasive monitoring with a pulmonary arterial catheter may be required for patients with congestive heart failure undergoing major procedures.

Valvular Heart Disease

The primary perioperative risks associated with valvular heart disease are congestive heart failure and bacterial endocarditis. It has been estimated that 20% of surgical patients who have significant valvular heart disease will develop new or worsening congestive heart failure perioperatively (38). Critical aortic stenosis is the valvular lesion most commonly associated with complications. Preoperative identification of this lesion by history and physical examination alone may be difficult. Clinical findings include a prolonged, harsh systolic murmur loudest at the right upper sternal border and radiating to the neck, which peaks late in systole and may obscure the second heart sound, diminished carotid pulses with delayed upstrokes (*pulsus parvus et tardus*), left ventricular hypertrophy on the electrocardiogram, and radiographic evidence of aortic valvular calcification.

If significant aortic stenosis is suspected, an echocardiogram can confirm the diagnosis. It has been suggested that patients with angina, heart failure, or syncope who have significant aortic stenosis established by echocardiography should undergo cardiac catheterization to assess the need for valve replacement prior to elective operations (39). Other types of valvular heart disease are not absolute contraindications to elective surgery. Nevertheless, patients with stenotic or incompetent valves require careful hemodynamic monitoring during perioperative fluid management.

Certain valvular and other cardiac conditions predispose the patient to endocarditis, and prophylactic antibiotics should be used in selected operative settings. Patients with a high risk of endocarditis are those with prosthetic cardiac valves, previous bacterial endocarditis, complex congenital heart disease, and surgically constructed systemic pulmonary shunts or conduits. Patients considered to be at moderate risk for endocarditis are those with most other congenital cardiac malformations, acquired valvular dysfunction, hypertrophic cardiomyopathy, and mitral valve prolapse with valvular regurgitation or thickened leaflets (40). The procedures for which prophylactic antibiotics are indicated are listed in Table 12.2 and the recommended antibiotic regimens are summarized in Table 12.3.

TABLE 12.2. Procedures for which endocarditis prophylaxis is recommended (40)

Dental procedures
Dental extractions
Periodontal procedures including surgery, scaling and root planing, probing, and recall
    maintenance
Dental implant placement and reimplantation of avulsed teeth
Endodontic (root canal) instrumentation or surgery only beyond the apex
Subgingival placement of antibiotic fibers or strips
Initial placement of orthodontic bands but not brackets
Intraligamentary local anesthetic injections
Prophylactic cleaning of teeth or implants where bleeding is anticipated
Respiratory, gastrointestinal, and genitourinary tract procedures
Tonsillectomy or adenoidectomy
Surgical procedures that involve respiratory mucosa
Bronchoscopy with a rigid bronchoscope
Sclerotherapy for esophageal varices
Esophageal stricture dilation
Endoscopic retrograde cholangiography with biliary obstruction
Biliary tract surgery
Surgical procedures that involve intestinal mucosa
Prostatic surgery
Cystoscopy
Urethral dilation

Source: Dajani AS, Taubert KA, Wilson W, et al. Prevention of bacterial endocarditis: recommendations of the American Heart Association. JAMA 1997;277:1794–1801. Copyright 1997, American Medical Association. All rights reserved.

TABLE 12.3. Regimens of prophylactic antibiotics for patients at risk for bacterial endocarditis (40)

Drug	Dosing Regimen
Dental, oral, respiratory tract or esophageal procedures	
Standard regimen	
Amoxicillin	2 g orally 1 h before procedure
Amoxicillin/penicillin-allergic patients	
Clindamycin	600 mg orally 1 h before procedure
or	
Cephalexin or cefadroxil	2 g orally 1 h before procedure
or	
Azithromycin or clarithromycin	500 mg orally 1 h before procedure
Patients unable to take oral medications	
Ampicillin	2 g IV or IM within 30 min before procedure
Penicillin-allergic patients unable to take oral medications	
Clindamycin	600 mg IV within 30 min before procedure
or	
Cefazolin	1 g IV or IM within 30 min before procedure
Genitourinary and gastrointestinal (excluding esophageal) procedures	
High-risk patients	
Ampicillin and gentamicin	IV or IM administration of ampicillin 2 g, plus gentamicin 1.5 mg/kg (not to exceed 120 mg), 30 minutes before the procedure; followed by ampicillin 1 g IM/IV or amoxicillin 1 g, orally 6 h after initial dose
High-risk patients allergic to ampicillin/amoxicillin	
Vancomycin and gentamicin	Intravenous administration of vancomycin 1 g, over 1–2 h plus gentamicin 1.5 mg/kg IM/IV (not to exceed 120 mg); complete injection/ infusion within 30 min of starting procedure
Moderate-risk patients	
Amoxicillin or ampicillin	Amoxicillin 2 g orally 1 h before procedure, or ampicillin 3 gm IM/IV within 30 min of starting procedure
Moderate-risk patients allergic to ampicillin/amoxicillin	
Vancomycin	1 g IV over 1–2 h; complete infusion within 30 min of starting procedure

Source: Dajani AS, Taubert KA, Wilson W, et al. Prevention of bacterial endocarditis: recommendations of the American Heart Association. JAMA 1997;277:1794–1801. Copyright 1997, American Medical Association. All rights reserved.

Rhythm Disturbances and Heart Block

A cardiac rhythm other than sinus rhythm is associated with an increased risk of cardiac complications, most commonly myocardial ischemia or congestive heart failure (39). If a patient is on an antiarrhythmic medication, this should be given on the day of surgery and restarted as soon as possible postoperatively. Parenteral forms of many of these drugs are available and can be used until the patient can tolerate oral medications. Supraventricular tachycardia is commonly encountered in older persons undergoing noncardiac surgery. Risk factors for developing perioperative supraventricular arrhythmia include male gender, age 70 years or older, significant valvular disease, history of a supraventricular arrhythmia, asthma, congestive heart failure, premature atrial complexes on preoperative electrocardiogram, ASA class III or IV, abdominal aortic aneurysm repair, and vascular or intrathoracic procedures (41).

The management of supraventricular and ventricular tachyarrhythmias in the postoperative period is generally the same as in the nonsurgical patient. In the management of atrial fibrillation, however, consideration should be given to the risk of postoperative anticoagulation.

The indications for a pacemaker are not influenced by an anticipated operative procedure. Patients with an asymptomatic chronic bifascicular block or left bundle branch block rarely progress to complete heart block in the perioperative period. Bradyarrhythmias can occur but are successfully managed with medications so that prophylactic insertion of a temporary pacemaker in such patients should be questioned (42).

Pulmonary Disease

Pulmonary problems are among the most common postoperative complications (43). Older persons may be particularly prone to pulmonary complications because of the age-related changes in the respiratory system. At the alveolar level, there is a decrease in elasticity due to alterations in collagen content and structure. There is also increased chest wall stiffness due to calcification of cartilage, arthritic changes, and diminished intervertebral space combined with insufficient respiratory muscle strength to match the added work load of breathing imposed by the increased chest-wall stiffness (44). These structural changes can increase residual volume and reduce the expiratory flow rates in older persons.

Considerable attention has been focused on pulmonary function tests to identify patients at high risk for respiratory complications (45,46). Functional and anatomic tests have proven helpful to clinicians in managing patients facing pulmonary resections. In such patients, the quantitative ventilation-perfusion scan can accurately predict postoperative flow rates; when the predicted postoperative forced expiratory volume in 1 second (FEV_1) is 0.8 L or greater, the operative risk is often considered acceptable (47,48). In contrast, the predictive value of pulmonary function tests for patients undergoing abdominal procedures is unproven (49,50).

Preoperatively, it is important to encourage abstinence from cigarettes, eradicate tracheobronchial infections, relieve airflow obstruction, and instruct the patient in lung expansion maneuvers. Intraoperative goals would include limiting the duration of the operation to less than 3 hours, using limited access surgical procedures when possible, and considering spinal or epidural anesthesia. Postoperatively, deep-breathing exercises and incentive spirometry should be encouraged, and consideration should be given to continuous positive airway pressure devices and regional analgesia via epidural or local nerve blocks (51).

Thromboembolic Disease

Thromboembolic complications are prevalent in the perioperative period. It has been estimated that between 20% and 30% of patients undergoing general surgery develop deep venous thrombosis, and the incidence is as high as 40% in hip and knee surgery, gynecologic cancer operations, open prostatectomies, and major neurosurgical procedures (52,53). The annual incidence of deep venous thrombosis (DVT) and pulmonary embolism (PE) at ages 65 to 69 is 1.3 and 1.8/1000, respectively. At ages 85 to 89, this incidence rises to 2.8 and 3.1/1000. The recommendations for prevention of venous thromboembolism of the Seventh American College of Chest Physicians Consensus Conference on Antithrombotic and Thrombolytic Therapy (52) related to older surgical patients are summarized in Table 12.4.

Renal, Fluid, and Electrolyte Disorders

The kidneys play a critical role in drug metabolism and fluid and electrolyte balance during the perioperative period. The age-related changes in kidney structure and function, combined with the effects of anesthesia and surgery, can have important consequences in the management of the older surgical patient. With aging, there is a loss of renal mass, primarily in the cortex, which results in a 30% to 50% decrease in the number of glomeruli by the seventh decade (54). This loss of filtering surface is associated with a fall in renal blood flow and reduction in glomerular filtration rate (GFR). The decrease in GFR is generally coincident with a decline in muscle mass, so that the serum creatinine levels may remain normal.

Intravenous fluid administration must be adjusted for the older surgical patient because there is a decline in both total body water and intracellular water with advancing age. For men between 65 and 85 years of age and weighing between 40 and 80kg, the intracellular volume represents 25% to 30% of body weight (55). For women of the same age and weight ranges, the intracellular volume is approximately 20% to 25% of body weight. In the absence of acute stress and conditions known to affect salt and water balance, the daily metabolic requirements per liter of intracellular fluid are water, =100mL; energy, =100kcal; protein, =3g; sodium, =3mmol; and potassium, =2mmol.

TABLE 12.4. Prevention of venous thromboembolism (52)

Clinical setting	Recommended prophylaxis
Medical conditions	
Acutely ill hospitalized patients with congestive heart failure (CHF) or severe respiratory disease, or who are confined in bed with additional risk factors	LDUH 5000 U b.i.d. or LMWH ≤3400 U daily
General surgery	
Moderate-risk patients undergoing nonmajor surgery and between 40 and 60 years old, or have additional risk factors	LDUH 5000 U b.i.d. or LMWH ≤3400 U daily
Higher-risk patients undergoing nonmajor surgery and are >60 years old; or patients undergoing major surgery who are >40 years or have additional risk factors	LDUH 5000 U t.i.d. or LMWH >3400 U daily
High-risk patients with multiple risk factors	LDUH 5000 U t.i.d. or LMWH >3400 U daily plus GCS and/or IPC
Higher-risk patients with a high risk of bleeding	GCS or IPC
Orthopaedic surgery	
Elective hip arthroplasty	LMWH >3400 U daily or fondaparinux 2.5 mg SQ daily or adjusted dose warfarin (INR target = 2.5; range 2–3)
Elective knee arthroplasty	LMWH >3400 U daily or fondaparinux 2.5 mg SQ or adjusted dose warfarin (INR target = 2.5; range 2–3)
Hip fracture surgery	Fondaparinux 2.5 mg SQ daily or LMWH >3400 U daily or adjusted dose warfarin (INR target = 2.5; range 2–3) or LDUH 5000 U t.i.d.
Neurosurgery	
Intracranial surgery	IPC with or without GCS

LDUH, low-dose unfractionated heparin; LMWH, low molecular weight heparin; GCS, graduated compression stockings; IPC, intermittent pneumatic compression; INR, international normalized ratio, tid, three times a day; bid, two times a day; SQ, subcutaneous.
Source: Reprinted from Geerts WH, Pineo GF, Heit JA, et al. Prevention of Venous Thromboembolism: the Seventh ACCP Conference on Antithrombotic and Thrombolytic Therapy. Chest 2004;126:338S–400S, with permission from the American College of Chest Physicians.

Endocrine Disorders

Diabetes mellitus, usually type 2, is common among older persons. It has been estimated that of the diabetic patients undergoing surgery, more than 75% are over the age of 50 (56). Diabetes not only complicates the management of surgical patients, but also predisposes the patient to an increased risk of morbidity and mortality from cardiovascular and infectious complications (57,58).

In all diabetic patients undergoing surgery, it is important to monitor blood sugar frequently. Values should be obtained preoperatively, during the procedure, and in the recovery room. Afterward, the frequency of monitoring will be determined by the treatment regimen, the patient's condition, and glucose control. For patients whose blood sugar can be maintained in the normal range by diet and exercise therapy, no special preoperative preparation is required. Hyperglycemia can be effectively treated with supplemental short-acting insulin preparations given subcutaneously. The patients receiving oral hypoglycemic medications should have these held on the day of the operation. Hyperglycemia can be treated with short-acting insulin. For patients receiving insulin, several management regimens are possible. Constant insulin infusions can be used successfully but require careful monitoring because of the rapid changes in glucose and potassium levels. More commonly, for patients normally treated with a single dose of insulin each day, one half to two thirds of the usual dose of insulin is given on the morning of surgery, and a glucose-containing intravenous solution is administered at a rate of 5 to 10 g of glucose per hour.

For patients who are normally managed with multiple doses of insulin throughout the day, one-third the usual morning dose is administered on the morning of surgery, and a glucose-containing solution is infused intravenously (59). Blood sugar control is easier if a constant rate of infusion of the glucose solution is maintained while non–glucose-containing intravenous fluids are used to adjust for changes in intravascular volume. Additional doses of regular insulin should be administered to control blood sugar levels; a 6-hour interval between glucose measurements is commonly used. In addition to meticulous attention to blood sugar levels, it is important to monitor diabetic surgical patients for infections and impaired wound healing (60). Cardiovascular complications are also common because diabetes is an important risk factor for atherosclerosis. Myocardial ischemia can be silent and may be detected unexpectedly on postoperative electrocardiograms.

Thyroid disease is not as prevalent as diabetes, but, if undetected, can result in major complications perioperatively. The consequences of operating on a patient with unsuspected hypothyroidism can be significant. These patients metabolize medications more slowly and their increased sensitivity to central nervous system depressants can result in respiratory insufficiency. In addition, cardiac reserve is diminished and the response to pressors may be blunted. Although the potential for these complications should be suspected and preventive measures instituted, hypothyroidism should not be considered an absolute contraindication to necessary operative procedures (61). Emergency surgery and trauma are indications for rapid replacement of thyroid hormone. When hypothyroidism is severe, an intravenous dose of 300 to 500 μg of L-thyroxine will significantly improve basal metabolic rate within 6 hours. Corticosteroids should also be given in the perioperative period because the acute rise in basal metabolic rate can exhaust adrenal reserves.

The increased perioperative risks associated with hyperthyroidism include hyperpyrexia, arrhythmias, and congestive heart failure. Older persons may be particularly prone to iodine-induced hyperthyroidism from nonionic contrast radiography (62). Elective operations should be delayed until treatment with thionamide medications render the patient euthyroid. When an emergency operation is necessary, the patient can be treated with 1000mg of propylthiouracil by mouth and a beta-blocker to control the increased catecholamine effects. Sodium iodide is often given to inhibit the release of thyroid hormone and transiently inhibit organification. Iodide can be given either by mouth or intravenously; administration should be delayed until at least 1 hour after the propylthiouracil to allow time for the latter to block organification. Supplemental corticosteroids are also recommended for hyperthyroid patients undergoing emergency operations. These are given to protect against the possibility of adrenal insufficiency related to the chronic hypermetabolic state and because corticosteroids may lower serum thyroxine and thyroid-stimulating hormone levels.

Nutrition

Physiologic dysfunctions, comorbid conditions, and a variety of psychosocial issues common to the elderly place this population at high risk for nutritional deficits. Malnutrition occurs in approximately 0% to 15% of community-dwelling elderly persons, 35% to 65% of older patients in acute care hospitals, and 25% to 60% of institutionalized elderly (24). Factors that may lead to inadequate intake and utilization of nutrients include the inability to get food (e.g., financial constraints, unavailability of food, limited mobility), the lack of desire to eat food (e.g., poor living situation, poor mental status, chronic illness), the inability to eat and absorb food (e.g., poor dentition, chronic gastrointestinal such as gastroesophageal reflux disease or diarrhea), and medications that interfere with appetite or nutrient metabolism (25).

Especially for older patients, there is no consensus on the best method for assessing nutritional status (63,64). However, simply measuring the *body mass index* (BMI = weight in kilograms/[height in meters]^2) is a useful guide. It is generally accepted that a BMI between 24 and 29 is appropriate for persons over age 65. The *Subjective Global Assessment* (SGA) is another relatively simple, reproducible tool for assessing nutritional status from the history and physical exam (26). The SGA ratings are most strongly influenced by loss of subcutaneous tissue, muscle wasting, and weight loss. In a study of patients undergoing elective gastrointestinal surgery, both SGA and serum albumin were predictive of postoperative nutrition-related complications (27).

In the face of stress from illness, injury, infection, or even elective surgery, the nutritionally compromised elderly patient may quickly develop protein-energy malnutrition. This metabolic response to the release of cytokines and hormones is characterized by increased requirements for energy and protein.

In the elderly surgical patient with protein-energy malnutrition, these changes are further aggravated by the increased energy requirements for wound healing. Additional deficits in vitamins, particularly A and C, and trace minerals such as zinc can adversely effect enzymes systems necessary for wound repair. Further, major tissue injury and sepsis is associated with large fluid shifts and sequestration of extracellular water in the interstitial space. Additional studies are needed in patients most likely to benefit from perioperative nutritional supplements: those who are severely malnourished before major surgery; and those who undergo operations resulting in prolonged periods of inadequate enteral intake. Until more is known, it is common to provide postoperative enteral tube feedings to patients with a functioning gastrointestinal tract who were malnourished preoperatively and who are unable to consume adequate calories orally. Total parenteral nutrition is indicated for malnourished patients who have a nonfunctioning gastrointestinal tract or for whom enteral feedings are contraindicated (65).

Swallowing Dysfunction

The most common and one of the most resource-intensive complications in the elderly in the postoperative period is pneumonia. Although the explanation for this increase is multifactorial, one factor that has only recently been studied is the effects of swallowing dysfunction on the incidence of postoperative aspiration. The majority of community-acquired bacterial pneumonias in the elderly are the result of microaspiration of oral flora (66). Alterations in deglutition secondary to stroke and other central nervous system disease, dementia, medications, and generalized decline predispose to the aspiration of oral contents.

Case (Part 4)

Three days postoperative, Mrs. Marlowe's pain and blood pressure are under better control. However, she remains disoriented and complains of not sleeping well.

What evaluation should be done to assess the cause of her continued delirium?

What can be done to minimize her disorientation?

What can you tell her daughter about the prognosis?

Neuropsychiatric Disorders

The most common psychiatric problem in the postoperative period is delirium. The major manifestation of this condition is an alteration in consciousness, and it is, by definition, a transient disorder (67). One prospective study reported delirium in 44% of older patients undergoing repair of hip fractures (66).

The differential diagnosis of delirium is very broad. A careful clinical assessment of the patient should focus on the possibility of infection, metabolic derangements, central nervous system events, myocardial ischemia, sensory deprivation, or drug intoxication. Lidocaine, cimetidine, atropine, aminophylline preparations, antihypertensives, steroids, and digoxin are medications commonly associated with delirium, but all drugs should be considered as possible causes.

The best management strategy is prevention; the incidence of delirium can be significantly reduced by meticulous attention to precipitating factors. A multicomponent intervention that addressed the six risk factors—cognitive impairment, sleep deprivation, immobility, visual impairment, hearing impairment, and dehydration—was successful in reducing the incidence of delirium from 15% to 9% (68). When it cannot be prevented, it is important to recognize the syndrome early, then identify and treat the underlying cause. When medications are necessary to protect the patient and others from agitated behaviors, haloperidol 0.5 mg can be given parenterally and repeated every 30 minutes as necessary. The minimum dose sufficient to control symptoms is recommended, and doses exceeding 6 mg over a 24-hour period are rarely indicated. (see Chapter 12: Depression, Dementia, Delirium, page 236.)

Alcoholism is another serious and common problem among older persons; it has been estimated that there are at least 1.5 million alcoholics in this country who are 65 years of age or older (69). The primary care consultant should carefully explore current ethanol use with all patients, and a screening tool such as the Michigan Alcoholism Screening Test may be useful in identifying alcohol abuse preoperatively (70).

Wound Healing

Wound healing is a complex constellation of coordinated events requiring adequate nutrition, adequate perfusion, and immunocompetence to support the cellular mechanism of tissue repair. Many of the processes involved in normal wound healing are susceptible to the changes of aging. Although it is generally thought that wounds in the elderly heal more slowly, this impression is largely unsubstantiated. Actual clinical differences in wound healing have been difficult to demonstrate because of myriad interacting and uncontrollable factors. Certain changes in the skin, subcutaneous tissue, muscle, and bones are documented, but the effect of these changes and others on the orchestrated process of tissue repair is more elusive. It is likely that comorbidity with poor perfusion, poor nutrition, and immune suppression rather than physiologic decline alone is responsible for most clinically relevant wound problems seen in elderly surgical patients.

Improving wound healing in the elderly is not primarily directed at the cellular event identified above but at the comorbid conditions that cause hypoperfusion and subsequent tissue hypoxia, immune suppression, and inadequate nutrition. Sufficient tissue perfusion to allow appropriate delivery of nutrients and oxygen to the wound is of paramount importance. In the elderly conditions such as diabetes, congestive heart failure, arteriosclerosis, and venous insufficiency commonly compromise this perfusion.

Infection

A leading cause of wound healing failure is infection. Older persons are potentially more susceptible to wound infection because of the changes in the nutrition, perfusion, and immune competence that accompany aging and the high prevalence of comorbid conditions, such as diabetes mellitus. Appropriate utilization of methodology to decrease wound infection, therefore, is particularly important when operating on elderly patients.

The Centers for Disease Control and Prevention provide excellent guidelines for the prevention of surgical site infection (64). According to these guidelines, antibiotic prophylaxis is "a critically timed adjunct used to reduce the microbial burden of intra-operative contamination to a level that cannot overwhelm the host." There are four basic principles that guide the use of antibiotic prophylaxis (64): (1) Prophylaxis should be used for all operations in which they have been shown to reduce the incidence of surgical site infections, or where the risk of infection would be catastrophic. (2) The agent used should be safe, inexpensive, and bactericidal, with an in vitro spectrum that covers the organisms that are likely to be encountered with that specific procedure. (3) The agent should be given before the skin is incised so the tissue and serum levels of the agent are adequate at the time the potential contamination might occur. (4) Therapeutic levels should be maintained throughout the operation by redosing until a few hours after the procedure is over and the skin is closed.

Postoperative Pain Management

Untreated or undertreated postoperative pain can have significant negative impact on the recovery of the elderly patient following surgery. Pain causes tachycardia, increases myocardial oxygen consumption, and may lead to myocardial ischemia. The anticipation of pain after major abdominal and thoracic procedures leads to splinting and poor inspiratory effort with subsequent atelectasis and increased risk of pneumonia. Because pain is exacerbated by moving, untreated pain results in immobility with all of the sequelae of prolonged bed rest including pressure ulcers, thromboembolic disorders, and the declines associated with deconditioning; depression and lethargy; anorexia and dehydration; neuromuscular instability, decreased bone density, muscular weakness, and incoordination; altered bladder and bowel function with retention and constipation; and urinary and fecal incontinence. (See Chapter 32: Principles of Pain Management, page 573.)

General Principles

- With newer advanced surgical techniques, surgical mortality in the elderly has declined. Thus appropriate surgical management of disease should not be denied solely because of advanced age but with consideration of the individual patient's risk factors and preferences.
- Perioperative risk increases with increasing number of comorbid conditions. When possible, risk should be lowered prior to elective surgery by optimizing the patient's status with respect to comorbid conditions based on established guidelines available to assist in perioperative risk assessment.
- Elderly patients require lower doses of medications used for anesthesia and postoperative pain management.
- Intra- and postoperative monitoring should be used when appropriate.
- Delirium is a common postoperative complication and its risk for development should be minimized by close attention to the patient's medications, clinical status, sleep cycle and environment.
- Elderly patients postoperatively are at higher risk for poor nutrition and wound healing.

Suggested Readings

ACC/AHA Guideline Perioperative Cardiovascular Evaluation for Noncardiac Surgery: ACC/AHA 2002 Guideline Update for Non-Cardiac Surgery. J Am Coll Cardiol 2002;39:542–553. *This guideline provides a clear, step-by-step algorithm for assessing cardiac risk for noncardiac surgery. In addition to the full guideline and the executive summary, a useful pocket version is also available on the American College of Cardiology Web site: http://www.acc.org.*
Pompei P. Preoperative assessment and perioperative care. In: Cassel CK, Leipzig RM, Cohen HJ, et al., eds. Geriatric Medicine, 4th. New York: Springer, 2003: 213–228.

Rosenthal RA. Surgical approaches to the geriatric patient. In: Cassel CK, Leipzig RM, Cohen HJ, et al., eds. Geriatric Medicine, 4th. New York: Springer, 2003: 239–258.

Silverstein JH. Anesthesia for the geriatric patient. In: Cassel CK, Leipzig RM, Cohen HJ, et al., eds. Geriatric Medicine, 4th. New York: Springer, 2003: 229–238.

References

1. Lawrence L, Hall MJ. 1997 Summary: National Hospital Discharge Summary. Advance Data from Vital and Health Statistics, No. 308. Hyattsville, MD: National Center for Health Statistics, 1999.
2. Mangano DT. Preoperative risk assessment: many studies, few solutions. Is a cardiac risk assessment paradigm possible? Anesthesiology 1995;83: 897–901.
3. Thomas DR, Ritchie CS. Preoperative assessment of older adults. J Am Geriatr Soc 1995;43:811–821.
4. Owings MF, Kozak LJ. Ambulatory and inpatient procedures in the United States, 1996. National Center for Health Statistics. Vital Health Stat 1998;13(139):1–9.
5. Maxwell JG, Taylor BA, Rutledge R, Brinker CC, Maxwell BG, Covington DL. Cholecystectomy in patients aged 80 and older. Am J Surg 1998;176(6): 627–630.
6. Valentin N, Lomholt B, Jensen JS, Hejgaard N, Kreiner S. Spinal or general anaesthesia for surgery of the fractured hip? A prospective study of mortality in 578 patients. Br J Anaesth 1986;58(3):284–291.
7. Djokovic JL, Hedley-Whyte J. Prediction of outcome of surgery and anesthesia in patients over 80. JAMA 1979;242(21):2301–2306.
8. Davis FM, Woolner DF, Frampton C, et al. Prospective, multi-centre trial of mortality following general or spinal anaesthesia for hip fracture surgery in the elderly. Br J Anaesth 1987;59(9):1080–1088.
9. Khuri, SF, Daley J, Henderson W. National Surgical Quality Improvement Program (NSQIP). Annual report. Fiscal Year 1999;A-5.
10. American Society of Anesthesiologists. New classification of physical status. Anesthesiology 1963;24:111.
11. Buxbaum JL, Schwartz AJ. Perianesthetic considerations for the elderly patient. Surg Clin North Am 1994;74:41–61.
12. Djokovic JL, Hedley-White J. Prediction of outcome of surgery and anesthesia in patients over 80. JAMA 1979;242:2301–2304.
13. Seymour DG, Pringle R. Post-operative complications in the elderly surgical patient. Gerontology 1983;29:262–270.
14. Narain P, et al. Predictors of immediate and 6 month outcome in hospitalized elderly patients. The importance of functional status. J Am Geriatr Soc 1988; 36:775–778.
15. Seymour DG, Pringle R. Post-operative complications in the elderly surgical patient. Gerontology 1983;29:262–270.
16. Older P, et al. Preoperative evaluation of cardiac function and ischemia in elderly patients by cardiopulmonary exercise testing. Chest 1993;103:701–705.

17. Charlson ME, Pompei P, Ales KL, MacKenzie CR. A new method of classifying prognostic comorbidity in longitudinal studies: development and validation. J Chron Dis 1987;40:373–383.
18. Krousel-Wood MA, Abdah A, Re R. Comparing comorbid-illness indices assessing outcome variation: the case of prostatectomy. J Gen Intern Med 1996;11:32–38.
19. Escarce JJ, Shea JA, Chen W, Qian Z, Schwartz JS. Outcomes of open cholecystectomy in the elderly: a longitudinal analysis of 21,000 cases in the prelaparoscopic era. Surgery 1995;117:156–164.
20. Gibbs J, Cull W, Henderson WG, Daley J, Hur K, Khuri SF. Preoperative serum albumin level as a predictor of operative mortality and morbidity: results from the National VA surgical risk study. Arch Surg 1999;134:36–42.
21. Zeldin RA, Math B. Assessing cardiac risk in patients who undergo noncardiac surgical procedures. Can J Surg 1984;27:402–404.
22. Jeffrey CC, Kunsman J, Cullen DJ, et al. A prospective validation of the cardiac risk index. Anesthesiology 1983;58:462–464.
23. Gerson MC, Hurst JM, Hertzberg VS, et al. Cardiac prognosis in noncardiac geriatric surgery. Ann Intern Med 1985;103:832–837.
24. Detsky AS, Abrams HB, McLaughlin JR, et al. Predicting cardiac complications in patients undergoing non-cardiac surgery. J Gen Intern Med 1986;1:211–219.
25. Goldman L. Multifactorial index of cardiac risk in noncardiac surgery: ten-year status report. J Cardiothoracic Anesth 1987;1:237–244.
26. Lee TH, Marcantonio ER, Mangione CM, et al. Derivation and prospective validation of a simple index for prediction of cardiac risk of major noncardiac surgery. Circulation 1999;11(10):1043–1049.
27. Eagle KA, Brundage BH, Chaitman BR, et al. Guidelines for perioperative cardiovascular evaluation for noncardiac surgery: a report of the American Heart Association/American College of Cardiology Taskforce on Assessment of Diagnostic and Therapeutic Cardiovascular Procedures. J Am Coll Cardiol 1996;27:910–948.
28. American College of Physicians. Clinical Guideline, Part I: Guidelines for assessing and managing the perioperative risk from coronary artery disease associated with major noncardiac surgery. Ann Intern Med 1997;127:309–312.
29. National Heart, Lung, and Blood Institute. The sixth report of the Joint National Committee on Prevention, Detection, Evaluation, and Treatment of High Blood Pressure. NIH publication No. 98–4080. Bethesda, MD: U.S. Department of Health and Human Services, National Institutes of Health, 1997.
30. Adler AG, Leahy JJ, Cressman MD. Management of perioperative hypertension using sublingual nifedipine: experience in elderly patients undergoing eye surgery. Arch Intern Med 1986;146:1927–1930.
31. Mangano DT. Perioperative cardiac morbidity. Anesthesiology 1990;72:153–184.
32. Palda VA, Detsky AS. Perioperative assessment and management of risk from coronary artery disease. Ann Intern Med 1997;127:313–328.
33. Mangano DT, Layug EL, Wallace A, Tateo I. Effect of atenolol on mortality and cardiovascular morbidity after noncardiac surgery. N Engl J Med 1996;335:1713–1720.

34. Wallace A, Layug EL, Tateo I, et al. Prophylactic atenolol reduces postoperative myocardial ischemia. Anesthesiology 1998;88:7–17.
35. Poldermans D, Boersma E, Bax JJ, et al. The effect of bisoprolol on perioperative mortality and myocardial infarction in high-risk patients undergoing vascular surgery. N Engl J Med 1999;341:1789–1794.
36. Ropper AH, Wechsler LR, Wilson LS. Carotid bruit and the risk of stroke in elective surgery. N Engl J Med 1982;307:1388–1390.
37. Limburg M, Wijdicks EFM, Li HZ. Ischemic stroke after surgical procedures: clinical features, neuroimaging, and risk factors. Neurology 1998;50: 895–901.
38. Goldman L, Caldera DL, Southwick FS, et al. Cardiac risk factors and complications in non-cardiac surgery. Medicine 1978;47:357–370.
39. Goldman L. Cardiac risks and complications of noncardiac surgery. Ann Intern Med 1983;98:513–514.
40. Dajani AS, Taubert KA, Wilson W, et al. Prevention of bacterial endocarditis: recommendations of the American Heart Association. JAMA 1997;277:1794–1801.
41. Polanczyk CA, Goldman L, Marcantonio ER, Orav EJ, Lee TH. Supraventricular arrhythmia in patients having noncardiac surgery: clinical correlates and effect on length of stay. Ann Intern Med 1998;129:279–285.
42. Hubner GA, Radermacher P, Schutz GM. Perioperative risk of bradyarrhythmias in patients with asymptomatic chronic bifascicular or left bundle branch lock: Does an additional first-degree atrioventricular block make any difference? Anesthesiology 1998;88:679–687.
43. Lawrence VA, Hilsenbeck SG, Mulrow CD, Dhanda R, Sapp J, Page CP. Incidence and hospital stay for cardiac and pulmonary complications after abdominal surgery. J Gen Intern Med 1995;10:671–678.
44. Mahler DA, Rosiello RA, Loke J. The aging lung. Geriatr Clin North Am 1986;2:215–225.
45. Tisi GM. Preoperative evaluation of pulmonary function: validity, indications, and benefits. Am Rev Respir Dis 1979;119:293–310.
46. Gass GD, Olsen GN. Preoperative pulmonary function testing to predict postoperative morbidity and mortality. Chest 1986;89:127–135.
47. Wernly JA, DeMEester TR, Kirchner PT, Myerowitz PD, Oxford DE, Golomb HM. Clinical value of quantitative ventilation-perfusion scans in the surgical management of bronchogenic carcinoma. J Thorac Cardiovasc Surg 1980; 80:835–843.
48. Boysen PG, Block AJ, Olsen GN, et al. Prospective evaluation for pneumonectomy using the technetium lung scan. Chest 1977;72:422–425.
49. Lawrence VA, Page CP, Harris GD. Preoperative spirometry before abdominal operations: a critical appraisal of its predictive value. Arch Intern Med 1989;149:280–285.
50. Zibrak JD, O'Donnell CR, Marton K. Indications for pulmonary function testing. Ann Intern Med 1990;112:763–771.
51. Smetana GW. Preoperative pulmonary evaluation. N Engl J Med 1999; 340:937–944.
52. Geerts WH, Pineo GF, Heit JA, et al. Prevention of Venous Thromboembolism: the Seventh ACCP Conference on Antithrombotic and Thrombolytic Therapy. Chest 2004;126:338S–400S.

53. Clagett GP, Anderson FA, Geerts W, et al. Prevention of venous thromboembolism. Chest 1995;108:312S.
54. Frocht A, Fillit H. Renal disease in the geriatric patient. J Am Geriatr Soc 1984;32:28–39.
55. Miller RD. Anesthesia for the elderly. In: Miller RD, ed. Anesthesia. New York: Churchill Livingstone, 1986:1801–1818.
56. Galloway JA, Shuman CR. Diabetes and surgery. A study of 667 cases. Am J Med 1963;34:177–191.
57. Hirsch IB, McGill JB, Cryer PE, White PF. Perioperative management of surgical patients with diabetes mellitus. Anesthesiology 1991;74:346–359.
58. Golden SH, Peart-Vigilance C, Kao WHL, Brancati FL. Perioperative glycemic control and the risk of infectious complications in a cohort of adults with diabetes. Diabetes Care 1999;22:1408–1414.
59. Jacober SJ, Sowers JR. An update on perioperative management of diabetes. Arch Intern Med 1999;159:2405–2411.
60. MacKenzie CR, Charlson ME. Assessment of perioperative risk in the patient with diabetes mellitus. Surg Gynecol Obstet 1988;167:293–299.
61. Ladenson PW, Levin AA, Ridgway EC, Daniels GH. Complications of surgery in hypothyroid patients. Am J Med 1984;77:261–266.
62. Martin FIR, Tress BW, Colman PG, Deam DR. Iodine-induced hyperthyroidism due to nonionic contrast radiography in the elderly. Am J Med 1993;95:78–82.
63. Detsky AS, Baker JP, O'Rourke K, Goel V. Perioperative parenteral nutrition: a meta-analysis. Ann Intern Med 1987;107:195–203.
64. Baker JP, Detsky AS, Wesson DE, et al. Nutritional assessment. A comparison of clinical judgment and objective measurements. N Engl J Med 1982;306:969–972.
65. Ellis LM, Copeland EM, Souba WW. Perioperative nutritional support. Surg Clin North Am 1991;71:493–507.
66. Berggren D, Gustafson Y, Eriksson B, et al. Postoperative confusion after anesthesia in elderly patients with femoral neck fractures. Anesth Analg 1987;66:497–504.
67. Tune L, Folstein F. Post-operative delirium. Adv Psychosom Med 1986;15:51–68.
68. Inouye SK, Bogardus ST, Charpentier PA, et al. A multicomponent intervention to prevent delirium in hospitalized older patients. N Engl J Med 1999;340:669–676.
69. Solomon DH. Alcoholism and aging. Ann Intern Med 1984;100:411–412.
70. Willenbring ML, Christensen KJ, Spring WD Jr, Rasmussen R. Alcoholism screening in the elderly. J Am Geriatr Soc 1987;35:864–869.

13
Depression, Dementia, and Delirium

RAINIER P. SORIANO

Learning Objectives

Upon completion of the chapter, the student will be able to:

1. State the epidemiology of depression, dementia, and delirium in older adults.
2. Describe the risk factors for the development of depression, dementia, and delirium.
3. Understand the diagnostic workup of depression, dementia, and delirium.
4. Develop a rational management plan for persons with depression, dementia, or delirium.

Case (Part 1)

Mrs. Martha Martin is a 76-year-old woman who, with her husband, George, managed a small restaurant for many years. George died about two years ago and now their son does most of the day-to-day work, but Martha remains involved—going to the restaurant each day, helping at the cash register and with seating the customers. You step out of the room and Martha's son, Leo is waiting to talk with you. He tells you that he is worried about Mom and that she just isn't the same as she used to be, that she really hasn't been the same since his father died. She now lives alone. She's very resistant to help and argues with him and his wife if they try to help her. He is afraid to let her work the register at the restaurant because he noticed a lot of her bills at home were unpaid. Some nights she goes home early and doesn't bother to cook or eat dinner. She forgets appointments. He tells you he thinks she has Alzheimer's disease.

Material in this chapter is based on the following chapters in Cassel CK, Leipzig RM, Cohen HJ, Larson EB, Meier DE, eds. Geriatric Medicine: An Evidence-Based Approach, 4th ed. New York: Springer, 2003: Kennedy GJ. Dementia, pp. 1079–1093. Inouye SK. Delirium, pp. 1113–1122. Koenig HG, Blazer DG II. Depression, Anxiety, and Other Mood Disorders, pp. 1163–1183. Selections edited by Rainier P. Soriano.

Dementia: General Considerations

Dementia is a syndrome of progressive, global decline in cognition, severe enough to degrade the individual's well-being and social function. Persons with dementia have learning and memory problems, plus at least one of the following: impairments in communication (*aphasia*), reasoning and planning (*executive function*), recognition and manipulation of objects in space (*agnosia, apraxia*), orientation, and the regulation of emotion and aggression.

The prevalence of dementia increases exponentially, doubling every 5 years at least to age 85, at which point the incidence may decline (1). Alzheimer's disease alone affects 8% to 15% of persons 65 and older.

Diagnostic Evaluation

The clinical history from patient and family, physical examination, mental status assessment, and laboratory procedures are carried out to detect reversible or partially reversible disease. Although few dementias are reversible, most have elements that will partially remit (2).

The use of a cognitive screening instrument allows the clinician to demonstrate the presence, and with longitudinal administrations, the course of deficits, objectively. Cognitive assessment should be conducted without the family present to avoid distractions and any potential embarrassment over failed items. Because the patient is asked to actively demonstrate errors, considerable care is required to place the person at ease and accurately administer the exam. A number of factors may influence cognitive performance yet not be indicative of dementia. These include inefficient learning strategies, slowed processing capacity, reduced attention, sensory deficits, and age-associated memory impairment (3). Age, education, and other demographic factors also alter performance (4).

Laboratory Evaluation

Diagnostic laboratory procedures include complete blood count, blood chemistries, liver function studies, and serologic test for syphilis, thyroid-stimulating hormone (TSH), vitamin B_{12} and folate levels, and electrocardiogram. In less than 1% of patients will these procedures detect a reversible cause of dementia. Chest x-ray, HIV test, and test of Lyme disease may also be included, based on the physical exam and history. A review of prescribed and over-the-counter medications, alcohol, and tobacco products intake is mandatory. Medications may be the most common cause of reversible dementia.

Computed tomography (CT) of the brain, without contrast, should be performed when focal neurologic signs are present, when change in mental status is sudden, or when trauma or mass effects are suspected. Magnetic resonance imaging (MRI) may be indicated when vascular dementia is suspected. However, the white matter changes seen on T2-weighted images are not necessarily indicative of dementia (5). Functional imaging studies with positron emission tomography (PET) or single photon emission computed tomography (SPECT) may detect the temporal-parietal metabolic deficits of Alzheimer's disease or the diffuse irregular deficits of vascular dementia when objective signs of memory impairment are equivocal (6). Persons with dementia require supervision to complete tasks of daily living, such as dressing and being safe from dangerous wandering. Severe dementia is evidenced by marked aphasia, loss of capacity to recognize family, incontinence, and dependency in all aspects of daily living.

Assessment

Mini–Mental State Examination

The mini–mental state examination (MMSE) is the most widely used screening exam for impaired cognition in the United States and has been translated to a number of languages and normed for age and education (Table 13.1). A perfect score is 30; mild impairment falls between 18 and 24; and persons with moderately advanced dementia have MMSE scores ranging between 10 and 19. For persons with less than 9 grades of education, a score of 17 or less is evidence of at least mild impairment. The average decline in MMSE scores among Alzheimer's patients is 2 to 4 points per year.

Clock Drawing Test

The clock drawing test is the briefest cognitive assessment tool, requiring less than 5 minutes to complete. The patient is asked to draw a clock face with all the numbers and hands and then to state the time as drawn. The number 12 must appear on top (3 points), there must be 12 numbers present (1 point), there must be two distinguishable hands (1 point), and the time must be identified correctly (1 point) for full credit. A score less than 4 is considered impaired (7). Other clock completion tests and clock drawing tests have been described in the literature with varying ease of administration and interpretations.

For those with higher educational attainment, and when decline is subtle, referral to a neuropsychologist is warranted. Like imaging studies, none of the cognitive screening or neuropsychological batteries can be considered diagnostic.

Differential Diagnosis

Although a histologic examination of brain tissues sets the criteria for *"definite"* Alzheimer's disease, the diagnosis of *"probable"* Alzheimer's dementia can be accurately made in 90% of cases by history from the patient and family and clinical examination (5). *"Possible"* cases may have atypical features but no identifiable alternative diagnosis. Alzheimer and Pick's disease represent cortical dementias in which there is primary neuronal degeneration (Table 13.2) (8). Huntington's and Parkinson's diseases represent the subcortical dementias. Dementia associated with Lewy bodies overlaps with both Parkinson's and Alzheimer's diseases in presentation and distribution of pathology. The secondary neuronal degeneration of the vascular dementias is due to angiopathic disorders, most commonly ischemic heart disease and arrhythmias, hypertension, and diabetes. Hemiparesis, gait disorder, and other signs of past stroke also suggest vascular dementia.

The rare dementias would be easy to overlook were it not for their distinctive features. Marked deficits in visual perception and praxis out of proportion to memory impairment suggest corticonuclear degeneration. Changes in affect, typically depression but also hypomania and irritability preceding signs of dementia, suggest a non-Alzheimer's diagnosis (9). Early deterioration in personality, loss of social inhibitions, and frontal lobe atrophy indicate Pick's dementia (10). Physical signs such as the tremor and bradykinesia of Parkinson's disease, the choreoathetoid movements of Huntington's disease, the myoclonic twitching of Creutzfeldt-Jakob disease, or the pseudobulbar palsy of vascular dementia may not present before intellectual deterioration is observed. Huntington's disease is typical of the subcortical dementias in that various cortical functions, including communication, praxis, and visual perception, are generally spared. Emotional disturbances and personality change are regular features of Huntington's disease and frequently the first signs of the illness (11). Normal pressure hydrocephalus is characterized by incontinence, gaitapraxia (magnetic gait) and ventricular atrophy out of proportion to cortical loss.

Delirium is perhaps the most common cognitive disorder and often complicates dementia. The hallmarks are fluctuating level of awareness, impaired attention, disorganized thinking, and demonstrable physiologic disturbance. Symptoms should remit once the disturbance is reversed, but recovery may be delayed in older persons. Delirium can also be chronic and difficult to distinguish from dementia. Cognitive impairment due to depressive disorders is distinguished by the patient's prominent complaints of difficulty with memory and concentration. Apathy, irritability, and reluctance to complete cognitive testing are apparent. Aphasia is usually absent.

Age-associated memory impairment (AAMI) is characterized by memory complaints in persons age 50 or older whose performance falls one standard deviation below the mean on tests normed for younger adults.

TABLE 13.1. The Standardized Mini–Mental State Examination (111)

Preparations

Ensure that the patient is willing and that vision and hearing aids, if needed, are in place. Ask, "Would it be all right to ask you some questions about your memory?" Ask each question a maximum of three times. If the patient does not respond, score the item as 0. If the answer is incorrect, score 0. Do not hint, prompt, or ask the question again once an answer has been given. If the patient answers, "What did you say?" do not explain or engage in conversation, merely repeat the same directions up to a maximum of three times. If the patient interrupts or wanders from the task, redirect the person by saying, "I will explain in a few minutes when we are finished. Now if we could just proceed please . . . we are almost finished."

Begin by saying, "I am going to ask you some questions and give you some problems to solve."

		Max Score
1.	(Allow no more than 10 seconds for each reply.)	
	a. "What year is this?" (Accept exact answer only.)	1
	b. "What season is this?" (In the last week of the old season or first of the new accept either.)	1
	c. "What month of the year is this?" (On the first day of the new month or last day of the previous, accept either month.)	1
	d. "What is today's date?" (The day before or after is acceptable, e.g., on the 7th accept the 6th or 8th.)	1
	e. "What day of the week is this?" (Exact day only.)	1
2.	(Allow no more than 10 seconds for each reply.)	
	a. "What county/borough are we in?"	1
	b. "What province/state/country are we in?"	1
	c. "What city/town are we in?"	1
	d. If in the clinic: "What is the name of this hospital/ building?" (Exact name of hospital/institution/building only.) If in the patient's home: "What is the street address of this house?" (Street name and house number or equivalent in rural areas.)	1
	e. If in the clinic: "What floor of the building are we on?" (Exact answeronly.) If in the home: "What room are we in?" (Exact only)	1
3.	"I am going to name three objects. After I have said all three, I want you to repeat them. Remember what they are because I am going to ask you to name then again in a few minutes." (Say the objects slowly at 1–second intervals.) "BALL (1 second), CAR (1 second), MAN. Please repeat the three items for me." (Score 1 point for each reply on the first attempt. Allow 20 seconds for the reply, if the patient cannot repeat all three on the first attempt, repeat until they are learned but no more than five times.)	3
4.	"Now please subtract 7 from 100 and keep subtracting 7 from what's left until I tell you to stop." (May repeat three times if the patient pauses; allow 1 minute for answer. Once the patient starts, do not interrupt until five subtractions have been completed. If the patient stops, repeat "keep subtracting 7 from what's left" for a maximum of three times.)	5
5.	"Now what were the three objects that I asked you to remember?" (Score 1 point each regardless of the order, allow 10 seconds.) BALL CAR MAN	3

TABLE 13.1. *Continued*

6. Show the patient a wristwatch and ask, "What is this called?" (Accept"wristwatch or "watch" but not "clock" or "time.")	1
7. Show a pencil and ask, "What is this called?" (Do notaccept "pen.")	1
8. "I'd like you to repeat a phrase for me: say 'no if's, and's, or but's.'" (Exact reply only.)	1
9. "Read the words on the page and then do what it says." (Hand the patient the sheet with CLOSE YOUR EYES on it. Instructions may be repeated three times but patient must close eyes for correct score.)	1
10. Ask if the patient is right or left handed. The paper held in front of the patient should be taken with the nondominant hand. "Take this paper in your right/left hand, fold it in half and place it on the floor." Takes paper with nondominant hand = 1 Folds it in half = 1 Places it on the floor = 1	3
11. Give the patient a pencil and paper and say, "Write any complete sentence on this piece of paper." (Allow no more than 30 seconds. Sentence should make sense. Ignore spelling.)	1
12. Place intersecting pentagons design, pencil, and paper in front of the patient. Say: "Please copy this design." Allow multiple attempts up to 1 minute. To be correct the patient's copy must show a four-sided drawing within two five-sided figures. Ignore rotation and distortions.)	1

Source: Adapted from Molloy DW, Alemayehu E, Roberts R. A standardized Mini-Mental State Examination (SMMSE): its reliability compared to the traditional Mini-Mental Sate Examination (MMSE). Am J Psychiatry 1991;148:102–105, with permission from American Psychiatric Publishing, Inc. Reprinted as appears in Kennedy GJ. Dementia, pp. 1079–1093. In: Cassel CK, Leipzig RM, Cohen HJ, et al., eds. Geriatric Medicine, 4th ed. New York: Springer, 2003.

Although lower memory scores are predictive of dementia, only 1% to 3% of these individuals will experience global cognitive decline in the ensuing 12 to 24 months.

Mild cognitive impairment (MCI) is characterized by performance between one and one-half standard deviations below the mean on tests of memory. As with AAMI, persons with MCI have memory complaints but do not meet diagnostic criteria for dementia. They exhibit slowed information retrieval, but orientation and communication are usually intact (12). Five percent to 15% of persons with MCI develop dementia within the year.

Management Considerations

The comprehensive approach to dementia care seeks to preserve the patient's independence by delaying disability to the end of the natural life span. There are five elements to the comprehensive approach: (1) accurate diagnosis of the specific dementia and recognition of other conditions

TABLE 13.2. Differential diagnosis of cognitive impairment in adults (113)

Condition	Distinguishing features
Dementia	Progressive decline, global cognitive impairment with learning and memory deficits (recent > remote) aphasia, apraxia, agnosia, executive dysfunction; patients tend to minimize deficits
Developmental disorder	Childhood onset without progressive decline; history of diminished educational and work attainment; attention unimpaired
Delirium	Sudden onset and fluctuating course with inattention, disorganized thinking, and altered level of awareness; impairment reversible but recovery may be prolonged by advanced age
Major depressive disorder with cognitive impairment	Memory and concentration complaints prominent; aphasia absent, apathy or irritability present; cooperation with testing difficult, risk of subsequent dementia elevated
Age associated	Age >50, memory complaints prominent; performance below 1 standard deviation from the mean on tests normed with young adults; information retrieval slowed; learning, orientation, communication intact; functional independence preserved
Mild cognitive impairment	Age >50, memory complaints prominent; performance below 1.5 standard deviation from the mean on tests compared to age mates; information retrieval slowed; learning, orientation, communication intact; functional independence preserved
Alzheimer's disease	Insidious onset with smooth, inexorable decline, cortical atrophy, apolipoprotein E ε4 allele and cardiovascular disease elevates risk; more rapid decline in middle-stage onset; mood disturbance early, psychosis and behavioral disturbance later in the course
Vascular dementia	Sudden onset, fluctuating course with temporary improvements or prolonged plateau; multiple infarcts, diffuse white matter lesions, diabetes, cardiovascular disease present; focal neurologic exam
Huntington's disease	Autosomal dominant but incomplete penetrance inheritance pattern; atrophic caudate nuclei: premorbid DNA testing quantifies risk, age of onset, severity
Parkinson's disease	Characteristic tremor with unilateral onset, bradykinesia, bradyphrenia, cognition may be spared
Acute cognitive impairment due to stroke, traumatic brain injury	Focal neurological exam; circumscribed rather than global cognitive deficits may improve significantly over 6 months
Frontal lobe degeneration, Pick's disease	Personality, sociability, executive function prominently impaired; disinhibition, impaired judgment and social indifference significant; aphasia, apraxia, amnesia, loss of calculation less notable
Lewy body dementia	Sudden onset, fluctuating level of awareness, psychosis (visual and auditory hallucinations more often than delusions) prominent, parkinsonian signs and falls; adverse response to typical antipsychotic drugs.

(Continued)

TABLE 13.2. *Continued*

Condition	Distinguishing features
Corticonuclear degeneration	Marked visual-spatial impairment, substantial apraxia, memory and behavior disturbance less prominent
Creutzfeldt-Jakob disease	Rapid progression, death in 6 to 12 months, characteristic EEG, myoclonic jerks
Alcohol-related dementia	Massive, prolonged abuse, may remit with abstinence
Normal pressure hydrocephalus	Gait disturbance ("magnetic gait"), incontinence, ventricular enlargement disproportionate to cortical atrophy
AIDS dementia	HIV positive, may present with behavioral disturbance, parkinsonian features

Source: Reprinted from Kennedy GJ. Geriatric Mental Health Care: A Treatment Guide for Health Professional. New York: Guilford, 2000:48, with permission from Guilford Publications.

that contribute excess disability; (2) caregiver education, counseling, and support; (3) pharmacologic palliation of cognitive impairment; (4) interventions, both pharmacologic and environmental, to lessen behavioral and psychological disturbances; (5) early advance-care planning in anticipation of late-stage and end-of-life care issues.

Reduction of Excess Disability

Beyond recognition of the specific dementia, the optimal treatment of associated conditions is critical. Of patients with dementia, half have a concurrent physical or mental illness that contributes to their functional impairments. Weight control, exercise, elimination of tobacco use, and minimizing alcohol intake represent good preventive health at any age, perhaps more so for individuals with dementia. For patients with suspected vascular dementia, the use of 325 mg of aspirin daily should be recommended (13).

Counseling and Coaching the Caregiver

The cornerstones of caregiver counseling are education, emotional support, and telephone availability. Rehabilitation of the patient should always include consultation with the family, and failure of the family to appear should alert the clinician to future problems. Most families are remarkably creative in providing care. Others seem enmeshed, trapped in maintaining conflict rather than resolving it (14). Clinical depression is a problem for 20% to 60% of the primary family caregivers (15,16).

Caregivers should be instructed to modify the physical environment so that it is safe and predictable. A regular schedule of activities including rising, meals, medications, and exercise lessens the burden on memory. Unfamiliar people, places, and events require accommodation for which the patient is ill equipped. Travel that disrupts the person's routine will be disorienting. Cherished holidays are better celebrated in the patient's home. The withdrawal of firearms, opportunities to cook or smoke unsupervised, and automobile driving requires compassion and at times imagination.

Pharmacologic Palliation of Impaired Cognition

In mild to moderately impaired persons, cholinesterase inhibitors may improve cognition, delay decline, lessen the disability in activities of daily living (17), improve psychological and behavioral disturbances including psychosis (18,19), and forestall nursing home admission (20). On average, cholinesterase inhibitors restore the person to a level of impairment seen 6 months previously. Although the effect is palliative, the less impaired time and delay in nursing home admission may be precious, particularly for patients whose improvement is marked. The side effects of cholinergic enhancement are nausea, diarrhea, sweating, bradycardia, and insomnia. They are most often transient, occurring in 10% to one third of patients at the initiation of treatment, depending on the agent. Roughly one patient in four experiences improvement readily noticeable to family and practitioner within weeks of beginning the drug. That number increases to one in three by the third month of treatment (21,22).

There are three cholinesterase inhibitors approved by the Food and Drug Administration (FDA) for mild to moderate Alzheimer's disease (Table 13.3). Donepezil (Aricept) has a prolonged action and specificity for brain tissue. The starting dose is 5 mg once daily and should be increased to 10 mg. Although it is metabolized by the cytochrome P-450 system, drug interactions are rare. Many practitioners find it has an alerting effect in late-stage patients. Rivastigmine (Exelon) is a brain-specific cholinesterase inhibitor administered twice daily. The dose ranges from 1.5 to 6 mg twice daily (23). Patients able to tolerate the gastrointestinal difficulties of higher doses may benefit more. It is not metabolized by the cytochrome P-450 system, and drug interactions are thought to be rare. Rivastigmine also inhibits butylcholinesterase, which may be more active in the latter stages of dementia, but the clinical significance of this property is uncertain (24). The acetylcholinesterase inhibitor galantamine (Razadyne) is a plant-derived alkaloid with nicotinic receptor modulating activities. Its capacity to allosterically modulate nicotinic receptors avoids the undesirable cardiovascular effects of direct nicotinic stimulation (25). However, the clinical significance of this property is uncertain. Galantamine is taken twice daily at doses ranging from 4 to 16 mg. Because multiple enzymes of the cytochrome P-450 system metabolize galantamine, drug interactions should be rare.

Memantine is an orally active N-methyl-D-aspartate (NMDA) receptor antagonist. Persistent activation of the central nervous system NMDA

TABLE 13.3. Agents used to palliate the cognitive impairment of dementia (26,113)

Generic name	Trade name	Initial dose	Final dose	Arrhythmia potential	Hypotensive potential	Sedative potential	Precautions	Advantages
Donepezil	Aricept	5 mg qd	10 mg qd	Bradycardia	Low	Low	Transient, initial GI upset, abrupt withdrawal leads to abrupt decline, may interact with paroxetine	Once a day dosing, safety
Rivastigmine	Exelon	1.5 mg b.i.d.	6 mg b.i.d.	Low	Low	Low	Transient, initial GI upset, titrated up at 2-week intervals, abrupt withdrawal leads to abrupt decline, b.i.d. dosing	Wider dose range, no drug interactions
Galantamine	Razadyne	4 mg b.i.d.	16 mg b.i.d.	Bradycardia	Low	Low	Transient, initial GI upset, titrated up at 4-week intervals, abrupt withdrawal leads to abrupt decline, b.i.d. dosing	Wider dose range, nicotinic receptor modulation
Memantine HCl	Namenda	5 mg qd	10 mg b.i.d.	Low	Low	Low	Adverse effects include fatigue, hypertension, dizziness, headache, constipation, back pain, and confusion	May have an important therapeutic role in advanced disease
Selegiline	Eldepryl	5 mg qd	5 mg b.i.d.	Low	Moderate	Low	Potentially life threatening diet and drug interactions are rare at recommended doses	Available as a transdermal patch
α-tocopherol	Vitamin E	30 IU qd	1000 IU b.i.d.	NA	NA	NA	Liver toxicity, coagulopathy	Low toxicity, OTC
Extract of Ginkgo biloba	Ginkgold tebonin forte	60 qd	60 q.i.d.	Low	Low	Low	q.i.d. dosing, an "herbal" not subject to FDA quality controls, little data available at max dose	Low toxicity, OTC

OTC, over the counter; FDA, Food and Drug Administration; NA, not applicable; AD, Alzheimer's disease; VaD, vascular dementia.
Source: Modified from Kennedy GJ. Geriatric Mental Health Care: A Treatment Guide for Health Professionals. New York: Guilford, 2000:48, with permission from Guilford Publications. Additional data from Reisberg B, Doody R, Stoffler A, et al. Memantine Study Group. Memantine in moderate-to-severe Alzheimer's disease. N Engl J Med 2003;348(14):1333–1341.

receptors by excitatory amino acid glutamate has been hypothesized to contribute to the symptomatology of Alzheimer's disease. Memantine is postulated to exert its therapeutic effect through its action as an NMDA receptor antagonist. The dosage shown to be effective in controlled trials is 20 mg daily (26).

Selegiline, a selective monoamine oxidase-B inhibitor, and vitamin E (α-tocopherol) reduce the rate of functional decline and delay nursing home placement in moderately impaired persons with dementia. However, cognitive performance is not enhanced, and the combination of the two agents is no more beneficial than vitamin E alone (27). Estrogen is associated with lesser prevalence of dementia among more highly educated women in epidemiologic studies, but in recent randomized controlled trials the use of estrogen to treat established cases of or prevent Alzheimer's disease has not yet been convincingly demonstrated (28).

Management of Behavioral and Psychological Symptoms

The causes of behavioral symptoms are usually multiple, including the caregiving context, the caregiver's capacities and tolerance, and the patient's disease. Intervention to make the disturbed behavior less disruptive is a more realistic goal than outright elimination. Characterization of the three-point sequence or ABCs of problematic behavior is central to the task of management (29). First, the caregiver is asked to identify the *antecedents* or triggering events such as changes in daily routine, interpersonal conflict, and emotional or physical stressors. The antecedents can then be removed or minimized as a preventive measure. The caregiver should describe the *behavior* in detail, how often it occurs, when and where it is most likely to happen, and how long it lasts. Caregivers may need to step back and observe or take note to provide sufficient detail and to set the baseline for objective measurement of improvement. This observation period also refines recognition of antecedents and how the problem behavior fits into other aspects of the patient's life. Then the caregiver identifies the *consequences* of the behavior, how the caregiver or others react to reinforce or deter the activity, and what happens when the activity ceases.

Preparations for Late-Stage and End-of-Life Care

In the early stage of the disease, when incapacity is minimal, the practitioner should anticipate the need for supportive services and urge referral before the need becomes acute. Arrangements for home health aides, day treatment, respite care, and residence in nursing facilities can be patched together with a good deal of continuity. However, providing these arrangements exceeds the capacity of any one individual and is best coordinated by a social worker or other professional functioning as a case manager.

Legal advice for the management of financial assets is another important area of consideration for the family. Nursing home placement devastates even substantial financial resources, and prolonged care at home is also expensive. Durable power of attorney assigned to a family member while the patient is still capable of exercising the necessary judgment will ensure adequate access to resources once the person is no longer able to manage financial decisions.

Case (Part 2)

You examine Mrs. Martin in the office. She is pleasant and cooperative and in no acute distress. Her blood pressure is 130/70 mmHg, her heart rate is 82/min and regular, respiratory rate is 12/min. She is afebrile. The rest of her exam including the neurologic examination is essentially within normal limits. During the course of the interview, she cries frequently about living without her husband. They were very happy together and she misses him. She tells you that her son is trying to run her life, and that sometimes she feels useless and hopeless.

Depression: General Considerations

Mood disorders are the most common reversible psychiatric conditions in later life, and the vast majority are usually treated by primary care physicians and geriatricians. While aging is often accompanied by loss and unwanted change, most elders do not suffer from depression. This is surprising given the many reasons why the elderly should be depressed, such as declining health, loss of function, death of family and loved ones, shrinking financial resources, and biologic changes in the brain that predispose them to emotional disorder.

Epidemiology

Major depressive disorder, a clinically significant and persistent depression associated with other symptoms like weight loss and insomnia, is less frequently diagnosed in old age than at other stages of the life cycle. Elders are (1) less likely to report depressive symptoms (due to the stigma of psychiatric illness), (2) less likely to recall symptoms (due to cognitive impairment), (3) less likely to have symptoms that fit nicely into diagnostic categories, and (4) more likely to express emotional symptoms as somatic complaints.

Although rates of depression among community-dwelling older adults are low, this is not true for those hospitalized with medical illness or living in nursing homes. Rates of major depression in acutely hospitalized elders are about 13% to 20%; moreover, an additional 30% of these patients experience minor depressive disorder (30,31). Likewise, rates of depression and other mood disorders are high among patients in nursing homes, where rates of major depression commonly exceed 15% and rates of minor depression range from 30% to 35% (32–35). Unfortunately, between 80% and 90% of depressed elders in acute medical settings go undiagnosed.

Etiology/Risk Factors

Mood disorders are nearly twice as common among women than among men, although this pattern may reverse in later life (36). Depression is more common in elders with lower incomes and less education (37–39), those who live in rural settings (39), and those who are divorced or separated (37,38). Persons with a prior history of psychiatric illness are especially vulnerable when facing the major adjustments required in later life, particularly with health problems (30). While many depressions in the elderly are of late onset (first episode after age 60), a significant minority represents recurrences of mood disorder first diagnosed in young adulthood or middle age (40). Depressive disorders in physically ill older adults are usually psychological reactions to progressive disability, chronic pain, side effects from drugs, financial insecurity, or feelings of guilt over being a burden.

High social support has been reported to buffer against depression in later life (37–39). Such support, particularly if perceived by the elder as helpful (high subjective support), may both prevent and facilitate recovery from depression. Religion, particularly when used regularly to cope with stressful life events, has been associated with greater well-being (41), lower rates of depression (42), and faster recovery from depression (43,44). Active involvement in the religious community and strong religious beliefs appear to reinforce each other and together enhance well-being (45). Most epidemiologic studies find physical health to be the strongest predictor of well-being and emotional health, regardless of age, sex, or race (37–39).

Diagnostic Evaluation

A patient's history should focus on the length of the current episode, any history of previous episodes, a history of drug or alcohol abuse, therapies tried in the past, and an assessment of the patient's suffering, particularly with respect to suicidal thoughts. If possible, confirmation of the patient's responses should be obtained from a relative or caregiver. In the physical examination, attention should be directed toward such neurologic findings as lateralization, tremor, muscle tone, and slowed reflexes.

Symptoms and Signs

Major Depressive Disorder

Major depression is defined in the American Psychiatric Association's Diagnostic and Statistical Manual of Mental Disorders, 4th edition (DSM-IV), as a depressed mood or a marked loss of interest that is experienced most of the day nearly every day during a 2-week period or longer. In addition, at least four of the following eight symptoms must be present: (1) weight loss (>5% of body weight in a month) or loss of appetite, (2) insomnia or hypersomnia, (3) psychomotor agitation or retardation, (4) fatigue or loss of energy, (5) feelings of worthlessness or guilt, (6) diminished concentration, (7) thoughts of suicide, or (8) loss of interest (including decreased sexual interest). According to DSM-IV, these symptoms must cause clinically significant distress or impairment in social, occupational, or other important areas of functioning.

The 30- or 15-item Geriatric Depression Scale (GDS) is currently the preferred screening tool for depression among primary care patients who care for older adults (Table 13.4). A score of greater than 5 in the 15-item GDS or greater the 15 in the 30-item GDS prompts further evaluation for the possibility of depression (46).

The symptoms of major depression can be divided into two groups: *vegetative* (or somatic) and *cognitive* (or psychological). Vegetative symptoms include insomnia, anorexia or weight loss, fatigue, concentration difficulties, and psychomotor agitation or retardation. Cognitive symptoms

TABLE 13.4. The Geriatric Depression Scale (Short-Form)

For each question, choose the best answer for how you felt over the past week.

1. Are you basically satisfied with your life?	Yes/NO
2. Have you dropped many of your activities and interests?	YES/No
3. Do you feel that your life is empty?	YES/No
4. Do you often get bored?	YES/No
5. Are you in good spirits most of the time?	Yes/NO
6. Are you afraid that something bad is going to happen to you?	YES/No
7. Do you feel happy most of the time?	Yes/NO
8. Do you often feel helpless?	YES/No
9. Do you prefer to stay at home, rather than going out and doing new things?	YES/No
10. Do you feel you have more problems with memory than most?	YES/No
11. Do you think it is wonderful to be alive now?	Yes/NO
12. Do you feel pretty worthless the way you are now?	YES/No
13. Do you feel full of energy?	Yes/NO
14. Do you feel that your situation is hopeless?	YES/No
15. Do you think that most people are better off than you are?	YES/No

*The scale is scored as follows: 1 point for each response in capital letters. A score of 0 to 5 is normal; a score above 5 suggests depression.
Source: www.stanford.edu/~yesavage/GDS.html

include depressed mood, irritability, hopelessness, guilt, feeling worthless or like a burden, loss of interest, social withdrawal, and suicidal thoughts. Cognitive symptoms can help identify depression in medically ill older patients whose somatic symptoms confuse the diagnostic picture. Somatic symptoms, however, cannot be ignored and may be important for recognizing severe forms of depression.

Minor Depression

Minor depression is defined as a less severe depressive episode than major depression and not as chronic as dysthymia. The diagnosis involves 2 weeks or more of depressed mood or loss of interest, together with between one and four of the traditional eight symptoms of depression (sleep disturbance, loss of sexual interest, guilt, loss of energy, difficulty concentrating, appetite disturbance, psychomotor agitation or retardation, suicidal thoughts). The frequency of minor depression in the elderly is 8% to 13% in community samples (47). Minor depression may actually be a prodrome or a residual of major depression, but the clinical significance of this syndrome has not been established, nor has the effectiveness of treatment.

Dysthymia

Dysthymia is a chronic depression lasting 2 years or longer that does not fulfill the criteria for major depression. Community data indicate that dysthymic disorder in the elderly is less frequent (48). Although chronic depressions are difficult to treat when they are related to character pathology, studies have shown a good response to adequate doses of tricyclics, or psychotherapy may be very helpful to these individuals who may have difficulty relating to others.

Bereavement

Bereavement, a universal human experience, cannot be classified as a psychiatric disorder. Normal symptoms of grief include sensations of somatic distress such as tightness in the throat, shortness of breath, sighing respirations, lassitude, and loss of appetite. The bereaved may be preoccupied with the image of the deceased. Pathologic grief may occur if the usual symptoms are delayed, persist beyond the expected period of time, or become unusually severe. Delayed grief can be distinguished from normal grieving by symptoms of overactivity without a sense of loss, frequently accompanied by psychosomatic complaints. When grief is unusually severe it may be associated with marked feelings of worthlessness, hopelessness, or suicidal ideation. Patients who fulfill the symptom criteria for major depression 2 months after bereavement, however, should be treated just like any other patient with major depression.

Laboratory Findings

Thyroid function studies [thyroxine (T_4), TSH)], complete blood cell count, serum electrolytes, B_{12} level, and drug levels are often helpful in identifying reversible organic causes of depression. Vitamin B_{12} deficiency may present with depressive symptoms, as well as dementia, in the face of a normal serum B_{12} level or hemogram; methylmalonic acid and homocystine levels should be checked in depressed patients with low normal serum B_{12} levels. A head CT scan or MRI scan can rule out brain tumors, although when the history is not suggestive and the neurologic exam is normal, the yield from these tests is very low. An electrocardiogram, as well as renal and liver function tests, can be helpful if psychopharmacologic treatment is contemplated.

Differential Diagnosis

Psychiatric conditions with depressive symptoms may be confused with depression. These include hypochondriasis, alcoholism, the organic mental disorders, delusional disorders, and schizophrenia. Hypochondriasis is both a symptom of depression and a separate disorder itself. The essential features are an unrealistic interpretation of physical sensations as abnormal and a preoccupation with the imagined physical illness underlying these sensations. Between 60% and 70% of depressed persons in one study were found to have hypochondriacal symptoms (49). It is a disorder that is usually distinguishable from depression by (1) the length of the episode (hypochondriasis persisting for years); (2) the degree of suffering by the patient (more among depressed patients); (3) and the waxing and waning course of symptoms in depression, which by nature is cyclical. Differentiating the older adult with hypochondriasis or generalized anxiety disorder from the one who is depressed has therapeutic implications; hypochondriacs often do not tolerate antidepressants because of real or imagined side effects.

Alcoholism, although less frequent in older than in younger persons, still occurs in about 5% to 8% of persons over age 60. A heavy alcohol intake may cause both physical and psychological symptoms that mimic depression. Conversely, many alcoholics drink to relieve the pain of depression that recurs when they become sober; in this case, depressive disorder has been masked by the alcohol problem. The same principles apply to elders who abuse prescription drugs.

The sudden appearance of a psychosis in later life, with paranoid or delusional thinking, may herald the onset of a major depression. Differentiating depression from late-life schizophrenia or delusional disorder may be difficult, but the latter two are not usually associated with profound depression. Late-life schizophrenia seldom begins suddenly;

instead, it is characterized by gradual withdrawal, bizarre complaints, and paranoia.

Finally, it may be difficult to distinguish an agitated depression from panic disorder with secondary depression. These can often be differentiated by determining which symptoms arose first; patients with a primary panic disorder report a history of anxiety symptoms that precede the onset of depression, whereas those with primary depression report that their depression came before the onset of panic.

Management Considerations

Once a diagnosis has been made and the patient's safety ensured, management includes one or more of the following specific treatments: psychotherapy, pharmacotherapy, or electroconvulsive therapy (ECT). Regardless of which modality is chosen, all depressed elders require psychological support, which involves listening, empathy, and demonstration of concern.

Psychotherapy

Psychotherapy avoids the side effects associated with psychoactive drugs. A wide variety of psychotherapies are available to the clinician for use in elderly depressed patients; only a few, however, have proven efficacy in late-life depression.

Cognitive therapy is designed to train patients to identify and correct the negative thinking in depression that contributes to its maintenance (50). Cognitive restructuring helps to break the vicious cycle of depressive thinking. Cognitive interventions may enable older persons to view their disabilities and other life-stressors in a more positive light, as well as disrupt negative ruminations. *Behavioral therapy* (BT), on the other hand, involves positive reinforcement of behaviors that alleviate depression (pleasurable activities) and the negative reinforcement of behaviors that lead to depression (withdrawal, etc.) (51). In BT, the patient is encouraged to keep weekly activity schedules, mastery and pleasure logs, and complete other homework assignments. A variant of cognitive/behavioral therapy is *interpersonal therapy* (IPT) (52), which is similar in approach to cognitive therapy, but the focus of therapy is on the interpersonal interactions of the patient. Group psychotherapy, using an educational problem-solving approach, may be a particularly effective, inexpensive, and acceptable form of treatment for older adults, especially those who are socially isolated (53,54).

Pharmacotherapy

Because of the excellent response of many depressed older adults to drug therapy, antidepressants should always be considered when depressive symptoms threaten the elder's ability to function. The five major classes of medications used to treat mood disorders are (1) selective serotonin reuptake inhibitors (SSRIs), (2) other novel antidepressants (venlafaxine, mirtazapine, bupropion, nefazodone), (3) tricyclic antidepressants, (4) monoamine oxidase (MAO) inhibitors, and (5) mood stabilizers (lithium carbonate, carbamazepine, and valproic acid).

Before starting therapy with an antidepressant, the older patient should undergo a thorough history and physical examination to identify contraindications. When using tricyclics, special effort should be employed to elicit a history of closed-angle glaucoma, difficulty with urination, severe dizziness with standing, seizure disorder, severe hypertension, recent myocardial infarction, or unstable angina. The physical examination should include measurement of orthostatic blood pressure changes, as well as examination of the liver and prostate for enlargement. Baseline liver and kidney function test results should also be obtained because most antidepressants are metabolized in the liver and excreted in the urine. An electrocardiogram should be obtained before starting therapy with antidepressants, especially tricyclics or tetracyclics; even patients on SSRIs may be at increased risk for developing cardiac complications, particularly in the presence of atrial arrhythmias.

Selective Serotonin Reuptake Inhibitors

Selective serotonin reuptake inhibitors such as fluoxetine, sertraline, paroxetine, or citalopram are now the drugs of first choice for geriatric depression. Initial doses must be small (10mg/day or 10mg every other day for fluoxetine, 12.5 or 25mg/day for sertraline, and 5 to 10mg/day for paroxetine) to reduce the likelihood of unpleasant side effects. The newer antidepressants, although generally void of orthostasis, anticholinergic, and the cardiac side effects of tricyclic antidepressants, have their own unpleasant effects that affect their use in older patients. These include weight loss, excessive stimulation and agitation, insomnia, gastrointestinal side effects, tremor, and disequilibrium. Because of its long half-life (10 to 14 days in frail elders), fluoxetine should be used cautiously in older patients. Sertraline, paroxetine, and citalopram with shorter half-lives are more quickly cleared from the body, but can create problems when the medication is abruptly discontinued.

Tricyclic Antidepressants

Until recently, nortriptyline, desipramine, and doxepin were popular drugs for treating older adults with endogenous depressions. If used today, lower doses than those for younger adults are preferred, because high blood levels may occur even at reduced dosages (55). Doses of 10 to 50mg of nortriptyline or 25 to 75mg of desipramine at bedtime are often adequate to relieve symptoms, although blood levels should be followed to ensure a therapeutic dose.

Other Novel Antidepressants

Venlafaxine and Mirtazapine

Patients who do not respond to traditional SSRIs, or who after being on these drugs for some time lose their responsiveness, may be tried on venlafaxine, which inhibits the reuptake of both serotonin and norepinephrine. Patients may be started on doses of 25 mg twice daily and increased gradually up to 150 mg twice daily if necessary. Blood pressure needs to be monitored, because this drug has been associated with worsening of hypertension. Mirtazapine is another novel antidepressant with relatively few side effects that may be tried either initially or after the patient has failed a trial with SSRIs. Mirtazapine has the benefit of being sedating, particularly at low doses. Patients should be started on 15 mg at bedtime, and then after a week or two increased to 30 mg, the dose at which most older adults respond.

Trazodone and Nefazodone

For patients with an agitated depression who need sedation, trazodone at doses from 50 to 300 mg/day or nefazodone at doses of 100 to 300 mg/day may be tried. Because they are virtually devoid of anticholinergic side effects, trazodone and nefazodone are attractive drugs for use in elderly patients. Nevertheless, their antidepressant potency is questionable at doses that elders can usually tolerate, and side effects such as excessive drowsiness, orthostasis, and priapism are reasons for caution (although less so for nefazodone than for trazodone).

Bupropion

Bupropion is another antidepressant that may have special advantages in certain patients. Older adults who have psychomotor retardation, or are unmotivated, fatigued, frail, and at high risk for falling, may find bupropion helpful. Doses beginning at 75 mg/day and increasing to 225 or 300 mg/day are recommended; any single dose should not exceed 150 mg, usually requiring a twice a day or three times a day dosing. Toxicity at the higher doses may be manifested by tremor, unpleasant gastrointestinal side effects, or visual hallucinations. Stopping or reducing the dose readily reverses these symptoms. Bupropion has also been associated with an increased risk of seizures, especially in patients with anorexia nervosa or bulimia; thus, a history of seizures should be ruled out before starting this drug.

St. John's Wort

St. John's wort is a natural herb that has been used for the treatment of depression, particularly in Europe. The preparations that can be bought in health food stores in the United States are of uncertain composition and purity. These preparations should not be used for a patient with a clinical diagnosis of depression, because there are known effective treatments that have been tested (the antidepressants described above), approved by the FDA, and have careful guidelines and requirements for their preparation.

Benzodiazepines

In general, benzodiazepines should not be used to treat geriatric depression. They can induce excessive sedation and may even worsen the depressive state (56,57). The possible exception is alprazolam, which has been reported to have antidepressant, as well as antianxiety, effects. At doses of 2 to 4 mg/d, the antidepressant effects of this drug have been reported to equal those of imipramine. Nevertheless, elders may easily become dependent on alprazolam, and it is difficult to get them off the drug once started.

Psychostimulants

Low-doses of stimulants like methylphenidate (5 to 15 mg two to three times/day) may enhance the appetite and mood of an apathetic older adult. At such doses, side effects are rare (especially if the last dose is given before 2 p.m.), and abuse or addiction is seldom encountered; nevertheless, blood pressure should be monitored and these drugs should be avoided in patients with unstable angina. Furthermore, tolerance may occur, requiring an escalation of dose to achieve the desired effect. Stimulants have been used to treat depression in medically ill older patients (30), although it remains unclear whether they actually treat the mood disorder or simply activate patients with psychomotor retardation.

Electroconvulsive Therapy

For severe depressions that are persistent and refractory to psychotherapy and pharmacotherapy, ECT is the most effective treatment (58). It is particularly effective in major depression with either melancholic or psychotic features. For an adequate therapeutic response, treatments are usually given three times per week for a total of eight to 12 times. This can be done on an inpatient or outpatient basis. The overall success rate for ECT in drug nonresponders is about 80%, a rate similar in both younger and older patients. In the absence of prophylactic drug therapy, the relapse rate 1 year following ECT exceeds 50%. Maintenance ECT (weekly or monthly) or concurrent use of antidepressants decreases the relapse rate to around 20% in the year following ECT.

Confusion following ECT varies from patient to patient, depending on the underlying level of cognitive impairment. Significant cognitive impairment is not a contraindication to ECT, because if due to depression, it may improve as the depression improves (59). Most memory impairment induced by ECT disappears by 6 months after treatment (60).

Prognosis

The natural history of major depression follows a pattern of remission and relapse. Until recently, most follow-up studies indicated that one third of depressed elders recovered completely from an index episode, one third experienced a partial recovery or relapsed soon after recovery, and one third remained continuously ill. Factors associated with better outcome are female sex, current employment, and high level of subjective social support (61). Other positive prognostic factors include an extroverted personality style, absence of severe symptomatology, a family history of depression, a history of recovery from previous episodes, no substance or alcohol abuse, no other comorbid major psychiatric illness, minimal intercurrent life changes, and religious coping style (42,62). On the other hand, poor outcomes have been associated with delusions, significant cognitive impairment, and physical illness (62–64).

Case (Part 3)

Four months later you get a call from the local hospital that Mrs. Martin is in the emergency room. She is confused, has fever and shaking chills, and complains of abdominal pain. Her white blood cell count is 20,000, her abdominal exam is remarkable for decreased bowel sounds, exquisite periumbilical tenderness, with rebound and guarding. She has traces of blood in her stool. She is on her way to the operating room (OR) for emergency surgery. You go to the hospital after Mrs. Martin's surgery. She did well in the procedure where her ruptured appendix was resected. The surgical resident reports that she has been sleeping a lot. When she is awake she is sometimes clear, but most of the time very confused. He asks whether her Alzheimer's disease is getting worse and he asks for advice on what he should do.

Delirium: General Considerations

Delirium, defined as an acute alteration in attention and cognition, is a common, serious, and potentially preventable source of morbidity and mortality for older persons. The incidence of delirium increases with age, cognitive impairment, frailty, illness severity, comorbidity, and other risk factors for delirium (see below). The emergency room and acute hospital have the highest overall rates of delirium. Previous studies have measured the prevalence of delirium, that is, cases present at the time of hospital admission, as 14% to 24%, and the incidence of delirium, that is, new cases arising during hospitalization, as 6% to 56% (65–77). The rates of postoperative delirium range from 10% to 52% (65–77). Hospital mortality rates in patients with delirium range from 25% to 33%, as high as mortality rates associated with acute myocardial infarction or sepsis (65,66,71,72,78–85).

Pathogenesis/Risk Factors

Predisposing or vulnerability factors for delirium include preexisting cognitive impairment or dementia, severe illness, high number of comorbid diseases, functional impairment, advanced age, chronic renal insufficiency, dehydration, malnutrition, depression, and vision or hearing impairment (69,74,85,88–91). Dementia is a leading risk factor for delirium. Patients with dementia have a two- to fivefold increased risk for delirium. Moreover, one third to one half of delirious patients have an underlying dementia.

Medications, the most common precipitating factors for delirium, contribute to at least 40% of delirium cases (75,92,93). Many medications can lead to delirium; the most common are those with recognized psychoactive effects, such as sedative-hypnotics, narcotics, H_2-blockers, and medications with anticholinergic effects. In previous studies, use of any psychoactive medication was associated with a fourfold increased risk of delirium (69,75). Sedative-hypnotic drugs have been associated with a three- to 12-fold increased risk of delirium; narcotics with a threefold risk; and anticholinergic drugs with a five- to 12-fold risk (85–87,89–91,94,95). Delirium increases in direct proportion to the number of medications prescribed, an effect that is likely due to adverse effects of the medications themselves, as well as the increased risk of drug–drug and drug–disease interactions.

Other precipitating factors for delirium include medical procedures or surgery, intercurrent medical illnesses, infections (pneumonia, urinary tract infection, endocarditis, abdominal abscess, or septic arthritis), immobilization, use of indwelling bladder catheters, use of physical restraints, dehydration, malnutrition, iatrogenic events, electrolyte or metabolic derangement (hyper- or hyponatremia, hypercalcemia, acid-base disorder, hypo- and hyperglycemia, thyroid or adrenal disorders), alcohol or drug intoxication or withdrawal, environmental influences, and psychosocial stress (71,80,83,87,96–102). Acute myocardial infarction or congestive heart failure commonly present as delirium in an elderly patient, without the expected symptoms of chest pain or dyspnea.

Diagnostic Evaluation

Symptoms and Signs

The key features of delirium are *acute onset* and *inattentiveness*. Determining the acuity of onset requires accurate knowledge of the patients' previous level of cognitive functioning. Another key feature is the *fluctuating course* of delirium, with symptoms tending to come and go or increasing and decreasing in severity over a 24-hour period.

Inattention is recognized as difficulty focusing, maintaining, and shifting attention. Delirious patients appear easily distracted, have difficulty following commands or maintaining a conversation, and often perseverate with an answer to a previous question. Attention should be assessed with simple tests, such as a forward digit span (inattention indicated by the inability to repeat five digits forward) or reciting the days of the week or the months backward.

Other key features include a *disorganization of thought* and *altered level of consciousness*. Disorganization of thought is a manifestation of underlying cognitive or perceptual disturbances, and is recognized by disorganized or incoherent speech, rambling or irrelevant conversation, unclear or illogical flow of ideas, or unpredictable switching from subject to subject.

Altered level of consciousness is typically manifested by lethargy, with reduced awareness of the environment. Clinically, delirium can present in either hypoactive or hyperactive forms. The hypoactive form of delirium—characterized by lethargy and reduced psychomotor activity—is the most common form in older patients. This form of delirium is often unrecognized, and is associated with a poorer overall prognosis (103–106). The hyperactive form of delirium, in which the patient is agitated, vigilant, and often hallucinating, is rarely missed. Importantly, patients can fluctuate between the hypoactive and hyperactive forms—the mixed type of delirium.

Confusion Assessment Method

Although the exact diagnostic criteria continue to evolve, the criteria for delirium appearing in the DSM-IV are widely used as the current diagnostic standard (107) (Table 13.5). However, these criteria were based on expert opinion, and their diagnostic performance has not been tested. The Confusion Assessment Method (CAM) (108,112) provides a validated tool, which is currently in widespread use for rapid identification of delirium (Table 13.5). The CAM algorithm, based on the presence of the features of acute onset and fluctuating course; inattention; and either disorganized speech or altered level of consciousness, has a sensitivity of 94% to 100%, specificity of 90% to 95%, positive predictive accuracy of 91% to 94%, and negative predictive accuracy of 90% to 100% for delirium (109).

TABLE 13.5. Diagnostic criteria for delirium (112)

DSM-IV diagnostic criteria

A. Disturbance of consciousness (i.e., reduced clarity of awareness of the environment) with reduced ability to focus, sustain, or shift attention.
B. A change in cognition (such as memory deficit, disorientation, language disturbance) or the development of a perceptual disturbance that is not better accounted for by a preexisting, established, or evolving dementia.
C. The disturbance develops over a short period of time (usually hours to days) and tends to fluctuate during the course of the day.
D. There is evidence from the history, physical examination, or laboratory findings that the disturbance is caused by the direct physiologic consequences of a general medical condition.

The Confusion Assessment Method (CAM) diagnostic algorithm*

Feature 1. Acute Onset and Fluctuating Course
    This feature is usually obtained from a family member or nurse and is shown by positive responses to the following questions: Is there evidence of an acute change in mental status from the patient's baseline? Did the (abnormal) behavior fluctuate during the day, that is, tend to come and go, or increase and decrease in severity?
Feature 2. Inattention
    This feature is shown by a positive response to the following question: Did the patient have difficulty focusing attention, for example, being easily distractible, or having difficulty keeping track of what was being said?
Feature 3. Disorganized Thinking
    This feature is shown by a positive response to the following question: Was the patient's thinking disorganized or incoherent, such as rambling or irrelevant conversation, unclear or illogical flow of ideas, or unpredictable switching from subject to subject?
Feature 4. Altered Level of Consciousness
    This feature is shown by any answer other than "alert" to the following question: Overall, how would you rate this patient's level of consciousness? (alert [normal], vigilant [hyperalert], lethargic [drowsy, easily aroused], stupor [difficult to arouse], or coma [unarousable]).

*The diagnosis of delirium by CAM requires the presence of features 1 and 2 and either 3 or 4.
Source: Adapted from Inouye SK. Delirium and other mental status problems in the older patients. In: Goldman L, Ausiello D, eds. Cecil Textbook of Medicine, 22nd ed. Philadelphia: WB Saunders, 2004;19–22, with permission from Elsevier. Reprinted as appears in Inouye SK. Delirium. In: Cassel CK, Leipzig RM, Cohen HJ, et al., eds., Geriatric Medicine, 4th ed. New York: Springer, 2003.

Laboratory Findings

Evidence-based strategies estimating the predictive value of laboratory tests in delirium assessment are lacking. Thus, the laboratory evaluation must be based on clinical judgment, and should be tailored to the individual situation. An astute history and physical examination, review of medications, targeted laboratory testing (e.g., complete blood count, chemistries, glucose, renal/liver function tests, urinalysis, oxygen saturation), and search for occult infection should assist with identification of the majority of potential contributors to the delirium. The need for further laboratory testing (such as thyroid function tests, B_{12} level, cortisol level, drug levels or toxicology screen, ammonia level) will be determined according to the individual patient's clinical picture. In patients with cardiac or respiratory diseases, or with related symptoms, an electrocardiogram, chest radiograph, or arterial blood gas determination may be warranted. The indications for cerebrospinal fluid examination, brain imaging, or electroencephalography remain controversial. Overall, the diagnostic yield for these procedures is low, and they are probably indicated in less than 10% of delirium cases. Cerebrospinal fluid examination is indicated for the febrile delirious patient where meningitis or encephalitis must be excluded. Brain imaging (such as CT or MRI) should be reserved for cases with new focal neurologic signs, with history or signs of head trauma, or without another identifiable cause of the delirium. Electroencephalography, which has a false-negative rate of 17% and false-positive rate of 22% for distinguishing delirious and nondelirious patients (105,106), plays a limited role and is most useful to detect occult seizure disorders and to differentiate delirium from nonorganic psychiatric conditions.

Differential Diagnosis

The paramount challenge in differential diagnosis is distinguishing dementia, a chronic confusional state, from delirium alone or delirium superimposed on dementia. These two conditions are distinguished by the acuity of symptom onset in delirium (dementia is much more insidious), and the impaired attention and altered level of consciousness associated with delirium. Disorientation and memory impairment, while commonly recognized features, are not useful in differential diagnosis, because they may be present with both conditions and may be absent in delirium. Differentiating depression and nonorganic psychotic disorders from delirium can pose other challenges for the clinician. Although paranoia, hallucinations, and affective changes can occur with delirium, the presence of key delirium features of acute onset, inattention, altered level of consciousness, and global cognitive impairment assists with the diagnosis of delirium.

Management Considerations

Nonpharmacologic Management

Nonpharmacologic approaches should be used for the management of every delirious patient. These approaches include strategies for reorientation and behavioral intervention, such as ensuring the presence of family members, orienting influences, use of sitters, and transferring a disruptive patient to a private room or closer to the nurse's station for increased supervision. Eyeglasses and hearing aids (if needed) should be worn as much as possible to reduce sensory deficits. Mobility, self-care, and independence should be enhanced; physical restraints should be avoided because of their adverse effects of immobility and increased agitation and their potential to cause injury. Clocks, calendars, and the day's schedule should be provided to assist with orientation. Room and staff changes should be kept to a minimum. A quiet environment with low-level lighting is optimal for the delirious patient. Allowing an uninterrupted period for sleep at night is of key importance in the management of the delirious patient.

Pharmacologic Management

Pharmacologic approaches should be reserved for patients with severe agitation, which may result in the interruption of essential medical therapies (e.g., intubation, intraaortic balloon pumps, dialysis catheters) or which may endanger the safety of the patient, other patients, or staff. However, clinicians must be aware that any drug used for the treatment of delirium will have psychoactive effects, and may further cloud mental status and obscure efforts to follow the patient's mental status. Thus, the drug should be given in the lowest possible dose for the shortest duration. Neuroleptics are the preferred agents of treatment, with haloperidol representing the most widely used and tested treatment for delirium. Although newer neuroleptics are available, fewer data are available to support their use. If parenteral administration is required, intravenous haloperidol results in rapid onset of action with short duration of effect, whereas intramuscular use will have a more optimal duration of action. The recommended starting dose of haloperidol is 0.5 to 1.0 mg orally or parenterally, repeating the dose every 20 to 30 minutes after vital signs have been checked, until sedation has been achieved. The end point should be *an awake but manageable patient, not a sedated patient*. The average elderly patient who has not previously been treated with neuroleptics should require a total loading dose not exceeding 3 to 5 mg of haloperidol. Subsequently, a maintenance dose of one half of the loading dose should be administered in divided doses over the next 24 hours, with tapering doses over the next few days. The leading side effects of haloperidol include sedation, hypotension, acute dystonias, extrapyramidal side effects, and anticholinergic effects (e.g., anticholinergic delirium, dry mouth, constipation, urinary retention).

Benzodiazepines are not recommended for treatment of delirium because of their tendency to cause oversedation, respiratory depression, and exacerbation of the confusional state. However, they remain the drugs of choice for treatment of withdrawal syndromes from alcohol and sedative-hypnotic drugs. For geriatric patients, lorazepam (starting dose 0.5 to 1.0 mg) is the recommended agent of this class, because of its favorable half-life (10 to 15 hours), lack of active metabolites, and availability of a parenteral form.

TABLE 13.6. Delirium risk factors and potential interventions (112)

Risk Factor	Interventions
Cognitive impairment	• Therapeutic activities program • Reality orientation program (reorienting techniques, communication)
Sleep deprivation	• Noise reduction strategies • Scheduling of nighttime medications, procedures, and nursing activities to allow uninterrupted period of sleep
Immobilization	• Early mobilization (e.g., ambulation or bedside exercises) Minimizing immobilizing equipment (e.g., bladder catheters)
Psychoactive medications	• Restricted use of PRN (as needed) sleep and psychoactive medications (e.g., sedative-hypnotics, narcotics, anticholinergic medications) • Nonpharmacologic protocols for management of sleep and anxiety
Vision impairment	• Provision of vision aids (e.g., magnifiers, special lighting) Provision of adaptive equipment (e.g., illuminated phone dials, large-print books)
Hearing impairment	• Provision of amplifying devices • Repair of hearing aids
Dehydration	• Early recognition and volume repletion

Source: Adapted from Inouye SK. Delirium and other mental status problems in the older patients. In: Goldman L, Ausiello D, eds. Cecil Textbook of Medicine, 22nd ed. Philadelphia: WB Saunders, 2004;19–22, with permission from Elsevier. Reprinted as appears in Inouye SK. Delirium. In: Cassel CK, Leipzig RM, Cohen HJ, et al., eds. Geriatric Medicine, 4th ed. New York: Springer, 2003.

Prevention

Primary prevention of delirium, that is, preventing delirium before it occurs, is the most effective strategy to reduce delirium and its attendant complications. Table 13.6 indicates well-documented delirium risk factors and tested preventive interventions for each risk factor (112). These risk factors were selected because current evidence supports both the clinical relevance and the remediable nature of each risk factor with practical interventions. A controlled clinical trial demonstrated the effectiveness of a delirium prevention strategy targeted to these risk factors. Implementation of these preventive interventions resulted in a 40% risk reduction for delirium in hospitalized older patients (114).

Prognosis

Delirium has been previously considered to be a transient, reversible condition; however, recent studies (109,110) have documented that delirium may be more persistent than previously believed. A delirium duration of 30 days or more is typical in older patients, and a prolonged transitional phase characterized by cognitive, affective, or behavioral abnormalities is quite common. Delirium appears to have greater deleterious effects on long-term cognitive functioning in patients with underlying cognitive impairment or dementia. Long-term detrimental effects are likely related to the duration, severity, and underlying cause(s) of the delirium. Whether delirium itself leads to permanent cognitive impairment or dementia remains controversial; however, previous studies document that at least some patients never recover their baseline level of cognitive functioning.

General Principles

- Dementia is a syndrome of progressive, global decline in cognition, severe enough to degrade the individual's well-being and social function.
- Persons with dementia have learning and memory problems, plus at least one of the following: impairments in communication (aphasia), reasoning and planning (executive function), recognition and manipulation of objects in space (agnosia, apraxia), orientation, and the regulation of emotion and aggression.
- The MMSE is the most widely used screening exam for impaired cognition in the United States. A perfect score is 30 with mild impairment falling between 18 and 24, and persons with moderately advanced dementia have MMSE scores ranging between 10 and 19.
- There are three cholinesterase inhibitors approved by the FDA for mild to moderate Alzheimer's disease: donepezil , rivastigmine and galantamine.
- Mood disorders are the most common reversible psychiatric conditions in later life. The five major classes of medications used to treat mood disorders are (1) selective serotonin reuptake inhibitors (SSRIs); (2) other novel antidepressants (venlafaxine, mirtazapine, bupropion, nefazodone); (3) tricyclic antidepressants; (4) MAO inhibitors; and (5) mood stabilizers (lithium carbonate, carbamazepine, and valproic acid).
- The key features of delirium are acute onset with a fluctuating course, inattentiveness, disorganization of thought, and altered level of consciousness.
- The Confusion Assessment Method (CAM) provides a validated tool that is currently in widespread use for rapid identification of delirium.
- Nonpharmacologic approaches should be used for management of every delirious patient, whereas pharmacologic approaches should be reserved for patients with severe agitation, which may result in the interruption of essential medical therapies or which may endanger the safety of the patient, other patients or staff.

Suggested Readings

Inouye SK. Delirium. In: Cassel CK, Leipzig RM, Cohen HJ, et al., eds. Geriatric Medicine, 4th ed. New York: Springer, 2003:1113–1122.
Kennedy GJ. Dementia. In: Cassel CK, Leipzig RM, Cohen HJ, et al., eds. Geriatric Medicine, 4th ed. New York: Springer, 2003:1079–1094.
Koenig HG, Blazer DG II. Depression, Anxiety and Other Mood Disorders. In: Cassel CK, Leipzig RM, Cohen HJ, et al., eds. Geriatric Medicine, 4th ed. New York: Springer, 2003:1163–1184.

References

1. Ritchie K, Kildea D. Is senile dementia "age-related" or "ageing related"?—evidence from meta-analysis of dementia prevalence in the oldest old. Lancet 1995;346:931–934.
2. Katzman R. Alzheimer's disease. N Engl J Med 1986;314:964–973.
3. Grober E, Lipton RB, Hall C, et al. Memory impairment on free and cued selective reminding predicts dementia. Neurology 2000;54:827–832.
4. Folstein M, Anthony JC, Parhad I, Duffy B, Gruenberg EM. The meaning of cognitive impairment in the elderly. J Am Geriatr Soc 1985;33:228–235.
5. Small GW, Rabins PV, Barry PP, et al. Diagnosis and treatment of Alzheimer disease and related disorders. JAMA 1997;278:1363–1371.
6. Cutler NR, Haxby JV, Duara R, et al. Brain metabolism as measured with serial assessment in a patient with familial Alzheimer's disease. Neurology 1985;35:184.
7. Stahelin HB, Monsch AU, Spiegel R. Early diagnosis of dementia via a two-step screening and diagnostic procedure. International Psychogeriatrics 1997;9:123–130.
8. Huber SJ, Paulson GW. The concept of subcortical dementia. Am J Psychiatry 1985;142:1313–1317.
9. Mahendra B. Depression and dementia: the multi-faceted relationship. Psychol Med 1985;15:227–236.
10. Heston LL, White JA, Mastri AR. Pick's disease; clinical genetics and natural history. Arch Gen Psychiatry 1987;44:409–411.
11. Folstein SE, Folstein MF. Psychiatric features of Huntington's disease. Psychiatr Dev 1983;2:193–206.
12. Peterson R, Smith G, Waring S, et al. Mild cognitive impairment; clinical characterization and outcome. Arch Neurol 1999;56:303–308.
13. Nyenhuis DL, Gorelick PB. Vascular dementia: a contemporary review of epidemiology, diagnosis, prevention, and treatment. J Am Geriatr Soc 1998;46:1437–1448.
14. Boss P, Caron W, Horbal J, Mortimer J. Predictors of depression in caregivers of dementia patients: boundary ambiguity and mastery. Family Process 1990;29:245–254.
15. Cohen D, Eisdorfer C. Depression in family members caring for a relative with Alzheimer's disease. J Am Geriatr Soc 1988;36:885–889.
16. Gallagher D, Rose J, Rivera P, et al. Prevalence of depression in family caregivers. Gerontologist 1989;29:449–456.

17. Rogers SL, Friedhof LT, Apter JT, et al. The efficacy and safety of donepezil in patients with Alzheimer's disease: results of a US multi-center, randomized, double-blind, placebo controlled trial. Dementia 1996;7:293–303.

18. Kaufer DI, Cummings JL, Christine D. Effect of tacrine on behavioral symptoms in Alzheimer's disease: an open label study. J Geriatr Psychiatry Neurol 1996;9:1–6.

19. Becker RE, Colliver JA, Markwell SJ, et al. Effects of metrifonate on cognitive decline in Alzheimer's disease: a double-blind, placebo-controlled, 6-month study. Alzheimer Dis Rel Disord 1998;12:54–67.

20. Knopman D, Schneider LS, Davis K, et al. Long term tacrine (Cognex) treatment effects on nursing home placement and mortality: the Tacrine Study Group. Neurology 1996;47:166–177.

21. Livingston G, Katona C. How useful are cholinesterase inhibitors in the treatment of Alzheimer's disease? A number needed to treat analysis. Int J Geriatr Psychiatry 2000;15:203–207.

22. Cameron I, Curran S, Newton P, et al. Use of donepesil for the treatment of mild-moderate Alzheimer's disease: an audit of the assessment and treatment of patients in routine clinical practice. Int J Geriatr Psychiatry 2000; 15:887–891.

23. Vellas B, Inglis F, Potkin S, et al. Interim results from an international clinical trial with rivastigmine evaluating a 2-week titration rate in mild to severe Alzheimer's disease patients. Int J Geriatric Psychopharm 1998;1:140–144.

24. Röseler M, Anand R, Cicin-Sain A, et al. Efficacy and safety of rivastigmine in patients with Alzheimer's disease: international randomized controlled trial. Br Med J 1999;318:633–638.

25. Maelicke A, Albequerque EX. Allosteric modulation of nicotinic acetylcholine receptors as a treatment strategy for Alzheimer's disease. Dement Geriatr Cogn Disord 2000;11(Suppl 1):11–18.

26. Reisberg B, Doody R, Stoffler A, et al. Memantine Study Group. Memantine in moderate-to-severe Alzheimer's disease. N Engl J Med 2003;348(14): 1333–1341.

27. Sano M, Ernesto C, Thomas RG, et al. A controlled trial of selegiline, alpha-tocopherol, or both as treatment or Alzheimer's disease. N Engl J Med 1997;336:1216–1222.

28. Marden K, Sano M. Estrogen to treat Alzheimer's disease: Too little, too late? So what's a woman to do? Neurology 2000;54:2035–2036.

29. Teri L, Rabins P, Whitehouse P, et al. Management of behavior disturbance in Alzheimer disease: Current knowledge and future directions. Alzheimer Dis Assoc Disord 1992;6:77–88.

30. Koenig HG, Meador KG, Shelp F, et al. Depressive disorders in hospitalized medically ill patients: a comparison of young and elderly men. J Am Geriatr Soc 1991;39:881–890.

31. Koenig HG, George LK, Peterson BL, et al. Depression in medically ill hospitalized older adults: prevalence, correlates, and course of symptoms based on six diagnostic schemes. Am J Psychiatry 1997;154:1376–1383.

32. Hyer L, Blazer DG. Depressive symptoms: impact and problems in long term care facilities. Int J Behav Geriatr 1982;1(3):33–35.

33. Parmelee PA, Katz IR, Lawton MP. Depression among institutionalized aged: assessment and prevalence estimation. J Gerontol 1989;44:M22–M29.

34. Weissman MM, Bruce ML, Leaf PJ, et al. Affective disorders. In: Robins LN, Regier DA, eds. Psychiatric Disorders in America: The Epidemiologic Catchment Area Study. New York: Free Press, 1991:53.
35. Rovner BW, German P, Brant LJ, et al. Depression and mortality in nursing homes. JAMA 1991;265:993–996.
36. Bebbington PE, Dunn G, Jenkins R, et al. The influence of age and sex on the prevalence of depressive conditions: report from the National Survey of Psychiatric Morbidity. Psychosom Med 1998;28:9–19.
37. Blazer DG, Hughes DC, George LK. The epidemiology of depression in an elderly community population. Gerontologist 1987;27:281–287.
38. Goldberg EL, Van Natta P, Comstock GW. Depressive symptoms, social networks and social support of elderly women. Am J Epidemiol 1985; 121:448–456.
39. Murrell SA, Himmelfarb S, Wright K. Prevalence of depression and its correlates in older adults. Am J Epidemiol 1983;117:173–185.
40. Meyers BS, Kalayam B, Mei-Tal V. Late-onset delusional depression: a distinct clinical entity? J Clin Psychiatry 1984;45:347–349.
41. Koenig HG, Kvale JN, Ferrel C. Religion and well-being in later life. Gerontologist 1988;28:18–28.
42. Koenig HG, Cohen HJ, Blazer DG, et al. Religious coping and depression in elderly hospitalized medically ill men. Am J Psychiatry 1992;149: 1693–1700.
43. Braam AW, Beekman ATF, Deeg DJH, et al. Religiosity as a protective or prognostic factor of depression in later life; results from the community survey in the Netherlands. Acta Psychiatr Scand 1997;96:199–205.
44. Koenig HG, George LK, Peterson BL. Religiosity and remission from depression in medically ill older patients. Am J Psychiatry 1998; 155:536–542.
45. Koenig HG. The Healing Power of Faith. New York: Simon & Schuster, 1999.
46. Sheikh JI, Yesavage JA. Geriatric Depression Scale (GDS): recent evidence and development of a shorter version. In: Clinical Gerontology: A Guide to Assessment and Intervention. New York: Haworth, 1986:165–173.
47. Beekman AT, Deeg DJ, Braam AW, Smit JH, Van Tilburg, W. Consequences of major and minor depression in later life: a study of disability, well-being and service delivery. Psychol Med 1997;27:1397–1409.
48. Weissman MM, Leaf PJ, Tischler GL, et al. Affective disorders in five United States communities. Psychol Med 1988;18:141–153.
49. De Alarcon R. Hypochondriasis and depression in the aged. Gerontology. 1964;6:266–277.
50. Beck AT, Rush J, Shaw B, et al. Cognitive Therapy of Depression. New York: Guilford, 1979.
51. Lewinsohn P. A behavioral approach to depression. In: Friedman R, Katz M, eds. The Psychology of Depression: Contemporary Theory and Research. New York: Wiley, 1974:157–176.
52. Klerman GL, Weissman MM, Rounsaville BJ, et al., eds. Interpersonal Psychotherapy of Depression. New York: Basic Books, 1984.
53. Arean PA, Perri MG, Nezu AM, et al. Comparative effectiveness of social problem-solving therapy and reminiscence therapy as treatments for depression in older adults. J Consult Clin Psychol 1993;61:1003–1010.

54. Myers WA. New Techniques in the Psychotherapy of Older Patients. Washington, DC: American Psychiatric Press, 1991.

55. Nies A, Robinson DS, Friedman MJ, et al. Relationship between age and tricyclic antidepressant pharmacokinetics and plasma levels. Am J Psychiatry 1977;134:790–793.

56. Tyrer P, Murphy S. The place of benzodiazepines in psychiatric practice. Br J Psychiatry 1987;151:719–723.

57. Greenblatt DJ, Shader RI, Abernathy DR. Current status of benzodiazepines: clinical use of benzodiazepines. N Engl J Med 1983;309:410–416.

58. Abrams R. Electroconvulsive Therapy, 2nd ed. New York: Oxford University Press, 1992.

59. Salzman C. Electroconvulsive therapy in the elderly. Psychiatr Clin North Am 1982;5:191–197.

60. Zervas IM, Calev A, Jandorf L. Age-dependent effects of electroconvulsive therapy on memory. Convulsive Ther 1993;9:39–42.

61. Baldwin RC, Jolley DJ. The prognosis of depression in old age. Br J Psychiatry 1986;149:574–583.

62. Post F. The management and nature of depressive illness in late life: a followthrough study. Br J Psychiatry 1972;121:393–404.

63. Murphy E, Smith R, Lindesay J, et al. Increased mortality rates in late-life depression. Br J Psychiatry 1988;152:347–353.

64. Murphy E. The prognosis of depression in old age. Br J Psychiatry 1983;142:111–119.

65. Black DW, Warrack G, Winokur G. The Iowa record-linkage study II: excess mortality among patients with organic mental disorders. Arch Gen Psychiatr 1885;42:78–81.

66. Fields SD, Mackenzie DR, Charlson ME, et al. Cognitive impairment: can it predict the course of hospitalized patients? J Am Geriatr Soc 1986;34:579–585.

67. Guze SB, Cantwell DP. The prognosis in "organic brain" syndromes. Am J Psychiatr 1964;120:878–881.

68. Guze SB, Daengsurisri S. Organic brain syndromes: prognostic significance in general medical patients. Arch Gen Psychiatr 1967;17:365–366.

69. Rabins PV, Folstein MF. Delirium and dementia: diagnostic criteria and fatality rates. Br J Psychiatry 1982;140:149–153.

70. Roth M. The natural history of mental disorder in old age. J Ment Sci 1955;101:281–303.

71. Trzepacz PT, Teague GB, Lipowski ZJ. Delirium and other organic mental disorders in a general hospital. Gen Hosp Psychiatr 1985;7:101–106.

72. Williams M, Campbell EB, Raynor WJ, et al. Predictors of acute confusional states in hospitalized elderly patients. Res Nurs Health 1985;8:31–40.

73. U.S. Bureau of the Census. Statistical Abstract of the United States, 116th ed. Washington, DC: 1996:165.

74. Elie M, Cole MG, Primeau FJ, Bellavance F. Delirium risk factors in elderly hospitalized patients. J Gen Intern Med 1998;13:204–212.

75. Foreman MD. Confusion in the hospitalized elderly: incidence, onset and associated factors. Res Nurs Health 1989;12:21–29.

76. Gustafson Y, Berggen D, Brannstrom B, et al. Acute confusional states in elderly patients treated for femoral fracture. J Am Geriatr Soc 1988;36:525–530.

77. Rogers MP, Liang MH, Daltroy LH, et al. Delirium after elective orthopedic surgery: risk factors and natural history. Int J Psychiatr Med 1989;19:109–121.
78. Schor J, Levkoff SE, Lipsitz LA, et al. Risk factors for delirium in hospitalized elderly. JAMA 1992;267:827–831.
79. Inouye SK. The dilemma of delirium: clinical and research controversies regarding diagnosis and evaluation of delirium in hospitalized elderly medical patients. Am J Med 1994;97:278–288.
80. Koponen H, Partanen J, Paakkonen A, et al. EEG spectral analysis in delirium. J Neurol Neurosurg Psychiatry 1989;52:980–985.
81. Foy A, O'Connell D, Henry D, et al. Benzodiazepine use as a cause of cognitive impairment in elderly hospital inpatients. J Gerontol Med Sci 1995;50A: M99–M106.
82. Marcantonio ER, Goldman L, Mangione CM, et al. A clinical prediction rule for delirium after elective noncardiac surgery. JAMA 1994;271:134–139.
83. Bates DW, Cullen DJ, Laird N, et al. Incidence of adverse drug events and potential adverse drug events: implications for prevention. JAMA 1995; 274:29–34.
84. Lindley CM, Tully MP, Paramsothy V, et al. Inappropriate medication is a major cause of adverse drug reactions in elderly patients. Age Ageing 1992;21:294–300.
85. Brook RH, Kamberg CJ, Mayer-Oakes A, et al. Appropriateness of acute medical care for the elderly: an analysis of the literature. Health Policy 1990;14:225–242.
86. Owens NJ, Sherburne NJ, Silliman RA, et al. The Senior Care Study: the optimal use of medications in acutely ill older patients. J Am Geriatr Soc 1990;38:1082–1087.
87. Millar HR. Psychiatric morbidity in elderly surgical patients. Br J Psychiatry 1981;38:17–20.
88. Flint FJ, Richards SM. Organic basis of confusional states in the elderly. Br Med J 1956;2:1537–1539.
89. Sirois F. Delirium: 100 cases. Can J Psychiatry 1988;33:375–378.
90. Seymour DG, Henschke RD, Cape T, et al. Acute confusional states and dementia in the elderly: the role of dehydration/volume depletion, physical illness and age. Age Ageing 1980;8:137–146.
91. Sier HC, Hartnell J, Morley JE, et al. Primary hyperparathyroidism and delirium in the elderly. J Am Geriatr Soc 1988;36:157–170.
92. Blackburn T, Dunn M. Cystocerebral syndrome: acute urinary retention presenting as confusion in elderly patients. Arch Intern Med 1990; 150:2577–2578.
93. Creditor MC. Hazards of hospitalization of the elderly. Ann Intern Med 1993;118:219–223.
94. Lazarus BA, Murphy JB, Colletta EM, et al. The provision of physical activity to hospitalized elderly patients. Arch Intern Med 1991;51: 2452–2456.
95. Becker PM, McVey LJ, Saltz CC, et al. Hospital-acquired complications in a randomized controlled clinical trial of a geriatric consultation team. JAMA 1982;257:2313–2317.
96. Steel K, Gertman PM, Crescenzi C, et al. Iatrogenic illness on a general medicine service at a university hospital. N Engl J Med 1981;304:638–642.

97. Trzepacz PT. Is there a final common neural pathway in delirium? Focus on acetylcholine and dopamine. Semin Clin Neuropsychiatry 2000;5:132–148.

98. Van der Mast RC. Pathophysiology of delirium. J Geriatr Psychiatry Neurol 1998;11:138–145.

99. McIntosh TK, Bush HL, Yeston NS, et al. Beta-endorphin, cortisol, and postoperative delirium: a preliminary report. Psychoneuroendocrinology 1985;10:303–313.

100. Blass JP, Gibson GE, Duffy TE, et al. Cholinergic dysfunction: a common denominator in metabolic encephalopathies. In: Pepeu G, Ladinsky H, eds. Cholinergic Mechanisms. New York: Plenum Press, 1981:921–928.

101. Flacker JM, Lipsitz LA. Large neutral amino acid changes and delirium in febrile elderly medical patients. J Gerontol Biol Sci 2000;55A: B249–B252.

102. Liptzin B, Levkoff SE. An empirical study of delirium subtypes. Br J Psychiatry 1992;161:843–845.

103. van Hemert AM, van der Mast RC, Hengeveld MW, et al. Excess mortality in general hospital patients with delirium: a 5-year follow-up of 519 patients seen in psychiatric consultation. J Psychosom Res 1994;38(4)339–346.

104. Murray AM, Levkoff SE, Wetle TT, et al. Acute delirium and functional decline in the hospitalized elderly patients. J Gerontol Med Sci 1993;48: M181–M186.

105. Rockwood K, Cosway S, Stolee P, et al. Increasing the recognition of delirium in elderly patients. J Am Geriatr Soc 1994;42:252–256.

106. Thomas RI, Cameron DJ, Fahs MC. A prospective study of delirium and prolonged hospital stay: exploratory study. Arch Gen Psychiatry 1988; 45:937–940.

107. American Psychiatric Association. Diagnostic and Statistical Manual of Mental Disorders (DSM-IV), 4th ed. Washington, DC: American Psychiatric Association, 1994.

108. Inouye SK, van Dyck CH, Alessi CA, Balkin S, Siegal AP, Horwitz RI. Clarifying confusion: the Confusion Assessment Method; a new method for detection of delirium. Ann Intern Med 1990;113:941–948.

109. Williams-Russo P, Urquhart BL, Sharrock NE, et al. Post-operative delirium: predictors and prognosis in elderly orthopedic patients. J Am Geriatr Soc 1992;40:759–767.

110. Brannstron B, Gustafson Y, Norberg A, et al. ADL performance and dependency on nursing care in patients with hip fractures and acute confusion in a task allocation care system. Scand J Caring Sci 1988;5:3–11.

111. Molloy DW, Alemayehu E, Roberts R. A standardized Mini-Mental State Examination (SMMSE): its reliability compared to the traditional Mini-Mental Sate Examination (MMSE). Am J Psychiatry 1991;148:102–105.

112. Inouye SK. Delirium and other mental status problems in the older patients. In: Goldman L, Ausiello D, eds. Cecil Textbook of Medicine, 22nd ed. Philadelphia: WB Saunders, 2004:19–22.

113. Kennedy GJ. Geriatric Mental Health Care: A Treatment Guide for Health Professionals. New York: Guilford, 2000:48.

114. Inouye SK, Bogardus ST, Charpentier PA, et al. A multicomponent intervention to prevent delirium in hospitalized older patients. N Engl J Med 1999; 340:669–676.

14
Insomnia and Other Sleep Disorders

Reena Karani

Learning Objectives

Upon completion of the chapter, the student will be able to:

1. List the most common sleep complaints in older adults.
2. Understand the definition, diagnostic features, and therapeutic options of common sleep disorders in older adults.
3. Know the rules of sleep hygiene for the elderly.

General Considerations

The prevalence of sleep complaints increases dramatically with age, and is estimated to be about 40% in the elderly population. These sleep problems are not a consequence of the aging process per se, but are strongly related to medical and psychiatric comorbidities as well as to psychosocial changes in later life.

The most common sleep complaints among older adults include:

- Waking up during the night
- Not feeling well rested and needing to take daytime naps
- Difficulty falling asleep

Sleep complaints are associated with coexisting health disorders, including poor self-perceived health, depressive symptoms, respiratory symptoms, physical disabilities, chronic medical conditions, and medication use.

Material in this chapter is based on the following chapter in Cassel CK, Leipzig RM, Cohen HJ, Larson EB, Meier DE, eds. Geriatric Medicine: An Evidence-Based Approach, 4th ed. New York: Springer, 2003: Shochat T, Ancoli-Israel S. Sleep and Sleep Disorders, pp. 1031–1042. Selections edited by Reena Karani.

TABLE 14.1. Definitions

Apnea: literally means "no breath." Complete pauses in respiration during sleep lasting at least 10 seconds.

Hypopnea: partial pauses in respiration during sleep lasting at least 10 seconds.

Myoclonus index (MI): Number of limb kicks with arousal per hour of sleep.

Non–rapid eye movement (NREM) sleep: Includes stages 1, 2, 3, and 4 sleep. Characterized by quiet sleep and little or no dream behavior; EEG shows slower and larger brain waves. Usually accounts for 75–80% of TST.

Rapid eye movement (REM) sleep: stage of sleep in which brain activity is extensive; dreams and rapid eye movements are common; electroencephalogram (EEG) shows low voltage, fast-frequency signals. Usually accounts for 20–25% of TST.

Respiratory disturbance index (RDI): Number of apneic and hypopneic episodes per hour of sleep.

Sleep efficiency: amount of time asleep relative to the total amount of time in bed.

Stage 1 sleep: NREM stage that is the transitional state between wakefulness and sleep. Characterized by slow rolling eye movements, low-voltage waves, and no sleep spindles on EEG. Usually accounts for approximately 4–6% of TST.

Stage 2 sleep: NREM stage that is characterized by mixed frequency EEG signals and sleep spindles. Usually accounts for approximately 50–55% of TST.

Stage 3 sleep: NREM stage defined by slow, delta waves on EEG, and along with stage 4, constitutes "deep NREM sleep." Usually appears only in the first third of the sleep period and accounts for 4–6% of TST.

Stage 4 sleep: NREM stage defined by slow, delta waves on EEG, and along with stage 3, constitutes "deep NREM sleep." Usually accounts for 12–13% of TST.

Total sleep time (TST): amount of actual sleep time or total rapid eye movement (REM) and non-REM (NREM) time.

Source: Adapted from Shochat T, Ancoli-Israel S. Sleep and Sleep Disorders. In: Cassel CK, Leipzig RM, Cohen HJ, et al., eds. Geriatric Medicine, 4th ed. New York: Springer, 2003:1031–1042.

Age Associated Changes in Sleep

Normal age-related changes that occur in sleep architecture include decreased sleep efficiency, decreased total sleep time, decreased stages 3 and 4 sleep, and increased stage 1 sleep (1). For definitions of common nomenclature, see Table 14.1.

Case A

Mr. Gonzalez, a 78-year-old man with diabetes, arthritis, and hypertension, comes to see you with his wife, who appears extremely concerned today. She tells you that over the past 2 months his snoring has gotten much worse and is keeping her up at night. In addition, she has noticed that Mr. Gonzalez often stops breathing at night for long periods of time and then suddenly wakes up "choking." Mr. Gonzalez is irritated about her complaining and informs you that his only new problem is the headache he has been waking up with every morning for the past several weeks.

Sleep-Disordered Breathing

Definition and Prevalence

Sleep-disordered breathing (SDB) or sleep apnea is characterized by complete or partial cessation of breathing, lasting at least 10 seconds, which occurs repeatedly throughout the night. The condition is defined by a respiratory disturbance index RDI >10, and the prevalence is 70% in elderly men and 56% in elderly women respectively, compared to only 15% and 5% of younger men and women, respectively (2,3).

Although there are two types of apnea, obstructive and central, many patients have a mixed picture, with both central and obstructive components (Table 14.2 and Fig. 14.1).

Sleep-disordered breathing is also an independent risk factor for hypertension (4), is associated with obesity and cardiac arrhythmias (5,6), and in severe cases may be linked to increased mortality (7,8).

Diagnostic Evaluation

Sleep-disordered breathing must be evaluated by an all-night sleep recording. Traditionally this is done in a sleep laboratory with equipment to measure airflow, oxyhemoglobin levels, RDI, and abdominal and chest movements. For elderly patients who may become confused or disoriented or simply uncomfortable while sleeping away from home, portable equipment can be set up in the patient's home.

TABLE 14.2. Characteristics of obstructive and central types of apnea

	Obstructive apnea	Central apnea
Causes	Anatomic obstruction of the airway during sleep	Failure of central nervous system (CNS) respiratory center neurons to fire
Commonly encountered patient features	Obesity Increased neck girth	History of congestive heart failure History of stroke
Symptoms	+ Loud snoring + Respiratory effort + Choking or gasping for air	+/− Loud snoring − Respiratory effort + Choking or gasping for air
Relation to body position	Yes; supine position may increase frequency and severity	No
Excessive daytime sleepiness	Yes	Yes

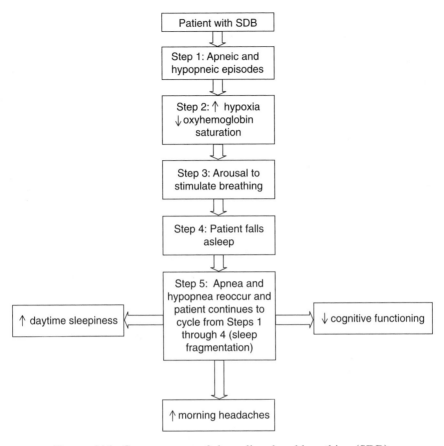

FIGURE 14.1. Consequences of sleep disordered breathing (SDB).

Management Considerations

General Interventions

Agents or activities that may exacerbate the severity of apnea should be avoided. These include alcohol, sedating medications (9,10), and smoking (11). For obese patients with SDB, weight loss can significantly reduce or eliminate the respiratory events (12). For positional apnea, sewing a pocket to the back of a nightshirt and placing a tennis ball inside the pocket is a simple, noninvasive method to avoid lying in a supine position (13).

Continuous Positive Airway Pressure

The continuous positive airway pressure (CPAP) machine continuously administers positive pressure through a hose connected to a face mask.

The mask is worn over the patient's nose. Air pressure is administered at a calculated level to act as a splint and keep the airway from collapsing during sleep. The CPAP mask must be worn every night, and compliance is therefore an important issue. This is the treatment of choice for obstructive sleep apnea (14). Although CPAP does not cure SDB, it is effective in decreasing

- apneic and hypopneic events,
- oxygen desaturation,
- snoring,
- excessive daytime sleepiness, and
- overall fatigue,

and in improving

- mood and
- general health.

Surgical Interventions

The most common anatomic obstructions causing obstructive sleep apnea are found in the nose, soft palate, or the base of the tongue. Surgical procedures for the correction of these abnormalities have been developed, but documented success rates are variable (Table 14.3).

Pharmacologic Agents

Pharmacologic treatments for SDB are only marginally successful. Commonly used agents include respiratory stimulants such as progesterone and acetazolamide for central sleep apnea, and tricyclic antidepressants for SDB associated with rapid eye movement (REM) sleep. Benzodiazepines must be avoided in patients with SDB because their sedative properties exacerbate the severity of the respiratory events.

TABLE 14.3. Indications for surgical intervention in sleep disordered breathing

Surgical intervention	Indication
Nasal reconstruction	Obstructed nasal airway
Pharyngeal reconstruction or	Excess tissue in the soft palate
uvulopalatopharyngoplasty (UPPP)	Enlarged uvula
	Enlarged tonsillar adenoidal tissue
Laser assisted uvulopalatoplasty (LAUP)	Excess tissue in the soft palate
	Enlarged uvula
	Enlarged tonsillar adenoidal tissue
Genioglossus advancement	Obstructed base of the tongue
Maxillomandibular advancement	Severe SDB, refractory to other treatments

Oral Appliances

Tongue retaining and mandibular advancement devices have been developed, and both are designed to enlarge the airway at the base of the tongue by advancing the tongue or the mandible forward. Although compliance rates are in the range of 50% to 100%, success rates (i.e., achieving a RDI <10) are only about 50% (15). Therefore, oral appliances are indicated for patients who do not respond to behavioral treatment such as weight loss or body position, who are intolerant to CPAP, or who are not candidates for surgery (16).

Case B

Mrs. Khan is a 65-year-old woman admitted for a chronic obstructive pulmonary disease (COPD) exacerbation. During morning rounds, she tells you that she has been having trouble falling asleep almost every night now for several weeks. When you review her chart, you notice the most recent nursing note: "Overnight patient appeared to be restless and kicking her legs in the bed. She awakened frequently in the early part of the night but subsequently fell asleep at 4 a.m."

Periodic Limb Movements in Sleep

Definition and Prevalence

Periodic limb movements in sleep (PLMS) is a disorder in which patients involuntarily kick their limbs (most often their legs) in short, clustered episodes lasting between 0.5 and 5 seconds. The kicks are often accompanied by arousals, and these episodes occur repeatedly throughout the night occurring about every 20 to 40 seconds. Periodic limb movements in sleep occurs most often in the first half of the night, during sleep stages 1 and 2. The condition is defined by myoclonus index (MI) >5, and the prevalence is approximately 45% in adults aged 65 years and older compared to only 5% to 6% in younger adults (17,18).

Although the nighttime arousals of PLMS are often too short to be recalled, patients may complain of insomnia, as they may have difficulty falling asleep as well as settling back to sleep following these episodes. In addition, patients present with complaints of excessive daytime sleepiness and may note that the bedding is very disorganized when they wake up in the morning. Bed partners often complain of the leg kicks disturbing their sleep.

Diagnostic Evaluation

Periodic limb movements in sleep must be evaluated by an all-night sleep recording. The MI is measured by recording movements of the anterior tibialis muscles and an EEG is used to measure signs of arousal, which may follow the limb jerks. As with SDB, portable equipment can also be set up in the patient's home.

Differential Diagnoses

Restless leg syndrome (RLS) is a related disorder that occurs during the relaxed, awake state often just prior to sleep onset. Patients report unpleasant, sometimes painful sensations and irresistible movements of their legs. The prevalence of RLS is not well defined, but most patients with RLS also suffer from PLMS, suggesting that these disorders may be related. Symptoms are alleviated by rubbing or squeezing the legs, or simply by walking.

Other movement disorders that must be differentiated from PLMS include hypnic myoclonus, and nocturnal leg cramps and jerks associated with long-term use of L-dopa (19).

Restless leg syndrome and PLMS may also be associated with medical conditions such as uremia, anemia, chronic lung disease, myelopathies, and peripheral neuropathies. In addition, medications such as tricyclic antidepressants and lithium carbonate, or withdrawal from benzodiazepines and anticonvulsants, may induce these disorders.

Management Considerations

Pharmacologic Agents

Periodic limb movements in sleep is treated with agents that reduce or eliminate leg jerks or arousals. Dopaminergic agents such as carbidopa/levodopa, pergolide (20), and pramipexole are the treatments of choice for PLMS, as they decrease both leg jerks and arousals. These medications are also successful for the treatment of RLS (20).

Benzodiazepines, such as clonazepam, decrease arousals but do not eliminate the limb movements (21). Due to age-related changes in pharmacokinetics and the need to avoid daytime sedation, these agents should only be used at lower doses and with great caution in older adults (22).

Opiates such as propoxyphene or acetaminophen with codeine are effective in decreasing the leg jerks, but the arousals may continue to occur.

Case C

Mr. Robinson is an 80-year-old nursing-home resident with hypertension and severe Parkinson's disease. His nighttime aide is afraid to continue watching over Mr. Robinson since he has become more aggressive and violent during the night. The aide tells you that the patient thrashes about at night kicking, punching, and scratching himself and anyone who comes to his assistance. The aide is very puzzled because Mr. Robinson does not act like this during the day.

Rapid Eye Movement Sleep Behavior Disorder

Definition and Prevalence

Rapid eye movement sleep behavior disorder (RBD) is a disorder in which the muscle atonia typical of the REM state is absent, causing vigorous movements that may be violent or aggressive toward the patient and/or the bed partner. It occurs most often in the second half of the night when REM sleep is most abundant, and may become more frequent over time. The condition is most often idiopathic but is considered a neuropathologic disorder and has been associated with neurodegenerative conditions such as dementia, parkinsonism, Guillain-Barré syndrome, olivopontocerebellar degeneration, and subarachnoid hemorrhage (23). It is also associated with depression, drug and alcohol abuse, and withdrawal syndromes. The prevalence of RBD is unknown, but predominately older men are diagnosed with the disorder.

A majority of RBD sufferers report ecchymoses, lacerations, and fractures to themselves and to their bed partners (24). Upon awakening, these patients remember vivid dreams that are consistent with their observed behavior during the night. In addition, some patients exhibit other sleep disorders such as narcolepsy and PLMS.

Diagnostic Evaluation

A detailed history of the sleep disorder, about the timing and frequency of the episodes and the types of behavioral disturbances, should be obtained from both the patient and the bed partner. One study suggests the following criteria for diagnosing RBD: a history or videotape recording of abnormal sleep behavior, and an electromyogram (EMG) recording showing elevated muscle tone or phasic limb twitching (25).

Differential Diagnosis

Night terrors and sleepwalking are disruptive behavioral enactments that occur during sleep. Unlike RBD, however, these occur during non-REM sleep, often in the early part of the night.

Another differential diagnosis is Parkinson's disease (PD). About 30% of PD patients treated with L-dopa exhibit a similar sleep disturbance (26).

Management Considerations

Pharmacologic Agents

Rapid eye movement sleep behavior disorder is treated with agents that reduce the vivid dreams and disruptive behaviors. Low-dose clonazepam, a benzodiazepine, is very effective in reducing both the vivid dreams and disruptive behaviors of RBD. When clonazepam is not well tolerated, alprazolam may be used. Due to age-related changes in pharmacokinetics and the need to avoid daytime sedation, these agents should only be used at lower doses and with great caution in older adults.

Other treatment options include tricyclic antidepressants such as desipramine (23) and antiepileptics such as carbamazepine (27).

Case D

Mrs. Chan is a 74-year-old widow who recently moved into an assisted living facility. She complains of difficulty falling asleep and decreased energy during the day as a result of poor sleep during the night. She recently read about melatonin for sleep and is wondering if it will help her problem.

Insomnia

Definition and Prevalence

Insomnia, unlike SDB, PLMS, or RBD, is not a sleep disorder but rather a complaint of insufficient and nonrestorative sleep. It is usually short lasting (several days to weeks) and is most often related to a specific stressful event such as taking an exam, starting a new job, or the loss of a loved one. Long-term insomnia can develop, and possible causes include medical, psychiatric, drug and medication use, and psychophysiologic issues. The prevalence of this complaint increases with age (28), and in one study over 50% of elderly patients complained of insomnia (29). Insomnia is associated with depressed mood, respiratory symptoms, poor perceived health, physical disabilities, widowhood, and the use of sedatives (30).

The most common insomnia-related complaints among the elderly include waking up too early in the morning and having difficulty getting back to sleep. Many older adults also suffer from advanced sleep phase syndrome (ASPS). Here, the timing of the sleep period is advanced to an earlier hour, and wake up time is correspondingly advanced as well.

Diagnostic Evaluation

A complete history is necessary to differentiate among the different types of insomnia, and a sleep diary provides additional information (Table 14.4). Three common types include:

- Sleep-onset insomnia or difficulty falling asleep: The patient may lie in bed without falling asleep anywhere from 30 minutes to a few hours.
- Sleep-maintenance insomnia or difficulty maintaining sleep throughout the night: The patient falls asleep easily, but awakens one to several times during the night and has difficulty falling back to sleep.
- Mixed-pattern insomnia or both sleep-onset and sleep-maintenance insomnia.

TABLE 14.4. Example of a sleep diary

Day: Date: Patient ID:

Complete before bedtime:

1. How many naps did you take today?
   Times: From:__:__ AM/PM To:__:__ AM/PM
          From:__:__ AM/PM To:__:__ AM/PM
2. How many cups of coffee or other beverages with caffeine did you drink?
   Times:__:__ AM/PM
         __:__ AM/PM
3. How many alcoholic beverages did you drink?
   Times:__:__ AM/PM
         __:__ AM/PM

Complete in the morning:

1. What time did you go to bed? __:__ AM/PM
2. What time did you turn out the lights and go to sleep? __:__AM/PM
3. How long did it take you to fall asleep? __ hours and __ minutes
4. How many awakenings did you have during the night? __
5. What time did you wake up in the morning? __:__ AM/PM
6. What time did you get out of bed? __:__ AM/PM
7. Did you feel refreshed when you got up? Yes/No

Source: Shochat T, Ancoli-Israel S. Sleep and sleep disorders. In: Cassel CK, Leipzig RM, Cohen HJ, et al., eds. Geriatric Medicine, 4th ed. New York: Springer, 2003.

Differential Diagnosis

The pain and discomfort associated with conditions such as cerebrovascular disease, arthritis, chronic obstructive pulmonary disease, and neurologic disorders can cause chronic insomnia (31). Alerting or stimulating agents such as central nervous system (CNS) stimulants, decongestants, beta-blockers, calcium channel blockers, corticosteroids, bronchodilators, and certain antidepressants may cause insomnia (13). Further, sedating medications that cause drowsiness and daytime napping can increase nighttime insomnia. Substances such as alcohol, caffeine, and nicotine can all cause insomnia.

Management Considerations

As many factors may contribute to insomnia, identifying and treating the underlying cause is the key for a successful outcome. A sleep diary completed by the patient can assist in determining optimal management interventions (Table 14.4). Nonpharmacologic or behavioral therapies are also essential in the management of insomnia-related complaints.

Nonpharmacologic Therapy

Sleep Hygiene

Sleep hygiene is aimed at maintaining healthy sleep habits and should be reviewed with all elderly patients suffering from insomnia. Guidelines include avoiding or limiting naps; avoiding substances that interfere with sleep such as alcohol, caffeine, and nicotine; changing the timing of medication administration based on whether the agent is stimulating or sedating; maintaining a stable sleep/wake pattern throughout the week; and exercising regularly (32). For a list of sleep hygiene rules see Table 14.5.

TABLE 14.5. Rules of sleep hygiene in the elderly (32)

1. Maintain a regular sleep/wake schedule.
2. Take no more than one nap per day.
3. Limit nap time to <60 minutes early in the day.
4. Exercise regularly.
5. Spend time in bright outdoor light.
6. Avoid caffeine, especially after lunch.
7. Avoid alcohol and nicotine.
8. Check the effects of medications on sleep.
9. Limit liquid intake in the evening.

Source: Reprinted from Marin J, Shochat T, Ancoli-Israel S. Assessment and treatment of sleep disturbances in older adults. Clin Psychol Rev 2000;20:783–805, with permission from Elsevier.

TABLE 14.6. Patient instructions for stimulus control therapy (33)

1. Patient goes to bed only when sleepy.
2. If not asleep within about 20 minutes, patient gets out of bed and engages in relaxing activity.
3. Patient returns to bed only when sleepy.
4. If patient again does not fall asleep within 20 minutes, repeat as necessary.
5. Wake-up time remains the same every day (regardless of number of hours asleep).
6. Daytime naps must be avoided.
7. Bed is used only for sleeping (not for reading, paying bills, or watching television).

Source: Reprinted from Bootzin RR, Nicassio PM. Behavioral treatments for insomnia. In: Hersen M, Eisler RM, Miller PM, eds. Progress in Behavior Modification, vol 6. New York: Academic Press, 1978;1–45, with permission from Elsevier.

Stimulus Control Therapy

Stimulus control therapy (33) is a behavioral technique designed to remove negative associations from the bedroom environment. It is appropriate for patients who feel stress, tension, or anxiety in the bed or bedroom. Patients are instructed to go to bed only when sleepy, and if they are unable to fall asleep in 15 to 20 minutes, they are told to leave the bedroom and engage in a relaxing activity, such as reading a magazine or writing a letter. Only when the patient feels sleepy again can he/she return to bed. For patient instructions for stimulus control therapy, see Table 14.6.

Sleep Restriction Therapy

Sleep restriction therapy (34) is designed to reduce time in bed in order to improve sleep efficiency. Patients are instructed to stay in bed only for the amount of time that they actually sleep (assessed by a subjective sleep log) plus 15 minutes (35,36). When sleep efficiency reaches ≥85%, time in bed may be increased by 15 minutes. The procedure is repeated until the desired amount of time in bed is reached. (For further details about sleep restriction therapy, see Chapter 70: Sleep and Sleep Disorders. In: Cassel CK, et al., eds. Geriatric Medicine, 4th ed., page 1037.)

Bright Light Therapy

Bright light therapy is used for the treatment of circadian rhythm sleep disorders. By changing the timing of light exposure, this therapy effectively shifts altered circadian rhythms to a more appropriate phase. For the elderly with advanced sleep phase syndrome, daily exposure to bright light in the evening hours delays the sleep episode to a later phase, so that they no longer experience the early morning awakenings.

Pharmacologic Therapies

These therapies should only be used in combination with nonpharmacologic or behavioral therapies. It is imperative to establish the type of sleep disturbance to determine the appropriative therapeutic agent.

Ultrashort-acting or short-acting, fast-absorbing sedative-hypnotics such as zolpidem or zaleplon are used to treat sleep-onset insomnia, whereas medium-acting sedative-hypnotics such as temazepam are used for sleep-maintenance insomnia. Long-acting hypnotics are generally contraindicated because they create excessive daytime sleepiness and diminished performance the following day (37). Due to age-related changes in pharmacokinetics and the need to avoid daytime sedation, these agents should be used only at lower doses and with great caution in older adults (22).

Melatonin, a natural hormone secreted by the pineal gland during the night, is associated with sleep promotion and circadian rhythm regulation. Melatonin secretion decreases in the elderly, and this has been associated with a decline in sleep quality (38). In those adults with low natural melatonin levels, melatonin supplementation has been found to improve sleep efficiency (39), but data about correct dosage and timing of administration are still unavailable. Moreover, melatonin is sold over-the-counter as a food supplement, and as such, lacks proper quality control.

Case E

Mr. Butler is an 84-year-old man with moderate Alzheimer's disease who has just been transferred to your nursing home. Prior to this, his family had been taking care of him at home. His son tells you that Mr. Butler no longer slept at night but wandered around the house confused and agitated. The family and Mr. Butler's doctor thought the problem would resolve, but when it continued over several months, the overwhelmed and exhausted family sought help.

Dementia and Sleep Disturbance

Dementia is highly associated with sleep disruption. Sleep/wake patterns in dementia are often polyphasic, with frequent nighttime awakenings and redistribution of sleep episodes throughout the day (40). Specifically, demented patients suffer from increased stage 1 sleep, decreased stage 3, 4, and REM sleep, and decreased sleep efficiency (41,42).

Circadian rhythm disorders are common in this population, resulting in nocturnal awakenings accompanied by agitation, confusion, and wandering. This pattern is often referred to as "sun downing," as it typically occurs at the same time of day (43). Bright light therapy has been found to be an effective treatment for this condition in older, institutionalized adults (44–46). The prevalence of SDB is also higher in demented older adults (33–70%) and there is a strong positive correlation between the severity of dementia and the severity of SDB (47,48). The causes of these sleep disturbances in demented patients may be due to neurodegenerative processes in areas of the brain that regulate sleep/wake mechanisms and respiratory effort.

General Principles

- The prevalence of sleep complaints increases with age, and the most common complaints are difficulty falling asleep, waking up at night, and not feeling well rested during the day.
- Sleep disordered breathing (SDB) or sleep apnea is characterized by complete or partial cessation of breathing that occurs repeatedly during the night.
- Periodic limb movements in sleep (PLMS) is a disorder in which patients kick their limbs involuntarily during the night, and these episodes result in arousals and poor sleep.
- Rapid eye movement sleep behavior disorder (RBD) causes vigorous and violent movements during the night that may be harmful to the patient and/or the bed partner.
- Insomnia, a complaint of insufficient or nonrestorative sleep, affects many older adults and impacts both their mood and general medical health.
- Sleep hygiene guidelines promote continuous and effective sleep and should be reviewed with all patients presenting with a sleep complaint.
- Dementia is highly associated with sleep disturbances.

Suggested Readings

American Thoracic Society. Indications and standards for use of nasal continuous positive airway pressure (CPAP) in sleep apnea syndromes. Am J Respir Crit Care Med 1994;150:1738–1745. *Reviews the use of CPAP in the various sleep apnea syndromes.*

Ancoli-Israel S. Epidemiology of sleep disorders. In: Roth T, Roehrs TA, eds. Clinics in Geriatric Medicine. Philadelphia: WB Saunders, 1989:347–362. *Broad review of sleep disorders including prevalence, diagnosis, evaluation and treatment.*

Shochat T, Ancoli-Israel S. Sleep and sleep disorders. In: Cassel CK, Leipzig RM, Cohen HJ, et al., eds. Geriatric Medicine, 4th ed. New York: Springer, 2003: 1031–1042.

Vitiello MV. Sleep disorders and aging: understanding the causes. J Gerontol 1997;52A:M189–M191. *Provides a comprehensive review of the causes of sleep disorders in older adults.*

References

1. Vitiello MV. Sleep disorders and aging: understanding the causes. J Gerontol 1997;52A:M189–M191.
2. Ancoli-Israel S, Kripke DF, Klauber MR, Mason WJ, Fell R, Kaplan O. Sleep disordered breathing in community-dwelling elderly. Sleep 1991;14(6): 486–495.
3. Young T, Palta M, Dempsey J, Skatrud J, Weber S, Badr S. The occurrence of sleep disordered breathing among middle-aged adults. N Engl J Med 1993; 328:1230–1235.
4. Lavie P, Herer P, Hoffstein V. Obstructive sleep apnea syndrome as a risk factor for hypertension: population study. BMJ (Clinical Research Ed.) 2000;320:479–482.
5. Wittels EH. Obesity and hormonal factors in sleep and sleep apnea. Med Clin North Am 1985;69:1265–1280.
6. Guilleminault C. Natural history, cardiac impact and long term follow-up of sleep apnea syndrome. In: Guilleminault C, Lugaresi E, eds. Sleep/Wake Disorders: Natural History, Epidemiology, and Long-term Evolution. New York: Raven Press, 1983:107–124.
7. Lavie P, Herer P, Peled R, et al. Mortality in sleep apnea patients: a multivariate analysis of risk factors. Sleep 1995;18:149–157.
8. Ancoli-Israel S, Kripke DF, Klauber MR, et al. Morbidity, mortality and sleep disordered breathing in community dwelling elderly. Sleep 1996;19: 277–282.
9. Guilleminault C, Silvestri R, Mondini S, Coburn S. Aging and sleep apnea: action of benzodiazepine, acetazolamide, alcohol, and sleep deprivation in a healthy elderly group. J Gerontol 1984;39:655–661.
10. Block AJ, Hellard DW, Slayton PC. Effect of alcohol ingestion on breathing and oxygenation during sleep. Analysis of the influence of age and sex. Am J Med 1986;80:595–600.
11. Wetter DW, Young TB, Bidwell TR, Badr MS, Palta M. Smoking as a risk factor for sleep-disordered breathing. Arch Intern Med 1994;154:2219–2224.
12. Loube DI, Loube AA, Mitler MM. Weight loss for obstructive sleep apnea: the optimal therapy for obese patients. J Am Diet Assoc 1994;94:1291–1295.
13. Ancoli-Israel S. Sleep problems in older adults: putting myths to bed. Geriatrics 1997;52:20–30.
14. American Thoracic Society. Indications and standards for use of nasal continuous positive airway pressure (CPAP) in sleep apnea syndromes. Am J Respir Crit Care Med 1994;150:1738–1745.
15. Schmidt-Nowara WW, Lowe A, Wiegand L, Cartwright R, Perez-Guerra F, Menn S. Oral appliances for the treatment of snoring and obstructive sleep apnea: a review. Sleep 1995;18:501–510.
16. An American Sleep Disorders Associations Report. Practice parameters for the treatment of snoring and obstructive sleep apnea with oral appliances. Sleep 1995;18:511–513.

17. Ancoli-Israel S, Kripke DF, Klauber MR, Mason WJ, Fell R, Kaplan O. Periodic limb movements in sleep in community-dwelling elderly. Sleep 1991; 14(6):496–500.
18. Bixler EO, Kales A, Vela-Bueno A, Jacoby JA, Scarone S, Soldatos CR. Nocturnal myoclonus and nocturnal myoclonic activity in a normal population. Res Commun Chem Pathol Pharmacol 1982;36:129–140.
19. Montplaisir J, Godbout R, Pelletier G, Warnes H. Restless leg syndrome and periodic limb movements during sleep. In: Kryger MH, Roth T, Dement WC, eds. Principles and Practice of Sleep Medicine, 2nd ed. Philadelphia: WB Saunders, 1994:589–597.
20. Earley CJ, Allen RP. Pergolide and carbidopa/levodopa treatment of the restless legs syndrome and periodic leg movements in sleep in a consecutive series of patients. Sleep 1996;19:801–810.
21. Mitler MM, Browman CP, Menn SJ, Gujavarty K, Timms RM. Nocturnal myoclonus: treatment efficacy of clonazepam and temazepam. Sleep 1986;9: 385–392.
22. Greenblatt DJ, Harmatz JS, Shapiro L, Engelhardt N, Gouthro TA, Shader RI. Sensitivity to triazolam in the elderly. N Engl J Med 1991;13: 1691–1698.
23. Schenck CH, Bundlie SR, Ettinger M, Mahowald MW. Chronic behavioral disorders of human REM sleep: a new category of parasomnia. Sleep 1986;9: 293–308.
24. Schenck CH, Mahowald MW. Polysomnographic, neurologic, psychiatric, and clinical outcome report on 70 consecutive cases with the REM sleep behavior disorder (RBD): sustained clonazepam efficacy in 89.5% of 57 treated patients. Cleve Clin J Med 1990;57:S10–S24.
25. Mahowald MW, Schenck CH. REM sleep behavior disorder. In: Kryger MH, Roth T, Dement WC, eds. Principles and Practice of Sleep Medicine, 2nd ed. Philadelphia: WB Saunders, 1994:574–588.
26. Sforza E, Krieger J, Petiau C. REM sleep behavior: clinical and physiopathological findings. Sleep Med Rev 1997;1:57–69.
27. Bamford CR. Carbamazepine in REM sleep behavior disorder. Sleep 1993;16: 33–34.
28. Mellinger GD, Balter MB, Uhlenhuth EH. Insomnia and its treatment. Prevalence and correlates. Arch Gen Psychiatry 1985;42:225–232.
29. Hohagen F, Kappler C, Schramm E, et al. Prevalence of insomnia in elderly general practice attenders and the current treatment modalities. Acta Psychiatr Scand 1994;90:102–108.
30. Foley DJ, Monjan A, Simonsick EM, Wallace RB, Blazer DG. Incidence and remission of insomnia among elderly adults: an epidemiologic study of 6,800 persons over three years. Sleep 1999;22:S366–S372.
31. Wooten V. Medical causes of insomnia. In: Kryger MH, Roth T, Dement WC, eds. Principles and Practice of Sleep Medicine. Philadelphia: WB Saunders, 1994:456–475.
32. Marin J, Shochat T, Ancoli-Israel S. Assessment and treatment of sleep disturbances in older adults. Clin Psychol Rev 2000;20:783–805.
33. Bootzin RR, Nicassio PM. Behavioral treatments for insomnia. In: Hersen M, Eisler RM, Miller PM, eds. Progress in Behavior Modification, vol 6. New York: Academic Press, 1978:1–45.

34. Glovinsky PB, Spielman AJ. Sleep restriction therapy. In: Hauri PJ, ed. Case Studies in Insomnia. New York: Plenum, 1991:49–63.
35. Friedman L, Bliwise DL, Yesavage JA, Salom SR. A preliminary study comparing sleep restriction and relaxation treatments for insomnia in older adults. J Gerontol 1991;46(1):P1–P8.
36. Friedman L, Benson K, Noda A, et al. An actigraphic comparison of sleep restriction and sleep hygiene treatments for insomnia in older adults. J Geriatr Psychiatry Neurol 2000;13:17–27.
37. Hemmelgarn B, Suissa S, Huang A, Boivin JF, Pinard G. Benzodiazepine use and the risk of motor vehicle crash in the elderly. JAMA 1997;2:27–31.
38. Haimov I, Laudon M, Zisapel N, et al. Sleep disorders and melatonin rhythms in elderly people. Br Med J 1994;309:167.
39. Haimov I, Lavie P, Laudon M, Herer P, Vigder C, Zisapel N. Melatonin replacement therapy of elderly insomniacs. Sleep 1995;18(7):598–603.
40. Prinz PN, Peskind ER, Vitaliano PP, et al. Changes in the sleep and waking EEGs of nondemented and demented elderly subjects. J Am Geriatr Soc 1982;30:86–92.
41. Bliwise DL. Sleep in dementing illness. Annu Rev Psychiatry 1994;13: 757–777.
42. Prinz PN, Vitaliano PP, Vitiello MV, et al. Sleep, EEG and mental function changes in senile dementia of the Alzheimer's type. Neurobiol Aging 1982;3: 361–370.
43. Bliwise DL, Carroll JS, Lee KA, Nekich JC, Dement WC. Sleep and sun downing in nursing home patients with dementia. Psychiatry Res 1993;48:277–292.
44. Satlin A, Volicer L, Ross V, Herz L, Campbell SS. Bright light treatment of behavioral and sleep disturbances in patients with Alzheimer's disease. Am J Psychiatry 1992;149:1028–1032.
45. Mishima K, Okawa M, Hishikawa Y, Hozumi S, Hori H, Takahashi K. Morning bright light therapy for sleep and behavior disorders in elderly patients with dementia. Acta Psychiatr Scand 1994;89:1–7.
46. Lovell BJ, Ancoli-Israel S, Gevirtz R. The effect of bright light treatment on agitated behavior in institutionalized elderly. Psychiatry Res 1995;57:7–12.
47. Ancoli-Israel S, Coy T. Are breathing disturbances in elderly equivalent to sleep apnea syndrome? Sleep 1994;17:77–83.
48. Ancoli-Israel S. Epidemiology of sleep disorders. In: Roth T, Roehrs TA, eds. Clinics in Geriatric Medicine. Philadelphia: WB Saunders, 1989:347–362.

15
Transient Ischemic Attack and Stroke

Daniel E. Wollman

Learning Objectives

Upon completion of the chapter, the student will be able to:

1. Differentiate between transient ischemic attack (TIA) and nonhemorrhagic and hemorrhagic stroke.
2. Understand the etiologies and diagnostic evaluation of stroke and cerebrovascular disease.
3. Appreciate the acute management, and primary and secondary preventive strategies in stroke.
4. Understand the principle behind the rehabilitation of the poststroke patient.

Case (Part 1)

G.W. is a 65-year-old man who comes to your office for an initial visit. He has recently retired and is new to the area. Many years ago he was told that he had "mild" diabetes and hypertension—both controlled with diet. He continues to smoke half a pack of cigarettes daily, a habit he has maintained for 30 years. His review of systems is negative for other symptoms. His physical examination is notable for height 5 feet 8 inches, weight 220 lb (body mass index, BMI = 33), blood pressure of 160/90 mmHg, mild arteriolar narrowing of the retinal vessels, and a serum glucose of 190 mg/dL.

Material in this chapter is based on the following chapters in Cassel CK, Leipzig RM, Cohen HJ, Larson EB, Meier DE, eds. Geriatric Medicine: An Evidence-Based Approach, 4th ed. New York: Springer, 2003: Brummel-Smith K. Rehabilitation, pp. 259–277. Tuhrim S. Cerebrovascular Disease and Stroke, pp. 1123–1137. Selections edited by Daniel E. Wollman.

General Considerations

Stroke is a major public health problem afflicting primarily older adults. It is the third-leading cause of death in the United States and is surpassed only by heart disease worldwide (1,2). In the United States over 700,000 new strokes occur annually (3). Stroke is also the leading cause of disability in the U.S., with an estimated 4 million stroke survivors living with stroke-related deficits (1). Over 70% of stroke survivors remain vocationally impaired, over 30% require help with activities of daily living, and 20% walk only with assistance (4). Approximately half of stroke survivors return to some form of employment, but this figure declines with age (5). The incidence of stroke doubles in each successive decade after age 55 and occurs approximately twice as often in African Americans as in whites at all ages. It is more common in men under age 75 but is equally common among older men and women (3,6).

Stroke Categories

Stroke is actually a heterogeneous group of diseases (Table 15.1). There are two main categories, nonhemorrhagic infarction and hemorrhagic infarction, which result from different pathophysiologic mechanisms, but both result in insufficient blood perfusing brain tissue.

Nonhemorrhagic Stroke

Nonhemorrhagic stroke (or infarction) accounts for about 80% of strokes. The subcategories of infarction include cardioembolic stroke, medium-large vessel atherothrombotic stroke, small vessel or lacunar stroke, and watershed stroke (Table 15.2).

Cardioembolic Stroke

Embolism from thrombi that form in the heart or that occur in large veins and pass through the heart via a right-to-left shunt account for approximately 30% of ischemic strokes. Atrial fibrillation is the most widely

TABLE 15.1. Categories of stroke

Nonhemorrhagic infarction	Hemorrhagic infarction
Cardioembolic	Subarachnoid
Lacunar (small vessel)	Intracerebral
Atherothrombotic	Primary
(medium-large)	Secondary
Watershed (hypoperfusion)	

TABLE 15.2. Risk factors/etiologies—nonhemorrhagic stroke

Specific diseases	Behaviors	Blood and blood vessel abnormalities
Hypertension	Smoking	Elevated homocysteine
Diabetes mellitus	Heavy alcohol use	Hypercoagulability
Congestive heart failure		Hyperlipidemia
Atrial fibrillation		Carotid stenosis
Vasculitis		Vessel dissection

recognized cardiac abnormality associated with ischemic stroke. It is a condition of the elderly, occurring in 0.1% of those 50 to 59 years of age but increasing gradually to 4% of those over age 80. The proportion of strokes attributed to atrial fibrillation also increases with age, rising from 7% of strokes in the sixth decade to 36% for those in the ninth decade (7). A variety of other cardiac sources of embolism have been identified including valvular lesions; hemostasis secondary to rhythm disturbances; hypokinesis of the left ventricle, either globally as in a cardiomyopathy or focally secondary to infarction; and rarely tumors.

Medium-Large Artery Occlusive Disease

The large vessels to the brain are prone to atherosclerotic narrowing most commonly at sites of origin or bifurcation, especially the bifurcation of the common carotid into the internal and external carotid arteries in the neck. Atherosclerotic stenosis leads to infarction by reducing blood flow distal to the point of stenosis and by acting as a nidus for adhesion and aggregation of platelets producing either thrombosis at that location or embolization to and occlusion of more distal, narrower arteries. The neurologic symptoms depend on the artery affected.

Lacunar Stroke

Lacunes are small, deep infarcts caused by degenerative changes within small penetrating arteries that bring blood to the internal capsule, basal ganglia, cerebral whiter matter, thalamus, and pons (8). Hypertension is the most important cause of *lipohyalinosis*, the most common mechanism of disease within the media of these microscopic arteries. Sometimes microatheroma originating at the orifice of these penetrating arteries leads to occlusion. Lacunar infarcts are the most common vascular lesions found within the brain at necropsy. In various series and registries, they account for at least 25% of ischemic strokes. The diagnosis of lacunar infarction is based on the presence of risk factors, the nature of the clinical signs and symptoms, and the results of neuroimaging tests. Most often, patients with lacunar infarction have a history of hypertension or diabetes. Lacunar infarction is unlikely in the presence of prominent headache, vomiting, or a decreased level of alertness. The clinical symptoms and signs should be compatible with a small, deep lesion. The presence of "cortical findings," such as aphasia, hemianopsia, or signs of anosognosia or inattention is strong evidence against lacunar disease. Computed tomography (CT) or magnetic resonance imaging (MRI) may show a small, deep infarct but may, in fact, be normal. In some cases, the clinical and neuroimaging tests are equivocal and do not establish a lacunar cause. In these patients, a search for other ischemic causes, such as coagulopathy, cardioembolism, and large artery ischemic disease, is warranted.

Watershed Infarction

Hypoperfusion secondary to a drop in systemic blood pressure or unilaterally as a consequence of carotid stenosis may result in infarction in the regions between two vascular territories. These are the regions most susceptible to ischemia following a decrease in perfusion, as they are the most distal regions from their respective blood supplies. Neuroimaging shows tissue damage spanning two adjacent vascular territories. Watershed infarction may be seen following prolonged cardiac arrest.

Hemorrhagic Stroke

Hemorrhagic stroke represents a clinically different entity from nonhemorrhagic infarction, both in presentation and management. The different categories of hemorrhage can be further subdivided pathophysiologically. Subarachnoid hemorrhage is leakage of blood at the brain surface into the cerebrospinal fluid, usually following the rupture of an aneurysm in an artery at the base of the brain (circle of Willis). Less often the bleeding may result from the rupture of a vascular malformation or trauma to a surface vessel. On the other hand, intracerebral hemorrhage (ICH) usually is caused by rupture of a small artery or arteriole with leakage of blood into the brain parenchyma. It accounts for 10% to 15% of all strokes and is associated with the highest mortality (9). It can be classified into primary and secondary, depending on the underlying etiology of bleeding. Primary ICH originates from spontaneous rupture of small vessels pathologically affected by chronic hypertension and accounts for 78% to 88% of all ICH (10). The basal ganglia, thalamus, brainstem, and deep white matter are common sites of primary ICH and may also occur in a minority of patients in association with cerebral amyloid angiopathy (11), structural vascular abnormalities, tumors, or impaired blood coagulation. A proportion of nonhemorrhagic infarctions "convert" to hemorrhagic infarction as the vessels in an infarcted territory rupture or leak. This diagnosis is suggested following a further deterioration in the neurologic examination after a period of stabilization from the initial stroke event, or may be seen incidentally in follow-up neuroimaging studies. Risk factors for hemorrhagic stroke are listed in Table 15.3.

TABLE 15.3. Risk factors—hemorrhagic stroke

Hypertension
Cerebral amyloid angiopathy
Structural vascular abnormalities (AVM, aneurysm,
    moyamoya)
Tumor
Thrombocytopenia and other coagulopathy

Case (Part 2)

Approximately 6 months later, G.W. was relaxing in front of the television with his wife when suddenly his speech became garbled, though comprehensible. He developed clumsiness of his right hand and a droop on the right side of his mouth. His wife called 911 and G.W. was transported to the hospital. A CT scan was performed and showed no hemorrhage or infarction; however, he continued to have dysarthria and weakness of his right arm. The rest of his examination, including electrocardiogram (ECG) and laboratory tests, was unremarkable. A diagnosis of lacunar stroke was made.

Symptoms and Signs

The key to stroke diagnosis rests in a careful history and physical examination, with particular attention to the neurologic evaluation. The clinician must gain an understanding of the temporal course and detailed neurologic dysfunction associated with the event. Knowledge of the cerebrovascular distributions and functional and structural anatomy permits a relatively accurate diagnosis, later confirmed by neuroimaging studies.

Temporal Course

Vascular causes of neurologic dysfunction are suggested by acute changes (sudden hemiparesis, sudden dysarthria, etc.) in comparison to the progressive weakness (sometimes occurring over the course of months) associated with a brain tumor, for example, expanding into the motor cortex. A resolved sudden neurologic deficit with symptoms referable to a discrete vascular territory is often diagnosed as a transient ischemic attack (TIA). In this case, the dysfunction is due to reversible tissue ischemia; however, there is no demonstrable tissue injury and recovery is usually complete (12). It is important to note there is a wide differential diagnosis for sudden neurologic deficit (e.g., seizure)—the most important distinguishing factors pointing to cerebrovascular disease are the presence of signs and symptoms referable to brain regions perfused by discrete vascular supplies. The

TABLE 15.4. Lacunar syndromes

Syndrome	Location	Symptoms
Pure motor stroke	Pons or internal capsule	Hemiparesis of face, arm, or leg
Pure sensory stroke	Lateral thalamus and/or posterior limb internal capsule	Hemisensory loss of face, arm, or leg
Ataxic hemiparesis	Subcortical white matter or pons	Incoordination and hemiparesis
Clumsy hand-dysarthria	Pons	Dysarthria and hand incoordination

TIA event is analogous to the acute anginal episode (reflecting reversible ischemia, without tissue injury, of the myocardium). A sudden, persistent deficit, on the other hand, is more likely stroke. Tissue injury ensues as a consequence of deprived blood flow. Continuing the analogy, ischemic stroke then would be comparable to myocardial infarction. The term *non-hemorrhagic cerebral infarction* is more descriptive and preferable to the term *cerebrovascular accident* (CVA). Lay terminology now refers to TIA and stroke as "brain attack."

Patterns of Neurologic Dysfunction

The symptoms of cerebral ischemia often lead to the localization of stroke (Tables 15.4 and 15.5). In general terms, symptoms of cerebral ischemia can be divided into those that arise from the anterior circulation, supplying the anterior three fourths of each hemisphere, and the posterior circulation, supplying the occipital lobes, posterior thalamus, cerebellum, and brainstem.

The anterior circulation consists of the paired internal carotid arteries that give off the ophthalmic arteries and then branch into anterior and middle cerebral arteries. Atherosclerotic lesions are most common at the

TABLE 15.5. Cortical infarction syndromes

Vascular distribution	Neurologic symptoms*
Middle cerebral artery (MCA)—dominant hemisphere, anterior division	Expressive aphasia, right hemiparesis
MCA (dominant hemisphere), posterior division	Receptive aphasia
MCA (nondominant)	Neglect
Anterior cerebral artery (ACA)	Contralateral lower extremity hemiparesis
Posterior cerebral artery (PCA)	Unilateral hemianopsia

*Assuming a right-handed individual with a left-dominant cerebral hemisphere.

origin of the internal carotid arteries in the neck and the bifurcations of the middle cerebral artery (13). The neurologic symptoms depend on the region of ischemia. The most common clinical presentations referable to the vascular territories supplied by deep penetrating arterioles arising from the anterior circulation include many of the lacunar syndromes, and likewise do not include cortical findings.

The posterior circulation consists of the paired vertebral arteries that give rise to the posterior inferior cerebellar arteries before joining to form the basilar artery that gives off the paired anterior inferior and superior cerebellar arteries and penetrating branches supplying the brainstem before bifurcating into paired posterior cerebral arteries. Symptoms and signs of posterior circulation ischemia are highly variable and overlap with those of the anterior circulation, but vertigo, diplopia, nausea, and vomiting are common complaints heard in brainstem or cerebellar disease; nystagmus, disconjugate eye movement abnormalities, gait or limb ataxia, crossed (i.e., ipsilateral face and contralateral limb or body) sensory or motor deficits, and hemianopic visual field loss are indicative of posterior circulation ischemia. Confusion and memory loss can be seen, especially in embolic occlusion of the basilar artery, blocking penetrating branches that supply the thalamus (14).

Diagnostic Evaluation

Following the history and physical examination, the clinician should have a clear understanding of the event, and an appreciation of the putative location resulting in the neurologic deficit. Initial neuroimaging studies assist with acute management, specifically in ruling out the presence of hemorrhage, but also serve to describe the vascular territory affected.

Neuroimaging

Computed axial tomography of the brain (CT) is the preferred diagnostic test in the immediate setting (15,16). This procedure, which uses circumferential x-ray to reconstruct an axial slice through the brain, can provide fairly sensitive information about gross structural abnormalities of the brain, such as mass effect or edema as well as the presence of acute blood, which appears radiodense, relative to brain tissue. It is important to note that the changes associated with infarction, in the absence of overt hemorrhage, may not be apparent for up to 24 hours. Subacute or chronic symptoms may be evaluated with magnetic resonance imaging (MRI). In the setting where hemorrhage has been excluded by CT, but when diagnosis remains elusive, MRI can be helpful as changes may be apparent as early as 6 hours following the onset. New techniques in MRI now permit obtaining information about tissue infarction as well as the state of the vascular supply—similar to myocardial perfusion imaging (17). Such information may soon prove critical in stratifying stroke revascularization techniques by identifying "territory at risk" versus infarcted tissue.

The general workup for stroke is based on a search for remediable factors associated with subsequent stroke events (Table 15.6).

Echocardiography and Carotid Ultrasound

The development of transesophageal echocardiography (TEE) has provided additional insight into the source of cerebral emboli. With this technique, it is possible to detect thrombus in the left atrial appendage. This is generally the site that harbors clot in a fibrillating atrium, but is not visible on transthoracic echocardiogram. Spontaneous echo contrast ("smoke") is often seen in a fibrillating atrium and is thought to represent platelet-fibrin aggregates that are a precursor to thrombus formation. A patent foramen ovale (PFO), the most common conduit for paradoxical emboli, is also readily diagnosed by this procedure. The TEE has also led to appreciation of atherosclerotic plaque in the ascending aorta and aortic arch, especially in elderly patients. These plaques can be ulcerated and serve as a nidus for clot formation or protrude into the lumen as a highly mobile peduncle, likely to embolize to more distal arteries. The thickness of this plaque has been correlated with the risk of stroke (7,18,19). Because it is a somewhat invasive procedure, TEE is not done routinely in most centers, but patients who have no obvious source of stroke should undergo TEE to determine if one of these embolic sources is present. Duplex ultrasound is used to determine the presence of a stenotic lesion or more rarely a dissection of the carotid arteries.

Other tests along with example findings are listed in Table 15.6. The purpose of performing these tests is to reduce the likelihood of a subsequent stroke.

TABLE 15.6. Stroke evaluation

Test/procedure	Example findings
Complete blood count	Thrombocytosis
Metabolic screen	Hypoglycemia
Electrocardiogram	Atrial fibrillation
Holter monitor	Paroxysmal atrial fibrillation
Echocardiogram	Patent foramen ovale, congestive heart failure, aortic atherosclerosis
Carotid ultrasound	Carotid stenosis
Magnetic resonance imaging/angiography	Lacunar infarct, intracranial stenosis
Erythrocyte sedimentation rate, hypercoagulability workup	Vasculitis, antiphospholipid antibody syndrome

Management Considerations

Despite recent advances in stroke treatment, prevention remains the most effective means of reducing the overall burden of stroke. Secondary prevention in patients who have experienced TIA or stroke targets those at highest risk, but primary prevention in individuals at high risk because of the presence of the factors discussed above is also of great importance. Even among those with no identified stroke risk factors, on a population basis lower salt intake [accompanied by increased dietary potassium and calcium (20)], a diet high in folic acid and low in saturated fats, and no more than moderate alcohol consumption can forestall the development of vascular disease risk factors and reduce stroke incidence.

Case (Part 3)

The total time elapsed from when G.W. was last seen asymptomatic to when the diagnosis of stroke was made was 4 hours. He was given aspirin and transferred to the general medical floor. Neurologic checks were ordered every 2 hours for the next 8 hours, followed by every 4 hours for the next 8 hours, then once per 8-hour shift. Occupational and speech therapy consultations were ordered. Blood pressure medication was deferred at this time. An echocardiogram, carotid ultrasound, and MRI were scheduled for the following morning.

Acute Stroke

Intravenous Thrombolytic Therapy

In June 1996, the Food and Drug Administration (FDA) approved the use of tissue plasminogen activator (t-PA) in acute ischemic stroke, if given within 3 hours of symptom onset. Clinical trials have demonstrated benefit of this procedure in some patients (21). Immediate transfer to a hospital upon symptom onset is critical. A CT scan should be performed as quickly as possible to exclude intracranial hemorrhage or a nonischemic cause of the patient's symptoms. When the diagnosis of acute nonhemorrhagic stroke is likely, most patients who arrive within 3 hours are candidates for intravenous thrombolysis. (For further details about the exclusion criteria for this procedure, see Chapter 77: Cerebrovascular Disease and Stroke. In: Cassel CK, et al., eds. Geriatric Medicine, 4th ed., page 1130.)

The major risk of treatment is intracerebral hemorrhage (ICH), which occurred in 6.4% of patients treated with t-PA in the trials. Mortality was similar in both groups (17% t-PA, 20% placebo). Given the relatively high rate of ICH following t-PA, it is important to consider the circumstances under which this modality should be sought. For example, the patient with mild weakness of one extremity may achieve a satisfactory therapeutic effect from physical therapy or may judge the degree of impairment insufficient to justify the exposure to the risk of ICH. On the other hand, the patient who suffers a dominant hemisphere stroke and is rendered aphasic may be left with a severe disability judged worthy of the risk of a therapeutic procedure. In all cases, careful, though timely, consultation with patient, family, and team members is crucial. Other thrombolytic treatment, currently available only at selected centers, includes intraarterial thrombolysis, in which a microcatheter is advanced to and sometimes through the obstructing clot (22).

Antithrombotic Therapy

Over the past 30 years, anticoagulation with continuous infusion of intravenous unfractionated heparin has probably been the most widely used acute stroke treatment, yet no clinical trial to date has adequately tested its efficacy. Recently, several trials of anticoagulation by different methods have reported conflicting results. The International Stroke Trial enrolled nearly 20,000 subjects and demonstrated no differences in the primary outcome measures (death at 14 days; death or dependency at 6 months) among any of the treatment groups (23). There was, however, an increased risk of hemorrhage in the high-dose heparin group. (For further details about this trial and other trials with mixed results, see Chapter 77: Cerebrovascular Disease and Stroke. In: Cassel CK, et al., eds. Geriatric Medicine, 4th ed., page 1130.)

Despite the lack of evidence supporting its use, intravenous unfractionated heparin remains in widespread use in patients not eligible for thrombolysis, especially those with presumed cardioembolic infarction, antiphospholipid-antibody syndrome, extracranial carotid or vertebral artery dissection, cerebral vein thrombosis, and impending large vessel thrombosis. It is usually given as a continuous intravenous infusion with a goal of maintaining the partial thromboplastin time at 1.5 to 2.0 times normal.

Antiplatelet Therapy

Early treatment with aspirin is commonplace for patients not treated with thrombolysis or anticoagulation. This practice arose because aspirin was of proven benefit in secondary stroke prevention and in the acute management of myocardial ischemia, but recently two trials evaluated its benefit in a total of more than 40,000 patients treated within 48 hours of stroke onset. In the International Stroke Trial, although there was no difference in the primary outcome measures among treatment groups, secondary analyses demonstrated a small (2.8% vs. 3.9%) decrease in the rate of recurrent ischemic stroke in patients treated with aspirin (23). The Chinese Acute Stroke Trial randomized 21,106 patients to aspirin 160 mg or placebo for 4 weeks, and demonstrated a slightly lower mortality rate (3.3% vs. 3.9%) and recurrent stroke rate (1.6% vs. 2.1%) in the aspirin group (24).

Other oral antiplatelet drugs effective in secondary prevention of stroke include clopidogrel, dipyridamole and ticlopidine (25).

Management of Blood Pressure

Elevated blood pressure, seen commonly after ICH, is associated with hematoma expansion and poor outcome (26). Elevated blood pressure may be secondary to uncontrolled chronic hypertension or occurs as a protective response to preserve cerebral perfusion. There is considerable controversy regarding treatment of blood pressure in the acute period after ICH. Most patients with ICH have chronic hypertension with cerebral autoregulation adapted for higher than normal blood pressures (27). Furthermore, cerebral perfusion pressure and autoregulatory capacity may be compromised due to elevated intracranial pressure (ICP) (28). American Heart Association (AHA) guidelines recommend antihypertensive treatment only when mean arterial pressure is ≥130 mmHg. Intravenous beta-blockers and vasodilators such as hydralazine or angiotensin-converting enzyme (ACE) inhibitors should be used because they have limited effect on cerebral circulation (29,30). It is important to recognize that the blood vessels in the infarcted territory may themselves be damaged, resulting in impaired regulation of blood flow, thus worsening tissue ischemia when systemic blood pressure is reduced (31). Some specialists recommend liberalization of blood pressure in the first 3 weeks following stroke, with recommendations for aggressive management during convalescence.

Neuroprotection

Ischemic neuronal death results from a cascade of events set in motion by insufficient supply of oxygen and nutrients. A number of agents have shown promise in laboratory models, but not in clinical trials (32). (For further details, see Chapter 77: Cerebrovascular Disease and Stroke. In: Cassel CK, et al., eds. Geriatric Medicine, 4th ed., page 1131.)

Case (Part 4)

An MRI obtained 18 hours after the start of G.W.'s symptoms showed a hyperintensity in the left internal capsule. This abnormality appeared on diffusion weighted imaging as well as in T2-weighted and in fast fluid-attenuated inversion-recovery (FLAIR) images and was thought consistent with an acute stroke. No embolic source or cardiac rhythm abnormality was found during the workup for G.W.'s stroke. A speech and swallow evaluation showed minimal abnormality. He continued to have some clumsiness in his arm and hand, but gross strength returned to 4 out of 5. He was discharged on aspirin and given a follow-up appointment for 1 week. A prescription referral for outpatient physical and occupational therapy was given to the patient.

Secondary Prevention

Antiplatelet Therapy

Antiplatelet therapy is the most commonly prescribed stroke prevention remedy and is usually appropriate for any symptomatic individual who does not require anticoagulation. Most patients are maintained on enteric-coated aspirin, with 325 mg daily the most commonly prescribed dose in the United States. However, much controversy exists. There is no consensus regarding the optimal dose, with recent recommendations suggesting a range of 50 to 325 mg (33), although other authorities suggest higher doses are more effective if tolerated (34). Newer medications such as Aggrenox (a combination of 25 mg of aspirin and 200 mg of dipyridamole in a sustained release formulation), and clopidogrel have been shown to have somewhat greater efficacy than aspirin in randomized trials, but maintenance on these medications currently costs in excess of $1000/year in the United States for an individual purchasing this drug at a retail pharmacy. Because the differences among various agents are small when compared with the effect of taking no antiplatelet agent and compliance has been shown to be a major problem, attention should be directed at ensuring patients are compliant with whatever regimen is prescribed (Table 15.7).

TABLE 15.7. Secondary stroke prevention

Condition	Treatment
Medium-large vessel atherosclerotic disease	Antiplatelet therapy (aspirin)
Atrial fibrillation	Anticoagulation (warfarin)
Hypertension/diabetes	Antiplatelet therapy (aspirin)
Carotid stenosis	Surgery, antiplatelet therapy
Congestive heart failure	Anticoagulation?
Antiphospholipid antibody syndrome	Anticoagulation

Specific Conditions

Atrial Fibrillation

Atrial fibrillation (AF) is a particularly important risk factor in the elderly. Chronic AF in association with valvular heart disease increases stroke risk 17-fold, whereas in the absence of valvular disease stroke risk is still increased fivefold (35). Recent studies have identified factors that increase stroke risk in nonvalvular AF including older age, hypertension, recent onset of congestive heart failure, diabetes mellitus, a history of systemic embolism, or cerebral ischemia. Poor left ventricular function and increased left atrial size on echocardiogram also increase stroke risk (36).

Chronic anticoagulation with warfarin has been shown to be very effective in reducing stroke risk in patients in AF with and without a history of stroke. Anticoagulation should be prescribed for all patients who have had cerebral ischemic symptoms in the setting of AF unless there is a specific contraindication, and prophylactically in most patients who have been asymptomatic but have the additional risk factors mentioned above, especially those over age 60 (37).

Carotid Stenosis

Narrowing of the lumen of the internal carotid artery is associated with an increased risk of stroke. A residual lumen of less than 20% of normal is highly correlated with the development of total occlusion of the internal artery or the development of symptoms related to that artery (13). Endarterectomy is the most widely used specific treatment for this condition. In the past decade, several large-scale randomized trials involving symptomatic and asymptomatic individuals have provided data that allow a rational selection of appropriate patients for this procedure (38,39).

The benefit of surgery must be balanced against the risk for each individual. Life expectancy also plays a role in the decision-making process because there is early morbidity including stroke and death associated with the procedure. This morbidity should be less than 3% in experienced hands. Given these caveats, endarterectomy can be performed safely even in the very elderly and should be recommended for appropriate individuals of any age whose life expectancy is great enough to anticipate benefit despite the risk of early perioperative morbidity.

Stroke Rehabilitation

Stroke is one of the most common conditions for which older people receive rehabilitation. Rehabilitation interventions begin during the acute hospital phase, primarily directed at preventing secondary complications.

The clinician needs to be involved in many aspects of the patient's care, in reducing ongoing risk factors, minimizing medications, providing the family with information, and care planning.

Most of the return of function is seen in the first month. In some cases, however, motor function may return as late as 6 months after the stroke. Sensory deficits or swallowing problems may improve later. In spite of these endogenous improvements, rehabilitation efforts following stroke are cost-effective and lead to higher functional levels (40). Patients and their families need accurate prognostic information soon after the stroke in order to make informed decisions about care. They should be told that most patients survive infarcts and that the highest mortality is in the first week. Many survivors have residual deficits longer than 6 to 12 months after the acute event. Rehabilitation interventions help survivors adjust to these disabilities even if they cannot be eliminated through therapy.

Acute Care Phase

Initially, rehabilitation efforts are geared toward preventing secondary disabilities and identifying patients who need more intensive rehabilitation. Prevention of secondary disabilities should begin soon after admission. The patient must be turned regularly to prevent the development of pressure ulcers. Sitting up, daily range of motion of the extremities, and exercise of the uninvolved limbs to prevent deconditioning should be provided. Constipation or dehydration must be avoided. Although most have some urinary incontinence initially, patients with persistent problems should receive appropriate investigation for treatable causes.

Predictions of eventual recovery are difficult during the acute phase. Factors associated with a poor prognosis include flaccid hemiplegia of greater than 2 months' duration, dementia, persistent bowel or bladder incontinence, severe neglect or sensory deficits, and global aphasia (41). Certain factors, such as a depressed caregiver, a caregiver not married to the patient, and family dysfunction, have been shown to predict which patients may not benefit from home rehabilitation (42).

The choice of which site—inpatient unit, nursing home, or home—to provide rehabilitation is complex. The most appropriate choice must often be negotiated between the clinician and the patient based on patient-specific desires and available resources (Fig. 15.1).

Rehabilitation Phase

It is in this phase that rehabilitation therapists play crucial roles. Physical therapists work with patients to develop strength, augment balance, enhance transfer ability, and increase endurance. When the lower extremities have good strength (i.e., ≥4/5 on manual muscle testing) and the patient can balance on the uninvolved side, gait training can be initiated.

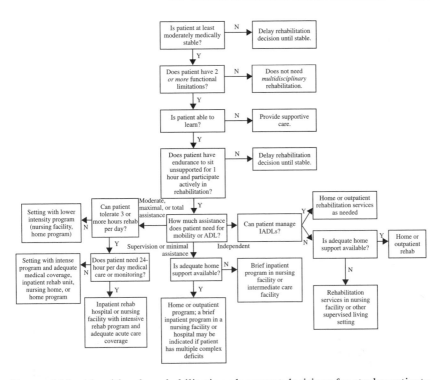

FIGURE 15.1. Algorithm for rehabilitation placement decisions for stroke patients. ADL, activities of daily living; IADL, instrumental activities of daily living. (Adapted from Johnston MV, Wood K, Statson B, et al. Rehabilitative placement of post stroke patients—reliability of the clinical practice guideline of the Agency for Health Care Policy and Research. Arch Phys Med Rehabil 2000;81:539–548, with permission from Elsevier. Reprinted as appears in Brummel-Smith K. Rehabilitation. In: Cassel CK, Leipzig RM, Cohen HJ, et al., eds. Geriatric Medicine, 4th ed. New York: Springer, 2003.)

For those patients with difficulty advancing the limb or maintaining stability, the patient should be evaluated for a brace and walking aid. For instance, a platform cane, or hemiwalker may be required (Fig. 15.2). Ankle-foot orthoses (AFO) are most commonly used in the elderly stroke patient (Fig. 15.3). Two types are commonly employed: the double adjustable upright metal AFO, used to stabilize a spastic ankle and provide some proprioceptive feedback to the knee; and the posterior plastic AFO, which prevents footdrop but requires a more stable ankle; 78% to 85% of patients will be able to walk after 6 months.

The occupational therapist works with the patient to provide training in daily self-care activities. Simple remedies may provide great self-care benefits. For instance, spasticity sometimes can be controlled with the use of weighted utensils. Other types of special utensils, such as rocker knives,

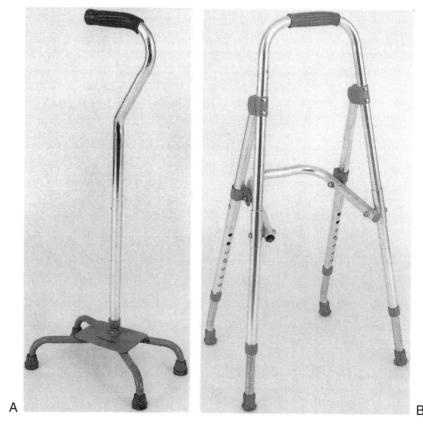

A   B

FIGURE 15.2. Walking aids used in stroke. A: A platform cane offers moderate stability on smooth, flat surfaces but can be unsafe when negotiating uneven ground. B: A hemiwalker offers much more stability for patients with more limited ambulation skills. (Brummel-Smith K. Rehabilitation. In: Cassel CK, Leipzig RM, Cohen HJ, et al., eds. Geriatric Medicine, 4th ed. New York: Springer, 2003.)

plate guards, and reachers, enable persons with hemiplegia to function more independently. A cognitive retraining program also may be provided by occupational therapists or sometimes by speech therapists. Early assessment for aphasia is critical to providing other team members with recommendations regarding communication needs. Approximately 24% to 53% of stroke survivors are partially or totally dependent 6 months after their strokes (43).

Special attention must be given to two common, and often related, problems. Poststroke depression is very common, affecting about 30% of sur-

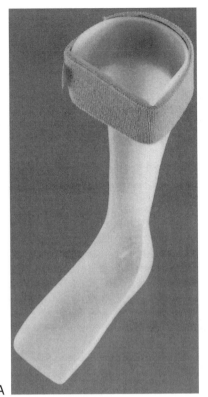
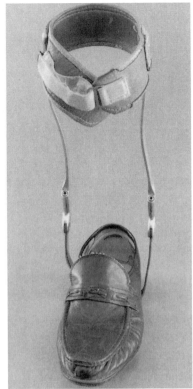

A   B

FIGURE 15.3. Lower extremity braces (ankle-foot orthoses, AFO). A: A plastic AFO provides some stability to a weak ankle but will usually not be appropriate when control of spasticity is required. B: A metal AFO is useful to control the effects of spasticity but is more difficult to don and is physically unattractive. (Brummel-Smith K. Rehabilitation. In: Cassel CK, Leipzig RM, Cohen HJ, et al., eds. Geriatric Medicine, 4th ed. New York: Springer, 2003.)

vivors. It is especially likely with left hemisphere damage. Depression is often recognized 2 to 3 weeks after the stroke. It retards functional recovery and may be misinterpreted as "poor motivation" (44). Treatment of depression facilitates the gains made in rehabilitation. Psychotherapy and the judicious use of antidepressant medication are usually needed. The choice of an antidepressant medication is usually made on the side-effect profile as all have more or less the same response rate. However, because most agents require at least 2 weeks to see a response, some have advocated early use of methylphenidate to accelerate the response (45,46). Depression must be distinguished from uncontrolled crying, which is also common after a stroke. This condition, thought to be due to "disinhibition," responds to selective serotonin reuptake inhibitors.

Malnutrition is another problem seen too often in rehabilitation. A bedside swallowing evaluation by a speech and language pathologist has been shown to be valuable (47), and early dietary consultation should be done on all persons after stroke. In some cases, short-term use of enteral feedings may be required.

Attention to premorbid problems must be especially vigilant in geriatric patients. Having access to one's dentures, eyeglasses, and clothing promotes self-esteem and may enhance the ability to participate in the rehabilitation program. The patient's family should be involved in the treatment program through training in caregiving skills. A bedside graph to document progress made by the patient and a chart that specifies goals to be achieved also can be helpful.

Chronic Phase

The chronic phase begins when the person who has suffered a stroke returns to society as a person with a disability. The home, especially the bathroom, usually needs modifications. Raised toilet seats with arm frames, grab bars, and a bathtub bench with a handheld shower hose are often required (Fig. 15.4). Kitchen modification also may be necessary. Prior to discharge, the home should be assessed for door widths to ensure passage of walkers or wheelchairs, the presence of steps and stairs, the need for ramps, the adequacy of lighting, and safety features that may need modifications.

Because the adjustment process to a major disability may take up to 2 years, ongoing psychological support often is necessary. The patient may benefit from individual or group psychotherapy, a day health center, or a stroke recovery group. Frank information should be provided regarding the fact that sexual activities following a stroke are quite safe, although new techniques are often needed.

Social activities should be strongly encouraged. A vocational rehabilitation counselor can assess and help with the return to employment if appropriate. Arrangements for transportation are particularly important, as many geriatric patients stop driving after a stroke. For patients with right hemisphere lesions and neglect, driving is inadvisable unless the neglect resolves.

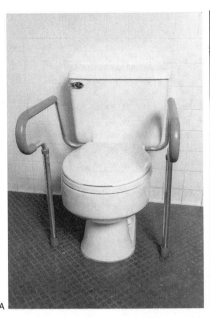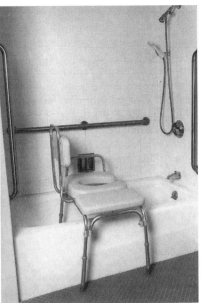

A   B

FIGURE 15.4. Bathroom modifications. A: Toilet arm attachments facilitate standing with weak hip extensors. B: A bath bench and hand-held shower hose allow
the patient to bathe independently. (Reprinted with permission from Brummel-
Smith K. Rehabilitation, pp. 259–277. In: Cassel CK, Leipzig RM, Cohen HJ,
et al., eds. Geriatric Medicine, 4th ed. New York: Springer, 2003.)

General Principles

- Primary prevention of cerebrovascular disease remains the ultimate, though difficult, goal.
- It is important to determine whether neurologic dysfunction is referable to stroke.
- Neurologic deficit should conform to a discrete vascular territory.
- Evaluation should be utilized to determine secondary prevention strategies.
- The patient's premorbid functional status, cognitive capabilities, and support system are strong predictors for success in rehabilitation interventions.

Suggested Readings

Albers GW, Easton JD, Sacco RL, Teal P. Antithrombotic and thrombolytic therapy for ischemic stroke. Chest 1998;114:6385–6985. *This paper provides an excellent overview of current treatment modalities in stroke.*

Brummel-Smith K. Rehabilitation. In: Cassel CK, Leipzig RM, Cohen HJ, et al., eds. Geriatric Medicine, 4th ed. New York: Springer, 2003:259–277.

Fisher CM. Lacunar strokes and infarcts: a review. Neurology 1982;32:871–876. *This is a classic paper describing much of what we continue to observe in the lacunar syndrome. Fisher also discusses the pathophysiology leading to small vessel thrombosis.*

Gilman S. Medical progress: imaging the brain—first of two parts. N Engl J Med 1998;338:812–820.

Gilman S. Medical progress: imaging the brain—second of two parts. N Engl J Med 1998;338:889–896. *These two papers provide an excellent overview of the appropriate use of neuroimaging in cerebrovascular disease and other neurological dysfunction.*

Tuhrim S. Cerebrovascular disease and stroke. In: Cassel CK, Leipzig RM, Cohen HJ, et al., eds. Geriatric Medicine, 4th ed. New York: Springer, 2003: 1123–1137.

References

1. American Heart Association. 1999 Heart and Stroke Statistical Update. Dallas: American Heart Association, 1998.
2. Murray CJL, Lopez AD. Mortality by cause for eight regions of the world: global burden of disease study. Lancet 1997;349:1269–1276.
3. Broderick J, Brott T, Kothari R, et al. The Greater Cincinnati/Northern Kentucky Stroke Study: preliminary first-ever and total incidence rates of stroke among blacks. Stroke 1998;29:415–421.
4. Gresham GE, Fitzpatrick TE, Wolf PA, et al. Residual disability in survivors of stroke—the Framingham Study. N Engl J Med 1975;293:954–956.
5. Black-Schaffer RM, Osberg JS. Return to work after stroke: development of a predictive model. Arch Phys Med Rehabil 1990;71:285–290.
6. Sacco RL, Boden-Albala B, Gan R, et al. Stroke incidence among white, black, and Hispanic residents of an urban community: the Northern Manhattan Stroke Study. Am J Epidemiol 1998;147:259–268.
7. Wolf PA, Abbott RD, Kannell AB. Atrial fibrillation as an independent risk factor for stroke: The Framingham Study. Stroke 1991;22:983–988.
8. Fisher CM. Lacunar strokes and infarcts: a review. Neurology 1982;32:871–876.
9. Bamford J, Sandercock P, Dennis M, Burn J, Warlow C. A prospective study of acute cerebrovascular disease in the community: the Oxfordshire Community Stroke Project—1981–86. 2. Incidence, case fatality rates and overall outcome at one year of cerebral infarction, primary intracerebral and subarachnoid haemorrhage. J Neurol Neurosurg Psychiatry 1990;53:16–22.
10. Foulkes MA, Wolf PA, Price TR, Mohr JP, Hier DB. The Stroke Data Bank: design, methods, and baseline characteristics. Stroke 1988;19:547–554.
11. Gilbert JJ, Vinters HV. Cerebral Amyloid Angiopathy: incidence and complications in the aging brain. Stroke 1983;4:915–923.
12. Albers GW, Caplan LR, Easton JD, et al. Transient ischemic attack—proposal for a new definition. N Engl J Med 2002;347:1713–1716.
13. Roederer GO, Langlois YE, Jager KA, et al. The natural history of carotid arterial disease in asymptomatic patients with cervical bruits. Stroke 1984; 15:605–613.

14. Caplan L. "Top of the basilar" syndrome. Neurology 1980;30:72–79.
15. Gilman S. Medical progress: imaging the brain—first of two parts. N Engl J Med 1998;338:812–820.
16. Gilman S. Medical progress: imaging the brain—second of two parts. N Engl J Med 1998;338:889–896.
17. Warach S, Dashe JF, Edelman RR. Clinical outcome in ischemic stroke predicted by early diffusion-weighted and perfusion magnetic resonance imaging: a preliminary analysis. J Cereb Blood Flow Metab 1996;16:53–59.
18. Alweiss GS, Goldman ME. Transesophageal echocardiography: diagnostic and clinical applications in the evaluation of the stroke patient. J Stroke Cerebrovasc Dis 1997;6:332–336.
19. Amarenco P, Cohen A, Tzoririo, et al. Atherosclerotic disease of the aortic-arch and the risk of ischemic stroke. N Engl J Med 1994;331: 1474–1479.
20. Sacks FM, Svetkey LP, Vollmer WM, et al. Effects on blood pressure of reduced dietary sodium and the Dietary Approaches to Stop Hypertension (DASH) diet. N Engl J Med 2001;344:3–10.
21. Hacke W, Brott T, Caplan L, et al. Thrombolysis in acute ischemic stroke: controlled trials and clinical experience. Neurology 1999;53(suppl 7):S3–S14.
22. Furlan A, Higashida R, Wechsler L, et al. Intra-arterial prourokinase for acute ischemic stroke: The PROACT II study. JAMA 1999;282:2003–2011.
23. The International Stroke Trial (IST): a randomized trial of aspirin, subcutaneous heparin, both, or neither among 19,435 patients with acute ischemic stroke. Lancet 1997;349:1569–1581.
24. CAST (Chinese Acute Stroke Trial) Collaborative Group. CAST: randomised placebo-controlled trial of early aspirin use in 20,000 patients with acute ischaemic stroke. Lancet 1997;349:1641–1649.
25. Adams HP, Bogousslavsky J, Baurathan E, et al. Abciximab in acute ischemic stroke—a randomized, double-blind, placebo-controlled, dose-escalation study. Stroke 2000;31:601–609.
26. Carlberg B, Asplund K, Hagg E. The prognostic value of admission blood pressure in patients with acute stroke. Stroke 1993;24:1372–1375.
27. Kuwata N, Kuroda K, Funayama M, Sato N, Kubo N, Ogawa A. Dysautoregulation in patients with hypertensive intracerebral hemorrhage. A SPECT study. Neurosurg Rev 1995;18:237–245.
28. Qureshi AI, Bliwise DL, Bliwise NG, Akbar MS, Uzen G, Frankel MR. Rate of 24–hour blood pressure decline and mortality after spontaneous intracerebral hemorrhage: a retrospective analysis with a random effects regression model. Crit Care Med 1999;27:480–485.
29. Broderick JP, Adams HP Jr, Barsan W, et al. Guidelines for the management of spontaneous intracerebral hemorrhage: a statement for healthcare professionals from a special writing group of the Stroke Council, American Heart Association. Stroke 1999;30:905–915.
30. Tietjan CS, Hurn PD, Ulatowski JA, Kirsch JR. Treatment modalities for patients with intracranial pathology: options and risks. Crit Care Med 1996; 24:311–322.
31. Goldstein LB. Should antihypertensive therapies be given to patients with acute ischemic stroke? Drug Saf 2000;22:13–18.
32. Lee J-M, Zipfel GJ, Choi DW. The changing landscape of ischaemic brain injury mechanisms. Nature 1999;399(suppl):A7–A14.

33. Albers GW, Easton JD, Sacco RL, Teal P. Antithrombotic and thrombolytic therapy for ischemic stroke. Chest 1998;114:6385–6985.
34. Dyken ML, Barnett HJ, Easton JD, Fields WS, Fuster V, et al. Low-dose aspirin and stroke. "It ain't necessarily so." Stroke 1992;23:1395–1399.
35. Wolf PA, Abbott RD, Kannel WB. Atrial fibrillation as an independent risk factor for stroke in the Framingham Study. Stroke 1991;22:983–988.
36. Atrial Fibrillation Investigators. Risk factors for stroke and efficacy of antithrombotic therapy in atrial fibrillation: analysis of pooled data from five randomized trials. Arch Intern Med 1994;154:1449–1457.
37. Ezekowitz MD, Levine JA. Preventing stroke in patients with atrial fibrillation. JAMA 1999;281:1830–1835.
38. European Carotid Surgery Trialist's Collaborative Group. MRC European Carotid Surgery Trial: interim results for symptomatic patients with severe (70–99%) or with mild (0–19%) carotid stenosis. Lancet 1991;337:1235–1243.
39. North American Symptomatic Carotid Endarterectomy Trial Collaborators. Beneficial effect of carotid endarterectomy in patients with high-grade carotid stenosis. N Engl J Med 1991;325:445–451.
40. Collaborative systematic review of the randomised trials of organised inpatient (stroke unit) care after stroke. Stroke Unit Trialists' Collaboration. BMJ 1997;314:1151–1159.
41. Dombovy M, Sandok B, Basford J. Rehabilitation for stroke: a review. Stroke 1986;8:651–656.
42. Evans RL, Bishop DS, Haselkorn JK. Factors predicting satisfactory home care after a stroke. Arch Phys Med Rehabil 1991;72:144–147.
43. Kojima S, Omura T, Wakamatsu W, et al. Prognosis and disability of stroke patients after 5 years in Akita, Japan. Stroke 1990;21:72–77.
44. van de Weg FB, Kuik DJ, Lankhorst GJ. Post-stroke depression and functional outcome: a cohort study investigating the influence of depression on functional recovery from stroke. Clin Rehabil 1999;13:268–272.
45. Lazarus LW, Winemiller DR, Lingam VR, et al. Efficacy and side effects of methylphenidate for poststroke depression. J Clin Psychiatry 1992;53:447–449.
46. Burns A, Russell E, Stratton-Powell H, Tyrell P, O'Neill P, Baldwin R. Sertraline in stroke-associated liability of mood. Int J Geriatr Psychiatry 1999;14:681–685.
47. Mann G, Hankey GJ, Cameron D. Swallowing disorders following acute stroke: prevalence and diagnostic accuracy. Cerebrovasc Dis 2000;10:380–386.
48. Johnston MV, Wood K, Statson B, et al. Rehabilitative placement of post stroke patients—reliability of the clinical practice guideline of the Agency for Health Care Policy and Research. Arch Phys Med Rehabil 2000:81: 539–548.

16
Parkinson's Disease and Related Disorders

Daniel E. Wollman

Learning Objectives

Upon completion of the chapter, the student will be able to:

1. Differentiate parkinsonism, Parkinson's disease, and other movement disorders.
2. Understand the diagnostic evaluation for movement disorders.
3. Appreciate the management considerations in parkinsonism and Parkinson's disease.

Case (Part 1)

R.M. is a 68-year-old man whom you have seen in your primary care practice for many years. He has been extremely healthy, and is currently on no medications. You see him once a year for his annual screening and influenza vaccination. At today's visit, he offers several new complaints. His friends are frequently asking him if things are okay and tell him he has a "sad look" on his face. In addition, many people have begun asking him to speak more loudly. He always prided himself on his fancy penmanship and notices now that his handwriting has become quite small.

General Considerations

Parkinson's disease (PD) is a common disorder among the elderly population. Its incidence increases with age from less than 10 per 100,000 at age 50 to more than 200 per 100,000 at age 80 (1). After the 9th decade, its

---

Material in this chapter is based on the following chapter in Cassel CK, Leipzig RM, Cohen HJ, Larson EB, Meier DE, eds. Geriatric Medicine: An Evidence-Based Approach, 4th ed. New York: Springer, 2003: Masdeu JC, Rodriguez-Oroz MC. Abnormalities of Posture and Movement, pp. 1139–1162. Selections edited by Daniel E. Wollman.

Table 16.1. Characteristics of movement disorders

Type	Distinguishing features
Resting tremor	Present when body part at rest
Postural tremor	Present with fixed posture or position (e.g., holding a teacup)
Action/kinetic tremor	Present during limb movement
Chorea	Arrhythmic, rapid, often jerky, purposeless movements
Dystonia	Involuntary sustained muscle contraction that produces twisting movements and abnormal postures in axial muscles and limbs. (e.g., focal dystonia—torticollis, retrocollis, "writer's cramp")
Myoclonus	Arrhythmic, asymmetric involuntary muscle contraction

incidence appears to decline but these data are likely to be an artifact derived from poor ascertainment and the smaller size of the population of this age. The gender distribution shows a slightly greater incidence in males, and there is no conclusive evidence for race differences. Epidemiologic studies have been conducted trying to identify risk factors for PD. Apart from increasing age, the strongest risk factor associated with PD is the presence of disease in a family member. Clinical manifestations in PD are caused by the loss of dopaminergic cells in the pars compacta of the substantia nigra (SNpc), and the subsequent loss of nigrostriatal dopaminergic modulation of the neural mechanism for movement control (2).

It is important to distinguish Parkinson's disease and parkinsonism from other movement disorders (Table 16.1). Excessive movements in the elderly may be rhythmic (*tremor*), arrhythmic (*myoclonus*), or hyperkinesias in all other cases. Abnormal hyperkinetic movements may have the speed of normal volitional, reaching movements and are called *chorea*. *Ballismus* or *hemiballismus* (usually unilateral) represents rapid, ballistic movements of the extremities. When the hyperkinesias are very slow and tend to present mainly as abnormal postures, they are called *dystonia* when predominantly proximal, and *athetosis*, when they involve the hand. However, particularly in adults, the term dystonia is often used to encompass both true dystonia as well as athetosis.

Symptoms and Signs

The cardinal manifestations of Parkinson's disease are tremor, rigidity, akinesia, and postural instability with associated gait disorder (Table 16.2). Postural and gait disturbances usually appear later in the course of typical Parkinson's disease, whereas they are an early manifestation of the other parkinsonian, or "Parkinson's plus" disorders, such as progressive supranuclear palsy (PSP), striatonigral degeneration, multisystem atrophy (MSA), and corticobasal-ganglionic degeneration (CBD) (2).

TABLE 16.2. Manifestations of Parkinson's disease

Common signs and symptoms	Less appreciated signs and symptoms
Resting tremor	Micrographia
Rigidity	Drooling
Bradykinesia	Decreased arm swing
Festinating or shuffling gait	Truncal rigidity
Masked facies	Hypophonia
	Orthostatic hypotension

The primary features of Parkinson's disease usually appear asymmetrically, affecting first one half of the body and spreading to the contralateral limbs and to the axial muscles in further stages. This pattern is of diagnostic importance, because other parkinsonian syndromes tend to cause rigidity and akinesia of both sides of the body from the inception of the disease.

Case (Part 2)

You perform a general physical and complete neurologic examination on R.M. Objective findings on examination includes normal mental status with neutral mood and normal range of affect. Throughout your examination and discussion, the patient demonstrates a paucity of facial expression; he does, however, smile at a joke you tell him. There is a fine tremor at rest involving his hands. His muscle tone appears somewhat increased with a ratchet-like quality to its movement. As the patient walks down the hallway, there is no swing of his right arm.

Tremor

The parkinsonian tremor is typically a resting tremor that disappears when a voluntary movement is performed. Electromyographic recording of the muscles involved shows a rhythmic alternating activity at 4 to 6 Hz between agonist and antagonist muscles. Distal joints are preferentially affected (i.e., metacarpophalangeal), and some distracting maneuvers, such as counting, induce an increment in its magnitude. In some patients there is also a postural tremor of higher frequency (7 to 12 Hz) with additional involvement of more proximal joints.

Rigidity

This consists of an involuntary increment in muscle tone in flexor and extensor muscle groups. This sign is clinically expressed by stiffness of the muscles at palpation and on passive range of motion, and by the spontaneous flexion of the joints in all extremities. It is due to continuous muscle activity that makes relaxation impossible. The most typical feature of rigidity is an augmented resistance to passive joint displacement on examination that can be smooth (lead pipe) or in the presence of underlying tremor, ratchet-like (cogwheel). Simultaneous movements in other body segments provoke an increment in rigidity (Froment's rigidity sign). It is more evident when the passive movement is slowly executed, a feature that separates it from spasticity, in which the tone increases with a higher velocity of motion. When rigidity is severe it may even restrict the range of passive displacement of a joint.

Akinesia

Although strictly speaking *akinesia* means absence of movements, this term includes both the slowness and clumsiness in the execution of movements and the reduction of spontaneous and induced movements. More specifically, *bradykinesia* refers to the slowness of the movement, which is more evident during complex tasks, when several muscle groups are working on a sequence of movements. *Hypokinesia* refers to the poverty of spontaneous movements, a reduction in their amplitude, and their occasional freezing. It is easily recognized in the reduction of the frequency and amplitude of automatic movements such as blinking, arm swing while walking, step length, reaching movements, and writing (*micrographia*).

Postural Instability and Gait Disturbance

These abnormalities begin at a later stage of the disease, usually after other signs have already appeared, and they are responsible to a great extent for the deterioration in the motor condition and quality of life of parkinsonian patients (3). If posture and gait disturbances start when the cardinal features of Parkinson's disease are already present, the diagnosis is not difficult. But even when gait is affected early, it has characteristics that can help the diagnosis, especially in the early stages (4). Initially, patients have a mildly flexed posture that slowly worsens, evolving to flexion of the knees, trunk, elbows, wrists, and metacarpophalangeal joints, with the arms adducted to the trunk. Loss of postural reflexes may occur soon after the diagnosis, but it is not disabling until intermediate or advanced stages, when the patient loses the capacity to make rapid postural adjustments and becomes prone to falling forward or backward. On clinical examination, postural reflexes can be tested by standing behind the patient and pulling him or her backward on the shoulders ("pull test"). Normally, this maneuver only elicits a contraction of the tibialis anterior muscle that will correct the backward tilt. With milder disease, patients may take one or two steps backward until catching themselves, but in more advanced stages they are unable to maintain their equilibrium, and the examiner has to keep them from falling.

As the disease progresses, stride length becomes progressively shortened. At this point shuffling is a common finding and turning is typically made up of several small steps ("en bloc"). In a more advanced stage, gait freezing appears. Initially it occurs when starting to walk (start hesitation), turning (turn hesitation), or passing through narrow spaces and in stressful situations. Eventually, this phenomenon may occur at any time, especially with environmental stimuli, such as sounds, or visual stimuli that attract patients' attention, making them stop (5). With gait freezing, the patients' feet seem to be stuck to the floor and they become unable to raise their legs. This is due to a simultaneous contraction of agonist and antagonist muscles in the leg, instead of the alternating sequence necessary for a plantar flexion followed by a dorsal flexion of the foot. The base of support is narrow and the patient does not accompany the attempt to move the feet with truncal or swing movement. Freezing can be overcome using sensory tricks, mainly visual, for instance by stepping on a piece of paper on the floor, or with a different motor strategy such as a military march (6). Once gait has been initiated, the first two or three steps are even shorter than usual. Sometimes patients may raise their feet a few millimeters, but instead of taking a normal step, they drag the foot forward a few centimeters, developing a shuffling gait. Once gait has been initiated, it is not infrequent that the forward flexor posture, shifting the center of gravity forward, and the failure of postural reflexes make patients walk faster in a shuffling way trying to restore their center of gravity (festinating gait) and finally falling forward. Forward falls are more frequent than backward falls in Parkinson's disease, whereas in parkinsonian disorders other than idiopathic Parkinson's disease the patient tends to fall backward.

Differential Diagnosis

A parkinsonian gait can be observed in conditions other than idiopathic Parkinson's disease. However, some subtle differences in posture and gait and the presence of signs not usually present in Parkinson's disease may help in the diagnosis. Because the disorder of gait and posture in Parkinson's disease is basically induced by a deficit in striatal dopaminergic modulation, any process disrupting the same mechanism can cause a similar disorder. There are several illnesses in which the degenerative process involves not only the substantia nigra, as in Parkinson's disease, but other structures as well (Table 16.3). These entities include multisystem atrophies (e.g., striatonigral degeneration, pontocerebellar atrophy, Shy-Drager syndrome), corticobasal ganglionic degeneration, progressive supranuclear palsy (PSP), Alzheimer's disease, diffuse Lewy-body disease, Creutzfeldt-Jakob disease, the rigid variant of Huntington's disease, and

TABLE 16.3. Other parkinsonian syndromes

Type	Distinguishing features
Drug-induced parkinsonism	History of neuroleptic use
Progressive supranuclear palsy	Impairment of vertical eye movements
Cortical basal ganglionic degeneration	Cortical signs, apraxia
Multisystem atrophy	Orthostatic hypotension
Cerebellopontine degeneration	Cerebellar dysfunction
Related disorders	
Lewy body disease	Dementia with fluctuating level of consciousness, prominent visual hallucinations
Huntington's disease	Dementia with chorea

some even less common disorders. (For further details, see Chapter 78: Abnormalities of Posture and Movement. In: Cassel CK et al., eds. Geriatric Medicine, 4th ed., page 1149.)

Neurologic Diseases

The differential diagnosis is based on the presence of clinical findings that are atypical for Parkinson's disease, such as cerebellar disturbances, severe autonomic failure, limb apraxia, supranuclear ophthalmoplegia, early cognitive impairment, marked postural instability, or absence of response to levodopa treatment. Besides these atypical findings, the characteristics of the parkinsonian syndrome itself often differ from typical Parkinson's disease. For instance, resting tremor is usually absent, and the syndrome conforms to the more rigid-akinetic forms of parkinsonism. Some of these disorders affect at onset both halves of the body, including the axial muscles. The facial expression has been compared to a "perplexed face," with a widened palpebral opening and a wrinkled forehead. Postural and gait disturbances occur earlier in the course than in Parkinson's disease, and consist mainly of a marked postural instability, with frequent falls forward and backward, and shuffling or freezing gait. The base of support is generally wider than in Parkinson's disease. Other differential diagnostic considerations include subcortical vascular disease and normal pressure hydrocephalus.

Systemic Disorders

In addition to these primarily neurologic diseases, there are some systemic disorders than can induce a clinical picture similar to that of Parkinson's disease, including gait abnormalities. This is the case with hypothyroidism, hypoparathyroidism and other endocrine disorders, and depression. Drugs easily induce parkinsonism among the geriatric population, so they have to be taken into consideration during the differential diagnosis. The most important ones are neuroleptics, antihypertensives (reserpine, α-methyl-dopa, some calcium-channel blockers), and other antidopaminergic drugs such as metoclopramide used as antiemetics. Parkinsonism may be also secondary to encephalitis and to toxins such as carbon monoxide, manganese, mercury, methane, cyanide, and N-methyl-4-phenyl-1,2,3,6-tetrahydropyridine (MPTP), but these are rarely seen in daily practice.

Progressive Supranuclear Palsy

Progressive supranuclear palsy (PSP) is a neurodegenerative illness that involves

1. the nigrostriatopallidal system producing rigidity, bradykinesia, and postural instability;
2. the cerebral cortex, mainly the frontal lobes, inducing cognitive and behavioral changes; and
3. the cholinergic nuclei of the pons and mesencephalon, as well as other areas of the brainstem, inducing supranuclear gaze palsies, axial motor abnormalities, sleep disturbances, dysarthria, and dysphagia (7,8).

Neuropathologically, it is characterized by neuronal loss and gliosis of the affected areas. Neurofibrillary tangles, of a type different from the ones found in Alzheimer's disease, appear in some neurons of the affected areas.

The average annual incidence rate (new cases per 100,000 person-years) for ages 50 to 99 years is about 5.3 (9). The age of onset (at the end of the sixth and the beginning of the seventh decades of life) and the initial symptoms are quite similar to those of Parkinson's disease. However, the course is quicker with survival of around 6 to 9 years. Although this entity shares a number of clinical signs with Parkinson's disease (bradykinesia, rigidity), there are some features that help in the differential diagnosis. Thus, in PSP the most frequent presenting sign (60%) is gait disturbance with instability and frequent falls, in contrast to Parkinson's disease in which this abnormality is prominent only after several years of evolution. Usually the patient does not have the flexed posture of Parkinson's disease and, on the contrary, there is often a dystonic hyperextension of the neck. Although the typical parkinsonian signs may be present to some extent from the beginning, the bilateral presentation with a more prominent involvement of axial musculature is a distinctive feature. Resting tremor is not a common finding, although it may be present in 5% to 10% of cases.

Another differential feature is that medicating with L-dopa has little effect on the parkinsonian signs of PSP. These patients usually have a contracted rather than flaccid face, dysphagia, spastic dysarthria rather than the hypophonia of Parkinson's disease, emotional incontinence, and cognitive decline in frontal and executive functions. Patients with atypical presentation may have a dementia suggestive of Alzheimer's disease. The eye findings are most characteristic. There is a supranuclear paresis of eye movements, with eyelid retraction. Saccades are slow and hypometric, with range limitation in both upward and downward directions. Limitation of upward gaze is not uncommon in Parkinson's disease, but in PSP downward gaze is often affected earlier and more prominently than upward gaze. The restriction of eye movements can be easily overcome by the doll's-eye maneuver, indicating damage of the supranuclear mechanisms of eye movement control.

In addition to the parkinsonian syndrome, nonspecific changes in personality with irritability, social withdrawal, and emotional lability are frequent in early PSP and very often they are the presenting features. Thus, an erroneous diagnosis of depression is frequent at this point of evolution and, for the geriatric specialist, it is important to bear this in mind. The diagnosis is based on the clinical features. There are no specific biologic markers of PSP; however, neuroimaging using magnetic resonance imaging (MRI) and positron emission tomography (PET) offer additional diagnostic guidance. (For further details, see Chapter 78: Abnormalities of Posture and Movement. In: Cassel CK, et al., eds. Geriatric Medicine, 4th ed., page 1152.)

Case (Part 3)

You obtain a metabolic screen and an MRI for R.M., all of which are normal. You diagnose R.M. with idiopathic Parkinson's disease and offer him a trial of carbidopa-levodopa, 100 mg three times a day. You explain to him the underlying problem in Parkinson's disease and how this medication attempts to restore dopamine levels. He begins the medication and telephones you to report significant improvements in his tremor and handwriting. You schedule a follow-up examination in 3 months.

Management Considerations

Pharmacologic Therapy

Levodopa, which is transformed into dopamine by the remaining nigral neurons, continues to be the "gold standard" in the treatment of Parkinson's disease. It is administered with a peripheral dopa-decarboxylase inhibitor (benserazide or carbidopa) to prevent its peripheral conversion to dopamine and increase its cerebral bioavailability. Dopamine in the systemic circulation causes a number of side effects, including nausea, vomiting, hypotension, and cardiac arrhythmias. Levodopa treatment, however, is not a panacea. After several years of levodopa treatment, and perhaps due to the natural evolution of the disease, the originally smooth response becomes less than satisfactory. Mobility begins to fluctuate depending on levodopa intake first ("wearing off") and in a random way later ("on-off"), and the patient may experience dyskinesias or involuntary movements during the phase of motor benefit, as well as psychiatric symptoms. The origin of these complications is not completely understood, but the pulsatile administration of levodopa is known to be a risk factor (10). Recently, therapeutic strategies have been developed to provide a more steady dopaminergic stimulation. Slow-release levodopa formulations and direct dopamine agonists, including bromocriptine, pergolide, lisuride, ropinirole, and pramipexole, maintain more stable striatal dopaminergic stimulation. Direct agonists are being used in the initial stages of the disease, alone or in association with low doses of levodopa, to prevent or delay the development of these complications (11). The most common side effects of these drugs are nausea, orthostatic hypotension, and psychiatric complications. Early in the disease, levodopa is generally more effective than direct agonists and, with selegiline (Table 16.4), tends to be preferred as the first-line drug. However, a clinical trial using a dopamine agonist as monotherapy in the early stages of the disease has shown a lesser incidence of motor complications than with the use of levodopa alone after 5 years of treatment (12). Another strategy to maintain steady dopaminergic stimulation involves the use of entacapone, a peripheral inhibitor of catechol-O-methyltransferase (COMT), an enzyme that accelerates the catabolism of levodopa (13). Its use in association with levodopa prolongs the elimination half-life of levodopa, increasing the time of pharmacologic benefit and providing more physiologic dopaminergic stimulation. At present it is mainly used in patients with motor complications.

TABLE 16.4. Pharmacotherapy in Parkinson's disease

Neuroprotection
Selegiline
Vitamin E

Dopamine receptor agonists
Pergolide
Pramipexole
Ropinirole
Bromocriptine

Dopamine replacement
Levodopa/carbidopa

Catechol-O-methyltransferase (COMT) inhibitors
Entacapone

Other pharmaceutical agents (less commonly used)
Anticholinergic
Amantadine

Gait freezing usually responds to levodopa therapy and dopamine agonists. However, sometimes the benefit is of less magnitude than for the rest of the parkinsonian features. The use of amantadine as coadjuvant therapy may also be useful in these cases. Its mechanism of action is not clear, but it has anticholinergic and antiglutamatergic activity. The main side effects are livedo reticularis and ankle edema, plus the usual anticholinergic side effects. In a few cases freezing can be aggravated by levodopa therapy and then it is extremely difficult to treat.

Anticholinergic therapy has no clear benefit for parkinsonian gait. These drugs were used mainly to treat sialorrhea and tremor. Tremor responds just as well to levodopa therapy. Their adverse effects, more pronounced in an older population (urinary retention, angle-closure glaucoma, constipation, and cognitive and psychiatric deficits), have contributed to making them obsolete.

Surgical Therapy

Until recently the only surgical indication in Parkinson's disease was disabling drug-resistant tremor, treated with thalamotomy or thalamic stimulation. Other surgical techniques used in the 1950s had been abandoned after dopamine became available, because they cause unacceptable side effects, partly because discrete target localization was difficult with the techniques then available. (Further review of this method of therapy, see Chapter 78: Abnormalities of Posture and Movement. In: Cassel CK, et al., eds. Geriatric Medicine, 4th ed., page 1150.)

Physical Therapy

Treatment of the parkinsonian gait at any stage of the disease should not be exclusively pharmacologic or surgical (4,14). There are specific rehabilitation programs with exercises directed to reduce rigidity and to increase the range of joint motion (15). Physical therapy, including passive and active mobilization exercises, walking, and range of motion exercises, when combined with medication treatment, may be superior to medication treatment alone (16). Many rehabilitative therapies, such as speech therapy and music therapy, have been studied in Parkinson's patients (17,18). All have shown improvements in functioning during treatment, but many report that the positive gains are not maintained once the treatment concludes. There have been no randomized, controlled trials that have shown long-term sustained effects on function due to rehabilitation alone. Hence, the physical treatment of Parkinson's disease can be considered an example of preventive geriatric rehabilitation.

The patient should be trained in techniques used to counter the effects of the disease. Strengthening and endurance training and proper use of assistive equipment also are important. Such training is best provided early in the course of the illness as an outpatient. Involvement in a support group may help to maintain newly learned skills.

Gait and balance training emphasizes a safe gait and improved balance. The patient should be taught to keep the head up, to counter the flexed posture consciously, and to lift the toes during the swing phase of the gait (19). It also may help to take longer steps and widen the base. The therapist often prescribes a home program of regular exercises to maintain or improve strength, range of motion, and flexibility.

Canes should be avoided when walking aids become necessary. Due to the posture of Parkinson's disease, protraction and internal rotation of the shoulder may place the tip of the cane between the legs, causing a fall. When the walker is prescribed, it should be fitted with front wheels, as pick-up walkers may induce a backward fall. In the home, shag or throw rugs should be removed, rails should be installed on all steps, and bathroom equipment (including raised toilet seats or arm frames and grab bars) should be prescribed.

Treatment of Other Movement Disorders

Parkinsonian Syndromes

Treatments based on the replacement of neurotransmitters or receptor stimulation have been of little benefit in the other parkinsonian syndromes. Dopaminergic stimulation with levodopa or, more reliably, with dopaminergic agonists at high doses, such as bromocriptine at more than 10 mg in three or four divided doses, often improves slightly the parkinsonian signs, often at the price of inducing complications such as agitation, confusion, or hallucinations. Anticholinergic, cholinergic, and noradrenergic drugs and antidepressants have been tested with even less benefit. Among them amantadine seems to be the second most efficient drug following dopaminergic medication. In some trials, it has been reported that gait improves with amitriptyline (100 mg/day in two doses), considered the third choice of drug. Fluoxetine and other blockers of serotonin reuptake have not proved beneficial. Local infiltration with botulinum toxin is useful in the treatment of dystonic features (retrocollis and blepharospasm). Physical therapy seems to be of little benefit against instability. It is important, however, to instruct relatives in the physical care these patients require. Surgical treatment is not currently an option for PSP.

Essential Tremor

Drug treatment of essential tremor may be very effective but not necessarily simple. At present there is no agreement about the drug of choice (20).

Propranolol has been classically considered the first-line drug at daily doses between 80 and 200 mg. It decreases tremor amplitude but the response is often incomplete. Other beta-blockers (metoprolol, nadolol, atenolol, timolol, and pindolol) are less effective than propranolol. In elderly people it is frequent to have concomitant disorders such as atrioventricular block, asthma, or diabetes that are relative contraindications for the use of beta-blockers, especially those blocking the β_2 subtype. Patients with bronchospasm may benefit from metoprolol (100–200 mg/day), a selective β_1-antagonist. Primidone (50–250 mg/day in a single dose at bedtime) has been demonstrated to be as effective as propranolol and it can be used as the drug of choice, particularly in the case of patients suffering from the previously mentioned disorders. However, the sedative effect sometimes constitutes a limiting factor that prevents the achievement of the dose needed for tremor control. Other useful drugs in some cases are phenobarbital (120 mg/day) and benzodiazepines such as diazepam, or clonazepam (1–3 mg/day). Recently, it has been suggested that when propranolol and primidone are not effective, alprazolam could be tried (20). If treatment with monotherapy does not control tremor, combinations of more than one drug may be considered. Other drugs such as gabapentin, carbonic anhydrase inhibitors (methazolamide), amantadine, clonidine, clozapine, flunarizine, nimodipine, etc., have not been proven effective in controlling essential tremor, although they have been reported to be helpful in isolated cases. Patients unsuccessfully controlled with pharmacologic treatments may improve with surgery (21).

Metabolic or toxic disorders that may be associated with postural tremor must always be taken into consideration (22). The most frequent are hyperthyroidism, pheochromocytoma, hypoglycemia, uremia, liver failure, alcohol withdrawal, hypothermia, and toxicity due to lithium, tricyclic antidepressants, valproic acid, neuroleptics, steroids, amiodarone, isoproterenol, theophyline, or cyclosporin A. (For further details, see Chapter 78: Abnormalities of Posture and Movement. In: Cassel CK, et al., eds. Geriatric Medicine, 4th ed., page 1156.)

Case (Part 4)

R.M. returns for his 3-month follow-up visit. His gait appears more fluid and there is less tremor present while he speaks with you. He reports having fallen about 2 weeks ago, without incurring any injury. You explain that although the medication is helpful, sometimes physical therapy provides an additional benefit. You also provide the patient with information regarding a health care proxy and living will.

Other Considerations

As with all degenerative diseases, it is important to address advance directives with patients to educate them about the natural course of the disease and to empower them with the opportunity to direct their care should they desire to do so. In the advanced stages of PD, like other neurologic diseases, individuals are at risk for aspiration pneumonia, dysphagia, and complications of immobility. Individuals should be educated about the therapeutic options for the terminal phases of these conditions (e.g., artificial ventilation or feeding and hydration).

General Principles

- Idiopathic Parkinson's disease is a common primary movement disorder of the elderly.
- Exclusion of secondary parkinsonism or other parkinsonian syndromes is important.
- Dopamine agonists and replacement remain the mainstay of therapy.
- Physical therapy can help with gait abnormalities that lead to falls and functional dependence.
- Education, counseling, and advance directives are important components in the management of this and other degenerative disorders.

Suggested Readings

Bower JH, Maraganore DM, McDonnell SK, Rocca WA. Incidence of progressive supranuclear palsy and multiple system atrophy in Olmsted County, Minnesota, 1976 to 1990. Neurology 1997;49:1284–1288. *This article focuses on the epidemiology of the less common "Parkinson's plus" syndromes associated with degenerative changes outside of the substantia nigra.*

Burleigh-Jacobs A, Horak FB, Nutt JG, Obeso JA. Step initiation in Parkinson's disease: influence of levodopa and external sensory triggers. Mov Disord 1997;12:206–215. *The complex interplay between motor and sensory information in Parkinson's disease is addressed here. The authors suggest how physical therapy in combination with pharmacotherapy may be beneficial in improving gait dysfunction in Parkinson's disease.*

Masdeu JC, Rodriguez-Oroz MC. Abnormalities of posture and movement. In: Cassel CK, Leipzig RM, Cohen HJ, et al., eds. Geriatric Medicine, 4th ed. New York: Springer, 2003:1139–1162.

Morens DM, Davis JW, Grandinetti A, Ross GW, Popper JS, White LR. Epidemiologic observations on Parkinson's disease: incidence and mortality in a prospective study of middle-aged men. Neurology 1996;46:1044–1050. *This article discusses the epidemiology of Parkinson's disease and its effect on mortality.*

References

1. Morens DM, Davis JW, Grandinetti A, Ross GW, Popper JS, White LR. Epidemiologic observations on Parkinson's disease: incidence and mortality in a prospective study of middle-aged men. Neurology 1996;46:1044–1050.
2. Obeso JA, Rodriguez MC, DeLong MR. Basal ganglia pathophysiology. A critical review. Adv Neurol 1997;74:3–18.
3. Klawans HL. Individual manifestations of Parkinson's disease after ten or more years of levodopa. Mov Disord 1986;1:187–192.
4. Pahwa R, Koller W. Gait disorders in parkinsonism and other movement disorders. In: Masdeu J, Sudarsky L, Wolfson L, eds. Gait disorders of aging. Falls and therapeutic strategies. Philadelphia: Lippincott Raven, 1997:209–220.
5. Mestre D, Blin O, Serratrice G. Contrast sensitivity is increased in a case of nonparkinsonian freezing gait. Neurology 1992;42:189–194.
6. Stern GM, Lander CM, Lees AJ. Akinetic freezing and trick movements in Parkinson's disease. J Neural Transm Suppl 1980;(16):137–141.
7. Litvan I. Progressive supranuclear palsy revisited. Acta Neurol Scand 1998;98:73–84.
8. Pahwa R. Progressive supranuclear palsy. Med Clin North Am 1999;83:369–379, v–vi.
9. Bower JH, Maraganore DM, McDonnell SK, Rocca WA. Incidence of progressive supranuclear palsy and multiple system atrophy in Olmsted County, Minnesota, 1976 to 1990. Neurology 1997;49:1284–1288.
10. Obeso JA, Rodriguez-Oroz MC, Chana P, Lera G, Rodriguez M, Olanow CW. The evolution and origin of motor complications in Parkinson's disease. Neurology 2000;55:S13–20; discussion S21–23.
11. Montastruc JL, Rascol O, Senard JM. Treatment of Parkinson's disease should begin with a dopamine agonist. Mov Disord 1999;14:725–730.
12. Rascol O, Brooks DJ, Korczyn AD, De Deyn PP, Clarke CE, Lang AE. A five-year study of the incidence of dyskinesia in patients with early Parkinson's disease who were treated with ropinirole or levodopa. 056 Study Group. N Engl J Med 2000;342:1484–1491.
13. Schapira AH, Obeso JA, Olanow CW. The place of COMT inhibitors in the armamentarium of drugs for the treatment of Parkinson's disease. Neurology 2000;55:S65–68; discussion S69–71.
14. Burleigh-Jacobs A, Horak FB, Nutt JG, Obeso JA. Step initiation in Parkinson's disease: influence of levodopa and external sensory triggers. Mov Disord 1997;12:206–215.
15. Schenkman M, Riegger-Krugh C. Physical intervention for elderly patients with gait disorders. In: Masdeu JC, Sudarsky L, Wolfson L, eds. Gait Disorders of Aging. Philadelphia: Lippincott Raven, 1997:327.
16. Formisano R, Pratesi L, Modarelli FT, et al. Rehabilitation and Parkinson's disease. Scand J Rehabil Med 1992;24:157–160.
17. Nagaya M, Kachi T, Yamada T. Effect of swallowing training on swallowing disorders in Parkinson's disease. Scand J Rehabil Med 2000;32:11–15.
18. Pacchetti C, Mancini F, Aglieri R, Fundaro C, Martignoni E, Nappi G. Active music therapy in Parkinson's disease: an integrative method for motor and emotional rehabilitation. Psychosom Med 2000;62:386–393.

19. Viliani T, Pasquetti P, Magnolfi S, Lunardelli ML, Giorgi C, Serra P, Taiti PG. Effects of physical training on straightening-up processes in patients with Parkinson's disease. Disabil Rehabil 1999;21:68–73.

20. Koller W, Busenbark K. Essential tremor. In: Watts R, Koller W, eds. Movement Disorders: Neurologic Principles and Practice. New York: McGraw-Hill, 1997:365–385.

21. Pahwa R, Lyons K, Koller WC. Surgical treatment of essential tremor. Neurology 2000;54:S39–44.

22. Manyam B. Uncommon forms of tremor. In: Watts R, Koller W, eds. Movement Disorders: Neurologic Principles and Practice. New York: McGraw-Hill, 1997:527–540.

17
Dizziness and Syncope

RAINIER P. SORIANO

Learning Objectives

Upon completion of the chapter, the student will be able to:

1. Describe the mechanisms that give rise to symptoms of dizziness and syncope among older adults.
2. Create a differential diagnosis for etiologies of dizziness and syncope in older adults utilizing key historical and physical examination data to create a differential diagnosis.
3. Identify and describe the prognosis and treatment of the common causes of dizziness and syncope in the elderly.

Case A (Part 1)

Mrs. Adams is a 69-year-old retired executive secretary. She is currently a hospital volunteer escorting newly admitted patients to their rooms and helping with patient transport around the hospital. She comes to your office with the following complaint: "Dr. Smith, I feel dizzy most of the time. What is causing this problem?"

Dizziness: General Considerations

Dizziness is a subjective sensation of postural instability or of illusory motion. It is one of the most common presenting complaints in primary care practice for persons aged 65 years and older. The prevalence of

---

Material in this chapter is based on the following chapters in Cassel CK, Leipzig RM, Cohen HJ, Larson EB, Meier DE, eds. Geriatric Medicine: An Evidence-Based Approach, 4th ed. New York: Springer, 2003: Kapoor WN. Syncope in the Elderly, pp. 957–966. Nanda A, Tinetti ME. Chronic Dizziness and Vertigo, pp. 995–1008. Selections edited by Rainier P. Soriano.

dizziness ranges from 4% to 30% in this age group. Dizziness is a word used by different people to describe many different phenomena. It is a nonspecific term that includes vertigo, dysequilibrium, lightheadedness, spinning, giddiness, faintness, floating, feeling woozy, and many other sensations.

Age-Associated Changes Related to Dizziness

Evidence suggests that age-related changes occur in each of the vestibular, visual, auditory, and proprioceptive systems. Although these age-related changes do not likely cause clinical disease, they may predispose older persons to the occurrence of dizziness by making them more vulnerable to the effects of superimposed impairments and diseases. Degenerative changes and reductions in the number of sensory cells (hair cells) in the semicircular canals, saccule, and utricle have been reported with aging. Age-related visual changes include a decrease in visual acuity, dark adaptation, contrast sensitivity, and accommodation. Age-related decline in proprioception has not been extensively studied.

Diagnostic Evaluation

Symptoms and Signs

An evaluation of dizziness begins with the clinical history. The patient should be asked to be as precise as possible about the sensations of dizziness, an often difficult task because patients may experience more than one manifestation or a vague sensation. The frequency and duration of dizziness, as well as any associated symptoms such as hearing loss, ear fullness, tinnitus, diplopia, dysarthria, and syncopal episodes, are all important. The physician should also ask about comorbid conditions, for example, cardiac diseases, diabetes, renal disorders, anxiety, or depression, which can predispose or exacerbate dizziness. A careful review of all medications, including over-the-counter drugs, is also important.

The physical examination should include measurements of orthostatic changes in blood pressure. One should look for cerebellar signs, for example, gait ataxia, truncal ataxia, or dysmetria, which suggest etiologies such as a cerebellar stroke or cerebellopontine angle tumors. A detailed history and physical examination should help the physician in identifying one or more causes responsible for dizziness. Although 50% of dizziness in older adults cannot be clearly assigned to one type, the most common specific symptoms that are vaguely labeled dizziness can be classified as shown in Table 17.1.

TABLE 17.1 Symptomatic categories of persons complaining of dizziness (26)

Vertigo: A definite rotational sensation or a sense of environmental motion. Vertigo is considered to result from a disturbance within the vestibular system or its connections. The patient may complain, "My head is spinning" or "The room is whirling."

(Pre) syncope: Actual loss of consciousness or the sensation that loss of consciousness is about to happen. Presyncope is usually considered to result from a hypoperfusion of the brain. Common complaints include "I might pass out" or "I feel faint."

Dysequilibrium: Sensation that balance (especially during ambulation) is impaired, but usually without the sensation of vertigo or near fainting. Dysequilibrium usually results from abnormalities in the proprioceptive system. Common complaints: "My balance is off" or "I might fall."

Lightheadedness: A vague term that refers to a head sensation that is nonvertiginous and nonsyncopal. The patient may describe, "floating," "wooziness," "spaciness," "whirling," and other nonspecific sensations. Commonly: "I'm just dizzy."

Source: Adapted from Reilly BM. Dizziness. In: Reilly BM, ed. Practical Strategies in Outpatient Medicine, 2nd ed. Philadelphia: WB Saunders, 1991; and Nanda A, Tinetti ME. Chronic Dizziness and Vertigo. In: Cassel CK, Leipzig RM, Cohen HJ, et al., eds. Geriatric Medicine, 4th ed. New York: Springer, 2003:995–1008.

Provocative Tests

Apart from the history and physical examination, certain provocative tests can be done at the bedside to evaluate the vestibular system. The most common causes of dizziness can be quickly diagnosed by reproducing a patient's symptoms. However, some of these maneuvers should be performed (if at all) cautiously.

To see if the vestibulo-ocular reflex (VOR), which helps to maintain visual stability during head movement, is intact, the following three tests can be done. The sensitivities, specificities, and predictive values of these tests for vestibular lesions in older persons have not been established.

Head-Thrust Test

In the head-thrust test, the patient is asked to fixate on the examiner's nose, and the head is moved rapidly by the examiner about 10 degrees to the left or right. In a normally functioning VOR, the eyes will be fixed on the target, whereas in patients with a vestibular deficit, the eyes are carried away from the target along with the head, followed by a corrective saccade back to the target. For example, in a patient with a right-sided vestibular lesion, head thrusts to the right produce a slipping away of the pupils from the target followed by a corrective movement back to the target, whereas head thrusts to the left produce a normal response of the eyes.

Post–Head-Shake Test

In the post–head-shake test, the head is rotated either passively by the examiner or actively by the subject at a frequency of about 2 Hz in the horizontal plane for about 10 seconds, and then the examiner looks for nystagmus when the head is stopped. In unilateral peripheral vestibular lesions, there will be a horizontal nystagmus with the fast phase usually beating toward the stronger ear, whereas in central lesions the nystagmus may be vertical.

Dynamic Visual Acuity Testing

This test is done by asking the patient to read a fixed eye chart while the examiner moves the head horizontally at a frequency of 1 to 2 Hz. A drop in acuity of two rows or more from the baseline is suggestive of an abnormal VOR. This test is sometimes difficult to perform, because patients may be able to read at times when the head is not in motion (i.e., at turnaround points or by resisting movements). These tests are more helpful in detecting unilateral than bilateral vestibular dysfunction. It is important to remember that compensatory mechanisms may mask a vestibular deficit when these maneuvers are used in patients with longstanding vestibular loss. If the findings of these tests are abnormal, then the patient can be referred for more sophisticated vestibular testing such as electronystagmography and rotational testing.

Stepping Test

This test is positive when there is a lesion in the vestibulospinal system. The patient is asked to stand at the center of a circle drawn on the floor. The circle is divided into sections by lines passing at 30-degree angles. The patient is blindfolded and is asked to outstretch both arms at 90 degrees to the body. The patient is then asked to flex and raise high first one knee and then the other, and to continue stepping forward at a normal walking speed for a total of 50 or 100 steps. The examiner notes body sway while the patient marches in place with the eyes closed. In a unilateral vestibular lesion or in acoustic neuroma, there will be a gradual rotation of the body (more than 30 degrees) toward the affected side.

Dix-Hallpike Maneuver (Nylan-Barany Test)

This test can definitively establish a diagnosis of benign paroxysmal positional vertigo (BPPV). In this maneuver, the patient is seated on an examination table with the head rotated 30 to 45 degrees to one side. The patient is asked to fix his/her vision upon the examiner's forehead. The examiner holds the patient's head firmly in the same position and moves the patient from a seated to a supine position with the head hanging below the edge of the table and the chin pointing slightly upward. The examiner should note the direction, latency, and duration of the nystagmus and the latency and duration of vertigo, if present.

Laboratory Findings

A small battery of laboratory tests should be performed on all patients with dizziness because the prevalence of undetected abnormalities is high and because results often lead to effective treatment. Hematocrit, glucose, blood urea nitrogen, electrolytes, thyroid function tests, and vitamin B_{12}

levels should be ordered in all patients complaining of dizziness. If a cardiovascular etiology is suspected, an electrocardiogram (ECG) to evaluate for the presence of cardiac arrhythmia is indicated. Holter monitoring and tilt table testing are indicated only if there is a strong suspicion of transient/intermittent cardiac arrhythmia or unexplained syncope. Audiometry, which includes pure tone assessment, speech discrimination, impedance measurement, and evoked responses, is recommended for evaluating dizzy patients with hearing loss. Gradual hearing loss is characteristic of acoustic neuroma, whereas Meniere's disease typically presents with fluctuating hearing loss.

Electronystagmography is the most established and widely used test. The procedure consists of a battery of tests designed to record eye movements in response to visual and vestibular stimuli. These include oculomotor evaluation, positional testing, and caloric testing. The oculomotor evaluation involves saccade testing, pursuit testing, optokinetic nystagmus, and spontaneous and gaze-evoked nystagmus. The positional testing is designed to detect nystagmus evoked when the head is held in different positions. The caloric testing assesses the symmetry of vestibular functions. This test can indicate the side of involvement in unilateral vestibular lesions. Each ear is stimulated first with warm (44°C) and then cool water (30°C), each instilled over 30 seconds. The temperature change stimulates or suppresses the respective horizontal semicircular canals, resulting in nystagmus. There will be a decreased response on the ipsilateral side in peripheral vestibular disorder.

Case A (Part 2)

You ask Mrs. Adams to elaborate on her complaint of dizziness. She replies that it started while she was getting ready for church one morning. Everything began to spin around and she felt nauseated, vomited once, and then went to bed. She slept for a few hours and woke up still dizzy. She has no history of head trauma, severe exertion, coughing, sneezing, or flu-like symptoms. She denies exposure to loud noises, taking new medications, or having emotional stress. She is generally healthy, does her own housework, has mild bilateral cataracts, and takes a beta-blocker daily. Mrs. Adams denies experiencing chest pain, loss of consciousness, slurred speech, prior falls or trauma, or gait problems. Upon further questioning, she tells you that when she arises in the morning, she usually needs some time to steady herself. She reports that the room does not spin but just moves back and forth. She also states that she usually gets this sensation when she looks quickly to one side.

Differential Diagnosis

Vertigo

Benign paroxysmal positional vertigo (BPPV) is characterized by brief bouts (seconds) of vertigo, of sudden onset that is provoked by certain changes in the head position (e.g., rolling over in bed into a lateral position, gazing upward, or leaning forward). Another characteristic feature of BPPV is an accompanying rotational nystagmus. The vertigo is often associated with nausea and/or vomiting.

Cerebrovascular diseases have been identified as a primary or contributing cause of dizziness in 4% to 70% of older patients. Vertebrobasilar ischemia results from an obstruction of the blood flow in the vertebrobasilar arteries most commonly caused by arteriosclerosis leading to either transient ischemic attacks (TIA) or infarction.

Meniere's disease is an idiopathic inner ear disorder characterized by episodic vertigo, tinnitus, fluctuating hearing loss, and a sensation of fullness in the inner ear. The frequency of this disease has been reported from 2% to 8% in dizziness cases (1–6). Males and females are affected equally, with onset usually occurring during the fifth decade of life. The main pathologic finding in patients with Meniere's disease is an excess of endolymph within the cochlea and vestibular labyrinth. The patient develops a varying degree of sensations of fullness and/or pressure, along with hearing loss, and tinnitus in the affected ear. Vertiginous episodes usually last from 1 to 24 hours. The patient may complain of a sense of unsteadiness after the acute episode. In the early stages, the hearing loss is completely reversible, but in later stages, partial or complete hearing loss occurs in about 90% of the patients (7).

An acoustic neuroma is a benign tumor of the eighth cranial nerve, characterized by tinnitus and progressive unilateral sensorineural hearing loss more for higher frequencies. This tumor has been reported in 2% to 3% of older persons with dizziness (3–5). Vertigo is a complaint of 19% of patients, whereas 48% complain of imbalance or disequilibrium (6). As the tumor grows, patients may complain of paresthesias or pain in the trigeminal nerve distribution.

Other diagnoses that may produce vertigo include acute/recurrent vestibular disease, cerumen against tympanic membrane, neurolabyrinthitis, neurosyphilis, stroke, and transient vertebrobasilar ischemia.

(Pre)syncope

Postural hypotension has been identified as a primary or contributing cause in 2% to 15% cases of dizziness. Postural hypotension has commonly been defined as a drop in systolic arterial blood pressure of at least 20 mmHg or a fall in diastolic blood pressure of 10 mmHg after standing up from a supine position. Commonly, the blood pressure is measured at 1 and 3 minutes after standing, but in some older persons, a significant orthostatic drop occurs only after 10 to 30 minutes (delayed orthostatic hypotension).

Situational syncope such as postprandial hypotension, usually defined as a decrease in systolic blood pressure of 20 mmHg or more in a sitting or standing posture within 1 to 2 hours of eating a meal, may also cause dizziness. Other causes include psychogenic, anemia, hypovolemia, hypothyroidism, cardiac dysrhythmia, systemic infection, acute myocardial infarction (MI), and vasovagal.

Dysequilibrium

Multiple neurosensory deficits/impairments can cause dizziness. Ocular diseases such as cataracts, glaucoma, and macular degeneration, which are common in older persons, may cause dizziness by impairing the visual functions. Others include Parkinson's disease and cerebellar atrophy.

Lightheadedness

Psychogenic causes of dizziness have been reported in the range of 0% to 57% in older persons with dizziness. Patients usually present with a vague sensation of dizziness along with other somatic complaints and with symptoms of psychological disorders such as anxiety (including panic disorder).

Adverse effects from medications have frequently been reported to cause or contribute to dizziness. Several classes of medications, such as anxiolytic drugs, antidepressants, antihypertensive drugs, aminoglycosides, chemotherapeutic agents, and nonsteroidal antiinflammatory drugs (NSAIDs), are known to produce dizziness as a side effect.

Case A (Part 3)

Examination reveals a pale woman with normal vital signs. Fine horizontal nystagmus is noted on physical examination and accentuated during examination in a fully darkened room with an ophthalmoscope. Ears, lungs, and heart are normal. Screening for hearing loss using a tuning fork and watch suggests equal function bilaterally. Cardiovascular and neurologic examination findings are normal. Rapid positional testing using the Dix-Hallpike maneuver reproduces her dizziness in the right head-hanging position. On further questioning, she admits having more difficulty rolling over to the right than to the left, when in bed. Mrs. Adams asks you if there's anything that could possible relieve her of the dizziness.

Management Considerations

Dizziness is a challenging problem for physicians who take care of older persons. The goal should be to eliminate the cause of the dizziness, if possible. If not, the goal should then be to alleviate the dizziness to the extent possible and to avoid the adverse consequences such as falls, functional disability, and increased depressive symptoms.

Pharmacologic Therapy

Vestibular suppressants, including antihistamines (e.g., meclizine) and anticholinergic agents (scopolamine), are commonly used for symptomatic relief. These agents are effective for acute dizziness but play little role in managing chronic dizziness. Meclizine is a weak antihistaminic agent usually taken orally in doses of 12.5 to 25 mg three times a day, as needed. Vestibular suppressants should not be used long term because of their central nervous system (CNS) side effects and because they suppress central and vestibular adaptation and thus may worsen or exacerbate dizziness (8). Benzodiazepines (e.g., diazepam) may be beneficial to patients with severe unilateral peripheral vestibular dysfunction. Scopolamine should not be used in older persons due to its anticholinergic side effects such as urinary retention and deficits in cognition.

Repositioning Maneuvers

The canalith repositioning procedure, introduced by Epley (9), is a currently recommended treatment for benign positional vertigo (10). The purpose of this bedside maneuver is to move free-floating debris by the effects of gravity from the posterior semicircular canal into the utriculus of the vestibular labyrinth, where it will no longer affect the dynamics of the semicircular canals (9). In this procedure, a Dix-Hallpike maneuver is performed with the patient's head rotated 45 degrees toward the affected ear and his/her head hanging below the edge of the table, and a vibrator is applied to the ipsilateral mastoid process. After the cessation of the provoked vertigo and nystagmus, the head, which is hanging below the edge of the table, is rotated 45 degrees to the opposite side. This maneuver may induce a brief episode of vertigo. The examiner should hold the patient's head in this position and wait for about 10 to 15 seconds or until the vertigo ceases. Then the head and body are further rotated until the head is in a face-down position. This maneuver may again induce a brief vertigo. The patient should be kept in the final face-down position for about 10 to 15 seconds or until the vertigo ceases. Then, with the head kept in the same position, the patient is brought to a seated position. Once the patient is upright, the head is turned forward with the chin tilted slightly downward. The patient should be instructed not to lie flat and to keep his/her head relatively upright for the next 24 to 48 hours. Another option would be to instruct the patient to wear a cervical collar and neither to lie supine nor to tilt the head upward, downward, or to the right or left more than 30 degrees (11). These strategies are to prevent the loose debris from gravitating back to the posterior semicircular canal. There are no data available to support these recommendations.

Surgery

Surgical excision is the treatment of choice for cerebellopontine angle tumors. Surgery is reserved for disabling unilateral peripheral disease unresponsive to medical therapy. Ablative procedures include transmastoid labyrinthectomy and partial vestibular neurectomy. The primary indication for either procedure is uncontrolled Meniere's disease or peripheral vestibulopathy (12). Nonablative procedures include endolymphatic sac decompression and posterior canal occlusion.

Patient Education

Patients should be given basic education concerning the functioning of the balance system and the pathophysiology of dizziness. This knowledge enables patients to understand the body movements responsible for these symptoms and also alleviates their anxiety about this problem. They should be instructed on modifying their activities; for example, if orthostatic hypotension is detected, patients should be instructed to rise slowly from a sitting or supine position. Movements such as looking up, reaching up, or bending down are to be avoided in part by storing items at home strategically. However, patients should be cautioned not to habitually avoid other movements such as head turning because doing so may compromise central adaptation, thereby exacerbating dizziness. Patients should also be instructed to avoid walking in the dark and to avoid over-the-counter drugs that may exacerbate dizziness.

Case B

Ms. Williams, Mrs. Adams's niece, called your office from the hospital emergency room (ER). She said that her aunt was currently in the ER after Ms. Williams witnessed a frightful episode last night. She saw her aunt go to the bathroom when all of sudden, she heard a loud thud. She ran to the bathroom and found her aunt lying unconscious next to the toilet bowl. Her aunt's pajama pants were still around her ankles. Mrs. Adams soon regained consciousness but not until the emergency medical service (EMS) was called for assistance. She was brought to the ER where she said that she couldn't remember what happened. The last thing she knew was that she was urinating in the bathroom when everything else turned black. She denied any chest pain or palpitations.

Syncope: General Considerations

Syncope is defined as a sudden transient loss of consciousness associated with loss of postural tone from which the patient recovers spontaneously. Syncope has a large differential diagnosis ranging from common benign problems to severe life-threatening disorders. As a result, the approach to this symptom frequently results in hospital admission and performance of many diagnostic tests. Although evaluation is often focused on explaining the symptom by a single disease process, this may not apply to the elderly since multiple physiologic processes and age-related changes may contribute to syncope.

Age-Associated Changes Related to Syncope

Elderly patients often have multiple comorbid conditions that interact with age-related physiologic derangements leading to a reduction in cerebral blood flow when even mild acute processes are superimposed. Physiologic changes related to aging may diminish the ability to adapt to a sudden drop in blood pressure (13). Baroreflex sensitivity diminishes with aging, manifesting as a reduction in vascular response to hypotensive stimuli. This may be due to a blunting of β-adrenergic–mediated vasodilation. As a result of decreased baroreceptor reflex sensitivity, older adults may not be able to maintain cerebral blood flow by increasing heart rate and vascular tone in the setting of hypotension. Thus, the elderly are more sensitive to the effects of vasodilators and other hypotensive drugs and are more likely to have exaggerated hypotension from volume loss, hemorrhage, and upright posture.

With aging, kidneys develop impairment of sodium conservation when salt intake is restricted. Basal plasma levels of renin and aldosterone are also decreased. These changes may increase the susceptibility of the elderly to orthostatic hypotension and syncope. As a result, the effects of diuretics, salt restriction, and upright posture may be more pronounced in the elderly.

Pathogenesis

Syncope is due to sudden decrease in cerebral blood flow to those areas of the brain that are responsible for consciousness (reticular activating system and both hemispheres). Elderly patients with hypertension and atherosclerotic vascular disease have baseline decreased cerebral blood flow that may be further reduced by multiple comorbid conditions. Additionally, elderly patients are often taking multiple medications, which may further reduce cerebral blood flow by altering vascular tone or volume.

Diagnostic Evaluation

The majority of the causes of syncope are identified by a careful history and physical examination (Table 17.2). Additionally, history and physical examination may suggest specific entities as possible causes (e.g., findings of aortic stenosis or neurologic signs and symptoms suggestive of a seizure disorder). In patients with a negative history, physical examination, and ECG, further testing can be approached by stratifying patients into those with and without heart disease.

Symptoms and Signs

The most important elements in the evaluation of syncope in the elderly are (1) determining whether the patient had syncope, (2) risk stratification,

TABLE 17.2. Etiologies of syncope

Neurally mediated syndromes	Decrease cardiac output
• Vasovagal	Obstruction to flow
• Situational	• Obstruction to LV outflow or inflow
Micturition	Aortic stenosis, IHSS
Cough	Mitral stenosis, myxoma
Swallow	• Obstruction to RV outflow or inflow
Defecation	Pulmonic stenosis
• Carotid sinus syncope	PE, pulmonary hypertension
• Neuralgias	Myxoma
• High altitude	Other heart disease
• Psychiatric disorders	• Pump failure
• Others (exercise, selected drugs)	MI, CAD, coronary spasm
Orthostatic hypotension	• Tamponade, aortic dissection
Neurologic diseases	Arrhythmias
• Migraines	• Bradyarrhythmias
• TIAs	Sinus node disease
• Seizures	Second and third degree
	atrioventricular block
	Pacemaker malfunction
	Drug-induced bradyarrhythmias
	• Tachyarrhythmias
	Ventricular tachycardia
	Torsades de Pointes (e.g., associated
	with congenital long QT
	syndromes or acquired QT
	prolongation)
	Supraventricular tachycardia

TIA, transient ischemic attack; LV, left ventricular; IHSS, idiopathic hypertrophic subaortic stenosis; RV, right ventricular; PE, pulmonary embolism; MI, myocardial infarction; CAD, coronary artery disease.
Source: Kapoor WN. Syncope in the elderly. In: Cassel CK, Leipzig RM, Cohen HJ, et al., eds. Geriatric Medicine, 4th ed. New York: Springer, 2003.

TABLE 17.3. Clinical features suggestive of specific causes of syncope (27)

Symptom or finding	Diagnostic consideration
After sudden unexpected pain, fear, unpleasant sight, sound, or smell	Vasovagal
Prolonged standing at attention	Vasovagal
Well-trained athlete after exertion (without heart disease)	Vasovagal
During or immediately after micturition, cough, swallow, or defecation	Situational syncope
Syncope with throat or facial pain (glossopharyngeal or trigeminal neuralgia)	Neurally mediated syncope with neuralgia
With head rotation, pressure on carotid sinus (as in tumors, shaving, tight collars)	Carotid sinus syncope
Immediately upon standing	Orthostatic hypotension
Medications that may lead to long QT or orthostasis/bradycardia	Drug induced
Associated with headaches	Migraines, seizures
Associated with vertigo, dysarthria, diplopia migraine	TIA, subclavian steal, basilar
With arm exercise	Subclavian steal
Confusion after spell or loss of consciousness more than 5 minutes	Seizure
Differences in BP or pulse in two arms	Subclavian steal or aortic dissection
Syncope and murmur with changing position (from sitting to lying, bending, turning over in bed)	Atrial myxoma or thrombus
Syncope with exertion	Aortic stenosis, pulmonary hypertension, mitral stenosis, hypertrophic cardiomyopathy, coronary artery disease
Family history of sudden death syndrome	Long QT syndrome, Brugada syndrome
Brief loss of consciousness, no prodrome, with heart disease	Arrhythmias
Frequent syncope, somatic complaints, no heart disease	Psychiatric illness

Source: Kapoor WN. Syncope. N Engl J Med 2000;343(25):1856–1862. Copyright 2000, Massachusetts Medical Society. All rights reserved.

and (3) selective use of diagnostic tests to define the etiology of the loss of consciousness.

A history from the patient and an eyewitness, if present, is needed to distinguish syncope from other entities such as dizziness, vertigo, drop attacks, coma, and seizure. Table 17.3 shows clinical presentations that may suggest specific entities. A particularly important issue is the distinction between syncope and seizure because videometric analysis of syncope has shown myoclonic activity in 90%, predominantly consisting of multifocal arrhythmic jerks both in proximal and distal muscles. Historical features are often sufficient to distinguish syncope from seizures. Seizures are associated with blue face (or not pale), frothing at the mouth, tongue biting, disorientation, aching muscles, sleepiness after the event, and duration of unconsciousness of more than 5 minutes. On the other hand, symptoms associated with syncope are sweating or nausea before the event and being oriented after the event. The best discriminatory symptom is disorientation after the episode, which often signifies a seizure (14).

Orthostatic hypotension is generally defined as a decline of 20 mmHg or more in systolic pressure upon assuming an upright position. However, this finding is reported in up to 24% of the elderly and is frequently not associated with symptoms. Thus, the clinical diagnosis of orthostatic hypotension should incorporate the presence of symptoms (e.g., dizziness and syncope) in association with a decrease in systolic blood pressure. In detection of orthostatic hypotension, supine blood pressure and heart rate should be measured after the patient has been lying down for at least 5 minutes. Standing measurements should be obtained immediately and for at least 3 minutes. Sitting blood pressures are not reliable for detection of orthostatic hypotension.

Several cardiovascular findings are crucial diagnostically. Differences in the pulse intensity and blood pressure (generally >20 mmHg) in the two arms are suggestive of aortic dissection or subclavian steal syndrome. Special focus on cardiovascular examination for aortic stenosis, idiopathic hypertrophic subaortic stenosis, pulmonary hypertension, myxomas, and aortic dissection may uncover clues to these entities.

Laboratory Evaluation

Initial laboratory blood tests rarely yield diagnostically helpful information. Hypoglycemia, hyponatremia, hypocalcemia, or renal failure is found in 2% to 3% of patients, but in most cases appears to result in seizures rather than syncope (15,16). These tests are often confirmatory of clinical suspicion of these laboratory abnormalities. In the elderly patients in whom a cause of syncope is not established by the initial history and physical examination, further evaluation should focus on the following issues: (1) arrhythmia detection, (2) tilt testing, and (3) multiple abnormalities causing symptoms.

Arrhythmia Detection

In diagnosing arrhythmias, every attempt should be made to attain symptomatic correlation. Arrhythmias are evaluated by prolonged electrocardiographic monitoring or electrophysiologic studies, although rarely (in 2–9%) the initial electrocardiogram or a rhythm strip may show an arrhythmia (15–18). One method of assessing the impact of ambulatory monitoring in syncope is to determine the presence or absence of arrhythmias in patients who develop symptoms during monitoring. Electrophysiologic studies are abnormal in approximately 50% of patients undergoing this test. The most common finding is inducible ventricular tachycardia. Electrophysiologic studies are more likely to be positive in patients with known heart disease, abnormal ventricular function, or abnormalities on electrocardiogram, or on ambulatory monitoring. Predictors of ventricular tachycardia by electrophysiologic studies include organic heart disease, premature ventricular contractions (PVCs) by ECG, and nonsustained ventricular tachycardia by Holter monitoring. Sinus bradycardia, first-degree atrioventricular (AV) block, and bundle branch block by ECG predict bradyarrhythmic outcome. Predictors of a negative electrophysiologic study in patients with syncope include the absence of heart disease, an ejection fraction >40%, normal electrocardiogram and Holter monitoring; absence of injury during syncope, and multiple or prolonged (>5 minutes) episodes of syncope.

Tilt Testing

The pathophysiologic mechanism of inducing syncope by upright tilt testing is poorly understood. One postulated mechanism centers around the stimulation of cardiac mechanoreceptors. Upright posture leads to pooling of blood in the lower limbs, resulting in decreased venous return. Normal compensatory response to standing upright is reflex tachycardia, more forceful contraction of the ventricles, and vasoconstriction. However, in individuals susceptible to vasovagal syncope, this forceful ventricular contraction in the setting of a relatively empty ventricle may excessively stimulate the cardiac sensory nerves (mechanoreceptors). Afferent impulses are relayed to the medulla, resulting in a decrease in sympathetic and increase in parasympathetic tone.

The American College of Cardiology Expert Consensus has recommended tilt testing methods and indications (19). Tilt testing methods generally involve the use of provocative agents such as isoproterenol or nitroglycerine because rates of positive responses without chemical stimulation appear to be low (19–21). In patients with unexplained syncope, positive responses occur in approximately 66% with isoproterenol protocols (21,22). The results with the use of nitroglycerine appear to be similar (23,24). The specificity of most currently used tilt testing approaches 90% with chemical stimulation (21,22).

Multiple Abnormalities Causing Symptoms

Skull films, lumbar puncture, radionuclide brain scan, and cerebral angiography have not yielded diagnostic information for a cause of syncope in the absence of clinical findings suggestive of a specific neurologic process (17). Electroencephalogram (EEG) shows an epileptiform abnormality in 1%, but almost all of these are suspected clinically. Head computed tomography (CT) scans are needed if subdural bleed due to head injury is suspected or in patients suspected to have a seizure as a cause of loss of consciousness.

Management Considerations

Management issues include hospitalization decision, treatment selection, and patient instructions and education. Because the treatment largely depends on the cause of syncope, a discussion of the treatment of all of the causes is beyond the scope of this review.

Neurally Mediated Syncope

Because of potential side effects, treatment should be reserved for elderly patients with frequent or disabling symptoms. Because psychiatric illnesses (especially depression and anxiety) probably lead to vasovagal reactions, screening for the psychiatric illnesses noted above should be performed. Treatment of the psychiatric illness often results in resolution of recurrent syncope.

The most commonly used drugs are beta-blockers (25) (e.g., metoprolol 50–200 mg/day, atenolol 25–200 mg/day, and propranolol 40–160 mg/day), which may inhibit the activation of cardiac mechanoreceptors by decreasing cardiac contractility. Other drugs include anticholinergic drugs, such as transdermal scopolamine one patch every 2 to 3 days, disopyramide (200–600 mg/day), paroxetine (20–40 mg/day) (26), theophylline (6–12 mg/kg/day), and measures to expand volume (increased salt intake, custom-fitted counterpressure support garments from ankle to waist, and fludrocortisone acetate at 0.1–1 mg per day).

Orthostatic Hypotension

The initial approach to treatment of orthostatic hypotension is to ensure adequate salt and volume intake and to discontinue drugs that cause orthostatic hypotension. Patients with orthostatic hypotension should be advised to raise the head of the bed at night, to rise from bed or chair slowly, and avoid prolonged standing. Compressive stockings applied up to thigh level may help decrease venous pooling. Frequent small feedings may be helpful for patients with marked postprandial hypotension. Pharmacologic agents of potential benefit include fludrocortisone (0.1–1 mg/day), in conjunction with increased salt intake. Various agents have been used including midodrine, ephedrine, phenylephrine, and others.

Patient Instructions and Education

Issues in patient education include instructions in prevention of syncope, nonpharmacologic treatment, and restriction of activities. Many patients with vasovagal syncope have precipitating factors or situations that should be identified, and the patient instructed to avoid these situations. Common triggers include prolonged standing, venipuncture, large meals, and heat (such as hot baths or sunbathing). Additionally, fasting, lack of sleep, and alcohol intake may predispose to vasovagal syncope and should be avoided. Postexercise vasovagal syncope may occasionally be related to chronic inadequate salt and fluid replacement. Syncope may be prevented with the use of electrolyte containing solutions and water in such instances. In other patients exercise may have to be curtailed.

General Principles

- Dizziness is a subjective sensation of postural instability or of illusory motion and is one of the most common presenting complaints in primary care practice for persons aged 65 years and older.
- Discrete causes of chronic dizziness can be divided into central nervous system disorders, vestibular disorders, psychogenic causes, systemic causes, medications, and miscellaneous.
- Apart from the history and physical examination, certain provocative tests can be done at bedside to evaluate the vestibular system including the head-thrust test, post–head-shake test, dynamic visual acuity test, stepping test, and the Dix-Hallpike maneuver.
- Dizziness is a challenging problem for physicians and the goal should be to eliminate the cause of the dizziness, if possible. If not, the goal should then be to alleviate the dizziness to the extent possible and to avoid the adverse consequences such as falls, functional disability, and increased depressive symptoms.

Suggested Readings

Kapoor WN. Syncope. N Engl J Med 2000;343(25):1856–1862. *An excellent review article on the approach to patients with syncope.*

Kapoor WN. Syncope in the elderly. In: Cassel CK, Leipzig RM, Cohen HJ, et al., eds. Geriatric Medicine, 4th ed. New York: Springer, 2003:957–966.

Nanda A, Tinetti ME. Chronic dizziness and vertigo. In: Cassel CK, Leipzig RM, Cohen HJ, et al., eds. Geriatric Medicine, 4th ed. New York: Springer, 2003: 995–1008.

Tinetti ME, Williams CS, Gill TM. Dizziness among older adults: A possible geriatric syndrome. Ann Intern Med 2000;132:337–344. *A cross-sectional population study on the predisposing characteristics and situational factors associated with dizziness.*

References

1. Kroenke K, Lucas CA, Rosenberg ML, et al. Causes of persistent dizziness: a prospective study of 100 patients in ambulatory care. Ann Intern Med 1992;117:898–904.

2. Drachman DA, Hart CW. An approach to the dizzy patient. Neurology 1972;22:323–334.
3. Sloane PD, Baloh RW. Persistent dizziness in geriatric patients. J Am Geriatr Soc 1989;37:1031–1038.
4. Lawson J, Fitzgerald J, Birchall J, Aldren CP, Kenny RA. Diagnosis of geriatric patients with severe dizziness. J Am Geriatr Soc 1999;47:12–17.
5. Davis LE. Dizziness in elderly men. J Am Geriatr Soc 1994;42:1184–1188.
6. Katsarkas A. Dizziness in aging. A retrospective study of 1194 cases. Otolaryngol Head Neck Surg 1994;110:296–301.
7. Sloane P, Blazer D, George LK. Dizziness in a community elderly population. J Am Geriatr Soc 1989;37:101–108.
8. Zee DS. Perspective on the pharmacotherapy of vertigo. Arch Otolaryngol 1985;111:609–612.
9. Epley JM. The canalith repositioning procedure: for treatment of benign paroxysmal positional vertigo. Otolaryngol Head Neck Surg 1992;107:399–404.
10. Furman JM, Cass SP. Benign paroxysmal positional vertigo (review article). N Engl J Med 1999;341:1590–1596.
11. Li JC. Mastoid oscillation: a critical factor for success in the canalith repositioning procedure. Otolaryngol Head Neck Surg 1995;112:670–675.
12. Goebel JA. Management options for acute versus chronic vertigo. Otolaryngol Clin North Am 2000;33:483–493.
13. Lipsitz LA. Altered blood pressure homeostasis in advanced age: clinical and research implications. J Gerontol 1989;44(6):M179–M183.
14. Hoefnagels WAJ, Padberg GW, Overweg J, et al. Syncope or seizure? The diagnostic value of the EEG and hyperventilation test in transient loss of consciousness. J Neurol 1991;54:953–956.
15. Linzer M, Yang EH, Estes NA, Wang P, Vorperian V, Kapoor WN. Diagnosing syncope. Part 1: Value of history, physical examination, and electrocardiography. The clinical efficacy assessment project of the American College of Physicians. Ann Intern Med 1997;126(12):989–996.
16. Linzer M, Yang EH, Estes NA, Wang P, Vorperian V, Kapoor WN. Diagnosing syncope. Part 2: Unexplained syncope. The clinical efficacy assessment project of the American College of Physicians. Ann Intern Med 1997;127(1):78–86.
17. Kapoor W. Evaluation and outcome of patients with syncope. Medicine 1990;69:160–175.
18. Kapoor W, Snustad D, Peterson J, et al. Syncope in the elderly. Am J Med 1986;80:419–428.
19. Benditt DG, Ferguson DW, Grubb BP, et al. Tilt table testing for assessing syncope. J Am Coll Cardiol 1996;28:263–275.
20. Grubb BP, Kosinski D. Current trends in the etiology, diagnosis and management of neurocardiogenic syncope. Curr Opin Cardiol 1996;11:32–41.
21. Kapoor WN. Using a tilt table to evaluate syncope. Am J Med Sci 1999;317(2):110–116.
22. Kapoor WN, Smith M, Miller NL. Upright tilt testing in evaluating syncope: a comprehensive literature review. Am J Med 1994;97:78–88.
23. Raviele A, Giada F, Brignole M, et al. Diagnostic accuracy of sublingual nitroglycerin test and low-dose isoproterenol test in patients with unexplained syncope. A comparative study. Am J Cardiol 2000;85:1194–1198.

24. Mahanonda N, Bhuripanyo K, Kangkagate C, et al. Randomized double-blind, placebo-controlled trial of oral atenolol in patients with unexplained syncope and positive upright tilt table test results. Am Heart J 1995;130: 1250–1253.

25. Di Girolamo E, Di Iorio C, Sabatini P, Leonzio L, Barbone C, Barsotti A. Effects of paroxetine hydrochloride, a selective serotonin reuptake inhibitor, on refractory vasovagal syncope: a randomized, double-blind, placebo-controlled study. J Am Coll Cardiol 1999;33(5):1227–1230.

26. Reilly BM. Dizziness. In: Reilly BM, ed. Practical Strategies in Outpatient Medicine, 2nd ed. Philadelphia: WB Saunders, 1991.

27. Kapoor WN. Syncope. N Engl J Med 2000;343(25):1856–1862.

18
Osteoarthritis

KATHLEEN R. SROCK

Learning Objectives

Upon completion of the chapter, the student will be able to:

1. Diagnose osteoarthritis (OA) by history, physical, and radiographic findings.
2. Differentiate OA from inflammatory arthritis, such as rheumatoid arthritis.
3. Implement patient appropriate treatments.
4. Know when to refer to the orthopedic surgeon for surgical evaluation.

Case (Part 1)

Ms. Creaky, a 72-year-old woman with a history of hypertension and gastroesophageal reflux disease (GERD), comes to your office and tells you that she must be getting old because her entire body hurts. She says that she has been having pain for years but that it has recently been getting worse, especially in her hands, knees, and left hip.

Material in this chapter is based on the following chapters in Cassel CK, Leipzig RM, Cohen HJ, Larson EB, Meier DE, eds. Geriatric Medicine: An Evidence-Based Approach, 4th ed. New York: Springer, 2003: Brauner DJ, Sorensen LB, Ellman MH. Rheumatologic Diseases, pp. 573–619. Pottenger LA. Orthopedic Problems with Aging, pp. 651–667. Selections edited by Kathleen R. Srock.

General Considerations

Osteoarthritis (OA) is the most common articular disorder and accounts for more disability among the elderly than any other disease. The commonly held notion that OA is an inevitable consequence of aging because of the normal "wear and tear" of the joint is much too simplistic. Cartilage does not simply wear out like the soles of one's shoes. Rather, the changes seen in OA involve the complex interaction of genetic susceptibility, joint mechanics and injury, chondrocytes that live a robust metabolic existence, biochemical alterations, and the complex interplay of mediators, as well as structures that surround the joint.

Definition and Prevalence

One useful way of understanding OA is as a final common pathway, a clinical and pathologic outcome of a range of disorders resulting in similar alterations in articular anatomy and function (1). Osteoarthritis occurs when the dynamic equilibrium between the breakdown and repair of joint tissues is overwhelmed. Factors that have been implicated include occupation, body weight, trauma, recreational activities, developmental abnormalities, collagen gene mutations, muscle weakness, alterations in proprioception, denervation of joints, and inherited and acquired errors of metabolism.

Epidemiologic studies have shown that the prevalence of OA increases progressively with age. In two studies, the prevalence of symptomatic knee OA was only 29% and 43% of radiologically defined disease (2,3). Radiologic findings frequently do not correlate with clinical symptomatology; thus, decisions regarding surgical intervention rely more upon functional limitations, especially in the elderly, than on radiographic findings. Until middle age, OA occurs with the same frequency in men and women, but after age 50, symptomatic OA is more common in women, and this difference in prevalence widens with increasing age.

Age-Related Changes Related to Osteoarthritis

Age-related changes in joints are different from those of other musculoskeletal tissues. Perhaps more than any other condition, the changes associated with OA are most strongly associated with images of aging, as in the gnarled hands and antalgic or painful, noisy gait of the old person with arthritis. But although OA is common in older people, it is not universal or inevitable. Many changes have been found to occur in cartilage with aging. The changes in cartilage proteoglycans are summarized in Table 18.1.

TABLE 18.1. Changes in cartilage proteoglycans with aging

1. Progressive decrease in the average length of the core protein of the aggrecan molecule
2. Decreased hydrodynamic size of the aggrecan molecule via decreased length of chondroitin sulfate chains and increase in number of keratin sulfate chains
3. Decreased proportion of aggrecans able to form aggregates with hyaluronic acid
4. Decreased size of aggregates from reduction of length of the hyaluronic acid molecule and smaller size of the aggrecan molecules

Source: Brauner DJ, Sorensen LB, Ellman MH. Rheumatologic diseases. In: Cassel CK, Leipzig RM, Cohen HJ, et al., eds. Geriatric Medicine, 4th ed. New York: Springer, 2003.

Case (Part 2)

Ms. Creaky is worried because she developed "bumps" on some of her fingers. She remembers her mother having similar bumps and eventually developing deformities. Although she has always been moderately obese she is frustrated with herself because she has gained 20 pounds over several months. She has never stuck to a regular exercise program but enjoyed walking on nice days. She blames her weight gain on her knee and hip pain, which prohibit her from extensive walking. She has started to spend most of her time in her apartment where she has groceries and meals delivered.

Pathogenesis/Risk Factors

Knowledge of risk factors is important in understanding OA to help identify those with higher likelihood of getting the disease, as well as for developing preventive strategies, both primary and secondary, and for therapeutic interventions. Factors that place increased stress on joints appear to be important risk factors for the later development of OA. This stress can take the form of repetitive stress and trauma as occurs in certain occupations. Many classic studies have implicated various occupations such as coal miners, pneumatic drillers, cotton operatives, ironworkers, and elite athletes.

Heavy physical activity in general has been implicated in the development of OA, and it appears that modulating factors such as type of activity, presence of obesity, and at what point in the life cycle the activity took place are all important. Although activities such as moderate running appear to be well tolerated in younger people, a stronger association of knee OA with physical activity has been found in women over the age of 50, compared with younger women.

Longitudinal studies have since found obesity to be a predictor for the development of OA. This association has been found to be the strongest for knee OA, less so for OA of the hands, and inconsistent for OA of the hip. The risk appears to be much stronger in women, though it also is present in men with severe obesity (highest quintile) (4,5). Even mild obesity (body mass index, BMI >25) has been found to put women at increased risk for the development of OA of the knee (6). Obesity appears to provide an additive risk when combined with heavy physical activity.

Crystals that are known to cause acute arthritis and periarthritis also play an important role in mediating the expression of OA. The class of crystals most commonly found in osteoarthritic joints is the calcium-containing crystals, of which calcium pyrophosphate and basic calcium phosphate are the best studied (7). Osteoarthritis is both more common and more severe in joints in which chondrocalcinosis and/or crystals have been demonstrated. Calcium pyrophosphate disease (CPPD) should be suspected when OA is seen in atypical joints such as the metacarpophalangeal (MCP) joints, wrists, elbows, and shoulders. Chondrocalcinosis can be seen on radiograph as linear calcified streaks within cartilage of the knee, triangular fibrocartilage of the wrist, and even in the cartilage of the symphysis pubis. Although chondrocalcinosis may suggest CPPD, it may also be an innocent bystander seen incidentally in unaffected joints.

Muscle weakness may play a large role in the age-related increase in incidence of OA, as aging is also frequently associated with generalized weakness related to deconditioning. Problems with proprioception, the conscious and unconscious perception of limb position and movement in space, have been implicated as a risk factor for OA. This has been studied most extensively in the knee, where proprioception derives from integration of afferents from receptors in muscles, tendons, joint capsule, ligaments, meniscal attachments, and skin. The hypermobility syndrome, a well-known risk factor for precocious OA, is associated with impaired proprioception, especially near full extension, and may result in mechanically unsound joint positions that could predispose to OA.

Inactivity is an important risk factor for OA that has been incompletely explored in humans, although there are excellent animal models that demonstrate immobilization leading to OA. Prolonged bed rest with lack of joint loading is a theoretical risk for the development of OA that should be included on the long list of adverse consequences of bed rest.

Case (Part 3)

Ms. Creaky denies trauma, swollen joints, weight loss, fever, and rashes. She describes having morning stiffness lasting for about 10 minutes especially in her hands and knees. Her knee pain is exacerbated by climbing stairs and prolonged standing.

On exam she has scattered bony enlargements at several distal interphalangeal (DIP) joints and proximal interphalangeal (PIP) joints. She has lateral deviation of her left third DIP and palmar deviation at her right fourth DIP. There is no synovitis of her PIPs, MCPs, or wrists. She has a small suprapatellar effusion of the left knee and bilateral crepitus. There is valgus deformity of her right knee. Quadriceps atrophy is seen bilaterally. She has good range of motion (ROM) of both hips but has pain along the lateral aspect of the left thigh at the level of the greater trochanter.

Diagnostic Evaluation

Symptoms and Signs

The most common pain described with OA is an achy type associated with use of the particular joint. Occasionally, the pain is described as sharp and fleeting, especially in the knees, where it can be associated with certain movements during weight bearing. When osteoarthritis involves the lower back or hips, the pain is often poorly localized. The pain is typically related to activity, but rest pain is present in approximately 50% and night pain in about 30%.

Stiffness is another commonly described symptom of OA. The stiffness associated with OA may be described as difficulty initiating movement in a joint or decreased or painful movement in a joint. Morning stiffness, commonly seen in the more inflammatory types of arthritis like rheumatoid arthritis, may be present but is usually of shorter duration (less than 30 minutes) and limited to fewer joints. More commonly, patients describe a gelling phenomena, in which particular joints, most commonly the knees and hands, become stiff after periods of inactivity. This is usually quite short-lived, lasting minutes, and improves after the joint is "worked out."

The older patient is also likely to have involvement of multiple joints in characteristic patterns. Even though trauma may have initiated problems in a joint in an older patient, OA is such an insidious condition that the trauma is usually not reported or remembered, as it may have occurred 20 to 30 years previously.

Upper Extremity Osteoarthritis

The joints most commonly involved in osteoarthritis are the distal and proximal interphalangeal joints of the hands, the first carpometacarpal joint, the first metatarsophalangeal joint, the knee, the hip, and the spine.

Heberden's nodes, characterized by bony enlargement of the dorsolateral and dorsomedial aspects of the distal interphalangeal (DIP) joints of the fingers, are extremely common in older patients, especially women. Heberden's nodes are 10 times more common in women than in men and they are familial. If a woman's mother has Heberden's nodes, then she is twice as likely to develop them. Flexor and lateral deviation of the distal phalanx are common. They may be single, but they usually are multiple. In most patients, they develop slowly over months or years, usually around the time of the menopause, giving rise to little or no pain. Similar nodes at the proximal interphalangeal (PIP) joints are known as *Bouchard's nodes*. Involvement of the first carpometacarpal (CMC) joint is common and is frequently symptomatic. Marked osteophytosis at this site leads to a characteristic squaring appearance of the hands. The relative frequency of joint involvement was similar in both sexes: DIPs, followed by the first CMC, PIPs, and rarely MCPs. Isolated involvement of any one or two MCP joints can occur as a result of trauma or in association with crystal disease.

Knee Osteoarthritis

Osteoarthritis of the knee, though not the most common site, probably has the greatest impact in terms of disability. Knee pain severity is the strongest risk factor for self-reported difficulty in performing tasks of upper and lower extremity function (8). The knee joint is composed of three compartments, the medial and lateral tibiofemoral and the patello-femoral. The medial compartment bears the greatest load during walking and is most commonly involved, followed by the patellofemoral, and lastly the lateral compartment. Osteoarthritis of the knee is usually in one compartment.

Persons affected with knee OA commonly complain of pain on walking, stiffness of the joint, difficulty rising from a seated position, and difficulty with ascending steps. Not uncommonly, joint effusions can be appreciated either by a positive bulge sign in which fluid is milked from the medial compartment and then seen to flow back when pressure is placed on the lateral compartment or, when more fluid is present by ballottement of the patella. Joint effusions in OA are noninflammatory, having a white blood cell count of less than 2000. If a joint aspiration has a white blood cell count greater than 2000, an alternative diagnosis should be considered (9).

Another common complaint associated with knee OA is a feeling that the knee is about to "give out." A thorough assessment for ligament stability should be performed. Increased varus-valgus movement documents laxity of the collateral ligaments. However, on examination, many of these patients do not have grossly unstable knees, and it is thought that the perceived instability is more related to muscle weakness and fatigue. The neighboring joints should be carefully examined, as they often exhibit decreased range of motion despite not being primarily involved with OA. Patients with knee OA may complain of joint pain in the opposite extremity because normal joints must compensate for the excess weight and strain not being applied to the affected joint. The physical examination should include observation of the gait, checking for an antalgic gait that is characterized by a short stance phase on the affected side, but when subtle, more easily recognized by a fast swing phase on the opposite side. Patients with cognitive impairment may not complain of pain but may instead present with antalgic gait, falls, or decreased mobility, causing them to spend more time in bed.

Hip Osteoarthritis

Osteoarthritis of the hip is less common but primarily confined to older individuals. It may be unilateral or bilateral. Hip joint pain is usually localized to the groin or along the inner aspect of the thigh. It may be referred to the buttock or along the obturator nerve to the knee. At times, the pain in the knee dominates the clinical presentation, and the diagnosis may be missed. Conversely, in the evaluation of pain in the hip area, other causes must be considered. Disorders of the lumbar spine at the L2-L3 level may refer pain into the groin, and at the L5-S1 level into the buttock. Trochanteric bursitis also may be confused with intraarticular hip disease. Patients with trochanteric bursitis complain of "hip" pain but on exam have good range of motion of the hip and pain along the superior lateral thigh at the area of the greater trochanter. Physical examination shows loss of internal rotation and abduction early in the disease process. Flexion contracture may be determined by using the *Thomas test*, in which the knee of the uninvolved leg is drawn to the chest to flatten the lumbar lordosis. If a flexion contracture exists, the involved leg flexes off the examining table. On gait examination, the patient may demonstrate an antalgic gait limp or a gluteus medius lurch, in which the torso leans over the involved weight-bearing hip.

Degenerative Joint Disease of the Spine

Degenerative joint disease of the spine results from involvement of the intervertebral disks, vertebral bodies, or the posterior apophyseal articulations. Narrowing of the disks may cause subluxation of the posterior apophyseal joints. The term *spinal osteoarthritis* describes the changes in the apophyseal joints, whereas *degenerative disk disease* applies to the changes in the intervertebral synchondrosis.

Acquired spinal stenosis is an important cause of low-back symptoms in the older patient, rarely seen in those younger than 50 years. Symptoms consist of back, buttock, or leg pain that usually worsens with ambulation, occasionally in combination with lower-limb sensory and motor deficits and rarely with problems with bowel and bladder control. Classically, pseudoclaudication is present, with pain and discomfort worsened with walking and relieved with stopping, sitting, or lying down and with symptoms eased in positions of flexion (bending forward, e.g., on a grocery cart) and exacerbated by positions of lumbar extension (walking uphill). The volume of the lumbar canal tends to decrease with age, with most individuals having at least an anatomic lumbar stenosis by age 80 relative to the volume of a younger population.

Laboratory and Radiographic Findings

Although the diagnosis of OA can be made without x-ray, the plain x-ray is still the most important imaging tool for investigating OA. The classic x-ray findings of OA include osteophytosis, joint space narrowing, subchondral sclerosis, and cysts. Cysts, varying in size from a few millimeters to several centimeters, are seen as translucent areas in juxtaarticular bone. Small age-related marginal osteophytes associated with some squaring of the joint margin should be differentiated from OA, in which the osteophytes are larger and have a more abnormal shape (10). X-rays are useful for confirming the diagnosis, assessing progression of disease, and determining the timing for joint replacement. It is important to remember that x-rays often do not correlate well with symptoms. However, when joint space narrowing, sometimes with "bone-on-bone" appearance, large osteophytes, and subchondral sclerosis, are present on a knee x-ray, there is little doubt that such changes represent severe OA.

Radiographic changes of OA of the spine are common in the older patient and are notorious for their lack of correlation with actual symptoms. Abnormal findings include decreased intervertebral space, end plate sclerosis, osteophyte formation, and *spondylolisthesis*—a slipping of one vertebra forward on the one below. The sclerotic bony changes associated with OA of the spine can give falsely elevated readings of bone mineral density (11). Because of the high frequency of osteoarthritic changes on radiologic examination of the lower spine, the main utility of plain x-rays in older patients is to rule out other processes such as infection, fracture, or malignancy.

Tailored magnetic resonance imaging (MRI) producing high spatial and/or contrast resolution images is proving to be an important tool in the early detection and surveillance of OA progression, as well as assessment of surrounding soft tissues (12). (For details on this and other modalities in the assessment of osteoarthritis, see Chapter 42: Rheumatologic Diseases. In: Cassel CK, et al., eds. Geriatric Medicine, 4th ed., page 578.)

Case (Part 4)

Ms. Creaky had routine blood work and x-rays prior to her appointment. The blood work is completely normal. Her hand x-rays show scattered osteophytes in the DIPs and PIPs corresponding to the Bouchard's and

Heberden's nodes felt on exam. There are no bony erosions, but several subchondral cysts are seen. She had bilateral standing knee films, which show medial compartment narrowing on the left and both severe medial and patellofemoral compartment narrowing on the right. There is spur formation bilaterally and chondrocalcinosis is seen on the left. Hip films show minimal spurring and normal joint spaces.

You diagnose her as having OA of her hands and knees and left trochanteric bursitis. You inject her left trochanteric bursa with 40 mg depo-methylprednisolone and 2 mL lidocaine. You also recommend physical therapy for quadriceps strengthening and gait aid evaluation. Finally, you encourage weight loss and regular physical activity.

Management Considerations

The goals of therapy for OA are to reduce pain, slow progression, and improve function and quality of life. Like many other chronic diseases, lifestyle modifications play an important part of the therapeutic approach of OA. Nonpharmacologic approaches are by far the most important therapies for OA. An important goal of therapy is to reduce stress on joints by weight reduction if indicated, strengthening of the muscles around involved joints, improving flexibility and proprioception, joint protection strategies, including improving joint mechanics, and the use of assistive devices and orthotics. In managing osteoarthritis, it is important to establish and communicate realistic objectives for each patient. It is critical to focus the patient's attention on enhancement and preservation of functional ability, such as walking, dressing, and living independently.

Nonpharmacologic Management

Exercise

There is a growing recognition that health and fitness are achievable with less intense regimens than previously thought, and that these regimens are feasible for people with variety of chronic and disabling conditions. Swimming is an especially good exercise that provides conditioning and strengthening without weight bearing that may exacerbate an already painful joint. Rehabilitation that increases muscle strength has been shown to be associated with decreased joint pain and disability without exacerbation of knee OA pain. Reeducation of neuromuscular skills can decrease reaction times and improve functional joint stability and proprioception, which are important in restoring shock-absorption function of muscle and protecting against further joint damage.

Osteoarthritis changes found in one joint frequently affect other joints with range of motion and strength deficits generally found in adjacent joints and bilaterally. Older people with knee OA have been found to decrease range of motion in all the major joints of the lower extremities (13). Decreased range of motion of the hip and knee increases the risk for injury and falls, in part because it becomes much more difficult to recover balance from a stumble. To prevent a fall after a stumble, one must produce rapid changes in hip and knee flexion angles while weight bearing (14). Maintaining or improving the compliance of periarticular soft tissue is also thought to protect joints from damaging peak forces as part of the neuromuscular protective system. Stretching and flexibility exercises are therefore key elements in exercise programs for people with OA (15).

Improved proprioceptive accuracy has also been demonstrated following muscle training. Knee orthoses have been shown to improve knee proprioception. Use of an elastic knee bandage improves proprioception, probably because the bandage stimulates superficial skin receptors, free nerve endings, and hair end organs that would react strongly to bandage movement on skin (16). This increase in proprioception may, in part, explain the improvement, especially the sense of safety patients report with elastic bandages, which do not provide significant mechanical support.

A modality intimately linked with exercise but also found to be an important adjunct in itself for the treatment of OA is education. Self-care education for OA resulted in notable preservation of function and control of resting knee pain in one large study (17). The cost of such a program was shown to be defrayed by a drop in the number of clinic visits but had no significant effects on the utilization and cost of pharmaceutical, laboratory, or radiology services (18).

Biomechanical Approaches

Simple interventions directed toward reducing the load in affected joints include the use of walking aids, wedged insoles that change the angle of the legs, shock absorbing footwear that reduce impact, and a heel lift if one leg is shorter than the other. Viscoelastic inserts may be effective in relieving pain and disease progression or even prevention, as they have been found to reduce the amplitude of the shock waves at heel strike with walking by 42% (19). If hip or knee involvement is unilateral, a cane held in the contralateral hand is helpful. If involvement is bilateral, crutches or a walker are more desirable. Biomechanical principles provide a rationale for prescribing adaptive devices such as an elevated toilet seat and high chairs. Knee cages around the knee may provide some stability when ligamentous laxity is pronounced. Pillows should never be placed under the knees at night because of the risk of developing flexion contracture. Flexion contracture of the hip may be prevented, and mild ones may be corrected by having the patient lie prone for 30 minutes twice daily. Occupational therapy to modify activities of daily living can reduce unnecessary over-loading of the joints of the upper and lower extremities. Other nonpharmacologic approaches include thermal modalities, transcutaneous electrical nerve stimulation (TENS), exercise programs, weight loss programs, patellar taping, tidal irrigation, and programs to improve coping skills and social support.

Pharmacologic Management

Although the future holds promise for the development of disease-modifying modalities for the treatment of OA, the current pharmacologic approach to treating OA is palliative rather than curative. The primary objective of drug therapy is to reduce pain. Pain is generally undertreated in older patients, and the pain of OA is no exception.

Acetaminophen

Guidelines for management of OA suggest a stepwise approach, starting with simple analgesic medication, which is usually acetaminophen. Despite its lack of antiinflammatory properties, acetaminophen has been shown to perform well against the nonsteroidal antiinflammatory drug ibuprofen (20). These data suggest that pure analgesics should be considered as first-line drugs in OA much more frequently than is the case today. For patients without liver disease, doses of 1 g of acetaminophen up to four times daily are recommended. Propoxyphene is no better than acetaminophen and should be avoided in older patients.

Nonsteroidal Antiinflammatory Drug and Cyclooxygenase-2 Inhibitors

For patients not receiving adequate relief, the addition or switch to a nonsteroidal antiinflammatory drug (NSAID) is the next step. The NSAIDs are among the most widely used therapeutic agents today, with nearly $2 billion spent in the United States yearly on prescription NSAIDs alone (21). These agents provide analgesia and suppress inflammation by inhibiting the cyclooxygenase enzymes that catalyze the formation of prostaglandins from arachidonic acid. Cyclooxygenase (COX) exists in two distinct isoforms: COX-1 is constitutively expressed in virtually all tissues; COX-1–mediated prostaglandins regulate renal and platelet function, protect the gastric mucosa, and promote hemostasis. COX-2–mediated prostaglandins play a role in pain, inflammation, and fever, and in the regulation of cell growth, apoptosis, and angiogenesis. It is a widely held view that the antiinflammatory properties of NSAIDs are mediated through COX-2 inhibition, whereas most of their adverse effects occur as a result of the inhibiting effects on COX-1. Conventional or traditional NSAIDs, such as ibuprofen and naproxen, suppress both COX-1– and COX-2–mediated prostaglandins.

Serious gastrointestinal toxicity such as bleeding, ulceration, and perforation can occur at any time, with or without warning symptoms, in patients treated chronically with conventional NSAIDs. Gastroduodenal ulcers can be demonstrated by endoscopy in 10% to 20% of patients who take NSAIDs on a regular basis, and the annual incidence of clinically important gastrointestinal (GI) complications approaches 2% (22). Advanced age has been consistently found to be a primary risk factor for adverse GI events. The risk increases linearly with age (23). Renal adverse effects of NSAIDs include reductions in glomerular filtration rate and renal blood flow, sodium retention, and increases in serum potassium. These effects can lead to fluid retention, edema, mild elevations of the blood pressure, and hyperkalemia (24).

In 1999, a class of NSAIDs termed COX-2 inhibitors (coxibs) was added to the therapeutic armamentarium for osteoarthritis (25). The actions of this class are more specific to COX-2. In contrast to the nonselective NSAIDs, the coxibs do not inhibit thromboxane B_2 levels or the antiplatelet effects of low-dose acetylsalicylic acid (ASA), nor do they increase bleeding time.

The initial two specific COX-2 inhibitors approved by the Food and Drug Administration (FDA) are rofecoxib and celecoxib. However in 2004, rofecoxib (Vioxx) was voluntarily withdrawn from the U.S. market because of safety concerns that led to early termination of a clinical trial involving patients taking the drug to prevent recurrent colon polyps (26,27). The Adenomatous Polyp Prevention on Vioxx (APPROVe) trial showed an increased risk of cardiovascular events (including myocardial infarction and stroke) in patients receiving rofecoxib compared with placebo, particularly for those patients who had been taking the drug for longer than 18 months (26). Two FDA committees recently evaluated whether the cardiovascular events associated with rofecoxib are a class effect and are associated with the other two selective COX-2 inhibitors in the class, celecoxib (Celebrex) and valdecoxib (Bextra). It was determined that the increased cardiovascular risk seen with rofecoxib is a class effect. Valdecoxib has since been withdrawn from the market and celecoxib's labeling now includes a black box warning about the increased risk of cardiovascular events (26). Due to these potential adverse outcomes, the use of COX-2 inhibitors has practically been mostly abandoned by both prescribers and patients.

Corticosteroids

Systemic adrenal corticosteroid analogues are not usually recommended in the management of osteoarthritis. Clinical results with these drugs are equivocal and are outweighed by their potential side effects. However, for the patient with severe debilitating pain in whom other therapies have not helped sufficiently, a brief course of low-dose prednisone (5 mg a.m.) may give remarkable palliation. An occasional intramuscular dose of depomethylprednisolone (40–80 mg) can also provide remarkable relief of symptoms without side effects and without contributing to polypharmacy.

Topical Medications

Topical application of creams containing a NSAID or capsaicin appears to have analgesic effects. Local application of capsaicin, which depletes substance P from sensory nerve endings, caused a 30% reduction in pain in OA of the knee (27). The lidocaine patch can also provide symptomatic relief when applied over a painful knee or shoulder.

Opioids

If pain relief is still not adequate, then acetaminophen with codeine or oxycodone, which has been shown to be effective in OA, should be tried in carefully selected patients. Controlled-release oxycodone or in fixed combination with acetaminophen added to NSAIDs has been compared in patients with OA with similar significant effectiveness in reducing pain and improving sleep found over placebo. The controlled release preparation was found to produce fewer side effects with significantly less nausea and dry mouth (28).

Glucosamine and Chondroitin Sulfate

Two compounds that are receiving increasing attention are the nutraceuticals—glucosamine and chondroitin sulfate. These compounds have been used in various forms for OA in continental Europe for more than a decade and have recently acquired substantial popularity in the United States because of several lay publications. The medical community in the United Kingdom and the United States has paid little attention to the potential benefits of these compounds, largely due to concerns about the validity of clinical trials.

The theoretical considerations for the possible effectiveness of glucosamine in OA stems from its status as a principal component of glycosaminoglycan (GAG), a key constituent of the matrix of all connective tissues. Glucosamine has a special tropism for cartilage and is incorporated by the chondrocyte into proteoglycans, which are secreted into the extracellular matrix (29).

In some preparations glucosamine is combined with chondroitin sulfate. Glucosamine and chondroitin are prepared by extraction from animal products, including bovine and calf cartilage. More than 90% of ingested glucosamine is absorbed, while less than 10% of chondroitin sulfate is absorbed. In short-term studies, glucosamine and chondroitin preparations have proven to be safe, but long-term toxicity studies remain to be done. A meta-analysis found that the clinical trials of glucosamine and chondroitin preparations for OA symptoms demonstrate moderate to large effects but exhibit methodologic problems (30). Given their excellent safety profile, glucosamine and chondroitin are likely to be useful in the treatment of OA even though they may be only modestly effective. Glucosamine and chondroitin are available in pharmacies and health food stores. The amounts generally administered are glucosamine 1500 mg/day and chondroitin sulfate 1200 mg/day, with an average cost of about $30 to $45 per month.

Joint and Bursa Injections

Aspiration and joint injections with corticosteroids have been one of the mainstays for the palliative therapy of painful joints. When effusions are large, especially in the knee, relief of symptoms often occurs with simple aspiration of the joint fluid. However, the fluid quickly reaccumulates unless corticosteroids are also injected. A single intraarticular injection of triamcinolone hexacetonide in knee OA provides short-term pain relief compared with placebo, with the best results seen in those with clinical evidence of joint effusion and successful aspiration of synovial fluid at the time of injection (31). The mechanism for alleviating pain besides decreasing inflammation, which is usually minimal in OA, is unclear. Because of earlier experience with frequent injections of corticosteroids leading to an accelerated rate of joint damage, it is recommended to limit the frequency of joint injections to once every 3 months and not to exceed three injections in a given joint per year.

In recent years, viscosupplementation has begun to emerge as an alternative or supplement to analgesics and NSAIDs in the management of patients with OA of the knee. (For details on viscosupplementation, the role of acupuncture, and other experimental therapies, see Chapter 42: Rheumatologic Diseases. In: Cassel CK, et al., eds. Geriatric Medicine, 4th ed., page 588.)

Case (Part 5)

Ms. Creaky returns to your office in 6 months using a cane. She no longer has pain at her left hip and feels that the pain in her hands and left knee has improved from the physical therapy. However, she says that her right knee pain is worse and she cannot even walk a block, much less do regular exercise, because of the pain. She has gained 5 more pounds and has hired an aide to do most of her shopping and cleaning. You inject her knee with 40 mg depomethylprednisolone and 2 mL lidocaine. You want to add tramadol to her medical regimen but she feels that she is on too many medications, so you give her a lidocaine patch as needed for the right knee pain. Despite these interventions, the patient returns in 3 months being pushed in a wheelchair by her aide. She feels that her knee pain has worsened considerably and she is distraught because she is unable to go out for dinner with her friends or walk around her apartment without pain. At this point you refer her to the orthopedic surgeon for evaluation for a possible right knee replacement.

Surgery for Osteoarthritis

Current surgical methods cannot restore damaged cartilage or re-create the original anatomy of the joint. Surgery is performed for four reasons: to replace the joint by attaching artificial surfaces to the ends of the bones comprising the joint (total joint replacement) (32); to debride areas of symptomatic cartilage (arthroscopic joint debridement) (33); to redirect the load bearing to a relatively unaffected part of the joint (realignment osteotomies) (34); and to fuse the joint (joint fusion).

Total Joint Arthroplasty

Arthroplasties of the hip and knee should not be considered unless the joint is irreversibly damaged and the patient's functional capacity is severely limited despite intensive medical treatment. Roentgenographic findings should provide a small role in the decision to have an arthroplasty except to indicate that the arthritic condition is irreversible because areas of the joint have completely lost their cartilage. Many patients have severe roentgenographic changes with only mild symptoms. Delaying surgery until symptoms become worse rarely makes the surgery more complicated. The best considerations for surgery are the amount of suffering and the degree that the patients have had to change their lifestyles because of the arthritis.

The most common severe complications include infections, pulmonary embolus, cardiac problems, and revision due to mechanical problems such as loosening and malalignment (35–37). Current hip and knee arthroplasties can be expected to last an average of 10 to 15 years. If the patient is active in sports or high-impact physical training, alternatives such as fusion or osteotomy must be considered. Arthroplasties are not capable of returning people to high-impact sports, and rarely do they make the joint feel completely normal. Patients who can barely function prior to surgery are usually extremely pleased with their arthroplasty, but those who have an arthroplasty because of mild pain are often unhappy.

(For further details on arthroscopic joint debridement, realignment osteotomies, and joint fusion, see Chapter 44: Orthopedic Problems with Aging. In: Cassel CK, et al., eds. Geriatric Medicine, 4th ed., page 654.)

General Principles

- Osteoarthritis is the most common articular disorder and accounts for more disability in the elderly than any other condition.
- Osteoarthritis is not a "normal" part of aging but develops from unclear complex interactions between cartilage, bone, ligaments, surrounding muscle, and inflammatory components of the immune system.
- Treatment needs to be individually tailored but should progress in a stepwise pattern starting with acetaminophen and NSAIDs.
- Physical therapy is a helpful adjuvant to medications because it can improve range of motion, quadriceps strength, and gait.
- Radiographic findings infrequently correlate with symptoms and should not alone be used to determine surgical intervention.
- Surgery is a legitimate option when patients have severe functional limitations despite aggressive medical treatment.

Suggested Readings

Altman RD. Criteria for classification of clinical osteoarthritis. J Rheumatology 1991;18(suppl 27):10. *An excellent review of the classification of osteoarthritis including underlying pathophysiology.*

Brauner DJ, Sorensen LB, Ellman MH. Rheumatologic diseases. In: Cassel CK, Leipzig RM, Cohen HJ, et al., eds. Geriatric Medicine, 4th ed. New York: Springer, 2003:573–619.

Buckwalter KA. Imaging of osteoarthritis and crystal deposition disease. Curr Opin Rheumatology 1993;5:503. *An important review of imaging modalities in the detection of osteoarthritis.*

Felson DT. Osteoarthritis. Rheum Dis Clin 1990;16:499. *A comprehensive review of the literature with a focus on the treatment modalities for this disease.*

Pottenger LA. Orthopedic problems with aging. In: Cassel CK, Leipzig RM, Cohen HJ, et al., eds. Geriatric Medicine, 4th ed. New York: Springer, 2003: 651–667.

References

1. Nuki G. Osteoarthritis: a problem of joint failure. Zeitschrift fur Rheumatologie 1999;58:142–147.
2. Felson DT. The epidemiology of knee osteoarthritis: results from the Framingham study. Semin Arthritis Rheum 1990;20:42–50.
3. Davis MA, Ettinger WH, Neuhaus JM. Obesity and osteoarthritis of the knee: evidence from the National Health and Nutrition Examination Survey (NHANES I). Semin Arthritis Rheum 1990;20:34–41.
4. Felson DT, Zhang Y, Hannan MT, et al. Risk factor for incident radiographic knee osteoarthritis in the elderly: the Framingham Study. Arthritis Rheum 1997;40:728–733.

5. Oliveria SA, Felson DT, Cirillo PA, et al. Body weight, body mass index, and incident symptomatic osteoarthritis of the hand, hip and knee. Epidemiology 1999;10:161–166.

6. Sahyoun NR, Hochberg MC, Helmick CG, et al. Body mass index, weight change, and incidence of self-reported physician-diagnosed arthritis among women. Am J Public Health 1999;89:391–394.

7. Ryan LM, Cheung HS. The role of crystals in osteoarthritis. Rheum Dis Clin North Am 1999;25:257–267.

8. Jordan J, Luta G, Renner J, et al. Knee pain and knee osteoarthritis severity in self-reported task specific disability: the Johnson County Osteoarthritis Project. J Rheum 1997;24:1344–1349.

9. Slemenda C, Heilman DK, Brandt KD, et al. Reduced quadriceps strength relative to body weight: a risk factor for osteoarthritis in women? Arthritis Rheum 1998;41:1951–1959.

10. Dieppe P, Peterfy C, Watt I. Osteoarthritis and related disorders: imaging. In: Klippel JH, Dieppe PA, eds. Rheumatology. London: Mosby, 1998: 8.4.1–8.4.10.

11. Liu G, Peacock M, Eilam O, et al. Effect of osteoarthritis in the lumbar spine and hip on bone mineral density and diagnosis of osteoporosis in elderly men and women. Osteoporosis Int 1997;7:564–569.

12. Pessis E, Auleley GR, et al. Quantitative MR imaging evaluation of chondropathy in osteoarthritic knees. Radiology 1998;208:49–55.

13. Messier SP, Loeser RF, Hoover JL, et al. Osteoarthritis of the knee: Effects of gait, strength and flexibility. Arch Phys Med Rehabil 1992;11:29–36.

14. Grabiner MD, Koh TJ, Lundin TM, et al. Kinematics of recovery from a stumble. J Gerontol 1993;48:M97–M102.

15. Ettinger WH, Burns R, Messier SP, et al. A randomized trial comparing aerobic exercise and resistance exercise with a health education program in older adults with knee osteoarthritis: The fitness arthritis and seniors trial (FAST). JAMA 1997;277:25–31.

16. Perleau R, Frank C, Fick G. The effect of elastic bandages on human knee proprioception in the uninjured population. Am J Sports Med 1995;23:251–255.

17. Mazzuca SA, Brandt KD, Katz BP, et al. Effects of self-care education on the health status of inner-city patients with osteoarthritis of the knee. Arthritis Rheum 1997;40:1466–1474.

18. Mazzuca SA, Brandt KD, Katz BP, et al. Reduced utilization and cost of primary care clinic visits resulting from self-care education for patients with osteoarthritis of the knee. Arthritis Rheum 1999;42:1267–1273.

19. Voloshin A, Wosk J. Influence of artificial shock absorbers on human gait. Clin Orthop Rel Res 1981;160:52–56.

20. Bradly JD, Brandt KD, Katz BP. Comparison of an antiinflammatory dose of ibuprofen, an analgesic dose of ibuprofen, and acetaminophen in the treatment of patients with osteoarthritis of the knee. N Engl J Med 1991;325:1807–1809.

21. Peterson WL, Cryer B. COX-1–sparing NSAIDs—is the enthusiasm justified? [editorial; comment]. JAMA 1999;282:1961–1963.

22. Lichtenstein DR, Wolfe MM. COX-2 selective NSAIDs: new and improved? [Editorial]. JAMA 2000;284:1297–1299.

23. Wolfe MM, Lictenstein DR, Singh G. Gastrointestinal toxicity of nonsteroidal antiinflammatory drugs. N Engl J Med 1999;340:1888–1899.
24. Swan SK, Rudy DW, Lasseter KC, Ryan CF, et al. Effect of cyclooxygenase-2 inhibition on renal function in elderly person receiving a low-salt diet. A randomized, controlled trial. Ann Intern Med 2000;133:1–9.
25. Golden BD, Abramson SB. Selective cyclooxygenase-2 inhibitors. Rheum Dis Clin North Am 1999;25:359–378.
26. FDA public health advisory: safety of Vioxx. http://www.fda.gov/cder/drug/infopage/vioxx/PHA_vioxx.htm.
27. FitzGerald GA. Coxibs and cardiovascular disease. N Engl J Med 2004; 351:1709–1711.
28. Deal CL, Schnitzer TJ, Lipstein E. Treatment of arthritis with topical capsaicin: a double-blind trial. Clin Ther 1991;13:383–395.
29. Caldwell JR, Hale ME, Boyd RE, et al. Treatment of osteoarthritis pain with controlled release oxycodone or fixed combination oxycodone plus acetaminophen added to nonsteroidal antiinflammatory drugs: a double blind, randomized, multicenter, placebo controlled trial. J Rheum 1999;26:862–869.
30. Deal CL, Moskowitz RW. Nutraceuticals as therapeutic agents in osteoarthritis: the role of glucosamine, chondroitin sulfate and collagen hydrolysate. Rheum Dis Clin North Am 1999;25:379–395.
31. McAlindon TE, LaValley MP, Gulin JP, Felson DT. Glucosamine and Chondroitin for treatment of osteoarthritis: a systematic quality assessment and meta-analysis. JAMA 2000;283:1469–1475.
32. Gaffney K, Ledingham J, Perry JD. Intra-articular triamcinolone hexactonide in knee osteoarthritis: factors influencing the clinical response. Ann Rheum Dis 1995;54:379–381.
33. Atlas SJ, Keller RB, Robson D, et al. Surgical and nonsurgical management of lumbar stenosis: four-year outcomes from the Maine lumbar spine study. Spine 2000;25:556–562.
34. Mc Ginley BJ, Cushner FD, Scott WN. Debridement arthroscopy. A 10–year followup. Clin Orthop 1999;367:190–194.
35. Naudie D, Bourne RB, Rorabeck CH, et al. Survivorship of the high tibial valgus osteotomy. Clin Orthop 1999;367:18–27.
36. Scheller AD, Turner RH, Lowell JD. Complications of arthroplasty and total joint replacement in the hip. In: Epps CH Jr, ed. Complications in Orthopaedic Surgery, 2nd ed., vol 2. Philadelphia: Lippincott, 1986;1059–1108.
37. Lonner JH, Lotke PA. Aseptic complications after total knee arthroplasty. J Am Acad Orthop Surg 1999;7:311–324.

19
Osteoporosis

Helen M. Fernandez

Learning Objectives

Upon completion of the chapter, the student will be able to:

1. Describe the modalities used to screen and diagnose osteoporosis.
2. Enumerate and describe the risk factors for osteoporosis.
3. Develop and implement a plan of care for a patient with osteoporosis.

Case (Part 1)

Mrs. Simon is a 69-year-old Caucasian woman with a history of hypertension and diabetes mellitus who presents to your practice for the first time. She had been followed intermittently at a local clinic but wants to transfer all her medical care to you. She has no complaints and has not had any surgeries or hospitalizations. Her family history includes hypertension and osteoporosis. Her medications include glyburide 5 mg every day and enalapril 5 mg every day.

Mrs. Simon does not smoke or use alcohol or drugs. She lives with her husband and has one grown daughter and two grandchildren. You decide you are going to focus on health maintenance issues, specifically Mrs. Simon's risk for osteoporosis.

What are Mrs. Simon's risk factors for osteoporosis?

What type of osteoporosis would Mrs. Simon most likely have?

Material in this chapter is based on the following chapter in Cassel CK, Leipzig RM, Cohen HJ, Larson EB, Meier DE, eds. Geriatric Medicine: An Evidence-Based Approach, 4th ed. New York: Springer, 2003: Inzerillo A, Iqbal J, Troen B, Meier DE, Zaidi M. Skeletal Fragility in the Elderly, pp. 621–650. Selections edited by Helen M. Fernandez.

General Considerations

Osteoporosis, the leading cause of serious morbidity and functional loss in old age, was once thought to be a natural part of the aging process. Although at times it is difficult to distinguish between the disease and normal skeletal aging per se in the clinical approach to osteoporosis management, progress in the scientific understanding of the underlying disease process has made it largely a preventable disease.

Epidemiology

Osteoporosis is the most common bone disease. The prevalence of low bone mass increases with advancing age in both men and women, reflecting age-associated bone loss. It is higher for women (approximately 80% of all cases) than for men because accelerated bone loss occurs in the immediate postmenopausal period (1).

Based on data from the National Health and Nutrition Examination Survey III (NHANES), 10 million people in the United States have osteoporosis at the hip and nearly 18 million more have low bone mass at the hip, placing them at risk for future hip fractures. It is anticipated that the prevalence of osteoporosis will increase as the population ages (2). The occurrence of osteoporotic fractures is even more striking. In the United States alone, these approximate 1.5 million per year. This includes 700,000 spine fractures, 300,000 hip fractures, 250,000 wrist fractures, and 300,000 other fractures. One in two women and 1 in 8 men over age 50 will have an osteoporotic fracture in her or his lifetime (2).

Although the incidence of osteoporotic fractures is high, when viewed in perspective with other common chronic ailments in the United States, the figures appear even more dramatic. For instance, after the age of 65, the incidence of hip fracture in white women is greater than the incidence of stroke, breast cancer, and diabetes (3). Among other chronic ailments, 28 million are affected with osteopenia and osteoporosis compared with 52 million and 42 million affected with hypercholesterolemia and hypertension, respectively (4). These figures are staggering and will increase as the population ages.

The economic burden this places on society is self-evident. The cost of all fractures in the United States is between $35 billion and $41 billion per year. The cost of all osteoporotic fractures totals between $10 billion and $15 billion per year. Hip fractures alone total between $4 billion and $6 billion per year (5). Expected costs for the year 2025 are $64 billion (6).

TABLE 19.1. Risk factors for osteoporotic fractures

Age
Female sex
Caucasian
Low bone density
Prior fracture after age 50
Hypogonadism
Smoking
Inactivity
Falls
Anticonvulsant therapy
Glucocorticoids
Hyperthyroidism
Alcoholism
Excess dietary protein
Family history

Source: Inzerillo A, Iqbal J, Troen B, et al. Skeletal fragility
in the elderly. In: Cassel CK, Leipzig RM, Cohen HJ, et al.,
eds. Geriatric Medicine, 4th ed. New York: Springer, 2003.

Risk Factors

The ability of clinical risk factors to predict fracture risk is good (7).
According to the 1998 National Osteoporosis Foundation (NOF) guidelines, family history, age, history of fracture, smoking, female sex, Caucasian race, estrogen deficiency, and low body weight are risk factors for the
development of osteoporosis (8). Smoking poses a major risk for the development of osteoporosis. Specifically, it increases the relative incidence of
hip fracture by 1.5 to 2.0 (9). This incidence may increase by as much as
15% over the next several decades. Low calcium intake below the recommended daily allowance (RDA) of 800 mg/day has been observed in about
75% of U.S. women (10). Even if the increased relative risk of hip fracture
due to this factor were small, the very large numbers of women affected
could ultimately lead to a high percentage of fractures due to low calcium
intake (11). Other major risk factors associated with hip fracture are maternal history of hip fracture, past fracture (particularly after age 50), glucocorticoids, anticonvulsants, and hyperthyroidism (Table 19.1).

Classification of Osteoporosis

There are a variety of causes of osteoporosis, meriting a classification into
primary and secondary forms. *Primary osteoporosis* occurs in association
with menopause or with aging. It is traditionally subdivided into types I

and II. Type I is referred to as postmenopausal osteoporosis and is due to estrogen deficiency. Type II, often called senile or involutional osteoporosis, is associated with aging. In contrast to type I, there is decreased bone turnover with a primary defect in osteoblastic activity and decreased bone formation.

Secondary osteoporosis is due to conditions other than aging or menopause. It may arise from a variety of causes (Table 19.2). All patients with unexplained bone loss should be considered candidates for laboratory evaluation for secondary causes that may also be superimposed on primary bone loss. To exclude common secondary causes, basic laboratory tests, thyroid function tests, immunoprotein electrophoresis (IPEP), 25-(OH)-vitamin D_3, 24-hour urine free cortisol, testosterone and/or estrogen, 24-hour urinary calcium, and intact parathyroid hormone (PTH) may be obtained. If these tests are negative or if further testing is warranted, a bone biopsy may be performed.

The most common cause of secondary osteoporosis is hypercortisolism, endogenous as in Cushing's syndrome, or, more commonly, iatrogenic from chronic glucocorticoid administration. Osteoporosis induced by glucocorticoid excess is characterized by decreased bone formation causing a relative increase in resorption and bone loss. Trabecular bone (as seen predominantly in the lumbar spine) is more affected than cortical bone.

TABLE 19.2. Secondary causes of systemic osteoporosis

Endocrine	*Gastrointestinal*	*Drugs*	*Genetic and other*
Hypogonadism	Low vitamin D	Anticonvulsants	Osteogenesis
Cushing's syndrome	intake	Heparin	imperfecta
Hyperthyroidism	Malabsorption	Glucocorticoids	Homocystinuria
Type 1 diabetes	Celiac disease	FK 506	Marfan's syndrome
Hyperparathyroidism	Crohn's disease	Levothyroxine	Rheumatoid
	Lactase deficiency	excess	arthritis
	Hepatic failure	Vitamin A excess	Ehlers-Danlos
	Small bowel	Methotrexate	syndrome
	resection	Cyclosporin A	
Malignancy	Anorexia nervosa	Alcohol	
Multiple myeloma	Gastrectomy		
Lymphoma			*Renal disease*
Leukemia			Renal failure
Malignancy induced	*Lifestyle*	*Immobilization*	RTA
PTHrP secretion	Smoking	Hip fracture	Idiopathic
Mastocytosis		Paralysis	hypercalciuria

PTHrP, parathyroid hormone related protein; RTA, renal tubular acidosis.
Source: Inzerillo A, Iqbal J, Troen B, et al. Skeletal fragility in the elderly. In: Cassel CK, Leipzig RM, Cohen HJ, et al., eds. Geriatric Medicine, 4th ed. New York: Springer, 2003.

Case (Part 2)

Mrs. Simon says that she usually drinks one glass of milk each day. She also takes calcium tablets to help with her frequent stomach upsets. She does remember breaking her arm once but she says that was from a nasty fall on the sidewalk a few years ago. She asks you how she could possibly have osteoporosis when she takes sufficient amounts of calcium.

How would you diagnose Mrs. Simon with osteoporosis?

What test(s) would you order to confirm a diagnosis of osteoporosis?

Diagnostic Evaluation

The clinical presentation of osteoporosis can vary from a symptomatic vertebral compression fracture to the observation of low bone mineral density (BMD) on a baseline dual-energy x-ray absorptiometry (DEXA), screening ultrasound, or a plain radiograph.

Symptoms and Signs

Vertebral fractures are the most common type of osteoporotic fracture. Their prevalence increases with age. Vertebral fractures often are asymptomatic and are detected on routine chest radiography. The most common sites for fractures are the lower thoracic and upper lumbar spine. Fractures occurring in the cervical and upper thoracic (above T6) vertebrae should suggest a secondary or pathologic cause, such as tumor or infection (Table 19.2).

An acute vertebral compression fracture may present with sudden onset of pain at the site of the fracture with associated radiation of pain laterally, paravertebral muscle spasm, and signs and symptoms of spinal cord compression. New crush fractures may result in substantial short-term pain and disability, but many patients with vertebral osteoporosis have chronic back discomfort, height loss, postural changes, or no symptoms at all (12). In the absence of radiographic evidence of fracture or bone scan evidence of microfracture, back pain should not be attributed to a diagnosis of osteoporosis. Sufficient numbers of wedge or crush fractures may lead to height loss and kyphosis with attendant back pain and impaired functional capacity (14). Associated abdominal distention, discomfort, and pulmonary restriction also may occur in severe cases of thoracic kyphosis.

Hip fractures are second in frequency and are associated with substantial morbidity and mortality and occur primarily in persons over age 75. Hip fractures are almost always associated with a fall, but whether the fracture precedes or follows the fall is not always clear. Occasionally, a patient with an impacted hip fracture retains the ability to walk but most hip fracture patients are unable to stand. The involved limb may appear shorter and externally rotated (see Chapter 21: Hip Fractures, page 374).

Distal radial fractures (Colles' fracture), the third most common osteoporotic fracture, usually occur in middle-aged women who attempt to break a fall with outstretched arms and hands (parachute reflex). Presentation with pain and deformity usually is straightforward. Rehabilitation exercises of the hand and forearm may be necessary.

Radiologic Evaluation

The World Health Organization (WHO) has defined osteoporosis in terms of BMD in postmenopausal Caucasian women. A BMD measurement of more than 2.5 standard deviations below the mean for young adult women, without fractures, is osteoporosis (13). Table 19.3 outlines these criteria for diagnosis and Table 19.4 identifies who should have BMD testing. Note that these criteria identify approximately 30% of postmenopausal women as having osteoporosis, using DEXA of the spine, hip, or forearm. It approximates equivalent lifetime fracture risk for spine, hip, and forearm as ~17% and lifetime fracture risk for any of the three fractures as ~40% (14).

TABLE 19.3. World Health Organization (WHO) diagnostic criteria for osteoporosis (13)

Normal	Bone mineral density (BMD) value within 1 standard deviation (SD) of the mean for young adult (T-score ≥ −1)
Osteopenia	BMD value between −1 and −2.5 SD below the mean for young adult (T score between −1 and −2.5)
Osteoporosis	BMD value of at least −2.5 SD below the mean for young adult (T-score ≤ −2.5)
Severe osteoporosis	BMD value of at least −2.5 SD below the mean for young adult, with a history of fracture (T-score ≤ −2.5)

Note: The diagnosis of osteoporosis and fracture risk assessment are based primarily on BMD. The WHO has defined low bone mass and osteoporosis on the basis of axial skeleton measurements of bone density to help facilitate screening and identify individuals at risk. The diagnosis of osteoporosis is based on T-score thresholds, but expert opinion holds that this classification was not meant to apply to individual patients. It may be reasonable to diagnose any patient with low bone density and a fragility fracture as having osteoporosis. *Source*: Adapted from Assessment of fracture risk and its application to screening for postmenopausal osteoporosis. Report of a WHO Study Group. World Health Organ Tech Rep Ser 1994;843:1–129, with permission from WHO Press.

TABLE 19.4. 2003 National Osteoporosis Foundation (NOF) recommendations for BMD testing (12)

1. All women age 65 and older regardless of additional risk factors
2. Younger postmenopausal women with one or more risk factors (other than being white, postmenopausal, and female)
3. Postmenopausal women who present with fractures (to confirm diagnosis and determine disease severity)

Source: Adapted from Physician's Guide to the Prevention and Treatment of Osteoporosis. Washington (DC): National Osteoporosis Foundation, 2003.

Dual-Energy X-Ray Absorptiometry

Dual-energy x-ray absorptiometry (DEXA) utilizes a beam of x-ray photons passing through the bone region of interest. This technique measures the sum of cortical and trabecular bone at the mid-radius (95% cortical bone), lumbar spine, femoral neck, total hip, and total body with a precision of approximately 1% to 3% depending on the operator and skeletal site measured (12).

For the diagnosis of osteoporosis with DEXA, measurement of at least two skeletal sites is preferable, usually the posteroanterior (PA) spine and hip. Reasons for falsely elevated BMD on DEXA include degenerative joint or disk disease, compression fractures, vascular calcifications, or scoliosis occurring in the path of the measurement beam. Use of femoral neck, total hip, and forearm measurement sites is usually preferable under these clinical circumstances (12).

Dual-energy x-ray absorptiometry values are reported by comparison to age and gender reference groups with *T scores* (standard deviations above or below values for young normals) and *Z scores* (standard deviations above or below age-matched values) (13). A T score more than 2 standard deviations below young normals indicates an increased risk of fracture and should lead to consideration of antiresorptive therapy to prevent further bone loss. A Z score of more than 1 to 2 standard deviations below the age-matched mean value should prompt a thorough evaluation for secondary causes of bone loss (Table 19.2).

Other Modalities

Other modalities including peripheral DEXA (pDEXA), quantitative computed tomography (QCT), and quantitative ultrasound (QUS). (For further details on these modalities in assessing osteoporosis, see Chapter 43: Skeletal Fragility in the Elderly In: Cassel CK, et al., eds. Geriatric Medicine, 4th ed., page 631.)

Case (Part 3)

You order a DEXA. The DEXA results are reported as a T score of –3.0 SD and a Z score +1.0. You discuss the results with Mrs. Simon, and she asks what she can do to prevent a future fracture. She says that her mother sustained a hip fracture and she eventually died, never regaining her functional status.

Prevention and Treatment of Osteoporosis

Osteoporosis therapy should ideally be aimed at the underlying type of osteoporosis, that is, involutional, postmenopausal, or due to secondary causes. Aside from calcium, the majority of agents available today are antiresorptive, exerting the most beneficial effect in high-turnover osteoporosis. They include estrogen, selective estrogen receptor modulators (SERMs), bisphosphonates, and calcitonins. Agents that increase formation would be most advantageous in age-related osteoporosis where the primary defect is decreased osteoblastic bone formation. These include PTH, vitamin D analogues, fluoride, and new osteoblastic stimulatory agents.

Calcium

The effects of calcium supplementation are maximized in patients in whom baseline intake is low, especially in the elderly (15). Nevertheless, there is continued controversy about whether calcium supplementation can prevent bone loss or restore bone mass.

How much calcium is enough? Total intakes, that is, diet plus supplemental, of 1.5 to 2 g of "elemental" calcium per day are recommended in postmenopausal women (16), although intake must be individualized. There is little evidence that one form of calcium supplementation is superior to another. Older persons have a high prevalence of gastric achlorhydria and should take their supplements with meals. Patients must be informed that calcium supplementation alone is not sufficient to prevent either menopausal or age-related bone loss. Risks of calcium supplementation are minimal, but persons with a personal or family history of nephrolithiasis must be screened with 24-hour urinary calcium determination. In addition, some older patients suffer from constipation or rebound gastric hyperacidity. Calcium citrate or calcium glubionate may be better tolerated in persons unable to tolerate other forms of calcium supplementation. Calcium supplements should be prescribed with care in patients with end-stage renal disease, mainly for phosphate control. Notably, calcium citrate should be avoided in renal failure as it enhances the absorption of aluminum, the excessive absorption of which could worsen the bone disease secondary to renal failure.

Exercise

It is evident from multiple studies that immobility and disuse leads to accelerated bone loss. Active individuals have higher bone mass than inactive individuals (17), as has been shown in several cross-sectional studies. Many researchers have proposed that the principal benefit of exercise in reducing fracture is its enhancement of muscle strength, balance, and coordination, and associated reduction in fall risk (18). Elderly patients may require pre-exercise stress testing before initiation of a new exercise program.

General recommendations include a duration of 30 minutes per day, 5 to 6 days per week, and maintenance of a high level of daily activity with adaptation according to age, lifestyle, strength, and agility.

Bisphosphonates

Bisphosphonates (BPs) are stable analogues of pyrophosphate that inhibit bone resorption. Their main effects include decreased osteoclast progenitor development, decreased osteoclast recruitment, and induction of osteoclast apoptosis leading to inhibition of bone resorption (19–21). The drug is tightly bound to the hydroxyapatite crystal and is retained in bone for many years. Only a small percentage of an oral dose is absorbed, mandating avoidance of food and other medications for several hours before and after a dose.

Alendronate sodium, a second-generation aminobisphosphonate, has been Food and Drug Administration (FDA) approved for the prevention and treatment of postmenopausal osteoporosis as well as the treatment of glucocorticoid-induced osteoporosis and Paget's disease. The dose of alendronate required to inhibit bone mineralization is 1000 times greater than that required to inhibit bone resorption, allowing daily administration. The recommended dose of alendronate for treatment of osteoporosis is 10 mg and that for prevention of osteoporosis is 5 mg. It is to be taken daily in the morning on an empty stomach with 8 oz of plain water. Patients are instructed to delay eating or taking other medications for a minimum of 30 minutes. Calcium supplements, at a different time of day, of at least 1500 mg per day must be given with bisphosphonates to reduce the risk of mineralization defects. A once weekly 70-mg dose of alendronate sodium (for the treatment of osteoporosis) and a 35-mg dose (for prevention) have also been FDA approved. Randomized controlled trial data using alendronate in postmenopausal women demonstrated significant reductions in both vertebral and nonvertebral fractures in association with significant gains in bone mineral density (22–27).

Another bisphosphonate, risedronate sodium, which is a potent third-generation bisphosphonate, has also been FDA approved for the prevention and treatment of postmenopausal osteoporosis and treatment of glucocorticoid-induced osteoporosis in men and women. The current dose is 5mg by oral administration daily. A weekly dose is also available.

Side effects have been generally minimal with both alendronate and etidronate, and include abdominal and musculoskeletal pain. Although tolerability profiles of alendronate are similar to those of placebo in the literature, there is a rare association of alendronate with erosive esophagitis. More commonly, patients experience nausea, dyspepsia, and other nonspecific gastrointestinal side effects prompting their discontinuation.

Estrogen

Evidence for the role of estrogen loss in osteoporosis is severalfold: bone loss is accelerated as ovarian function ceases (28), such loss is inhibited with initiation of estrogen replacement therapy (29,30), and is resumed when estrogen replacement is terminated (31).

The Women's Health Initiative (WHI) estrogen-plus-progestin trial is the first randomized clinical trial demonstrating that combination postmenopausal hormone therapy reduces the risk of fractures at the hip, vertebrae, and wrist (32). The WHI analysis shows that after an average of 5.6 years, there was a 24% reduction in all fractures and a 33% reduction in hip fractures in women assigned to estrogen plus progestin (33,34). Hip bone density increased 3.7% after 3 years of taking estrogen plus progestin compared to 0.14% in the placebo group. The combination therapy reduced the risk of fracture to a similar degree in women who were considered to be at high or low risk of fracture.

However, the overall risks of the combination therapy outweighed the benefits, including the fracture benefits. Even in the group of women at increased risk of fracture, who would benefit most from the prevention of fractures, the risks of estrogen plus progestin outweigh the benefits. Therefore, treatment with estrogen plus progestin should not be recommended for the prevention and treatment of osteoporosis in women who do not have menopausal symptoms. Other medications for osteoporosis should be considered. If the combination therapy is prescribed to prevent osteoporosis, women need to be informed of the risks (35).

Selective Estrogen Receptor Modulators

The selective estrogen receptor modulators (SERMs) currently include tamoxifen, raloxifene, and droloxifene. They have been shown to bind with high affinity to estrogen receptors. By binding differently from parent estrogens to the same receptor, SERMs can confer a conformation that enables the receptor to interact with a different second messenger. Thus, they act as agonists at bone and with respect to lipoproteins, but in contrast to estrogen, which is an antagonist at the breast and uterus (36,37).

Raloxifene is FDA approved for the prevention and treatment of osteoporosis, at the 60-mg dose. Studies on raloxifene have demonstrated a BMD increase of 2.4% at the spine and the hip at 3 years (38). Results from the Multiple Outcomes of Raloxifene Evaluation (MORE) study demonstrated a significant reduction, about 30% to 50%, in vertebral fractures, but no change in nonvertebral fractures (39). Its side effects include venous thromboembolism and lack of relief of postmenopausal vasomotor symptoms (40).

The SERMs have failed, however, in clinical trials, in part due to such adverse effects as urinary incontinence and uterine prolapse. Three other SERMs—arzoxifene, bazedoxifene, and lasofoxifene—are currently in clinical trials.

Calcitonin

Calcitonin is a 32 amino acid peptide hormone synthesized and secreted from the C cells of the thyroid. The main action of calcitonin is on bone, although it may, at pharmacologic concentrations, increase renal calcium and phosphate excretion and 1,25-dihydroxycholecalciferol production. In bone sections, calcitonin application results in a rapid loss of ruffled borders. When applied for a longer term, there is a reduction in the number of osteoclasts in bone. In osteoclasts, calcitonin inhibits bone resorption. This occurs by the inhibition of cell motility and enzyme secretion (41–48).

Salmon calcitonin has a 40-fold greater potency than human calcitonin, but long-term use is associated with a high rate of development of neutralizing antibodies (49). Resistance to human calcitonin has also been observed, presumably due to receptor downregulation. Resistance can be minimized by the use of lower doses, intranasal or rectal administration, or intermittent administration of the drug. The major drawbacks of calcitonin therapy include its high cost and the need for parenteral, nasal, or rectal administration. As of 1996 both parenteral and nasal calcitonin have been FDA approved for treatment of osteoporosis in the United States. Analgesic effects of calcitonin have also been documented in multiple studies of vertebral fracture patients, but these results are compromised by failure to utilize appropriate control groups (50).

Nasal calcitonin is generally well tolerated, but its use may be associated with local irritation and rhinitis, which usually subside with continued therapy. There is no evidence of any serious or long-term side effects in studies of up to 5 years' duration.

Other Treatment Strategies

Fluoride remains an experimental drug; it has not been shown to decrease fracture risk, and it is not approved by the FDA for treatment of osteoporosis (51–53). *Parathyroid hormone* acts on osteoblasts to modulate the expression of a variety of growth factors and certain cytokines (54,55). The precise mechanism underlying the anabolic effects of PTH on bone is just beginning to be unraveled (56–58). When administered at a low dose, intermittently, PTH stimulates bone formation. Although results to date show promise, PTH remains experimental until larger controlled clinical trials evaluating fracture rate are completed. The major drawbacks to utilizing PTH are its need to be given parenterally and achieving the pulses in the circulation necessary to enable bone formation (59). *Vitamin D* may indirectly stimulate bone resorption, but it also enhances gastrointestinal calcium absorption, promotes mineralization, and inhibits PTH-induced bone resorption (60). Because of the risk of hypercalcemia and hypercalciuria with calcium, pharmacologic doses of active vitamin D metabolites must be considered experimental. *Hepatic hydroxymethylglutaryl coenzyme A (HMG CoA) reductase inhibitors* (statins) activate osteoclast apoptosis, reduce osteoclast recruitment, and promote osteoblastic bone formation (62,63). Further controlled studies are necessary to determine the clinical applicability statins will have in the treatment of osteoporosis. *Growth factors* (insulin-like growth factors I and II, and transforming growth factor-β) act to increase proliferation of osteoblasts and are currently undergoing evaluation for methods of localizing their effects to the skeleton. *Anabolic steroids* are potent antiresorptives, but androgenic side effects, adverse lipid changes, and hepatotoxicity limit their use. *Flavonoids* (61) are common plant metabolites with some indirect estrogenic properties, and *ipriflavone* has been shown in animal and human studies to prevent bone loss or increase bone mass in diverse research settings. It has not yet been shown to reduce fracture rates, and long-term evaluation of both efficacy and toxicities are needed.

General Principles

- There are few clinical symptoms, but the presence of certain signs and symptoms in a high-risk patient (e.g., height loss, dowager's hump, and back pain) warrants a high level of suspicion for the possibility of osteoporosis.
- The World Health Organization has defined osteoporosis as a bone density measurement of more than 2.5 standard deviations below the mean for young adult women without fractures.

- A T score more than 2 standard deviations below that of young normals indicates an increased risk of fracture and should lead to consideration of antiresorptive therapy to prevent further bone loss.
- A Z score of more than 1 to 2 standard deviations below the age-matched mean value should prompt a thorough evaluation for secondary causes of bone loss.
- The first-line treatments for osteoporosis are calcium with vitamin D and bisphosphonates.

Suggested Readings

Hodgson SF, Watts NB, Bilezikian JP, et al. American Association of Clinical Endocrinologists 2001 Medical Guidelines for Clinical Practice for the Prevention and Management of Postmenopausal Osteoporosis. Endocr Pract 2001;7(4):293–312. *A comprehensive clinical practice guideline for clinicians taking care of patients with osteoporosis.*
Inzerillo A, Iqbal J, Troen B, et al. Skeletal fragility in the elderly. In: Cassel CK, Leipzig RM, Cohen HJ, et al., eds. Geriatric Medicine, 4th ed. New York: Springer, 2003:621–650.

References

1. Looker AC, Orwoll ES, Johnston CC Jr, et al. Prevalence of low femoral bone density in older US adults from NHANES III. J Bone Miner Res 1997; 12:1761–1768.
2. Lindsay R, Meunier PJ. Osteoporosis: review of the evidence for prevention, diagnosis and treatment and cost effectiveness analysis. Osteoporosis Int 1998;8:S1–S88.
3. Melton LJ III. Epidemiology of hip fractures: implications of the exponential increase with age. Bone 1996;18(3 suppl):121S–125S.
4. Melton LJ III. How many women have osteoporosis now? J Bone Miner Res 1995;10:175–177.
5. Ray NF, Chan JK, Thamer M, et al. Medical expenditures for the treatment of osteoporotic fractures in the United States in 1995: report from the National Osteoporosis Foundation. J Bone Miner Res 1997;12:24–35.
6. Cooper C, Campion G, Melton LJ III. Hip fractures in the elderly: a worldwide projection. Osteoporosis Int 1992;2:285–289.
7. Cummings SR, Nevitt MC, Browner WS, et al. Risk factors for hip fracture in white women. Study of Osteoporotic Fractures Research Group. N Engl J Med 1995;332:767–773.
8. Williams AR, Weiss NS, Ure CL, et al. Effect of weight, smoking, and estrogen use on the risk of hip and forearm fractures in post-menopausal women. Obstet Gynecol 1982;60:695–699.
9. Heaney RP, Gallagher IC, Johnston CC, et al. Calcium nutrition and bone health in the elderly. Am J Clin Nutr 1982;36:986–1013.
10. Slemenda CW, Hui SL, Longcope C, et al. Predictors of bone mass in perimenopausal women. Ann Intern Med 1990;112:96–101.

11. Ryan PJ, Blake G, Herd R, et al. A clinical profile of back pain and disability in patients with osteoporosis. Bone 1994;15:27–30.
12. Physician's Guide to the Prevention and Treatment of Osteoporosis. Washington (DC): National Osteoporosis Foundation, 2003.
13. Assessment of fracture risk and its application to screening for postmenopausal osteoporosis. Report of a WHO Study Group. World Health Organ Tech Rep Ser 1994;843:1–129.
14. Kanis JA, Melton LJ III, Christiansen C, et al. The diagnosis of osteoporosis. J Bone Miner Res 1994;9:1137–1141.
15. Heaney RP. Nutritional factors in osteoporosis. Annu Rev Nutr 1993;13: 287–316.
16. Heaney RP, Rocker RR, Saville PD. Calcium balance and calcium requirement in middle aged women. Am J Clin Nutr 1977;30:1603–1611.
17. Chestnut CH. Bone mass and exercise. Am J Med 1993;95(5A):34S–36S.
18. Drinkwater BL. Exercise in the prevention of osteoporosis. Osteoporosis Int 1993;1:S169–171.
19. Boonekamp PM, Lowik CW, van der Wee-Pals LJ, et al. Enhancement of the inhibitory action of APD on the transformation of osteoclast precursors into resorbing cells after dimethylation of the amino group. J Bone Miner Res 1987;2:29–42.
20. Hughes DE, Wright KR, Uy HL, et al. Bisphosphonates promote apoptosis in murine osteoclasts in vitro and in vivo. J Bone Miner Res 1995;10:1478–1487.
21. Watts NB, Harris ST, Genant HK, et al. Intermittent cyclical etidronate treatment of postmenopausal osteoporosis. N Engl J Med 1990;332:75–79.
22. Liberman UA, Weiss SR, et al. Effect of treatment with oral alendronate on bone mineral density and fracture incidence in postmenopausal osteoporosis. N Engl J Med 1995;333:1437–1443.
23. Eastell R. Treatment of postmenopausal osteoporosis. N Engl J Med 1998;338: 736–746.
24. Black DM, Cummings SR, Karpf DB, et al. Randomized trial effect of alendronate on risk of fracture in women with existing vertebral fractures. Lancet 1996;348:1535–1541.
25. Hosking D, Chilvers CE, Christiansen C, et al. Prevention of bone loss with alendronate in postmenopausal women under 60 years of age. Early postmenopausal intervention study group. N Engl J Med 1998;338;8:485–492.
26. Tonino RP, Menunier PJ, Emkey RD, et al. Long-term (seven year) efficacy and safety of alendronate in the treatment of osteoporosis in postmenopausal women. Osteoporos Int 2000;(suppl 2):S209.
27. Struys A, Snelder AA, Mulder H. Cyclical etidronate reverses bone loss of the spine and proximal femur in patients with established corticosteroid-induced osteoporosis. Am J Med 1995;99:235–242.
28. Heaney RE, Recker RR, Saville PD. Menopausal changes in bone remodeling. J Lab Clin Med 1978;92:964–970.
29. Lindsay R. Osteoporosis. Clin Geriatr Med 1988;4:411–430.
30. Nactigall LE, Nactigall RH, Nachtigall RD. Estrogen replacement therapy I: a 10 year prospective study in the relationship of osteoporosis. Obstet Gynecol 1979;53:277–284.
31. Lindsay R, Hart DM, MacLean A, et al. Bone response to termination of estrogen treatment. Lancet 1978;1:1325–1327.

32. Writing Group for the Women's Health Initiative Investigators. Risks and benefits of estrogen plus progestin in healthy postmenopausal women. JAMA 2002;288:321–333.

33. Cauley JA, Robbins J, Chen Z, et al. Effects of estrogen plus progestin on risk of fracture and bone mineral density: the Women's Health Initiative Randomized Trial. JAMA 2003;290:1729–1738.

34. National Heart, Lung, and Blood Institute Women's Health Initiative Web site. http://www.nhlbi.nih.giv/whi/.

35. Fletcher SW, Colditz GA. Failure of estrogen plus progestin therapy for prevention. JAMA 2002;288:366–368.

36. Sillero-Arenas M, Delgado-Rodriguez M, Rodigues-Canteras R, Bueno-Cavanillas A, Galvez-Vargas R. Menopausal hormone replacement therapy and breast cancer: a meta-analysis. Obstet Gynecol 1992;79:286–294.

37. Balfour JA, Goa KL. Raloxifene. Drugs Aging 1998;12:335–341.

38. Spencer CP, Morris EP, Rymer JM. Selective estrogen receptor modulators: Women's panacea for the next millennium? Am J Obstet Gynecol 1999; 180:763–770.

39. Delmas PD, Bjarnason NH, Mitlak BH, et al. Effects of raloxifene on bone density, serum cholesterol concentrations, and uterine endometrium in postmenopausal women. N Engl J Med 1997;337:1641–1647.

40. Kuehn BM. Longer-lasting osteoporosis drugs sought. JAMA 2005;293: 2458.

41. Cummings SR, Black D, Barrett-Connor E, et al. The effect of raloxifene on risk of breast cancer in postmenopausal women: results from the MORE randomized trial. Multiple outcomes of Raloxifene Evaluation. JAMA 1999;281: 2189–2197.

42. Anderson RE, Schraer H, Gay CV. Ultrastructural immunocytochemical localization of carbonic anhydrase in normal and calcitonin-treated chick osteoclasts. Anat Rec 1982;204:9–20.

43. Akisaka T, Gay CV. Ultracytochemical evidence for a proton-pump adenosine triphosphatase in chick osteoclasts. Cell Tissue Res 1986;24:507–512.

44. Chambers, TJ, Fuller K, and Darby JA. Hormonal regulation of acid phosphatase release by osteoclasts disaggregated from neonatal rat bone. J Cell Physiol 1987;132:92–96.

45. Moonga BS, Moss DW, Patchell A, et al. Intracellular regulation of enzyme release from rat osteoclasts and evidence for a functional role in bone resorption. J Physiol 1990;429:29–45.

46. Yumita S, Nicholson GC, Rowe DJ, et al. Biphasic effect of calcitonin on tartrate-resistant acid phosphatase activity in isolated rat osteoclasts. J Bone Miner Res 1991;6:591–597.

47. Offermanns S, Iida-Klein A, Segre GV, et al. G alpha q family members couple parathyroid hormone (PTH)/PTH-related peptide and calcitonin receptors to phospholipase C in COS-7 cells. Mol Endocrinol 1996;10: 566–574.

48. Zaidi M. Calcium "receptors" on eukaryotic cells with special reference to the osteoclast. Biosci Rep 1990;10:493–507.

49. Moonga BS, Alam AS, Bevis PJR, et al. Regulation of cytosolic free calcium in isolated osteoclasts by calcitonin. J Endocrinol 1992;132:241–249.

50. Muff R, Dambacher MA, Fischer IA. Formation of neutralizing antibodies during intranasal synthetic salmon calcitonin treatment of postmenopausal osteoporosis. Osteoporosis Int 1991;1:72–75.

51. Reginster JY. Calcitonin for prevention and treatment of osteoporosis. Am J Med 1993;95(suppl 5A):44S–47S.

52. Overgaard K, Hansen MA, Jensen SB, et al. Effect of salmon calcitonin given intranasally on bone mass and fracture rates in established osteoporosis: a dose response study. Br Med J 1992;305:56–61.

53. McDermott MT, Kidd GS. The role of calcitonin in the development and treatment of osteoporosis. Endocr Rev 1987;8:377–390.

54. Kanis IA, Johaell O, Gullberg B, et al. Evidence for efficacy of drugs affecting bone metabolism in preventing hip fracture. Br Med J 1992;305:1124–1128.

55. Rico H, Hernandez ER, Revilla, et al. Salmon calcitonin reduces vertebral fracture rate in post-menopausal crush fracture syndrome. J Bone Miner Res 1992;16:131–138.

56. Silverman SL, Chesnut C, Andriano K, et al. Salmon calcitonin nasal spray reduces risk of vertebral fracture(s) in established osteoporosis and has continuous efficacy with prolonged treatment accrued 5 year world wide data of the PROOF study. Bone 1998;23(suppl 5):S174.

57. Riggs BL, Hodgson SF, O'Fallon WM, et al. Effect of fluoride treatment on the fracture rate in postmenopausal women with osteoporosis. N Engl J Med 1990;322:802–809.

58. Kleerekoper M, Peterson EL, Nelson DA, et al. A randomized trial of sodium fluoride as a treatment for postmenopausal osteoporosis. Osteoporosis Int 1991;1:155–161.

59. Pak CYC, Sakhaee K, Adams-Huet B, et al. Treatment of postmenopausal osteoporosis with slow-release sodium fluoride: final report of a randomized controlled trial. Ann Intern Med 1995;123:401–408.

60. Finkelstein JS, Klibanski A, Arnold A, et al. Prevention of estrogen deficiency related bone loss with human PTH: a randomized controlled trial. JAMA 1998;280:1067–1073.

61. Brandi ML. New treatment strategies: ipriflavone, strontium, vitamin D metabolites and analogs. Am J Med 1993;95(suppl 5A):69S–74S.

62. Fisher JE, Rogers MJ, Halasy JM, et al. Alendronate mechanism of action: geranylgeraniol, an intermediate in the mevalonate pathway, prevents inhibition of osteoclast formation, bone resorption, and kinase activation in vitro. Proc Natl Acad Sci USA 1999;96(1):133–138.

63. Mundy G, Garrett R, Harris S, et al. Stimulation of bone formation in vitro and in rodents by statins. Science 1999;286:1946–1949.

20
Instability and Falls

HELEN M. FERNANDEZ

Learning Objectives

Upon completion of the chapter, the student will be able to:

1. Identify the prevalence of falls in older adults.
2. Identify predisposing risk factors for falls among older adults.
3. Develop and implement a plan of care for a patient with history of recurrent falls.

Case (Part 1)

Sara Romero calls you to make an appointment for her mother, Bertha Perez. Ms. Romero tells you that her mother is falling at home. You have not seen Mrs. Perez for about 2 years. Her medical history consists of diabetes mellitus type 2 and hypertension. During this new encounter, Mrs. Perez tells you that she moves slowly but is relatively healthy for her age. Her daughter disagrees and tells you that her mother has had several near falls and one serious fall, which resulted in a right 5th rib fracture. Mrs. Perez admits that she is afraid of being alone because she feels unsteady on her feet. Her daughter comments that her mother only leaves the house with a family member.

General Considerations

Falling is an important clinical marker of frailty, as evidenced by its association with other functional problems, such as incontinence, and with a high mortality rate that is not directly attributable to fall-related injuries

---

Material in this chapter is based on the following chapter in Cassel CK, Leipzig RM, Cohen HJ, Larson EB, Meier DE, eds. Geriatric Medicine: An Evidence-Based Approach, 4th ed. New York: Springer, 2003: Thomas DC, Edelberg HK, Tinetti ME. Falls, pp. 979–994. Selections edited by Helen M. Fernandez.

(1). As a consequence of its associated morbidity, falling is also an important health problem in its own right among frail, as well as healthier, older persons.

Prevalence

Each year, approximately one third of community-living adults over age 65 years and 50% of persons over age 80 years sustain a fall (2–4). Half of these individuals experience multiple falls. Among individuals under age 75, women fall more frequently than men do. This gender difference in prevalence lessens, however, among adults over age 75 (5).

Unintentional injury is the sixth leading cause of death in persons over the age of 65 years; the majority of these deaths are attributed to falls and their complications, especially among persons 85 years of age and older (6). Although women are about twice as likely to suffer a serious injury during a fall (7,8), the rates for fall-related deaths are consistently higher among men, who are 22% more likely than women to sustain a fatal fall (9).

About 7% of persons over 75 years visit emergency rooms for a fall injury event each year; more than 40% of these visits result in hospitalizations (10). As many as 10% of falls in this age group are complicated by serious injury, such as a fracture, joint dislocation, or severe head trauma (11). An estimated 5% of falls by community-living elderly persons result in a fracture, fewer than 1% in a hip fracture (10). In persons over age 75, fractures of the lower extremity are about twice as common as fractures of the upper extremity. An additional 5% of falls result in serious soft tissue injuries requiring medical attention (4,6). These injuries include hemarthroses, joint dislocations, sprains, and hematomas. Subdural hematomas and cervical fractures are devastating, but rare. About 30% to 50% of falls by elderly persons result in minor injuries such as bruises, lacerations, and abrasions.

Fear of falling is common among community-living older adults, particularly among older women. Many older women express concern over the loss of independence and quality of life resulting from a fall and hip fracture (12). One in four fallers report that he or she avoids activities because of fear of falling (4,13). As a result of this fear, patients report a poorer quality of life with a loss of function and independence (14).

Falling has been associated with an increased likelihood of hospitalization, nursing home placement, and death (15–17). Much of this relationship, however, may be accounted for by older age, chronic conditions, and activities of daily living (ADL) disabilities (17). Noninjurious as well as injurious falls have been found to be independent predictors of nursing home placement, after adjusting for other known risk factors, and falls with serious injury were twice as likely as noninjurious falls to result in nursing home placement (18).

> **Case (Part 2)**
>
> On examination, Mrs. Perez has mild quadriceps muscle weakness (4/5), normal joint range of motion, +1 ankle reflexes, slightly diminished but present proprioception, no obviously decreased sensation, and slight hesitancy when arising from a chair. Her Romberg test is normal. She walks without an assistive device.

Pathogenesis

Nonsyncopal falls occur when environmental hazards or demands exceed the individual's ability to maintain postural stability. Specific diseases such as Parkinson's syndrome, normal pressure hydrocephalus, white matter disease, and high cervical myelopathy may result in severe postural instability. Some authors also describe a gait disturbance of unknown central nervous system etiology, referred to as senile or essential gait disorder. Overall, these central nervous system diseases account for a relatively small percentage of falls by older persons.

Investigators have attempted, through a careful review of fall circumstances, to identify the most likely immediate cause of falls. Summarizing the results of several studies, Rubenstein et al. (19) reported that an environmentally related factor was the most likely cause of 41% (range 23–53%) of falls, gait or balance disturbance or weakness of 13% (2–29%), drop attack of 13% (0–25%), dizziness or vertigo of 8% (0–19%), confusion of 2% (0–7%), and postural hypotension of 1% (0–6%), whereas visual disorder, syncope, acute illness, drugs, and other factors accounted for an additional 17% of falls (19). The cause was unknown for 6% (0–16%) of falls. The relative frequency of the various causes varied widely among the studies.

A related and clinically useful method for explaining fall etiology is to consider both predisposing as well as situational factors. *Predisposing risk factors* are those intrinsic characteristics of the individual that chronically impair stability and render the individual vulnerable to new insults. *Situational factors* are those host, activity, and environmental factors that are present at the time of the fall.

Predisposing Risk Factors

Stability depends on the intricate functioning of sensory, central integrative, and musculoskeletal effector components. Accumulated impairments and diseases affecting these components, superimposed on age-related physiologic changes or lifestyle factors (e.g., past physical activity), result in a predisposition to falling (20). Table 20.1 lists the common risk factors for falls.

The major sensory modalities responsible for orienting the individual in space and identifying hazards include the visual, auditory, vestibular, and proprioceptive systems. These modalities have multiple interconnections with one another. Age-related visual changes include decreased visual acuity, contrast sensitivity, dark adaptation, and accommodation. In addition, ocular diseases that are common in older persons, such as macular degeneration, glaucoma, and cataracts, may adversely affect visual functioning. Visual acuity, contrast sensitivity, and depth perception, a visual function involved in spatial orientation, have been shown to be especially relevant to postural stability and falling (21–23). Hearing contributes directly to stability through the detection and interpretation of auditory stimuli, which help localize and orient the individual in space, particularly when other sensory modalities are impaired. More than 50% of elderly persons have some hearing loss (24).

An age-related decline in vestibular function has been suggested as an explanation for increased postural sway as well as dizziness and perhaps falling in elderly persons (25). Predisposing factors include past aminoglycoside use as well as present use of aspirin, furosemide, quinine, quinidine, and perhaps tobacco and alcohol. Head trauma, mastoid or ear surgery, and middle-ear infections are other possible predisposing factors. Elderly persons with vestibular problems complain of worsening stability in the dark because of increased reliance on visual input.

The proprioceptive system provides spatial orientation during position changes, while walking on uneven ground, or when other modalities are impaired. The proprioceptive system includes peripheral nerves, apophyseal joint mechanoreceptors, the posterior columns, as well as multiple central nervous system connections. Older adults with proprioceptive problems complain of worsening difficulties in the dark or on uneven ground. They may complain of true vertigo. Gait often improves in these individuals with even minimal support.

Specific diseases such as Parkinson's disease, normal pressure hydrocephalus, and stroke are associated with an increased risk of falling. Central nervous system processes that adversely affect cognition further impede stability because problem solving and judgment are needed to interpret and respond appropriately to environmental stimuli. Individuals with impaired mental status or dementia have consistently been found to have an increased incidence of falling, even in the absence of a clinical gait disorder. Additional studies have demonstrated the relationship between white matter disease, even in the absence of cognitive impairment, and gait disorders (26). Any impairment within the musculoskeletal system, including joints, muscles, and bones, will decrease stability and increase fall risk.

Systemic diseases may contribute to instability by impairing sensory, neurologic, or musculoskeletal functioning, or by causing a reduction in

TABLE 20.1. Predisposing and situational factors associated with risk of falling

Predisposing factors with contribution to falling	Possible interventions
Sensory	
Vision: acuity, perception, impaired hazard recognition; distorted environmental signals; spatial disorientation	Medical: refraction; cataract extraction Rehabilitative: balance and gait training Environmental: good lighting; home safety assessment; architectural design that minimizes distortions and illusions
Hearing: spatial disorientation; balance impairment; distorted environmental signals (auditory)	Medical: cerumen removal; audiologic evaluation with hearing aid if appropriate Rehabilitative: training in hearing aid use Environmental: decrease background noise
Vestibular dysfunction: Spatial disorientation at rest; impaired visual fixation; balance impairment especially with head or body turning	Medical: avoid vestibulotoxic drugs; surgical ablation Rehabilitative: habituation exercises Environmental: good lighting (increased reliance on visual input); architectural design that minimizes distortions and illusions
Proprioceptive-cervical disorders; peripheral neuropathy: spatial disorientation during position changes or while walking on uneven surfaces or in dark	Medical: diagnose and treat specific disease (e.g., spondylosis, B_{12} deficiency) Rehabilitative: balance exercises; correct walking aid Environmental: good lighting (increased reliance on visual input); appropriate footwear; home safety assessment
Central neurologic	
Central nervous system diseases: impaired problem solving, strength, sensation, balance, gait, tone, or coordination	Medical: diagnose and treat specific diseases (e.g., Parkinson's syndrome, normal pressure hydrocephalus) Rehabilitative: physical therapy; balance and gait training; correct walking aid Environmental: home safety assessment; appropriate adaptations (e.g., high, firm chairs, raised toilet seats, grab bars in bathroom)
Dementia/cognitive impairment: impaired problem solving, impaired gait	Medical: minimize sedating or centrally acting drugs Rehabilitative: supervised exercise and ambulation Environmental: safe structure, supervised environment
Musculoskeletal	
Muscle weakness: upper and lower extremity impaired postural stability Arthritides: impaired postural stability Feet: impaired proprioception; impaired postural instability; altered gait pattern	Medical: diagnose and treat specific diseases Rehabilitative: balance and gait training; Tai Chi; muscle strengthening exercises; back exercises; correct walking aid; correct foot wear; good foot care (nails, bunions) Environmental: home safety assessment; appropriate adaptations

TABLE 20.1. *Continued*

Predisposing factors with contribution to falling	Possible interventions
Back: impaired ability to regain stability	
Other	
Postural hypotension: impaired cerebral blood flow leading to fatigue, weakness, postural instability; syncope if severe	Medical: diagnose and treat specific diseases; avoid offending drugs; rehydrate; replenish salt Rehabilitative: tilt table if severe; reconditioning if component of deconditioning; graded pressure stockings; dorsiflexion and hand flexion exercises prior to arising Environmental: elevate head of bed
Depression: ? accident-proneness; ? poor concentration	Medical: ? antidepressants associated with increased risk of falling; ? select least anticholinergic
Medications: especially sedatives, phenothiazines, antidepressants; total number and dose of medications Impaired alertness; postural hypotension; postural instability; fatigue	Medical: lowest effective dose of essential medications; readjust or discontinue when possible

Situational factors	Possible interventions
Acute host factors	
Acute illness; new or increased medications Transiently impaired alertness; postural hypotension; fatigue	Medical: diagnose and treat specific diseases; start medications low and increase slowly Environmental: increase supervision during illnesses or with new medication
Displacing activity	
Increased opportunity to fall	Rehabilitative: recommend avoiding only clearly hazardous and unnecessary activities (e.g., climbing on chairs); balance and gait training
Environmental hazards	
Slipping or tripping hazards (e.g., loose rugs, wet floors, ice, small objects) stairs, lighting, and furniture Nursing home: movable tables; inappropriate bed or chair height; ill fitting shoes or pants; restraints	Environmental: home safety assessment with appropriate adaptive or structural changes

Source: Thomas DC, Edelberg HK, Tinetti ME. Falls. In: Cassel CK, Leipzig RM, Cohen HJ, et al., eds. Geriatric Medicine, 4th ed. New York: Springer, 2003.

cerebral oxygenation or perfusion, fatigue, or confusion. Common examples include anemia, electrolyte disturbances, hypoglycemia or hyperglycemia, acid-base disturbances, or hypothyroidism.

Postural hypotension may result in instability by compromising cerebral blood flow (27). The prevalence of postural hypotension ranges from 10% to 30% in community-dwelling persons over age 65 years. Like falling, postural hypotension is frequently multifactorial. Contributing factors include age-related autonomic changes, decreased baroreceptor sensitivity, decreased renin-angiotensin response to upright position, decreased venous and lymphatic return, and salt and water depletion. The effects of diseases such as diabetes or Parkinson's disease and medications, such as antidepressants, neuroleptics, antihypertensives, nitrates, and diuretics, are further contributing factors. Postural hypotension should be considered if the fall occurred while moving from a lying or sitting to a standing position, after prolonged standing, or during exertion. Another abnormality in blood pressure homeostasis is postprandial hypotension (27). The mechanisms and mediators of postprandial hypotension remain unknown, although inability to compensate for splanchnic blood pooling after the meal has been postulated as a possible etiology.

Medications may contribute to gait instability through a variety of mechanisms, including impairment of cognitive functioning, postural hypotension, dehydration, impaired balance, fatigue, or electrolyte disturbance. Centrally acting medications, including sedative-hypnotics, tranquilizers, antidepressants, and neuroleptics, have repeatedly been associated with an increased risk of falls and injuries (28,29). Both selective serotonin reuptake inhibitors (SSRIs) and tricyclic antidepressants have been implicated in falls and hip fractures (30). Other classes of medications associated with falls in older adults include diuretics, type 1A antiarrhythmics, and digoxin (31). In addition to specific medications, recent changes in dose and the total number of medications have been associated with an increased risk of falling (32). Conversely, evidence suggests that postural instability, as manifested by impaired balance, dizziness, and falling, is one of the most frequent presentations of adverse drug effect in an older population (33,34).

Situational Factors

Falling is well recognized as a nonspecific presentation of acute illness in older adults. Acute febrile illnesses (e.g., pneumonia or urinary tract infections) and chronic disease exacerbations (e.g., congestive heart failure or diabetes mellitus) likely precipitate falls by temporarily impairing stability (4). Some cardiac dysrhythmias cause a decrease in cerebral blood flow and loss of consciousness, resulting in a fall (35). Carotid baroreceptor hypersensitivity may contribute to syncopal, as well as nonsyncopal, falls. One type of fall, mentioned most frequently in the British literature, is the drop attack (36), which refers to a sudden loss of postural tone without loss of consciousness. Drop attacks may occur while walking, while turning the neck, while looking up, or without an obvious precipitating movement. Some individuals note that their knees buckled or "just gave out." It is likely that at least some of those who report their knees buckling have impaired mechanoreceptors secondary to arthritic joint changes. Difficulty getting up is often reported. The etiology and frequency of drop attacks are unknown.

The majority of falls by community-dwelling elderly persons occur during the course of usual, relatively nonhazardous activities such as walking, changing position, or performing basic ADLs. Only a small percentage of falls occur during clearly hazardous activities such as climbing on chairs or ladders or participating in sports activities (4).

Although major environmental hazards account for few falls, environmental factors probably contribute to the majority of falls by community-dwelling older adults. The precise role of environmental factors is difficult to ascertain because studies lack control data on nonfallers or fallers at times other than their fall. Over 70% of falls by community-dwelling older adults occur at home. About 10% of falls occur on stairs—well out of proportion to the time spent on them, with descending being more hazardous than ascending (4,37). The most commonly mentioned environmental hazards include carrying heavy or bulky objects, and negotiating obstacles that can be tripped over, slippery floors, and poor lighting (34). Slippery or improperly fitting shoes are another potential hazard. Finally, patterns on floors or walls, depending on their quality, may either distort or improve visual perception (38).

Diagnostic Evaluation

The first step in evaluating individuals who have experienced a fall or who are at risk for falling is to identify possible contributing factors (39,40). The following components of the evaluation provide complementary information: a thorough assessment of predisposing risk factors and diseases including a complete history and physical exam and laboratory workup; a balance and gait assessment; and a review of previous fall situations.

Symptoms and Signs

The risk assessment begins with a careful history and physical examination aimed at identifying all predisposing risk factors. It is important to bear in mind that the multiple diseases and disabilities suffered by many older individuals may render the signs and symptoms of specific conditions obscure, vague, or nonspecific. Therefore, a thorough systematic assessment of all possible contributing factors is essential. The governing concept in fall assessment is that it may be possible to decrease fall risk by ameliorating as many contributing factors as possible.

The neurologic diseases that predispose to falls can be diagnosed from a thorough neurologic history and examination. Although most neurologic diseases associated with falling result in postural instability and pathologic gait patterns, these findings are not disease specific.

Simple screening tests such as the Snellen chart can be used to measure near and distant visual acuity. If there are any questions concerning visual function, the individual should be referred to an ophthalmologist or optometrist for a full evaluation. Portable audiometry or the whisper test (41) can be used to screen for hearing problems. Although vestibular dysfunction is difficult to diagnose from simple clinical tests, a vestibular contribution to instability should be suspected if the individual complains of vertigo, worsening stability in the dark or with specific head positions, or provides a history of predisposing factors including past aminoglycoside use; use of aspirin, furosemide, quinine, or quinidine; or head trauma, mastoid or ear surgery, or middle ear infections.

Individuals with proprioceptive impairments complain of worsening stability in the dark, on uneven ground, on inclines, or on thick rugs. Decreased position and vibration sense are noted on examination. Although postural hypotension has not been identified as a frequent risk factor for falls among community-dwelling elderly persons, this is likely because it is not feasible to assess blood pressure change at the time of a fall. Blood pressure change with position change should be part of the risk factor assessment.

The screen for depressive symptoms may reveal vegetative complaints, poor concentration, or apathy. Finally, a careful medication review is an essential component of a fall risk assessment. The assessment should involve the direct recording of all prescription medications from the original containers and verification of the dose and timing of each medication. Over-the-counter medications, particularly sedative hypnotics, cold preparations, and nonsteroidal antiinflammatory agents, must be ascertained as well. In addition, possible medication side effects including confusion, lightheadedness, fatigue, weakness, or postural hypotension should be elicited from the patient.

Carotid hypersensitivity should be suspected if the individual gives a history of "just going down" or falling with head turning or with looking up. Carotid sinus massage should be performed if carotid sinus syndrome is suspected, if there is no evidence of cerebrovascular disease or cardiac conduction abnormality, and if the procedure is judged safe for the individual patient. The *carotid sinus syndrome* is defined as greater than a 3-second sinus pause or more than a 5mmHg drop in systolic blood pressure.

Laboratory Evaluation

All elderly persons who have experienced falls should undergo routine laboratory screening including a complete blood count, thyroid function tests, electrolytes, including serum blood urea nitrogen (BUN) and creatinine, serum glucose, as well as a determination of vitamin B_{12} levels. These tests are warranted to screen for anemia, thyroid dysfunction, electrolyte abnormalities, dehydration, hyperglycemia or hypoglycemia, and B_{12} deficiency because of the prevalence, nonspecific presentation, and potential for modification of underlying diseases by these diagnoses. Drug levels, for example, should be measured in individuals taking anticonvulsants, tricyclic antidepressants, antiarrhythmics, and high-dose aspirin. History and examination should guide other laboratory investigations.

As noted above, in approximately 10% of cases, falls by community-dwelling older adults are a nonspecific manifestation of an acute illness. In these situations the laboratory and diagnostic evaluation in these situations should be dictated by the suspected etiology. Examples of potentially useful tests include the electrocardiogram, cardiac enzymes, chest x-ray, urine analysis and culture, and blood cultures.

Brain imaging with computed tomography or magnetic resonance imaging is indicated only when focal abnormalities are noted on the neurologic examination. Cervical spine films may be helpful for individuals with impaired gait, lower extremity spasticity, and hyperreflexia suggestive of cervical spondylosis. A lateral dimension of the spinal canal of less than 12mm is suggestive of a significant encroachment on the cervical cord. Magnetic resonance imaging should be pursued to confirm this finding only if the individual is deemed a candidate for neurosurgery.

A 24-hour ambulatory cardiac monitor (Holter) is not warranted for the routine evaluation of nonsyncopal falls. The yield of ambulatory electrocardiographic monitoring is very low in these individuals. In addition, the results may be difficult to interpret due to the high prevalence of asymptomatic arrhythmias in older adults.

Case (Part 3)

You asked Mrs. Perez to perform a timed "up-and-go" test: You asked her to stand from her armless chair without using her hands for assistance and to walk 10 feet out and back. She was concerned when you told her to do it as fast—but as safely—as possible. Mrs. Perez started to get up but had to rock back and forth in her seat several times to give her momentum to get off her chair. Her walking is slow and cautious, with shortened steps and a slightly widened base of support. She completed the test in 32 seconds.

Balance and Gait Evaluation

Balance and gait represent end products of the accumulated effects of disease, age-related and lifestyle changes, and impairments in sensory, neurologic, and musculoskeletal functioning. Therefore, a careful assessment of balance and gait is an essential component of the fall evaluation. There is strong epidemiologic evidence to support balance and gait assessment as the single best means of identifying individuals at increased risk of falling (4,5,8,13). Simple but reliable methods for observing an individual's balance and gait performance are available for use in clinical practice (42,43). The "up-and-go" test and the Performance-Oriented Assessment of Mobility are two examples of clinical observation tests of balance and gait that have been used extensively in clinical practice (42,43). Both assessments involve observing the individual perform various combinations of maneuvers such as getting up from a chair, reaching up, turning, bending over, assuming various narrowed stances, walking at a usual and rapid pace, and sitting in a chair. The examiner watches for instability or difficulty with performing each maneuver (Table 20.2). The assessment may help to identify not only the individuals at risk for falling, but also the circumstances in which falls are most likely to occur. As discussed below, combinations of medical, rehabilitative, and environmental interventions can be recommended based on the simple observations of balance and gait.

Review of Fall Situations

The fourth component of the fall evaluation is a careful review of recent fall situations. In determining the contribution of possible intrinsic factors, the clinician should obtain information on premonitions; feelings of lightheadedness, vertigo, or unsteadiness; recent medications, particularly focusing on recent changes; preceding alcohol consumption; or symptoms of acute illness, postural hypotension, or dysrhythmias. A precise description of activity at the time of the fall is important as well (44).

Environmental details that should be ascertained include obstacles in the immediate area of the fall; the volume and intensity of lighting; the floor or ground surface; objects being carried; footwear, including the fit, heel height, and type of sole; and walking aids used at the time of the fall. A home safety evaluation as well as careful review of specific fall situations may reveal remedial environmental hazards. While common sense dictates eliminating obvious hazards such as throw rugs and obstacles, these have not been shown to be independent risk factors. Still, a recent Cochrane Review supports interventions to reduce home hazards, particularly by a trained professional for patients in the immediate posthospitalization period.

TABLE 20.2. Position changes, balance maneuvers, and gait components included in performance-oriented mobility assessment (50)

Position change or balance maneuver	Observation: fall risk if:
Getting up from chair*	Does not get up with single movement; pushes up with arms or moves forward in chair first; unsteady on first standing
Sitting down in chair	Plops in chair; does not land in center
Withstanding nudge on sternum or pull at waist	Moves feet; begins to fall backward; grabs object for support; feet not touching side by side
Side-by-side standing with eyes open and shut	Same as above (eyes closed tests patient's reliance on visual input for balance)
Neck turning	Moves feet; grabs object for support; feet not touching side by side; complains of vertigo, dizziness, or unsteadiness
Bending over	Unable to bend over to pick up small object (e.g., pen) from floor; grabs object to pull up on; requires multiple attempts to arise

Gait component or maneuver	Observation: fall risk if:
Initiation	Hesitates; stumbles; grabs object for support
Step height (raising feet with stepping)	Does not clear floor consistently (scrapes or shuffles); raises foot too high (more than 2 inches)
Step continuity	After first few steps, does not consistently begin raising one foot as other foot touches floor
Step symmetry	Step length not equal (pathologic side usually has longer step length-problem; may be in hip, knee, ankle, or surrounding muscles)
Path deviation	Does not walk in straight line; weaves side to side
Turning	Stops before initiating turn, staggers; sways; grabs object for support

*Use hard, armless chair.

Note: Other more difficult balance maneuvers include tandem, semi-tandem, and one leg standing. Patient walks down hallway at "usual pace," turns and comes back using usual walking aid. Repeat at "rapid pace." Examiner observes single component of gait at a time (analogous to heart examination). Other gait observations include heel-toe sequencing; arm swing; trunk sway; stepping over objects.

Source: Modified with permission in Tinetti ME, Ginter SF. Identifying mobility dysfunctions in elderly patients. Standard neuromuscular examination or direct assessment? JAMA 1988;259:1190–1193. Copyright 1988, American Medical Association. All rights reserved. Reprinted as appears in Thomas DC, Edelberg HK, Tinetti ME. Falls. In: Cassel CK, Leipzig RM, Cohen HJ, et al., eds. Geriatric Medicine, 4th ed. New York: Springer, 2003.

Case (Part 4)

Mrs. Perez's daughter is quite concerned about your evaluation. She asks you what she could do to minimize the risks of her mother having an injurious fall again. You recommend an increase in physical activity for her mother. Ms. Romero says that there are activities offered at a senior center nearby, such as Tai-Chi, swimming, aerobics, stationary bicycling, and resistance training. She asks you which one would be best for her mother to assist in preventing her from falling.

Prevention and Management Considerations

The goal of a fall evaluation and prevention strategy is to minimize the risk of falling without compromising mobility or functional independence. Given the inherent trade-offs between safety and independence, this goal may be difficult to achieve for some individuals. Perhaps a better goal, rather than to prevent all falls, would be to prevent relevant fall-related morbidities such as serious injury, fear, and the inability to get up. As the ability to identify the subset of fallers at risk for these fall sequelae improves, evaluative and preventive efforts can be better targeted.

The appropriate intervention strategy depends on the health status and fall history of the individual. For healthy individuals who have not suffered falls, the treatment goal is to maintain or improve balance, gait, flexibility, and endurance in order to decrease the risk of falls and to maintain mobility and functional independence. Evidence is emerging that among "healthier," less impaired persons, exercise seems to have as strong an effect on falls as does the multifactorial approach in the less healthy (45). The aim of treatment in older individuals who have already experienced falls or who suffer from chronic diseases and impairments is to reduce the rate of subsequent falls and decrease the incidence of fall-related morbidity such as injury, fear, inability to get up, functional decline, and immobility. The treatment strategy should be guided by the results of the assessment (46–48). The governing concept should be that it is possible to reduce the risk of falls and fall sequelae by eliminating or modifying as many contributing factors as possible. Because of the overlapping, compensatory nature of the systems affecting stability as described earlier, simple interventions may result in major improvements, even if the interventions are not targeted at the systems believed to be most impaired.

As most of the factors contributing to fall risk are chronic diseases or impairments that may be modifiable, but only rarely curable, the treatment strategy should combine appropriate combinations of medical, surgical, rehabilitative, and environmental interventions. Rather than targeting one area of risk, an individualized, interdisciplinary, multifactorial approach to modifying all risk factors was shown to be most beneficial in reducing falls among older adults.

Physical therapy is an integral part of any fall assessment and treatment program (47). A home safety evaluation with recommendations for modification and adaptation, prescription of and training in the appropriate use of assistive devices, transfer and gait training, and instruction in muscle strengthening and balance exercises are examples of fall preventive interventions carried out by a trained physical therapist (47). The physical therapist may also help in treating the consequences of falls by teaching strategies for how to fall, or getting up from the floor after a fall, and by encouraging confidence in performance of ADLs without falling. Recent evidence suggests that a home exercise program may reduce falls, but further evidence is needed to determine the long-term effects of this intervention (49).

Suggested Readings

Guideline for the prevention of falls in older persons. American Geriatrics Society, British Geriatrics Society, and American Academy of Orthopaedic Surgeons Panel on Falls Prevention. J Am Geriatr Soc 2001;49(5):664–672. *A user-friendly approach for the prevention of falls in all older adults.*

Thomas DC, Edelberg HK, Tinetti ME. Falls. In: Cassel CK, Leipzig RM, Cohen HJ, et al., eds. Geriatric Medicine, 4th ed. New York: Springer, 2003: 979–994.

References

1. Tinetti ME, et al. Shared risk factors for falls, incontinence, and functional dependence. Unifying the approach to geriatric syndromes. JAMA 1995;273: 1348–1353.
2. Campbell AJ, et al. Falls in old age: a study of frequency and related clinical factors. Age Ageing 1981;10(4):264–270.
3. Prudham D, Evans JG. Factors associated with falls in the elderly: a community study. Age Ageing 1981;10(3):141–146.
4. Tinetti ME, Speechley M. Risk factors for falls among elderly persons living in the community. N Engl J Med 1988;36:1701–1707.
5. Tinetti ME, Liu WL, Claus EB. Predictors and prognosis of inability to get up after falls among elderly persons. JAMA 1993;269:65–70.
6. Sattin RW. Falls among older persons: a public health perspective. Annu Rev Public Health 1992;13(7):489–508.

7. O'Loughlin JL, et al. Incidence of and risk factors for falls and injurious falls among the community-dwelling elderly. Am J Epidemiol 1993;137(3): 342–354.

8. Nevitt MC, Cummings SR, Hudes ES. Risk factors for injurious falls: a prospective study. J Gerontol 1991;46:M164–M170.

9. Stevens JA, et al. Surveillance for injuries and violence among older adults. MMWR CDC Surveill Summ 1999;48(8):27–50.

10. Sattin RW, et al. The incidence of fall injury events among the elderly in a defined population. Am J Epidemiol 1990;131:1028–1037.

11. Tinetti ME, et al. Risk factors for serious injury during falls by older persons in the community. J Am Geriatr Soc 1995;43(11):1214–1221.

12. Salkeld G, et al. Quality of life related to fear of falling and hip fracture in older women: a time trade off study [see comments]. BMJ 2000;320(7231): 341–346.

13. Nevitt MC, et al. Risk factors for recurrent nonsyncopal falls. A prospective study. JAMA 1989;261(18):2663–2668.

14. Cumming RG, et al. Prospective study of the impact of fear of falling on activities of daily living, SF-36 scores, and nursing home admission. J Gerontol A Biol Sci Med Sci 2000;55(5):M299–M305.

15. Wolinsky FD, Johnson RJ, Fitzgerald JF. Falling, health status, and the use of health services by older adults. A prospective study. Med Care 1992;30(7): 587–597.

16. Kiel DP, et al. Health care utilization and functional status in the aged following a fall. Med Care 1991;29:221–228.

17. Dunn JE, et al. Mortality, disability, and falls in older persons: The role of underlying disease and disability. Am J Public Health 1992;82(3): 395–400.

18. Tinetti ME, Williams CS. Falls, injuries due to falls, and the risk of admission to a nursing home. N Engl J Med 1997;337(18):1279–1284.

19. Rubenstein LZ, Josephson KR, Robbins AS. Falls in the nursing home. Ann Intern Med 1994;121:442–451.

20. Wolfson LI, et al. Gait and balance in the elderly. Two functional capacities that link sensory and motor ability to falls. Clin Geriatr Med 1985;1(3): 649–659.

21. Lord SR, et al. Physiological factors associated with falls in older community-dwelling women. J Am Geriatr Soc 1994;42(10):1110–1117.

22. Glynn RJ, et al. Falls in elderly patients with glaucoma. Arch Ophthalmol 1991;109(2):205–210.

23. Tobis JS, et al. Visual perception dominance of fallers among community-dwelling older adults. J Am Geriatr Soc 1985;33(5):330–333.

24. Woolf SH, et al. The periodic health examination of older adults: the recommendations of the U.S. Preventive Services Task Force. Part II. Screening tests. J Am Geriatr Soc 1990;38(8):933–942.

25. Hazell JW. Vestibular problems of balance. Age Ageing 1979;8(4):258–260.

26. Masdeu JC, et al. Brain white-matter changes in the elderly prone to falling. Arch Neurol 1989;46(12):1292–1296.

27. Lipsitz LA. Orthostatic hypotension in the elderly. N Engl J Med 1989;321: 952–957.

28. Ray WA, Griffin MR. Prescribed medications, and the risk of falling. Top Geriatr Rehabil 1990;5:12–20.
29. Leipzig RM, Cumming RG, Tinetti ME. Drugs and falls in older people: a systematic review and meta-analysis: I. Psychotropic drugs. J Am Geriatr Soc 1999;47(1):30–39.
30. Liu B, et al. Use of selective serotonin-reuptake inhibitors of tricyclic antidepressants and risk of hip fractures in elderly people. Lancet 1998;351(9112): 1303–1307.
31. Leipzig RM, Cumming RG, Tinetti ME. Drugs and falls in older people: a systematic review and meta-analysis: II. Cardiac and analgesic drugs. J Am Geriatr Soc 1999;47(1):40–50.
32. Robbins AS, et al. Predictors of falls among elderly people. Results of two population-based studies. Arch Intern Med 1989;149(7):1628–1633.
33. Gray SL, Mahoney JE, Blough DK. Adverse drug events in elderly patients receiving home health services following hospital discharge. Ann Pharmacother 1999;33(11):1147–1153.
34. Stevens M, Holman CDJ, Bennett N. Preventing falls in older people: impact of an intervention to reduce environmental hazards in the home. J Am Geriatr Soc 2001;49:1442–1447.
35. Kapoor WN. Syncope in older persons. J Am Geriatr Soc 1994;42(4):426–436.
36. Sheldon JH. On the natural history of falls in old age. Br Med J 1960;2: 1685–1690.
37. Startzell JK, et al. Stair negotiation in older people: a review. J Am Geriatr Soc 2000;48(5):567–580.
38. Owen DH. Maintaining posture and avoiding tripping. Optical information for detecting and controlling orientation and locomotion. Clin Geriatr Med 1985;1(3):581–599.
39. Tinetti ME, Speechley M. Prevention of falls among the elderly. N Engl J Med 1989;320:1055–1059.
40. Vellas BJ, et al. A two-year longitudinal study of falls in 482 community-dwelling elderly adults. J Gerontol A Biol Sci Med Sci 1998;53:M264–M274.
41. MacPhee GJ, Crowther JA, McAlpine CH. A simple screening test for hearing impairment in elderly patients. Age Ageing 1988;17(5):347–351.
42. Tinetti ME, Williams TF, Mayewski R. Fall risk index for elderly patients based on number of chronic disabilities. Am J Med 1986;80(3):429–434.
43. Mathias S, Nayak US, Isaacs B. Balance in elderly patients: the "get-up and go" test. Arch Phys Med Rehabil 1986;67(6):387–389.
44. Berg WP, et al. Circumstances and consequences of falls in independent community-dwelling older adults. Age Ageing 1997;26(4):261–268.
45. Buchner DM, et al. The effect of strength and endurance training on gait, balance, fall risk, and health services use in community-living older adults. J Gerontol A Biol Sci Med Sci 1997;52(4):M218–M224.
46. Tinetti ME, et al. A multifactorial intervention to reduce the risk of falling among elderly people living in the community. N Engl J Med 1994;331(13): 821–827.
47. Koch M, et al. An impairment and disability assessment and treatment protocol for community-living elderly persons. Phys Ther 1994;74(4):286–294; discussion 295–298.

48. Lipsitz LA. An 85-year old woman with a history of falls. JAMA 1996;276(1): 447–454.

49. Lord SR, et al. The effect of a 12-month exercise trial on balance, strength, and falls in older women: a randomized controlled trial. J Am Geriatr Soc 1995;43(11):1198–1206.

50. Tinetti ME, Ginter SF. Identifying mobility dysfunctions in elderly patients. Standard neuromuscular examination or direct assessment? JAMA 1988;259: 1190–1193.

21
Hip Fractures

Rengena E. Chan-Ting

Learning Objectives

Upon completion of the chapter, the student will be able to:

1. Identify the major risk factors for hip fractures in the geriatric population.
2. Recognize the signs and symptoms of hip fractures in the elderly.
3. Understand the consequences of hospitalization of an older adult with a hip fracture.
4. Explain postoperative complications in the elderly after a surgical hip procedure.

Case (Part 1)

Ms. Hope is a petite, 86-year-old Caucasian woman who lives independently in a three-story walkup apartment. She has not seen a physician for many years because she feels that she is in "good health." One evening, as she was on her way to the bathroom, she tripped and fell on her left side. She was unable to stand due to excruciating pain. Luckily, she was able to pull the telephone close enough to her and call for an emergency ambulance. The emergency medical service brought Ms. Hope to the emergency room with a diagnosis suspicious for a left hip fracture.

What is Ms. Hope's chances for a full recovery?

Material in this chapter is based on the following chapters in Cassel CK, Leipzig RM, Cohen HJ, Larson EB, Meier DE, eds. Geriatric Medicine: An Evidence-Based Approach, 4th ed. New York: Springer, 2003: Pottenger LA. Orthopedic Problems with Aging, pp. 651–667. Morrison RS, Siu AL. Medical Aspects of Hip Fracture Management, pp. 669–680. Selections edited by Rengena E. Chan-Ting.

General Considerations

Hip fractures are an important cause of mortality and functional dependence in the United States. Approximately 250,000 hip fractures occur annually in this country, and this number is expected to increase to over 650,000 by the year 2040 (1,2). For adults over age 65, the annual incidence of hip fracture is 818 per 100,000 persons (3), and women are two to three times more likely to experience a fracture than are men (4,5). Indeed, it is estimated that a white woman with an average life expectancy of 80 years has a 15% lifetime risk of fracture and by age 80, she has a 1% to 2% annual risk (6). The mortality seen in the Medicare population following fracture is 7% at 1 month, 13% at 3 months, and 24% at 12 months (7). For those patients who survive to 6 months, 60% have recovered their prefracture walking ability, 50% have recovered their prefracture ability to perform their activities of daily living (ADLs), and about 25% have recovered their prefracture ability to perform instrumental activities of daily living (IADLs) (8). However, after 1 year, only 54% of surviving patients are able to walk unaided, and only 40% are able to perform all physical ADLs independently (8). Furthermore, it is estimated that these total annual costs will increase to $16 billion by the year 2040 as a result of the projected increase in the number of adults over age 65.

Case (Part 2)

In the emergency room, Ms. Hope is seen by an orthopedic surgeon, who notes on physical exam that her left foot is externally rotated and that her left hip is shorter and tender to slight passive range of motion. Radiographs and physical exam confirm that she sustained a left femoral intertrochanteric neck fracture.

What is the leading factor that places Ms. Hope at an increased risk for a hip fracture?

Diagnostic Evaluation

Symptoms and Signs

The majority of hip fractures are easily diagnosed on the basis of history, physical exam, and standard radiographs. Ninety percent of hip fractures result from a simple fall, and the characteristics of the fall (direction, site of impact, and protective response), as well as certain patient characteristics, are recognized as important factors influencing the risk of fracture (9).

A diagnosis of osteoporosis is the leading factor that places patients at increased risk for hip fracture (9). Other patient characteristics that have been shown to be associated with hip fracture include female sex, white race, maternal history of hip fracture, physical inactivity, low body weight, consumption of alcohol, previous hip fracture, nursing home residence, visual impairment, cognitive impairment, and psychotropic medication use (9). Patients with hip fracture typically report hip pain on weight bearing following a fall, and on physical exam the involved leg is often foreshortened and externally rotated.

Ancillary Tests

Plain radiographs (an anteroposterior view of the pelvis and a lateral view of the femur) hip confirm the diagnosis in the majority of circumstances. Occasionally, however, plain films do not reveal evidence of a fracture despite a high clinical suspicion (e.g., pain with weight bearing after a fall). In these cases, an anteroposterior view obtained with the hip internally rotated 15 to 20 degrees may reveal a fracture by providing an optimal view of the femoral neck (9). In circumstances in which all plain films are negative but clinical suspicion is still high, either a technetium-99m bone scan or magnetic resonance imaging (MRI) should be undertaken to rule out an occult fracture. The MRI appears to be a more sensitive test to detect early fractures as the bone scan can be normal within the first 72 hours following a fracture. If all tests or imaging studies are unrevealing, other diagnoses to consider include fractures of the pubic ramus, acetabulum, or greater trochanter, trochanteric bursitis, or trochanteric contusion.

Classification of Hip Fractures

Femoral Neck Fractures

Femoral neck fractures occur distal to the femoral head but proximal to the greater and lesser trochanters and are thus located within the capsule of the hip joint. The location of the fracture has important implications for healing and operative repair. Fractures in this region can disrupt the blood supply to the femoral head and can result in complications such as nonunion and avascular necrosis of the femoral head. Thus, although nondisplaced and minimally displaced femoral neck fractures can often be treated by insertion of cannulated screws, displaced femoral neck fractures typically require a hemiarthroplasty procedure to ensure appropriate fracture healing.

Intertrochanteric Fractures

Intertrochanteric fractures are located lateral to the femoral neck. These fractures occur in a well-vascularized metaphyseal region between the greater and lesser trochanters, and although intertrochanteric fractures can be associated with considerable blood loss, they typically are not associated with the healing complications associated with femoral neck fractures. Intertrochanteric fractures are typically repaired by open reduction and internal fixation (ORIF) with a compression screw device.

Subtrochanteric Fractures

Subtrochanteric fractures occur just below the lesser trochanter and account for only 5% to 10% of hip fractures. These fractures behave clinically like long bone fractures and are repaired either by insertion of an intramedullary device or by placement of a compression screw and long side plate.

Case (Part 3)

Ms. Hope is diagnosed as having a left femoral intertrochanteric neck fracture. The orthopedic surgeon had a lengthy discussion involving the risks and benefits of an ORIF surgical procedure, which will repair her femoral intertrochanteric neck fracture.

What are Ms. Hope's management considerations and options at this point?

Management Considerations

Nonoperative Management

Nonoperative management should be considered for nonambulatory patients with advanced dementia. One recent study suggested that mortality following fracture in patients with end-stage dementia exceeds 50% at 6 months (10). For such patients, aggressive pain management and a return to their previous home environment may be the most optimal treatment plan given the burdens associated with routine hospitalization (e.g., delirium, restraints, and painful therapeutic interventions, such as phlebotomies, arterial blood gas monitoring, intravenous catheter insertions) (10,11).

Timing of Surgery

The timing of surgical repair of hip fracture may affect patients' outcomes in two ways. Delay in surgical repair, and hence delay in return to weight bearing, could affect functional recovery. Conversely, failure to stabilize medical problems before surgery could increase the risk of preoperative complications. Although the scheduling of surgery is set by the orthopedist, the rate-limiting step in this process is often the internist's preoperative medical evaluation.

For patients who are medically stable without active comorbid illness (e.g., active heart failure), surgical repair of hip fracture within the first 24 to 48 hours of admission is associated with a lower 1-year mortality as compared to patients whose surgery is delayed. Patients who would benefit from delay and further medical evaluation have not been well characterized. Until further data are available, it seems reasonable to attempt surgical repair for the majority of patients with hip fracture within 24 to 48 hours of admission to the hospital. Patients with active comorbid medical illness such as congestive heart failure, active infection (e.g., pneumonia), unstable angina, or severe chronic obstructive pulmonary disease probably would benefit from a more extensive preoperative evaluation and medical management of their comorbid condition prior to repair of their fracture.

Case (Part 4)

Ms. Hope wants to return to her apartment, and continue to live independently; therefore, she decides to give consent for an ORIF surgical procedure.

What can be done to minimize preoperative and postoperative complications for Ms. Hope?

Antibiotic Prophylaxis

Antibiotic prophylaxis has become the standard of care for major surgical operations to prevent postoperative wound complications. In hip fracture, the timing of administration, the duration of antibiotic therapy, and the effectiveness of antibiotic prophylaxis have been the subject of some debate in the literature.

Available evidence supports the use of a single dose of an intravenous antibiotic with a long half-life to reduce the incidence of deep wound infection, superficial wound infection, urinary tract infections, and respiratory tract infections. Given that the major pathogen appears to be *Staphylococcus aureus*, administration of a first-generation cephalosporin (e.g., cefazolin 1 to 2 g intravenously) is recommended. For patients allergic to penicillin and cephalosporin and for patients admitted to hospitals in which methicillin-resistant *S. aureus* and *Staphylococcus epidermidis* are frequent causes of postoperative wound infections, vancomycin is probably the most appropriate prophylactic agent (1 g intravenously) (12). Prophylactic antibiotic therapy should probably be initiated within 2 hours prior to surgery and continued for 24 hours following surgery.

Thromboembolic Prophylaxis

Venous thromboembolism is an important cause of morbidity and mortality in postoperative hip fracture patients. Although thromboembolic prophylaxis is becoming a routine aspect of the care of the patient with hip fracture, a number of questions remain as to the choice of the optimal agent, the timing of prophylaxis, and the duration of prophylaxis post–fracture repair. Studies to date have focused on four classes of agents: heparinoids, antiplatelet agents, warfarin sodium, and the use of compression stockings.

Patients receiving epidural/spinal anesthesia and receiving concurrent low molecular weight heparin should be monitored frequently for signs and symptoms of neurologic impairment. Aspirin has been found to significantly reduce the risk of deep venous thrombosis and pulmonary embolism by about one third, with much of this benefit appearing to occur after the first postoperative week. Aspirin also appears to have some benefit, but to a lesser extent, and may be considered for patients at high risk for hemorrhagic complications (13).

Overall, low-dose warfarin appears to be an effective agent for thromboembolic prophylaxis. It appears more effective than aspirin but is probably less effective than low molecular weight heparin. The required international normalized ratio (INR) monitoring required for appropriate treatment with warfarin to prevent either over- or under-anticoagulation is a potential drawback. Conversely, it might be a better tolerated agent for patients wishing to avoid the discomfort of a twice-daily injection (14–17).

It is recommended that intermittent pneumatic compression devices be routinely used until the patient is ambulating on a routine basis. They have been shown to decrease the incidence of postoperative deep vein thrombosis in urologic, neurosurgical, and general surgical patients (13). Compression stockings have also been evaluated in patients with hip fracture and have been shown to significantly reduce the incidence of thromboembolic events as compared to no treatment (18).

There is strong evidence supporting the use of either low-dose heparin or low molecular weight heparin as prophylaxis for deep venous thrombosis. The latter may be slightly more effective but is more expensive and has been associated with bleeding or hemorrhage in the spinal cord following epidural anesthesia in non–hip fracture populations. For these reasons, and until further data are available, low-dose heparin is probably the preferred agent. At present, it seems reasonable to begin anticoagulation on admission and continue prophylaxis until the patient is fully ambulatory and to extend prophylaxis further in patients in whom the risk of deep venous thrombosis may be increased (patients who experienced prolonged immobility postrepair or patients for whom surgery was delayed).

Case (Part 5)

Ms. Hope underwent left ORIF and is now 3 hours postoperative and in the postoperative recovery unit. She is slowly weaned from breathing support and is now breathing on her own, as well as voiding urine after the indwelling catheter was discontinued. She continues to receive morphine for pain.

What are some postoperative management strategies that Ms. Hope could benefit from?

Nutritional Management

Malnutrition has been associated with increased surgical morbidity and mortality (19,20), increased hospital length of stay (20), and poorer functional outcomes (20). It has been reported that as many as 20% of patients experiencing a hip fracture suffer from severe malnutrition (21). Interventions to improve nutritional status, therefore, might improve outcomes and decrease complications.

Oral protein supplementation appears to be beneficial in reducing minor postoperative complications, preserving body protein stores, and reducing overall length of stay. They also have significantly fewer complications at 6 months, significantly higher albumin levels, and significantly shorter overall lengths of stay than nonsupplemented subjects. Patients with evidence of moderate-severe malnutrition may benefit from nocturnal enteral tube feeding if tolerated (see Chapter 11: Nutrition, page 189).

Urinary Tract Management

Urinary retention, incontinence, and urinary tract infections are commonly observed in postoperative hip fracture patients (22). Because of the frequency of postoperative bladder problems, successful strategies to reduce voiding problems might lead to decreased morbidity.

Indwelling catheters should probably be removed within 24 hours of surgery. Evidence does not exist regarding the management of patients who continue to experience urinary retention following 48 hours of intermittent catheterization. In one study, those postoperative patients who had the indwelling catheter removed the morning after surgery had significantly lower rates of urinary retention (23).

Case (Part 6)

On postoperative day 2 Ms. Hope is stable enough to be transferred to the ward, where she can accept visitors for an extended period of time. Her family and friends notice that Ms. Hope is not at her baseline

mental status. She appears to have a short attention span and has acute and fluctuating symptoms of disorganized thinking. A computed tomography (CT) scan of the brain reveals no acute pathology. Ms. Hope's mental status improves over the next 72 hours.
What could account for Ms. Hope's change in mental status?

Delirium

Delirium is a transient global disorder of cognition and attention characterized by concurrent disorders of attention, perception, thinking, memory, psychomotor behavior, and the sleep-wake cycle (24,25), which may be the most frequent medical complication observed following hip fracture (26). Delirium occurs in an estimated 11% to 30% of elderly general medical patients (27) and in 13% to 61% of patients with hip fracture (28). The occurrence of delirium in hospitalized patients has been shown to increase length of stay, risk of complications, mortality, and institutionalization (29–33). Furthermore, the majority of patients who develop delirium have at least some persistent symptoms that may linger as much as 6 months later.

In patients with a hip fracture, delirium has been associated with poorer functioning in physical, cognitive, and affective domains 6 months postfracture and with slower rates of recovery (34,35).

Baseline risk factors for delirium appear to be fairly consistent across most studies. Advanced age, history of cognitive impairment, greater illness severity, and history of alcohol use appear to place hospitalized medical and surgical patients at increased risk for the development of confusion. A number of recurring potentially modifiable risk factors for developing delirium include electrolyte and metabolic laboratory abnormalities, medications with psychoactive properties, and infection. Environmental manipulation and supportive reorientation appear to reduce the incidence of delirium and benefit the acutely delirious patient, although more research addressing the optimal symptomatic management is needed. A more thorough review of delirium may be found in Chapter 13: Depression, Dementia, and Delirium, page 236.

Case (Part 7)

On postoperative day 6, Ms. Hope is seen by her primary care physician, who diagnoses her delirium, and medical therapy is initiated. A rehabilitation consult has been made to help facilitate a discharge plan. The physiatrist recommends that Ms. Hope be transferred to a subacute rehabilitation facility for approximately 5 weeks prior to returning to her three-story walkup apartment. She agrees, and a transfer to the subacute rehabilitation facility is initiated.
Why was rehabilitation to a subacute facility initiated?

Rehabilitation

Rehabilitative services for hip fracture patients may include limb and joint mobilization and progressive exercises, physical and occupational therapy to regain mobility and independence in ADL, physician oversight of the therapy, psychological counseling, social work, restorative nursing services, and recreational services.

Rehabilitation is a shared responsibility with the surgeon who, depending on the fracture and type of surgery, may have specific recommendations about mobilization and weight bearing. Available data suggest that early mobilization can be done safely in selected patients, although the potential benefits of early mobilization have not been well studied and quantified. In the case of interdisciplinary rehabilitation featuring geriatric assessment, there is some suggestion from randomized trials that these programs can improve functional outcome and increase the likelihood of patients returning to the community (36–47) (see Chapter 10: Exercise and Rehabilitation, page 168).

Case (Part 8)

Ms. Hope is now at the subacute rehabilitation facility and has worked hard over the past 5 weeks at regaining her strength and mobility. In addition, she has been adherent to her osteoporosis medical therapy which was started before her hospital discharge. Prior to discharge, from the subacute rehabilitation facility all patients undergo a fall assessment. This fall assessment involves an occupational therapist, who inspects the patient's home environment and then makes recommendations. Ms. Hope's home assessment revealed that her hallway to the bathroom was filled with clutter including a loose rug that could have attributed to her fall. Recommendations from the fall risk assessment were followed through and Ms. Hope returned home.

Given that Ms. Hope has osteoporosis, what are her chances of falling and fracturing herself for a second time?

Fall Assessment

Patients who have fractured a hip have an increased risk of a subsequent fracture (48). Interventions to reduce the likelihood and number of subsequent falls therefore might have beneficial effects on outcome. Studies suggest that interventions to reduce the incidence of falls are more likely to be beneficial if they focus on persons at risk for falls and if the interventions target specific risk factors or behaviors. Exercise and balance training also appear to be somewhat effective in decreasing fall risk. Because persons who have sustained hip fractures are at higher risk of subsequent falls, these findings may be generalizable to this population (49–54). A comprehensive review of fall assessment and prevention may be found in Chapter 20: Instability and Falls, page 366.

General Principles

- The mortality seen in the Medicare population following fracture is 7% at 1 month, 13% at 3 months, and 24% at 12 months. For those patients who survive to 6 months, 60% have recovered their prefracture walking ability, 50% have recovered their prefracture ability to perform their activities of daily living, and about 25% have recovered their prefracture ability to perform instrumental activities of daily living. However, after 1 year, only 54% of surviving patients are able to walk unaided, and only 40% are able to perform all physical activities of daily living independently.
- The risks and benefits of a surgical procedure for hip fractures in the elderly must be thoroughly considered. If surgery is the option, then other considerations include prophylactic antibiotics, thromboembolic prophylaxis, nutritional management, and prevention of delirium.
- A diagnosis of osteoporosis is the leading factor that places patients at increased risk for hip fracture. Others include female sex, white race, maternal history of hip fracture, physical inactivity, low body weight, consumption of alcohol, previous hip fracture, nursing home residence, visual impairment, cognitive impairment, and psychotropic medication use. It is imperative that an etiology of the hip fracture be sought as to prevent further risks of fracture.

Suggested Readings

Anderson BC. Office Orthopedics for Primary Care: Diagnosis and Treatment, 2nd ed. Philadelphia: WB Saunders, 1999. *Provides treatment care for common disorders including hip pain, low back pain, cervical spine pain, as well as repetitive motion syndromes for nonsurgeons.*

Morrison RS, Siu AL. Medical aspects of hip fracture management. In: Cassel CK, Leipzig RM, Cohen HJ, et al., eds. Geriatric Medicine, 4th ed. New York: Springer, 2003:669–680.

Pottenger LA. Orthopedic problems with aging. In: Cassel CK, Leipzig RM, Cohen HJ, et al., eds. Geriatric Medicine, 4th ed. New York: Springer, 2003:651–668.

Zuckerman JD, Schon LC. Hip fractures. In: Zuckerman JD, ed. Comprehensive Care of Orthopedic Injuries in the Elderly. Baltimore: Urban & Schwarzenberg, 1990. *Describes the principles and practices involved in proper care of orthope-*

dic injuries in the elderly including fractures and soft tissue injuries, from the most common "classic" injuries to the distinctly uncommon injuries that would be more frequently encountered in younger patients.

References

1. Barrett-Connor E. The economic and human cost of osteoporotic fracture. Am J Med 1995;98:3S–8S.
2. Schneider IL, Guralnik JM. The aging of America: impact on health care costs. JAMA 1990;263:2335–2340.
3. Vital and Health Statistics, Healthy People 2000 Review, Bethesda: National Center for Health Statistics, 1997.
4. Hedlund R, Lindgren U. Trauma type, age, and gender as determinants of hip fracture. J Orthop Res 1987;5(2):242–246.
5. Gallagher JC, Melton LJ, Riggs BL, Bergstrath E. Epidemiology of fractures of the proximal femur in Rochester, Minnesota. Clin Orthop 1980;150: 163–171.
6. Cummings S, Kelsey J, Nevitt M, O'Dowd K. Epidemiology of osteoporosis and osteoporotic fractures. Epidemiol Rev 1985;7:178–208.
7. Lu-Yao G, Baron J, Barrett J, Fischer E. Treatment and survival among elderly Americans with hip fractures: a population based study. Am J Public Health 1994;84:1287–1291.
8. Magaziner J, Simonsick E, Kashner M, Hebel J, Kenzora J. Predictors of functional recovery one year following hospital discharge for hip fracture: a prospective study. J Gerontology 1990;45:M101–M107.
9. Zuckerman J. Hip fracture. N Engl J Med 1996;334:1519–1525.
10. Morrison RS, Siu AL. Survival in end-stage dementia following acute illness. JAMA 2000;284(1):47–52.
11. Morrison RS, Siu AL. A comparison of pain and its treatment in advanced dementia and cognitively intact patients with hip fracture. J Pain Symptom Manage 2000;19:240–248.
12. Abramowicz M, ed. Handbook of Antimicrobial Therapy. New Rochelle, NY: Medical Letter, 1998.
13. Fisher CG, Blachut PA, Salvian AJ, Meek RN, O'Brien PJ. Effectiveness of pneumatic leg compression devices for the prevention of thromboembolic disease in orthopaedic trauma patients: a prospective, randomized study of compression alone versus no prophylaxis. J Orthop Trauma 1995;9(1):1–7.
14. Morrison R, Chassin M, Siu A. The medical consultant's role in caring for patients with hip fracture. Ann Intern Med 1998;128:1010–1020.
15. Powers P, Gent M, Jay R, et al. A randomized trial of less intense postoperative warfarin or aspirin therapy in the prevention of venous thromboembolism after surgery for fractured hip. Arch Intern Med 1989;149:771–774.
16. Morris G, Mitchell J. Preventing venous thromboembolism in elderly patients with hip fractures: studies of low-dose heparin, dipyridamole, aspirin, and fluriprofen. Br Med J 1977;1:535–537.
17. Gerhart TN, Yett HS, Robertson LK, Lee MA, Smith M, Salzman EW. Low-molecular-weight heparinoid compared with warfarin for prophylaxis of deep-vein thrombosis in patients who are operated on for fracture of the hip. A prospective, randomized trial. J Bone Joint Surg [Am] 1991;73(4):494–502.

18. Coe NP, Collins RE, Klein LA, et al. Prevention of deep vein thrombosis in urological patients. A controlled, randomized trial of low-dose heparin and external pneumatic compression boots. Surgery 1978;83:230–234.
19. Patterson BM, Cornell CN, Carbone B, Levine B, Chapman D. Protein depletion and metabolic stress in elderly patients who have a fracture of the hip. J Bone Joint Surg [Am] 1992;74(2):251–260.
20. Koval KJ, Maurer SG, Su ET, Aharonoff GB, Zuckerman JD. The effects of nutritional status on outcome after hip fracture. J Orthop Trauma 1999; 13(3):164–169.
21. Bastow M, Rawlings J, Allison S. Undernutrition, hypothermia, and injury in elderly women with fractured femur; an injury response to altered metabolism? Lancet 1983;1983(i):143–146.
22. Smith NK, Albazzaz MK. A prospective study of urinary retention and risk of death after proximal femoral fracture. Age Ageing 1996;25(2):150–154.
23. Michelson JD, Lotke PA, Steinberg ME. Urinary-bladder management after total joint-replacement surgery. N Engl J Med 1988;319(6):321–326.
24. Lipowski Z. Delirium in the elderly patient. N Engl J Med 1989;320: 278–303.
25. Lipowski Z. Transient cognitive disorders (delirium, acute confusional states in the elderly). Am J Psychiatry 1983;140:1426–1436.
26. Gillick M, Serell N, Gillick L. Adverse consequences of hospitalization in the elderly. Soc Sci Med 1982;16:1033–1038.
27. Rummans T, Evans J, Krahn L, et al. Delirium in elderly patients: evaluation and management. Mayo Clin Proc 1995;70:989–998.
28. Gustafson Y, Berggren D, Brannstrom B, et al. Acute confusional states in elderly patients treated for femoral neck fracture. J Am Geriatr Soc 1988; 36(6):525–530.
29. Cole M, Primeau F, McCusker J. Effectiveness of interventions to prevent delirium in hospitalized patients: a systematic review. Can Med Assoc 1996;155:1263–1268.
30. Francis J, Kapoor WN. Prognosis after hospital discharge of older medical patients with delirium. J Am Geriatr Soc 1992;40(6):601–606.
31. Levkoff S, Evans D, Liptzin B, et al. Delirium: the occurrence and persistence of symptoms among elderly hospitalized patients. Arch Intern Med 1992; 152:334–340.
32. Murray AM, Levkoff SE, Wetle TT, et al. Acute delirium and functional decline in the hospitalized elderly patient. J Gerontol 1993;48(5): M181–M186.
33. Rockwood K. Delays in the discharge of elderly patients. J Clin Epidemiol 1990;43:971–975.
34. Dolan MM, Hawkes WG, Zimmerman SI, et al. Delirium on hospital admission in aged hip fracture patients: prediction of mortality and 2-year functional outcomes. J Gerontol A Biol Sci Med Sci 2000;55(9):M527–M534.
35. Marcantonio ER, Flacker JM, Michaels M, Resnick NM. Delirium is independently associated with poor functional recovery after hip fracture. J Am Geriatr Soc 2000;48(6):618–624.
36. Zuckerman J, Sakales S, Fabian D, Frankel V. Hip fractures in geriatric patients: results of an interdisciplinary hospital care program. Clin Orthop 1992;274:213–225.

37. Stromqvist B, Hansson LI, Nilsson LT, Thorngren KG. Hook-pin fixation in femoral neck fractures. A two-year follow-up study of 300 cases. Clin Orthop 1987;218:58–62.

38. Arnold WD. The effect of early weight-bearing on the stability of femoral neck fractures treated with Knowles pins. J Bone Joint Surg [Am] 1984;66(6): 847–852.

39. Jarnlo GB. Hip fracture patients. Background factors and function. Scand J Rehabil Med Suppl 1991;24:1–31.

40. Ceder L, Stromqvist B, Hansson LI. Effects of strategy changes in the treatment of femoral neck fractures during a 17-year period. Clin Orthop 1987; 218:53–57.

41. Karumo I. Intensive physical therapy after fractures of the femoral shaft. Ann Chir Gynaecol 1977;66(6):278–283.

42. Skinner P, Riley D, Ellergy J, Beaumont A. Displaced subcapital fractures of the femur: a prospective randomized comparison of internal fixation, hemiarthroplasty and total hip replacement. Injury 1989;20:291–293.

43. Sorenson J, Varmarken J, Bomler J. Internal fixation of femoral neck fractures. Dynamic hip and Gouffon screws compared in 73 patients. Acta Orthop Scand 1992;63:288–292.

44. Elmerson S, Andersson G, Irstam L, et al. Internal fixation of femoral neck fracture. No difference between Rydell four-flanged nail and Gouffon's pin. Acta Orthop Scand 1988;59:372–376.

45. Olerud C, Rehnberg L, Hellquist E. Internal fixation of femoral neck fractures. Two methods compared. J Bone Joint Surg [Br] 1991;73:16–19.

46. Nungu S, Olerud C, Rehnberg L. Treatment of intertrochanteric fractures: comparison of ender nails and sliding screw plates. J Orthop Trauma 1991; 5:452–457.

47. Dalen N, Jacobsson B, Eriksson P. A comparison of nail-plate fixation and Enders nailing in pertrochanteric fractures. J Trauma 1988;28:405–406.

48. Finsen V, Benum P. The second hip fracture: an epidemiologic study. Acta Orthop Scand 1986;57:431–433.

49. Wagner EH, LaCroix AZ, Grothaus L, et al. Preventing disability and falls in older adults: a population-based randomized trial. Am J Public Health 1994;84(11):1800–1806.

50. Tinetti M, Baker D, McAvay G, et al. A multifactorial intervention to reduce the risk of falling among elderly people living in the community. N Engl J Med 1994;331:315–320.

51. Mulrow CD, Gerety MB, Kanten D, et al. A randomized trial of physical rehabilitation for very frail nursing home residents [see comments]. JAMA 1994;271(7):519–524.

52. Hornbrook M, Stevens V, Wingfield D, Hollis J, Greenlick M, Ory M. Preventing falls among community dwelling older persons: results from a randomized trial. Gerontologist 1994;34:16–23.

53. Reinsch S, Macrae P, Lachenbruch P, Tobis J. Attempts to prevent falls and injury: a prospective community study. Gerontologist 1992;32:450–456.

54. Vetter N, Lewis P, Ford D. Can health visitors prevent fractures in elderly people. BMJ 1992;304:888–890.

22
Hypertension

Olusegun A. Apoeso

Learning Objectives

Upon completion of the chapter, the student will be able to:

1. Identify and understand the age-related changes associated with hypertension.
2. Accurately diagnose and evaluate hypertension in older adults.
3. Understand hypertension management principles and practice.

Case (Part 1)

M.B., a 67-year-old African-American man who recently moved to your state from Florida, was referred to your geriatric practice for follow-up. He has a past medical history significant for diet-controlled diabetes mellitus type 2. He also reports previous elevated blood pressure readings averaging 150/85 mmHg. He has not been on any medication because he was told that his blood pressure is not unusual for his age. He denies any history of heart or kidney diseases. He has a 20-pack-year smoking history and does not use alcohol or recreational drugs. He lives alone independently and has a family history of hypertension and stroke.

General Considerations

The classification of blood pressure outlined by the Joint National Committee on Detection, Evaluation, and Treatment of High Blood Pressure (JNC-VII), shown in Table 22.1, is the same for all adults irrespective of

---

Material in this chapter is based on the following chapter in Cassel CK, Leipzig RM, Cohen HJ, Larson EB, Meier DE, eds. Geriatric Medicine: An Evidence-Based Approach, 4th ed. New York: Springer, 2003: Supiano MA. Hypertension, pp. 545–559. Selections edited by Olusegun A. Apoeso.

TABLE 22.1. Classification of blood pressure (1)

Category*	Systolic (mmHg)		Diastolic (mmHg)
Normal	<120	and	<80
Prehypertension	120–139	and	80–89
Stage 1	140–159	or	90–99
Stage 2	≥160	or	≥100

*Treatment determined by highest blood pressure category.
Source: Reprinted from Chobanian AV, Bakris GL, Black HR, et al. The Seventh Report of the Joint National Committee on Prevention, Detection, Evaluation, and Treatment of High Blood Pressure: the JNC VII report. JAMA 2003;289(19):2560–2572.

age (1). Contrary to a former viewpoint that held that high blood pressure is an expected normal aspect of aging, it is now evident that hypertension in older individuals defined according to these blood pressure levels should be viewed as a disease state that is associated with an increased risk for adverse outcomes (e.g., coronary heart disease, congestive heart failure, stroke, peripheral vascular disease, and renal disease) and mortality.

Age-Associated Changes Related to Blood Pressure

Many age-related changes in physiology contribute to the increase in blood pressure. As is the case in younger individuals, the etiology of essential hypertension in older humans is not known. An increase in peripheral vascular resistance is one pathognomonic feature of hypertension in the elderly.

An age-associated increase in arterial vascular stiffness has been demonstrated, particularly in the larger arteries (2). Several alterations in vessel structure contribute to the decrease in distensibility, such as an increase in smooth muscle cell size and number, an increase in medial collagen deposition, and a decrease in elastin content (3). Arterial compliance and stroke volume are the major determinants of pulse pressure. Because stroke volume does not vary significantly with age, the decline in arterial compliance produces an increase in pulse pressure, which contributes to a disproportionate increase in systolic pressure. This finding may account for the age-associated increase in the prevalence of isolated systolic hypertension, as well as an increase in pulse pressure.

Prevalence

Epidemiologic studies such as the National Health and Nutrition Examination Surveys have shown that the overall prevalence of hypertension in noninstitutionalized individuals above the age of 65 is between 50% and 70%. The prevalence is highest among African Americans relative to whites and Mexican Americans. Unlike the younger hypertensive population in which there is a male predominance, there is no marked gender difference in the overall prevalence of hypertension in the elderly older adults.

Case (Part 2)

On physical examination, M.B. is 5 feet 10 inches tall (1.78 m) and weighs 197 lb (86 kg). His sitting blood pressure is 162/88 mmHg. His pulse is 76/min regular and of full volume. Even though you carefully listened for bruits and looked for signs of target organ damage, M.B.'s complete examinations was otherwise normal.
Can you make a diagnosis of hypertension at this time?

Diagnostic Evaluation

The statement that "hypertension should not be diagnosed on the basis of a single measurement" (1) is especially relevant to the older patient. It is critically important to make an accurate diagnosis of hypertension in this population. To do so requires careful attention to correct measurement of blood pressure with respect to utilizing the proper cuff size, measuring the blood pressure in both arms, having the patient appropriately positioned (sitting comfortably following 5 minutes of quiet rest with the arm supported at heart level), palpating the systolic blood pressure level at the radial artery to avoid the auscultatory gap, and taking two blood pressure measurements separated by at least 2 minutes (more if there is greater than 5 mmHg difference between the first two readings) at each of three visits. The average of these measurements is used to define an individual's blood pressure, which determines the presence or absence of hypertension according to the classification scheme given in Table 22.1. Careful adherence to these measurement techniques minimizes the likelihood that older individuals will be misdiagnosed as hypertensive and inappropriately placed on an antihypertensive medication.

Although not directly pertinent to the diagnosis of hypertension, another critically important aspect of blood pressure measurement in the older hypertensive patient is obtaining baseline postural or orthostatic blood pressure measurements. *Orthostatic hypotension* is usually defined as a decline in blood pressure from the supine baseline of greater than 20 mmHg systolic and/or 10 mmHg diastolic after 1 to 2 minutes of standing. Aging per se is not associated with an increased prevalence of orthostatic hypotension (4). The supine systolic blood pressure has been identified as the best predictor of the postural decrease in systolic blood pressure (5). Accordingly, the presence of supine hypertension is an important risk factor for orthostatic hypotension (4). Baseline orthostatic blood pressure readings, therefore, are required in every patient to avoid adverse events related to further declines in postural blood pressure that may result from antihypertensive therapy.

Case (Part 3)

M.B.'s blood pressure measurements were not orthostatic and were similar in both arms. His electrocardiogram was normal. You decide to run some laboratory tests and obtain a chest x-ray.
   What is your differential diagnosis?
   What tests are indicated at this time?
   Will you start M.B. on an antihypertensive medication at this time?
   What will be your follow-up plans?

Differential Diagnosis

As is the case in younger hypertensive populations, the overwhelming majority (greater than 90%) of older hypertensive patients have essential or primary hypertension. Secondary forms of hypertension may be even more rare in the older population. Renal disease and renovascular hypertension are the most frequent causes of secondary hypertension in the elderly; endocrinologic causes are generally less common.

   The approach to the evaluation for secondary and potentially reversible factors that may account for the increase in blood pressure in older individuals is similar to that recommended for younger hypertensive patients. Thus, a standard clinical evaluation consisting of a complete history and physical exam, chemistry profile (to assess electrolytes, renal function, and glucose), electrocardiogram (ECG), and chest x-ray is recommended to identify these factors. Further evaluation is normally not needed unless there are abnormal symptoms or signs elicited from this evaluation that would be consistent with renal disease (elevated serum creatinine or abnormal urinalysis), renovascular disease (e.g., presence of abdominal bruit), hyperaldosteronism (hypokalemia), hypercortisolism (hyperglycemia, cushingoid appearance), hyperparathyroidism (hypercalcemia), or pheochromocytoma (symptoms of headache, palpitations, diaphoresis, and paroxysmal elevations of blood pressure). A careful review of medications is warranted to determine if medication-related increases in blood pressure (e.g., due to corticosteroids or nonsteroidal antiinflammatory drugs) could be contributing to the elevated blood pressure. Other clinical situations that might lead to an evaluation for secondary hypertension in the older patient include malignant hypertension, the abrupt development of diastolic hypertension (which is unusual in light of the general decrease in diastolic blood pressure with age above the age of 60 years), worsening of blood pressure control, or blood pressure that remains uncontrolled on a regimen of three antihypertensive medications.

Case (Part 4)

You choose to bring M.B. back for a repeat blood pressure check and follow-up, rather than start him on any medication. You put in place a mechanism by which his blood pressure can be reliably measured at home pending his next appointment. You emphasize the importance of reporting to you if his systolic blood pressure measurement at home rises above 160mmHg, or his diastolic blood pressure above 100mmHg.

You are now seeing M.B. on follow-up 3 weeks after his initial visit. He has no symptoms to report. The average value of blood pressure readings from home is 158/89mmHg. His weight is unchanged from his last visit. His carefully repeated blood pressure measurement reading is 160/88mmHg. His other examination findings were essentially unchanged from previous visit. The chest x-ray was reported as normal. Fasting blood glucose was 156mg/dL and hemoglobin (Hgb)A$_{1c}$ was 8.2%. Total cholesterol was 185mg/dL, triglyceride 230mg/dL, high-density lipoprotein 48mg/dL, and low-density lipoprotein 114mg/dL. He also has microalbuminuria. His other serum chemistries, liver function test, and complete blood count were within normal limits. You conclude that M.B. does have stage 1 or 2 hypertension and diabetes mellitus type 2.

How do you evaluate for target organ damage secondary from hypertension?

What other cardiovascular risk factors does M.B. have?

Target Organ Damage and Risk Factor Assessment

Once the diagnosis of hypertension has been appropriately made and secondary causes considered, the remainder of the evaluation should be directed toward the identification of target organ damage, an assessment of other cardiovascular risk factor, and identification of comorbid conditions that may influence the therapeutic decision-making process. In the older hypertensive patient, it may be more difficult to detect the manifestations of target organ damage that are directly attributable to elevated blood pressure due to concurrent age- or disease-associated changes in organ function. It is useful, however, to determine if there is any previous history consistent with coronary artery disease, cardiac failure, cerebrovascular disease (transient ischemic attack or stroke), or peripheral vascular disease. The patient should be assessed for any physical signs consistent with these conditions, as well as for evidence of hypertensive retinopathy or left ventricular hypertrophy. In addition to identifying the presence of hyperlipidemia or diabetes mellitus, information concerning smoking history, dietary intake of salt and fat, alcohol intake, and level of physical activity should be obtained to aid in a determination of overall cardiovascular risk. This information will affect the patient's risk stratum assignment and the approach to his or her treatment and will also be needed to advise the patient about lifestyle modifications that may be recommended as nonpharmacologic approaches to blood pressure control. Finally, knowledge of comorbid conditions is necessary to identify special clinical situations where a given class of antihypertensive medication would be either recommended or contraindicated (Table 22.2).

Management Considerations

As is the case in the approach to treatment of other chronic diseases in an older patient, it is important to define goals of antihypertensive therapy that are individualized to a given patient. In this context, the benefits as well as the potential risks of any therapeutic intervention need to be balanced to achieve an overall goal of preventing the morbidity and mortality associated with high blood pressure without adversely affecting the patient's functional performance or quality of life.

Another general approach to therapy is to continually assess not only the response to therapy, but also the development of adverse effects of treatment. For example, the development of orthostatic hypotension is an adverse effect that may occur with any antihypertensive medication and the symptoms may be atypical; rather than providing a history of postural unsteadiness, the older patient may cite generalized weakness or fatigue.

Case (Part 5)

M.B. has no obvious evidence of target organ damage. Considering his multiple cardiovascular risk factors, that is, age, diabetes, smoking history, overweight, and high low-density lipoproteins, you want to start a management plan to lower his blood pressure over the next few months.

What nonpharmacologic lifestyle modifications will you initiate?

What will be your goal for weight reduction?

TABLE 22.2. Potential advantages, disadvantages, and special clinical considerations in the older hypertensive related to the major antihypertensive classes recommended for initial treatment

Antihypertensive class	Potential advantages	Potential disadvantages	Clinical situations to recommend use	Clinical situations to recommend against use, or which require monitoring
Diuretics	Benefit documented in clinical trails Produce greater reduction in SBP than DBP Inexpensive	Metabolic abnormalities Urinary incontinence	Systolic hypertension	Glucose intolerance, gout, hyperlipidemia
Calcium antagonists	Benefit documented in clinical trails Absence of CNS or metabolic effects	Peripheral edema, constipation, heart block	Systolic hypertension Coronary artery disease	Left ventricular dysfunction
β-antagonists	Benefit documented in clinical trails	May increase peripheral vascular resistance Metabolic abnormalities CNS effects	Coronary artery disease and post–myocardial infarction	COPD, peripheral vascular disease, heart block, glucose intolerance, type 2 DM, hyperlipidemia, depression
ACE inhibitors	Absence of CNS or metabolic effects	Hyperkalemia, renal insufficiency, cough	Congestive heart failure, type 2 DM	Renal insufficiency or renal artery stenosis

ACE, angiotensin-converting enzyme; CNS, central nervous system; COPD, chronic obstructive pulmonary disease; DM, diabetes mellitus; DBP, diastolic blood pressure; SBP, systolic blood pressure.
Source: Supiano MA. Hypertension. In: Cassel CK, Leipzig RM, Cohen HJ, et al., eds. Geriatric Medicine, 4th ed. New York: Springer, 2003.

Nonpharmacologic Treatments

There are a number of lifestyle modifications that may be recommended: weight reduction; an aerobic exercise program; dietary alterations to decrease sodium, saturated fat, and cholesterol while maintaining adequate intake of potassium, calcium, and magnesium; smoking cessation; and moderation of alcohol intake.

Nonpharmacologic therapies may be effective initial therapy; individuals with stage 1 hypertension (systolic blood pressure less than 160 mmHg) who do not have diabetes should complete a 6-month trial of nonpharmacologic therapy before adding an antihypertensive medication if the target blood pressure is not achieved. In addition, these therapies may be adjunctive in combination with pharmacologic treatments, they may result in concurrent improvements in other cardiovascular risk factors, and there are minimal associated risks.

Weight reduction is recommended for hypertensive individuals who are greater than 10% above their ideal body weight, and weight loss on the order of 5 kg has been shown to result in small (generally less than 5 mmHg), but significant decreases in blood pressure (6–8).

Case (Part 6)

You educate M.B. on necessary lifestyle modifications, especially weight reduction, smoking cessation, and a low sodium, saturated fat, and cholesterol diet. You decide to start a low-dose oral hypoglycemic agent.

In what risk group is M.B.?

Will you start antihypertensive medications at this time? If so, what are your possible options?

Pharmacologic Treatments

The general approach to pharmacologic treatment of hypertension is outlined in JNC-VII (1) (italics indicate a direct quotation from JWC-VII). *Individuals with a systolic BP of 120 to 139 mmHg or a diastolic BP of 80 to 89 mmHg are considered as prehypertensive and require health-promoting lifestyle modifications to prevent cardiovascular disease (CVD). Most patients with hypertension require two or more antihypertensive medications to achieve the BP goal (<140/90 mmHg, or <130/80 mmHg for patients with diabetes or chronic kidney disease). If BP is more than 20/10 mmHg above the BP goal, consideration should be given to initiating therapy with two agents, one of which usually should be a thiazide-type diuretic.*

The choice of initial antihypertensive drug class should be based on an individualized patient assessment. *Thiazide-type diuretics should be used in drug treatment for most patients with uncomplicated hypertension, either alone or combined with drugs from other classes.* One should consider whether the patient has simple hypertension or if the hypertension is complicated by the coexistence of other conditions (e.g., diabetes, coronary artery disease, heart failure, or prostatism) that may influence drug selection. *Certain high-risk conditions are compelling indications for the initial use of other antihypertensive drug classes (angiotensin-converting enzyme inhibitors, angiotensin-receptor blockers, beta-blockers, calcium channel blockers).* Each of the antihypertensive drug classes has been shown to be effective in reducing blood pressure in the older patient population. For those with simple hypertension, the initial drug selection based on the evidence available to date is either a thiazide diuretic or a long-acting dihydropyridine calcium channel antagonist (1). Beyond this general recommendation, selection of a particular antihypertensive drug needs to be an individualized decision for each patient, taking into account the drug's potential advantages and disadvantages (Table 22.2), together with the patient's comorbidities. In general, irrespective of the initial agent that is selected, the starting dose should be reduced and dose titration done more gradually in an older hypertensive patient. If the target blood pressure goal is not obtained at a maximal dose of the initial agent following several months of treatment, therapy may either be switched to an alternative class or a second drug from another class may be added.

Diuretics

Therapy with low-dose thiazide diuretics has demonstrated significant benefits in mortality, stroke, and coronary events in randomized clinical trials in older hypertensive patient populations. These beneficial effects combined with their relative safety, favorable side effect profile (their adverse metabolic effects—hypokalemia, hyperuricemia, and glucose intolerance—are attenuated at lower doses), once-daily dosing, and low cost have led to the recommendation that thiazide diuretics are preferred for initial therapy (9). Another advantage is that diuretic therapy leads to a disproportionate reduction in systolic relative to diastolic blood pressure and is better at achieving a reduction in systolic blood pressure compared to other agents (9,10). Thiazide diuretics are also well suited for use in combination therapies due to synergistic effects with other antihypertensive drug classes. It is worth noting that, despite these recommendations, this class of therapy is being underutilized (11).

Calcium Channel Antagonists

Each of the three chemical classes of calcium channel antagonists, phenylalkylamines, dihydropyridines, and benzothiazepines, has been shown to be effective in treating hypertension in older patient populations (12–14). There are significant age-associated alterations in the pharmacokinetics of each of the three classes of calcium channel antagonists (a decrease in clearance and an increase in plasma levels) such that lower doses of these agents should be used in older patients (15,16). Based on their mechanism of action, which leads to a reduction in peripheral vascular resistance, and their lack of significant central nervous system (CNS) or metabolic effects, the calcium channel antagonist family of medications is well matched to the pathophysiology of the older hypertensive patient. The dihydropyridine class (e.g., nifedipine) has more potent direct vasodilator effects and may be more likely to produce peripheral edema and reflex tachycardia. Members of the phenylalkylamine (e.g., verapamil) and benzothiazepine (e.g., diltiazem) classes have more potent effects on suppressing atrioventricular (AV) conduction and may produce heart block and also appear to be more commonly associated with the development of constipation.

β-Adrenergic Antagonists

The primary mechanism of action of β-adrenergic antagonists is a reduction in cardiac output without significant reduction in peripheral vascular resistance (and less reduction in systolic blood pressure compared to other agents). Based on the physiologic characteristics of the older hypertensive (Table 22.3), there are several reasons to question whether β-adrenergic antagonists would be the appropriate choice for the older hypertensive patient. Several reports have concluded that antagonist therapy is less effective as monotherapy with respect to blood pressure reduction and in the prevention of cardiovascular events and death in comparison with low-dose thiazide diuretics. In addition, there was a higher discontinuation rate due to adverse side effects. The current recommendation is that β-receptor antagonists should not be considered as first-line monotherapy for simple

TABLE 22.3. Pathophysiologic alterations which may contribute to or are associated with elevated blood pressure in aging

Increased arterial stiffness
Decreased baroreceptor sensitivity
Increased sympathetic nervous system activity
Decreased α- and β-adrenergic responsiveness
Decreased endothelial cell derived relaxing factor function
Sodium-sensitivity
Low plasma renin activity
Insulin resistance

Source: Supiano MA. Hypertension. In: Cassel CK, Leipzig RM, Cohen HJ, et al., eds. Geriatric Medicine, 4th ed. New York: Springer, 2003.

hypertension in older patients. However, due to their effectiveness in the management of symptomatic coronary artery disease, in secondary prevention following myocardial infarction, and in certain congestive heart failure settings, β-receptor antagonists should be considered for older patients whose hypertension is complicated by these comorbid conditions.

Angiotensin Converting Enzyme Inhibitors and Angiotensin Receptor Blockers

Because older hypertensive individuals are in general characterized as having low renin levels (Table 22.3), one might predict that angiotensin converting enzyme (ACE) inhibitors and angiotensin receptor blockers (ARBs) would not be effective therapeutic agents in this population. Nevertheless, this antihypertensive class has been shown to be effective in treating the older hypertensive (13,14). The ACE inhibitors and ARBs are generally well tolerated by older patients (with the exception of cough), and their lack of CNS and metabolic (glucose, electrolyte, and lipid) effects may be a particular advantage. There are compelling indications to use ACE inhibitor therapy in patients with coexisting left ventricular systolic dysfunction as well as in diabetic patients who have microalbuminuria.

The major limitations to the use of ACE inhibitors in older hypertensive patients are the development of hyperkalemia (especially in those with renal insufficiency) and the potential for development of renal failure in the setting of bilateral renal artery stenosis. Fortunately, ACE inhibitor–mediated renal failure is not a common occurrence and is generally reversible. The use of ACE inhibitors with short duration of action and frequent monitoring of renal function will aid in the detection and prevention of this adverse outcome. Other potential adverse effects of ACE inhibitors are the development of a nonproductive cough (occurring in up to 10% of patients), rash, and angioneurotic edema, and they may necessitate discontinuation of therapy. The ARBs (candesartan, irbesartan, losartan, valsartan) are reasonable alternatives for those with ACE inhibitor–associated cough. Generally, it is recommended to avoid ARBs in patients with a history of ACE inhibitor–related angioedema, although there are case reports of this being done safely (17).

α_1-Adrenergic Receptor Antagonists

Although the reduction in peripheral vascular resistance that occurs with α-receptor antagonist therapy is particularly appropriate for the pathophysiologic profile of geriatric hypertension, and although these agents are effective in blood pressure reduction (18), the development of postural hypotension has limited the widespread use of this class of antihypertensive in the geriatric population. One clinical situation in which α-receptor antagonist therapy may be considered is in older hypertensive men with prostatism, because these drugs have been shown to be efficacious in improving obstructive urinary symptoms (16).

Case (Part 7)

Based on M.B.'s medical history, age, and comorbidities, you classify him into risk group C and decided to start him on an ACE inhibitor. You reemphasize the need to continue nonpharmacologic lifestyle modifications and educate him about possible medication side effects.

What steps can you take to encourage medication adherence?

What will be your goal for blood pressure reduction and your plan for follow-up?

Patient Adherence and Resistant Hypertension

Effective management of hypertension in an older individual requires an approach that promotes the patient's adherence to its long-term treatment. There are several specific methods to enhance adherence to the long-term medical therapy of this condition. Written information describing the specific treatment and an agreed-upon blood pressure goal should be given to the patient. In general, a simpler regimen promotes patient adherence. The use of calendar or pillbox systems may be recommended to further assist patient adherence. Blood pressure self-monitoring by patients is another approach to involve them in the management of their hypertension and perhaps enhance adherence to therapy. Patient education regarding the significant benefits to be gained from adequate blood pressure control is of particular importance because hypertension is usually asymptomatic. The interdisciplinary geriatric team is well suited to promoting this approach. To this end, it may be useful to involve nurses to provide reinforcement and feedback on the degree of blood pressure control during visits for blood pressure monitoring, dietitians to review dietary information and adherence, pharmacists to promote adherence to the medical regimen, and social workers to solicit the assistance of family members, if needed, and to review the financial burden associated with the cost of medical therapy.

The frequency of follow-up visits should be adjusted to reflect the patient's degree of blood pressure elevation at presentation, with closer follow-up indicated for those with stage 3 hypertension. With the exception of hypertensive urgencies, attempts to reduce the patient's blood pressure to target levels too rapidly are unnecessary and likely deleterious. For most patients, an interval of 1 to 2 months is appropriate between visits to determine the need for dose titration. Given the age-related changes in systems that regulate blood pressure and impaired blood pressure homeostasis, overtreatment of hypertension may result in situational (postural or post-prandial) hypotension. At all follow-up visits, it is imperative to determine the supine and standing blood pressure. It is good practice to titrate antihypertensive drug doses to achieve the target (seated) blood pressure only with the knowledge of whether this increase in dose could exacerbate preexisting postural hypotension. It is also prudent to assess the patient's adherence to his or her antihypertensive medication prior to recommending an increase in its dosage or to consider switching to an alternative medication. For some patients, it is important to obtain additional information derived from home or non-office setting blood pressure measurements.

Patients who fail to achieve adequate control of their blood pressure despite the use of three antihypertensive medications at maximal doses should be evaluated for causes of resistant hypertension. This evaluation should include an assessment of their adherence to the medical therapy, a review focused on potential drug interactions (e.g., nonsteroidal antiin-flammatory agents, corticosteroids, sympathomimetics, and alcohol), and an assessment for volume overload. Other potential explanations for resistant hypertension are the presence of a secondary cause (renovascular hypertension in particular) or pseudohypertension, which should be evaluated as outlined above.

Case (Part 8)

You see M.B. 4 weeks later and he has no complaints. He denies any medication side effects. His blood pressure readings at home have a systolic and diastolic average of 142 mmHg and 85 mmHg, respectively. His monitored blood glucose levels and serum chemistries were within the normal range. His blood pressure in your clinic is 138/80 mmHg nonorthostatic.

What are the possible explanations for uncontrolled hypertension in older adults?

What are the consequences of uncontrolled hypertension and their possible management strategies?

Hypertensive Urgencies and Emergencies

Hypertensive urgencies and emergencies are defined by the necessity to reduce blood pressure quickly to prevent target organ damage, not by an absolute blood pressure level. Elevated blood pressure in and of itself without symptoms or signs of target organ damage does not usually require aggressive therapy.

Hypertensive urgencies are more common than true hypertensive emergencies (19). They are defined as situations where blood pressure should be lowered within 24 hours to prevent the risk of target organ damage, such as accelerated or malignant hypertension without symptoms or evidence of ongoing target organ damage (1). The majority of these situations may be managed as with oral administration of antihypertensive medications but generally necessitate a hospitalized setting for frequent blood pressure monitoring. The medications recommended for this situation include nifedipine, clonidine, labetalol, and captopril. Because no additional benefit has been noted with the use of sublingual administration of any of these agents and the more rapid onset of action may unpredictably produce a deleterious reduction in blood pressure, the oral dosage forms, which are effective within 15 to 30 minutes, are recommended (20). It should be noted that the blood pressure does not need to be reduced to normal levels within 24 hours; indeed, an attempt to do so carries with it the risks of complications from coronary or cerebral hypoperfusion.

Examples of true hypertensive emergencies in older patients include hypertensive encephalopathy, intracranial hemorrhage, acute heart failure with pulmonary edema, dissecting aortic aneurysm, and unstable angina. The goal of treatment in these emergent clinical situations is immediate reduction in blood pressure, although again not necessarily to a normal level. The management of these conditions usually requires an acute hospital setting to permit the parenteral administration of an antihypertensive agent and continuous blood pressure monitoring. Intravenous nitroprusside has been the most widely utilized of these medications. Its onset of action is essentially immediate, it has a very short duration of action, and its rate of infusion may be titrated to result in a carefully controlled reduction in blood pressure over a 30- to 60-minute period. Prolonged nitroprusside administration is limited by the accumulation of a thiocyanate metabolite and the risk of cyanide toxicity. Intravenous nitroglycerine is an alternative for longer duration of therapy. Additional parenteral alternatives include labetalol, enalaprilat, and hydralazine. Once the hypertensive emergency or urgency has been managed, a workup for secondary causes, paying particular attention to the possibility of renovascular hypertension, assessment of adherence with the antihypertensive regimen, and evaluation of resistant hypertension, should be pursued with appropriate close patient follow-up and monitoring.

General Principles

- No age adjustment is necessary in setting the threshold value that defines high blood pressure and hypertension in older individuals, as defined according to JNC-VII, and hypertension should be viewed as a disease state that is associated with an increased risk for adverse outcomes and mortality.

- Overall prevalence of hypertension in noninstitutionalized individuals above the age of 65 is between 50% and 70%. The prevalence is highest among African Americans.
- An increase in peripheral vascular resistance is a pathognomonic feature of hypertension in the elderly.
- Hypertension should not be diagnosed on the basis of a single measurement and it is critically important to obtain a baseline postural or orthostatic blood pressure measurement.
- The overwhelming majority (greater than 90%) of older hypertensive patients have essential or primary hypertension. Renal diseases and renovascular hypertension are the most frequent causes of secondary hypertension in the elderly.
- The approach to the evaluation for secondary and potentially reversible factors that may account for the increase in blood pressure in older individuals is similar to that recommended for younger hypertensive patients.
- It is important to define goals of antihypertensive therapy and the choice of initial antihypertensive drug class that are individualized to a given patient.
- Nonpharmacologic therapies may be effective initial therapy.
- Patients who fail to achieve adequate control of their blood pressure despite the use of three antihypertensive medications at maximal doses should be evaluated for causes of resistant hypertension.
- With the exception of hypertensive urgencies, attempts to reduce the patient's blood pressure to target levels too rapidly are unnecessary and likely deleterious.
- Postprandial hypotension is common among long-term-care residents, affecting about one third of the population.

Suggested Readings

Chobanian AV, Bakris GL, Black HR, et al. The Seventh Report of the Joint National Committee on Prevention, Detection, Evaluation, and Treatment of High Blood Pressure: the JNC VII report. JAMA 2003;289(19):2560–2572. *This recent report provides a revised guideline for hypertension prevention and management. One of the key messages: in persons older than 50 years, systolic blood pressure (SBP) of more than 140mmHg is a much more important cardiovascular disease (CVD) risk factor than diastolic BP (DBP).*
Supiano MA. Hypertension. In: Cassel CK, Leipzig RM, Cohen HJ, et al., eds. Geriatric Medicine, 4th ed. New York: Springer, 2003:545–559.

Thacker HL, Jahnigen DW. Managing hypertensive emergencies and urgencies in the geriatric patient. Geriatrics 1991;46:26–37. *Hypertension urgency and emergency are distinguished from each other by the clinical decision of how quickly the blood pressure must be lowered with the goal being a smooth and safe reduction in blood pressure.*

Wright JM, Lee C-H, Chambers GK. Systematic review of antihypertensive therapies: Does the evidence assist in choosing a first-line drug? Can Med Assoc J 1999;161:25–32. *A review of available evidence about the effectiveness of specific first-line antihypertensive drugs in lowering blood pressure and preventing adverse outcomes.*

References

1. Chobanian AV, Bakris GL, Black HR, et al. The Seventh Report of the Joint National Committee on Prevention, Detection, Evaluation, and Treatment of High Blood Pressure: the JNC VII report. JAMA 2003;289(19):2560–2572.
2. Cooper LT, Cooke JP, Dzau VJ. Minireview: the vasculopathy of aging. J Gerontol Biol Sci 1994;49(5):B191–B196.
3. Lakatta E. Mechanisms of hypertension in the elderly. J Am Geriatr Soc 1989;37:780–790.
4. Mader SL, Josephson KR, Rubenstein LZ. Low prevalence of postural hypotension among community-dwelling elderly. JAMA 1987;258(11):1511–1514.
5. Harris T, Lewis A, Kleinman JC, Cornoni-Huntley J. Postural changes in blood pressure associated with age and systolic blood pressure. J Gerontol Med Sci 1991;46(5):M159–M163.
6. The Trials of Hypertension Prevention Collaborative Research Group. Reducing blood pressure by nonpharmacologic interventions. JAMA 1992;267:1213–1220.
7. Cutler JAK. Combinations of lifestyle modification and drug treatment in management of mild-moderate hypertension: a review of randomized clinical trials. Clin Exp Hypertens 1993;15(6):1193–1204.
8. Schotte DE, Stunkard AJ. The effects of weight reduction on blood pressure in 301 obese patients. Arch Intern Med 1990;150:1701–1704.
9. Wright JM, Lee C-H, Chambers GK. Systematic review of antihypertensive therapies: Does the evidence assist in choosing a first-line drug? Can Med Assoc J 1999;161:25–32.
10. Ekbom T, Dahlof B, Hansson L, Lindholm LH, Schersten B, Wester P-O. Antihypertensive efficacy and side effects of three beta-blockers and a diuretic in elderly hypertensives: a report from the STOP-Hypertension study. J Hypertens 1992;10:1525–1530.
11. Moser M. Why are physicians not prescribing diuretics more frequently in the management of hypertension? JAMA 1998;279:1813–1816.
12. Vidt DG, Borazanian RA. Calcium channel blockers in geriatric hypertension. Geriatrics 1991;46:28–38.
13. Materson BJ, Reda DJ, Cushman WC, et al. Single-drug therapy for hypertension in men. N Engl J Med 1993;328:914–921.
14. Applegate WB, Phillips HL, Schnaper H, et al. A randomized controlled trial of the effects of three antihypertensive agents on blood pressure control and quality of life in older women. Arch Intern Med 1991;151:1817–1823.

15. Donnelly R, Reid JL, Meredith PA, Ahmed JH, Elliott HL. Factors determining the response to calcium antagonists in hypertension. J Cardiovasc Pharmacol 1988;12(suppl 6):S109–S113.
16. Oesterling JE. Benign prostatic hyperplasia: medical and minimally invasive treatment options. N Engl J Med 1995;332:99–109.
17. Gavras I, Gavras H. Are patients who develop angioedema with ACE inhibitors at risk of the same problem with AT 1 receptor blockers? Arch Intern Med 2000;160:685–693.
18. Neaton JD, Grimm RH Jr, Prineas RJ, et al. Treatment of mild hypertension study; final results. JAMA 1993;270:713–724.
19. Thacker HL, Jahnigen DW. Managing hypertensive emergencies and urgencies in the geriatric patient. Geriatrics 1991;46:26–37.
20. Zeller KR, Kuhnert LV, Matthews C. Rapid reduction of severe asymptomatic hypertension: A prospective, controlled trial. Arch Intern Med 1989;149:2186–2189.

23
Cardiovascular and Peripheral Arterial Diseases

Anna U. Loengard

Learning Objectives

Upon completion of the chapter, the student will be able to:

1. Describe the age-related physiologic changes in the cardiovascular system.
2. Explain and identify clinical features of cardiovascular and peripheral vascular diseases in the older adult.
3. Recognize and be familiar with a variety of testing modalities used in the workup of cardiovascular and peripheral vascular diseases.
4. Identify and describe the treatments for cardiovascular and peripheral arterial diseases.

Case A (Part 1)

Mr. Jones, an 82-year-old man, comes to your office with a complaint of increasing shortness of breath while walking. He tells you it began about 3 weeks ago and he now has to stop while climbing the flight of stairs to his apartment. His medical problems are significant for hypertension and diabetes mellitus for which he has been using insulin for 3 years. He also complains of swelling in his legs and once last week he woke up in the middle of the night and says he could not breathe. He got up and opened the window for some air and then felt better. He denies any history of prior myocardial infarction (MI) or angina.

Material in this chapter is based on the following chapters in Cassel CK, Leipzig RM, Cohen HJ, Larson EB, Meier DE, eds. Geriatric Medicine: An Evidence-Based Approach, 4th ed. New York: Springer, 2003: Wenger NK. Cardiovascular Disease, pp. 509–543. Hiatt WR, Nehler MR, Peripheral Arterial Disease, pp. 561–571. Selections edited by Anna U. Loengard.

Cardiovascular Disease: General Considerations

Cardiovascular disease increases dramatically with aging and is the major cause of mortality and disability in elderly persons; 83% of all cardiovascular deaths in the United States occur in patients older than 65 years of age (1). Cardiovascular disease is also a major contributor to the need for hospital, ambulatory, and custodial care. Coronary heart disease is the most prevalent cardiac problem, followed by hypertensive cardiovascular disease (2), with valvular and pulmonary heart disease other important etiologies. Despite these statistics, the scarcity of scientific studies involving very elderly patients is striking. Age-based exclusions from most clinical trials limit the generalizability of data to the characteristically high-risk geriatric population.

Age-Associated Changes Related to the Cardiovascular System

The presentation of cardiovascular disease in elderly patients is complicated by its superimposition on the physiologic and structural cardiovascular changes of aging. These variables influence the response of elderly patients both to specific cardiac illnesses and to their therapies. Both the physiologic and the structural changes that occur in the cardiovascular system with aging decrease cardiac functional reserve capacity, limit the performance of physical activity, and lessen the ability to tolerate a variety of stresses, including cardiovascular disease (3).

Maximal heart rate and maximal aerobic capacity decrease progressively with age, independent of habitual physical activity status, owing in part to decreased catecholamine responsiveness. Nonetheless, the maximal oxygen uptake of sedentary elderly individuals is 10% to 20% less than that of their physically active counterparts, with maximal work capacity comparably decreased. Peak exercise cardiac output and peak exercise ejection fraction also decrease at elderly ages. Cardiac dilation, enabling an increase in stroke volume, compensates for the diminished heart rate response to maintain the increase in cardiac output required for exercise. Aortic and large artery thickness and vascular stiffness increase with aging, with a resultant increase in arterial systolic pressure and impedance to left ventricular ejection. This increased afterload of aging is likely the stimulus for left ventricular hypertrophy, even in normotensive elderly persons. Both systolic blood pressure and mean blood pressure increase with aging with widening of the pulse pressure.

Aging changes in the heart also include the following features: an altered geometric contour; a decrease in ventricular compliance, with substantial reduction in the early diastolic filling rate; the diastolic dysfunction of aging, with increased dependence on the contribution of atrial contraction to late left ventricular filling to maintain cardiac output; a prolonged duration of myocardial contraction and relaxation times; and lessened chronotropic and inotropic responses to sympathetic (catecholamine) stimulation.

Baroreceptor responsiveness decreases with aging, due in part to loss of vascular distensibility. The number of pacemaker cells in the sinoatrial (SA) node and number of bundle branch fibers decrease with age, with the loss of SA pacemaker cells more pronounced. The sick sinus syndrome is due to loss of sinus node pacemaker cells and fatty infiltration around the SA node with aging. Atrioventricular block, intraventricular conduction delay, and bundle branch blocks may be caused by fibrosis and calcium deposition in the cardiac skeleton. The combination of atrial dilation and atrial fibrosis may underlie the increased prevalence of atrial arrhythmias.

Thickening of the aortic and mitral valve leaflets and the circumference of all four cardiac valves increase at elderly age. Collagen degeneration and secondary calcium deposition are common at elderly age; one third of patients aged 70 and older have calcium deposition in either the aortic or mitral valve (4). Calcific degeneration is the major cause of aortic valve disease in elderly patients.

Case A (Part 2)

Mr. Jones's electrocardiogram (ECG) shows Q waves in leads V1 to V3, but no evidence of acute ischemia. His blood pressure is 150/80 and pulse is 80 and regular. You instruct him to take an aspirin each day and prescribe furosemide as well as a beta-blocker. He was already taking an angiotensin-converting enzyme (ACE) inhibitor due to his combination of hypertension and diabetes. You refer him for a stress test the next day and give him a return appointment to see you a few days later.

Diagnostic Evaluation

Symptoms and Signs

The coexistence of multiple diseases hinders the accurate evaluation of symptoms and may obscure or complicate the patient's clinical history. Habitual activity levels differ substantially but often decrease with progressive aging, so that many symptoms do not retain their activity-precipitated characteristics. See the later sections on the specific cardiovascular diseases and peripheral arterial diseases for details.

Because orthostatic hypotension is common in elderly persons, it is essential to document the effect of postural change when measuring blood pressure. Disease and medications, rather than aging per se, account for the preponderance of postural hypotension. However, in frail elderly nursing-home residents, orthostatic hypotension is often encountered postprandially and when first arising in the morning (5).

Frequent findings in elderly individuals include the early-peaking basal systolic murmur of aortic sclerosis, typically accompanied by a fourth heart sound at the cardiac apex as evidence of reduced ventricular compliance. Neither the S_4 nor the increased ventricular filling pressure reflects ventricular systolic dysfunction, whose counterpart is an S_3. S_2 may be single at elderly age or the inspiratory splitting may be less prominent. A combination of dorsal kyphosis, emphysema, or chest wall alterations may limit palpation of the apical impulse, even when left ventricular hypertrophy is present. Data from the Cardiovascular Heath Study suggest the importance of the ankle-arm index (see page 422), a noninvasive assessment for peripheral arterial disease; a normal value is inversely related to the risk of cardiovascular disease (6).

Noninvasive Diagnostic Tests

Because of difficulties in obtaining a clinical history and in interpreting findings at physical examination, diagnostic tests assume greater importance. Noninvasive methods should initially be selected since elderly patients are at increased risk for complications of most diagnostic procedures. However, many noninvasive tests have limitations unique to an elderly population.

Resting Electrocardiogram

About 50% of elderly individuals have abnormalities of the resting electrocardiogram (ECG). Aging changes in the cardiac conduction system and the age-related increase in left ventricular mass underlie the ECG changes, most commonly PR and QT interval prolongation, intraventricular conduction abnormalities, reduction in QRS complex and T-wave voltage, nonspecific ST-segment and T-wave changes, and a leftward shift of the frontal plane QRS axis. QT prolongation is more common in elderly women than in elderly men. Both lung hyperinflation and dorsal kyphosis accentuate the diminution in QRS voltage, despite the increase in left ventricular mass. Electrocardiographic evidence of myocardial infarction occurs far more frequently than reported in the clinical history.

Long-Term (24-Hour) Ambulatory Electrocardiogram

The 24-hour ambulatory electrocardiogram or use of an event recorder is the most useful diagnostic technique to identify symptomatic arrhythmias, particularly when diary evidence is available to correlate symptoms with these spontaneously occurring arrhythmias. The test is indicated to identify cardiac rhythm disturbances as etiologic of otherwise unexplained lightheadedness, dizziness, falls, frank syncope, or uncomfortable palpitations. The limitation of utility of this study is the high prevalence of both supraventricular and ventricular arrhythmias in the absence of cardiac disease or cardiac symptoms, even arrhythmias as potentially serious as nonsustained ventricular tachycardia (7). The increase in both supraventricular and ventricular ectopic beats with aging is more likely a consequence of aging changes in the aorta and ventricles than of intrinsic abnormalities of the conduction system. Most asymptomatic arrhythmias in the absence of cardiac disease do not warrant therapy.

Echocardiogram

The echocardiogram is far more accurate than the chest roentgenogram in the assessment of cardiac chamber size because the kyphoscoliotic chest deformity and sternal depression common in elderly persons may cause a factitious increase in heart size on the chest roentgenogram. The echocardiogram is also more accurate for the determination of left ventricular hypertrophy, a powerful marker for coronary risk, than is the ECG; in addition to identifying left ventricular wall thickness and mass, cardiac chamber size, and valvular abnormalities, wall motion abnormalities and ventricular ejection fraction can be determined, as can pericardial effusion. Doppler echocardiography is reliable for determining the aortic valve area and estimating the pressure gradient in elderly patients with significant aortic stenosis.

Exercise Tests and Exercise Radionuclide Studies

Among elderly patients able to perform an adequate treadmill test, exercise testing can be undertaken with comparable safety and efficacy as in younger patients. The exercise test can help determine if the chest discomfort represents myocardial ischemia, can characterize risk status in the patient with angina pectoris or following myocardial infarction, can guide recommendations for a physical activity regimen, and can assess the suitability for return to work when appropriate. A normal response to exercise testing has the same favorable prognosis as in a younger population, and an abnormal response to exercise imparts comparable risk as in younger individuals. Few data however, are available regarding exercise testing in patients older than 75 years of age. The Naughton protocol or a modification of the standard Bruce protocol is preferable for treadmill exercise testing of elderly patients with limited exercise capability.

Exercise thallium scintigraphy is helpful when conduction abnormalities or repolarization changes on the resting ECG limit the interpretation of the exercise ECG. The presence and extent of exercise-induced reversible abnormalities permit effective risk stratification in elderly patients (8,9). Myocardial perfusion scintigraphy after intravenous administration of dipyridamole (Persantine) is well tolerated by older patients and may help identify myocardial ischemia in elderly patients who are unable to exercise. The sensitivity, specificity, and safety appear comparable in populations older and younger than 70 years of age (10). Ventricular function can be assessed by radionuclide ventriculography; although it is more expensive than echocardiography, it is applicable to elderly patients in whom adequate echocardiographic images cannot be obtained.

Case A (Part 3)

Mr. Jones returns to your office after having his exercise thallium study. He reports feeling better on his new medications and says that he can walk a full flight of stairs before having to rest. His test shows an ejection fraction of 30% and evidence of an old anterior MI. It also shows evidence of ischemia with exercise in the lateral aspect of his left ventricle. You explain his options, and Mr. Jones elects to have a cardiac catheterization. The cath shows disease in his left main artery, as well as 80% stenosis of his right coronary artery and his left circumflex artery. He is referred to a cardiothoracic surgeon and elects bypass surgery.

Mr. Jones does well during surgery. Postoperatively he has a few episodes of rapid atrial fibrillation with systolic blood pressures in the 70s. On postoperative day 5 he is found to be delirious, pulling at his nasal canula and trying to climb out of bed. His oxygen saturation is 88% on room air and a chest x-ray shows a new left lower lobe infiltrate. He is started on antibiotics. His delirium resolves and on postoperative day 8 the physical therapist recommends subacute rehabilitation due to the patient's inability to get out of bed without assistance. After 3 weeks in rehab, Mr. Jones is discharged home with a functional level close to baseline.

Invasive Diagnostic Tests

Transesophageal echocardiography (TEE), used to evaluate for aortic dissection, infective endocarditis, and valvular heart disease, among others, appears to be well tolerated in the elderly, as are cardiovascular catheterization and coronary arteriography. Precise diagnosis may enable more successful medical and surgical therapies. Procedure-related morbidity and mortality, although relatively infrequent, are increased two- to threefold in the elderly. (For further details on other invasive diagnostic tests, see Chapter 39: Cardiovascular Disease. In: Cassel CK, et al., eds. Geriatric Medicine, 4th ed., page 512.)

Manifestations of Cardiovascular Disease

Heart Failure

Most of the 5 million patients with heart failure in the United States are elderly, and heart failure is the most frequent hospital discharge diagnosis for patients older than 65 years of age (11). Heart failure is more common in men than in women until about age 80 (12). During the past two decades, heart failure deaths have almost doubled in the over-75 population. The prevalence of heart failure increases with increasing age and is estimated to involve 5% of the population aged 65 to 74 years and 10% of those older than 75 years.

Heart failure tends to be both underdiagnosed and overdiagnosed in elderly patients. Many elderly patients fail to report progressive easy fatigability, dyspnea, cough, and ankle edema, considering these a consequence of aging. Early manifestations of heart failure may be masked by the sedentary lifestyle of many elderly patients, whereas exertional dyspnea may reflect another common problem, chronic pulmonary disease, rather than cardiac failure. Owing to activity limitations, profound fatigue rather than exertional dyspnea may be the presenting feature. On occasion, only anorexia, insomnia, nocturnal cough, or frequent nocturnal urination may herald heart failure. Many elderly patients with heart failure may have disordered mental function and behavior consequent to diminished cerebral blood flow.

Coronary atherosclerotic heart disease, hypertensive cardiovascular disease, and hemodynamically significant calcific aortic stenosis are the most prevalent causes. Mitral regurgitation is also contributory. Heart failure is more frequently precipitated or exacerbated by associated medical problems than in younger patients. These include atrial fibrillation and other arrhythmias, acute myocardial infarction, uncontrolled hypertension, intercurrent infections and fever, fluid overload (13), acute blood loss, pulmonary embolism, anemia, occult thyrotoxicosis, renal insufficiency, acute lower urinary tract obstruction in men, and major dietary indiscretions. Drugs causing myocardial depression (beta-blocking drugs, calcium-blocking drugs, and a number of antiarrhythmic agents) or poor compliance with the medical regimen is also contributory. Frequent use of nonsteroidal inflammatory agents by elderly patients, often as nonprescription drugs, can precipitate heart failure by a combination of sodium and water retention and the induction of renal dysfunction. Echocardiography has substantially improved the recognition of heart failure in elderly patients and is the most useful noninvasive test to differentiate systolic and diastolic ventricular dysfunction (14).

Diastolic Dysfunction

Although ventricular systolic dysfunction with cardiac enlargement is a frequent finding in elderly patients with heart failure, diastolic dysfunction is a prominent cause of heart failure in this population. This is the case in more than half of octogenarians with heart failure (14). Clues to diastolic dysfunction as the mechanism for heart failure include a normal or near-normal heart size and a cause for left ventricular hypertrophy such as hypertension or hypertrophic cardiomyopathy. The characteristics of the aging heart and associated diabetes mellitus may impair ventricular diastolic distensibility. Ventricular diastolic dysfunction may be present in as many as half of all elderly patients with clinical manifestations of heart failure and has a more favorable prognosis than systolic dysfunction when correctly treated (15).

Systolic Dysfunction

Patients with left ventricular systolic decompensation present with cardiac enlargement, tachycardia, gallop sounds, lung rales, or pulmonary edema. Dependent edema, jugular venous distention, hepatomegaly, and ascites occur when right-sided heart failure supervenes. Weight gain may be evident. The skin, particularly of the extremities, may be cool as a result of peripheral vasoconstriction. Restlessness and agitation are due, in part, to increased sympathetic activity; control of heart failure more effectively limits these symptoms than does sedation.

Management of Heart Failure

Vasodilator therapy, beta-blockade, and spironolactone have improved the outlook for elderly patients with ventricular systolic dysfunction. Vasodilator drugs—angiotensin-converting enzyme (ACE) inhibitors, angiotensin receptor blocking drugs, and hydralazine plus nitrates (16–20)—favorably alter the loading conditions of the heart, improve symptoms of reduced cardiac output, improve functional status, retard the spontaneous worsening of heart failure, and improve survival. Angiotensin-converting enzyme inhibitors are superior to hydralazine plus nitrates (18), which can be used for patients intolerant to ACE inhibitors. Although experience with beta-blocking drugs in elderly patients is less extensive than in younger patients, with trials excluding patients over age 75 to 80 years, both carvedilol and metoprolol given to patients with class II and III heart failure improved ventricular systolic function, exercise tolerance, and survival (21–23). Spironolactone in patients up to age 80 with severe heart failure improved symptoms and prognosis (24).

Digitalis improves myocardial contractility and remains an important component of management of ventricular systolic dysfunction, even when sinus rhythm is present (25). In the Digitalis Investigation Group (DIG)

Trial (26), although survival was not altered, the combined end point of heart failure death or hospitalization was reduced in patients treated with digitalis. Lower doses are appropriate for elderly patients (0.125 mg of digoxin daily) because of the reduced glomerular filtration rate at elderly age, which lessens drug elimination rate. Digitalis toxicity should be suspected when altered mental status, fatigue, or anorexia occur, in addition to the usual nausea and vomiting.

Elderly patients with severe systolic dysfunction, particularly in association with atrial fibrillation, are candidates for oral anticoagulant therapy to limit thromboembolic complications.

Reversion of atrial fibrillation or atrial flutter to sinus rhythm can substantially augment the cardiac output and improve heart failure because of the importance of the atrial contribution to ventricular filling in the poorly compliant aged ventricle.

Sodium restriction improves diuresis and limits the resultant hypokalemia; however, major dietary alterations require assistance and encouragement in elderly patients. Difficulties with food purchasing and preparation, lack of interest in meals when eating alone, dental problems that impair chewing, and financial constraints often hamper dietary alterations. Preprocessed convenience foods, which have high sodium content, are often a sizable component of the diet of elderly individuals. Although physical activity limitation is advisable when heart failure is decompensated, protracted immobilization predisposes to deep vein thrombosis and pulmonary embolism. Resumption of a regular physical activity regimen is recommended once compensation is achieved.

Because of the significant morbidity and mortality from cardiac failure at elderly age, patients require frequent and meticulous surveillance. An intensive multidisciplinary treatment strategy for heart failure involving specialized education, assessment, and management in a randomized clinical trial decreased readmissions and improved medication compliance. This approach has proved cost-effective in elderly populations by limiting rehospitalizations (27,28). Intensive home care surveillance resulted in improved functional status (29).

Case B

Mrs. Rivera is a 75-year-old woman you are seeing in the emergency room (ER). She has a medical history significant for hypertension and atrial fibrillation. Her medications include a beta-blocker and warfarin. She tells you that she had been feeling fatigued for the last few weeks, and as she was walking to her house today, she passed out. She said she had no warning and thinks she was out for a "minute or so." Her husband saw her from the house and came outside immediately. He says she regained consciousness as he approached and denies seeing any seizure activity. In the ER her BP is 90/60 mmgH and pulse is 50/min and irregular. Her ECG shows third-degree heart block. She is admitted to the coronary care unit (CCU) and arrangements for pacemaker placement are made.

Arrhythmias and Conduction Abnormalities

Both arrhythmias and conduction abnormalities increase in prevalence with increasing age, reflecting age-related changes in specialized conducting tissue and in atrial and ventricular myocardium. The prevalence of single supraventricular premature beats increases with aging. They are present in virtually all individuals older than 80 years of age, even in the absence of heart disease, are typically asymptomatic, and do not require treatment.

Although arrhythmias may present as syncope or altered consciousness, many elderly patients have significant arrhythmias in the absence of these symptoms or of palpitations. Syncope may result from either tachyarrhythmias or bradyarrhythmias. Because syncope of cardiovascular origin entails an enormous 1-year mortality rate of 24%, identification of its mechanism is urgent to enable appropriate therapy; elderly patients with syncope of a noncardiac cause have a more favorable outlook, with their annual mortality approximating 3% (30,31).

Atrial fibrillation also increases in prevalence with increasing age, being present in almost 10% of the population older than 80 years (32); it is a major contributor to stroke in elderly patients, even in the absence of valvular disease (33). In the Cardiovascular Health Study (34), a history of heart failure, valvular heart disease, or stroke; left atrial enlargement on echocardiogram; abnormal mitral or aortic valve function; and treated hypertension and advanced age all were independently associated with an increased prevalence of atrial fibrillation in community-dwelling elderly men and women. Chronic atrial fibrillation is associated with an increased incidence of stroke that accelerates with age. Anticoagulation can reduce stroke risk by almost 70% (35). Reduction in stroke and stroke mortality has been documented with warfarin treatment, even in patients older than 75 years so treated. However, elderly patients remain undertreated with warfarin based on clinical practice guidelines for atrial fibrillation.

Ambulatory electrocardiography in elderly persons who are presumably free of cardiac disease shows that ventricular arrhythmias are pervasive, including frequent multiform premature ventricular ectopic complexes (PVCs) and nonsustained ventricular tachycardia (VT). Asymptomatic ventricular arrhythmias do not impart excess risk in healthy elderly patients and rarely require treatment in the absence of significant myocardial ischemia or ventricular dysfunction.

Elderly patients with symptomatic, refractory life-threatening ventricular tachyarrhythmias tolerate electrophysiologic testing well; this procedure can identify patients who require drug therapy or surgical intervention including coronary artery bypass graft (CABG) surgery, endocardial resection, aneurysmectomy, or cardioverter-defibrillator implantation. Radiofrequency catheter ablation therapy is effective and safe to treat tachyarrhythmias at elderly age (36). (For further details regarding ventricular arrhythmias, see Chapter 39: Cardiovascular Disease. In: Cassel CK, et al., eds. Geriatric Medicine, 4th ed., page 515.)

Bradyarrhythmias, both the sick sinus syndrome and complete atrioventricular block, occur frequently in an elderly population symptomatic bradyarrhythmias are the major indications for pacemaker implantation. Sick sinus syndrome does not generally require treatment in the absence of symptoms or extreme bradycardia. In elderly patients with the bradycardia-tachycardia subset of the sick sinus syndrome, pacemaker implantation may be required to permit pharmacologic treatment of the tachyarrhythmias with digitalis, beta-blocking drugs, or calcium-blocking drugs.

Management of Arrhythmias and Conduction Abnormalities

Pacemaker implantation is appropriate at all ages, because pacemakers can improve symptoms and both the quantity and quality of life. Before permanent pacing, more than half of all patients with complete atrioventricular block died within 2 years. Even in octogenarians and nonagenarians, normal relative survival occurred in those without other heart disease (37).

Pacing mode should be determined not by patient age but by the etiologic electrophysiologic problem. Sinus bradycardia is a common rhythm in elderly patients; when asymptomatic, it is not an indication for pacemaker implantation or other intervention. Similarly, asymptomatic complete atrioventricular block does not warrant pacing if escape rhythm is greater than 40 bpm.

Limited data are available about use of implantable cardioverter-defibrillators in elderly patients. Although these devices can be placed with minimal risk and are equally effective in preventing sudden death in older as in younger patients, nonsudden cardiac death was increased threefold in one series of patients older than 75 years (38).

Case C

Mrs. Berger is a 90-year-old woman with a history of hypertension, severe dementia, and hypothyroidism. She is bed-bound and usually minimally verbal at baseline. You get a call from her daughter who reports that her mother is more confused and is not eating. She reports no fever, cough, or foul-smelling urine. Mrs. Berger does not complain of chest pain and does not appear short of breath. She is brought to the ER where her ECG shows ST elevations in the inferior leads. She is given aspirin and a beta-blocker, and a discussion is begun regarding catheterization and thrombolytics.

Atherosclerotic Coronary Heart Disease

Atherosclerotic coronary heart disease (CHD) is the most prevalent cardiac disease at elderly age, involving an estimated 3.6 million patients. Coronary disease is responsible for more than two thirds of all cardiac deaths among the elderly U.S. population, and morbidity and mortality from CHD increase progressively with age. In the U.S., most patients with CHD, with new episodes of acute myocardial infarction, and with chronic heart failure secondary to CHD, are older than 65 years of age (39). For those men and women above 75 with CHD, 85% and 55%, respectively, experience activity limitation.

Angina Pectoris

The presentation of angina pectoris, both as an isolated event and following myocardial infarction, is more likely to be atypical, owing to a combination of a habitually decreased activity level, associated diseases, and possibly an altered sensitivity to pain in elderly persons. Angina is less likely to be activity induced in that arthritis, claudication, or musculoskeletal problems limit activity for many elderly patients before angina occurs. This angina may be misinterpreted as unstable because it occurs at rest in predominantly inactive patients. Furthermore, angina is more likely to be precipitated by a concurrent medical or surgical problem such as infection, blood loss, hypertension or hypotension, thyrotoxicosis, or arrhythmias. Dyspnea and fatigue and change in mental state may be the prominent manifestations of myocardial ischemia, and eating may precipitate angina. Additionally, patients with memory loss may not remember transient chest pain. Silent ischemia is highly prevalent at elderly ages, with the risks greatest in the early morning hours or on awakening.

Myocardial Infarction

Elderly patients have a significantly different presentation, clinical course, and prognosis of myocardial infarction (MI) than is the case in younger patients. There is a marked increase in morbidity and mortality (40), with 80% of all MI deaths occurring after age 65. Functional disability prior to MI importantly predicts MI severity and postinfarction survival (41).

Chest pain as the presenting manifestation of acute MI is less frequent in elderly individuals (42,43). Classic chest pain is reported by only one third of patients older than 85 years of age. Elderly patients have an increased prevalence of comorbid illness associated with painless infarction such as diabetes and hypertension. Additionally, there may be less or altered sensitivity to pain with aging. Although the MI may be painless, the clinical presentation is often symptomatic and may include acute dyspnea, exacerbation of heart failure, or pulmonary edema; syncope, cerebrovascular accident, vertigo, palpitations, peripheral arterial

TABLE 23.1. Atypical manifestations: acute myocardial infarction in elderly patients

Presentation
Painless infarction more common
Acute symptoms
Dyspnea
Exacerbation of heart failure
Pulmonary edema
Syncope
Stroke
Vertigo
Acute confusion
Palpitations
Peripheral arterial emboli
Nausea and vomiting
Acute renal failure
Subtle manifestations
Altered mentation
Excessive weakness or fatigue
Changes in eating pattern
Changes in other usual behaviors
Common precipitating factors
Hypovolemia
Blood loss
Infection
Hypotension

Source: Wenger NK. Cardiovascular disease. In: Cassel CK, Leipzig RM, Cohen HJ, et al., eds. Geriatric Medicine, 4th ed. New York: Springer, 2003.

embolism, nausea and vomiting, or acute renal failure; more subtle changes involve altered mentation, including acute confusion or agitation, profound weakness or fatigue, and changes in eating pattern or in other usual behaviors (Table 23.1). Asymptomatic or atypical presentations of MI commonly exclude elderly patients from the potential benefits of thrombolytic therapy or acute coronary angioplasty. Acute MI in elderly patients is often a non–Q-wave MI and, as is the case with angina pectoris, is more often precipitated by an intercurrent medical or surgical problem associated with hypovolemia, blood loss, infection, hypotension, and the like.

Management of Atherosclerotic Coronary Heart Disease

Medication Management

Drug management of acute MI is comparable to that of a younger population. There is an increased propensity to adverse effects from narcotic analgesic medications; half the usual dosage for younger individuals is recommended for the elderly (44). In general, adverse responses to drug therapy are more likely to occur and can be exacerbated by coexisting medical illnesses and related multiple-drug therapy. All drugs should be introduced at lower doses than in younger patients, with gradual dosage increases as tolerated. Comparable reduction in mortality occurred in patients with MI older and younger than 70 years treated with aspirin during acute MI in the International Study of Infarct Survival (ISIS-2) trial (45). Virtually no patients older than 75 years were enrolled in other clinical trials of aspirin use. Aspirin use was associated with a 22% decrease in 30-day mortality risk in this Medicare population. Aspirin was not prescribed at discharge to 24% of eligible elderly patients in the Cooperative Cardiovascular Project.

Intravenous administration of beta-blocking drugs in acute MI improved survival only in older patients (46–50), although data are not available for patients older than 75 years. Beta-blocker use was associated with a 43% decreased mortality rate and 22% decreased rehospitalizations in a Medicare cohort, with benefit also evident in patients older than age 75. Diltiazem and verapamil appear to provide comparable benefits in younger and older patients with non–Q-wave MI and preserved ventricular function, although calcium-channel blocking drugs have not improved survival and may worsen outcome in patients with ventricular dysfunction (51). Angiotensin-converting enzyme inhibitors likely provide comparable benefit in elderly and younger patients, particularly those with large infarctions and ventricular dysfunction. Angiotensin-converting enzyme inhibitor therapy in patients with a decreased ejection fraction following MI resulted in decreased fatal and nonfatal cardiovascular events, including the development of heart failure and recurrent infarction; relative risk reduction was greater for the 35% of patients older than 65 years. Nitrate drug use requires attention to orthostatic hypotension because of diminished baroreceptor responsiveness; elderly patients must be cautioned to sit when taking sublingual nitroglycerin for relief of angina. Among eligible patients recently hospitalized for MI, lipid-lowering drugs were used by only one third. Age greater than 74 years was independently related to lack of lipid-lowering drug use (52).

Advanced age alone (up to age 75) should not exclude patients from treatment with thrombolytic therapy. The American College of Cardiology/American Heart Association (ACC/AHA) clinical practice guidelines for acute MI cite a class I recommendation for this treatment for patients up to age 75 and a class IIa for those 75 and older (53). Statistically significant reduction in mortality was more prominent at older than at younger age, despite the increased risk of bleeding, and in particular intracerebral bleeding, in the elderly (54–57).

A substantial number of elderly patients have an essentially uncomplicated MI with an excellent prognosis for recovery and rehabilitation. They are ideal candidates for early ambulation to prevent the deleterious effects of prolonged immobilization. Education and counseling are important components of care. At discharge, there should be a careful review of medications, with written recommendations for diet, activity, and coronary risk reduction. Exercise test data can be used to recommend the intensity of physical activity that can be performed with safety following discharge from the hospital. Many elderly patients can exercise safely without supervision; predischarge exercise testing can identify the high-risk subset of patients for whom initially supervised exercise is appropriate (see Preventive and Rehabilitative Approaches To Care, page 418).

Myocardial Revascularization

Elderly patients with chronic angina unresponsive or poorly responsive to medical management, or those with persisting chest pain following MI, are candidates for coronary arteriography to assess their suitability for myocardial revascularization. Older patients with evidence of myocardial ischemia at low workloads at exercise testing also constitute a high-risk group for early recurrent coronary events and should be evaluated for myocardial revascularization.

Older patients now constitute more than half of the population undergoing cardiac catheterization, percutaneous transluminal coronary angioplasty (PTCA), and CABG surgery. As in younger populations, use of at least one internal mammary artery graft improved symptoms and event-free survival in patients 70 years and older (58). The symptomatic improvement and favorable late sustained improvement and quality of life among elderly survivors of CABG suggest that an optimistic approach to the management of symptomatic elderly patients with advanced obstructive CHD is reasonable (59).

Patients older than 70 years of age sustain a higher operative mortality from elective CABG than do younger individuals, as well as higher rates of postoperative cardiac and noncardiac complications, which occur in as many as 30% to 50%. These complications include greater need for prolonged ventilatory support for respiratory failure; for implanted pacemakers; for inotropic support and use of the intraaortic balloon pump; greater reoperation for bleeding; stroke; delirium; renal failure; perioperative infarction; and sepsis. In elderly patients with preserved ventricular function and without major associated medical problems, 5-year survival following successful CABG approximates 90%. These results were comparable to those in patients younger than age 65.

Case D

Mr. Morgan is a 76-year-old man with a history of MI, hypertension and osteoarthritis. He comes to see you for an annual checkup and wants to know what he can do to be sure he lives as long as possible. He takes a beta-blocker, aspirin, and occasional nonsteroidal antiinflammatory drugs (NSAIDs) for his arthritis pain. He exercises by walking 3 miles twice a week and swims in the summer. He tries to follow a low-fat, low-cholesterol diet but admits he cheats quite frequently. He is currently 30 lb above the upper limit of ideal weight for his height and frame. You counsel him on the benefits of exercise and eating well. He has not eaten breakfast yet and a fasting lipid profile is obtained. He has a total cholesterol of 250 mg/dL, with a low-density lipoprotein (LDL) of 160 mg/dL and a high-density lipoprotein (HDL) of 40 mg/dL. Because of his history of heart disease you start him on a statin for secondary prevention with an LDL goal of <100 mg/dL.

Preventive and Rehabilitative Approaches to Care

Preventive strategies are increasingly applied to the elderly population, as modifiable coronary risk factors are highly prevalent in elderly patients (60) and continue to predict the occurrence and recurrence of coronary events and mortality in old age (61). Preventive approaches include control of hypertension, weight reduction or control, dietary sodium and fat restriction, regular modest intensity physical activity, and emphasis on smoking cessation.

Recommendations for recognition and management of hyperlipidemia are comparable in younger and elderly populations, as hypercholesterolemia continues to confer increased coronary risk at elderly age. The Adult Treatment Panel of the National Cholesterol Education Program (NCEP) recommends that all adults with total blood cholesterol values above 200 mg/dL be evaluated and that those with elevated LDL cholesterol levels be treated (62). About one third of elderly men and one half of elderly women have elevated cholesterol levels warranting intervention, based on NCEP guidelines. Recommendations for cholesterol lowering in the elderly population are based predominantly on extrapolation of data derived from younger populations. Few elderly patients were enrolled in most secondary prevention studies, and virtually none older than 75 years. Although intervention outcome data are limited for geriatric populations, statin drugs appear to have similar efficacy and safety in nonelderly and elderly populations (63–66). Dietary therapy is recommended for the aged adult; this consists of a diet restricted in saturated fat and cholesterol and high in fruits, vegetables, and grains; additional dietary components include lean meats, fish, and low-fat dairy products.

Cigarette smoking continues to be associated with an increased risk of sudden cardiac death and fatal reinfarction, and smoking cessation decreases cardiovascular risk to that of nonsmoking individuals, independent of the age at smoking cessation (67). Smoking cessation decreased the risk of mortality or MI in older men and women with angiographically documented coronary disease (68).

Because deconditioning due to inactivity occurs more rapidly at elderly age, a physically active lifestyle should be encouraged for elderly patients, incorporating a planned regimen of modest intensity physical activity, designed to improve functional status and minimize or delay subsequent disability and dependency. A physical activity regimen, even in previously sedentary elderly patients, can enhance endurance and functional capacity. Rehabilitative exercise training can limit the high risk of disability of elderly patients after a coronary event and encourage coronary risk reduction (69). Walking is an ideal exercise regimen after discharge from the hospital, with gradual increases in the pace and distance of walking. Because the energy expenditure of walking often entails a significant proportion of the aerobic capacity of elderly patients, walking even as slowly as 3.5 miles an hour is an excellent physical conditioning stimulus. Additional benefits of exercise training include improved neuromuscular coordination, joint mobility, coordination and flexibility, and the potential to limit bone demineralization.

Case E (Part 1)

Mr. Sherman is a 78-year-old man with a history of long-standing diabetes, hypertension, and history of angioplasty and stenting of his right coronary artery. He comes to your office with a complaint of leg pain. He says it started gradually and now he is unable to walk more than a block without stopping. When he rests the pain goes away. He says it is mainly in his calves. It has limited his exercise tolerance and he is no longer able to walk on the treadmill he has at home. He denies ever having pain at rest.

Peripheral Arterial Disease: General Considerations

Peripheral arterial disease (PAD) involves the atherosclerotic occlusion of the arterial circulation to the lower extremities. The disease may be asymptomatic (identified only by a reduced blood pressure in the ankle), or it may manifest symptoms of intermittent claudication or severe chronic leg ischemia. The typical patient with PAD presents a decade later than the patient with coronary artery disease and experiences a profound limitation in exercise capacity and quality of life. In addition to affecting the limbs, PAD is a manifestation of systemic atherosclerosis affecting other major circulations involving the cerebral and coronary circulations. Thus, all patients with PAD are at an increased risk of cardiovascular morbidity and mortality. The treatment goals are directed at providing symptom relief and at reducing the risk of systemic cardiovascular morbidity and mortality.

Epidemiology

Symptoms underestimate the true incidence and prevalence of the disease. Using the ankle/brachial index (ABI), the prevalence of PAD is quite high, affecting 12% of the adult population and 20% of individuals over the age of 70 (70).

The natural history of PAD has been evaluated in several studies (71–75). These studies have shown that elderly control subjects had an all-cause mortality rate of 1.6% per year. This rate was increased to 4.8% per year among patients with PAD, a 2.5-fold increased risk. Cardiovascular mortality rates are similarly affected, with three- to fourfold increased risk for patients with PAD. Importantly, women are at approximately the same risk as men, and even asymptomatic individuals, who are identified solely based on an abnormal ABI, have a markedly increased risk of cardiovascular events.

Pathogenesis/Risk Factors

The most potent risk factors for PAD are age, diabetes mellitus, and cigarette smoking. In addition, hyperlipidemia, hypertension, and elevations in plasma homocysteine levels play an important role in promoting peripheral atherosclerosis (Table 23.2). The underlying disease process in PAD is the

TABLE 23.2. Risk factors for peripheral arterial disease (PAD) (70,76–79)

Age	Risk of PAD increases twofold with every 10 years of increased age.
Diabetes mellitus	Risk of claudication increased four to five times over that of nondiabetics, particularly when associated with hypertension, smoking, hyperlipidemia.
Cigarette smoking	Risk increased three- to fourfold for PAD. In addition, current cigarette smoking also significantly affects PAD outcomes. For example, progression from intermittent claudication to ischemic rest pain with risk of amputation occurs significantly more frequently in patients who continue to smoke than those who are abstinent.
Hyperlipidemia	Independent risk factors for PAD include a reduced HDL cholesterol level, and elevations of total cholesterol, LDL cholesterol, triglycerides, and lipoprotein$_{(a)}$. For every 10mg/dL increase in total cholesterol concentration, the risk of PAD increases approximately 10%.
Hypertension	The presence of hypertension increases risk of PAD approximately two- to threefold.
Homocysteine	Alterations in homocysteine metabolism are a recognized independent risk factor for PAD.

Source: Data from Hiatt WR, Hoag S, Hamman RF. Effect of diagnostic criteria on the prevalence of peripheral arterial disease. The San Luis Valley diabetes study. Circulation 1995;91:1472–1479. Murabito JM, D'Agostino RB, Silbershatz H, Wilson WF. Intermittent claudication. A risk profile from The Framingham Heart Study. Circulation 1997;96:44–49. Quick CRG, Cotton LT. The measured effect of stopping smoking on intermittent claudication. Br J Surg 1982;69(suppl):S24–S26. Stewart CP. The influence of smoking on the level of lower limb amputation. Prosthet Orthot Int 1987;11:113–116. Malinow MR, Kang SS, Taylor LM, et al. Prevalence of hyperhomocyst(e)inemia in patients with peripheral arterial occlusive disease. Circulation 1989;79:1180–1188.

result of atherosclerosis in the arterial circulation of the lower extremity, due to similar pathogenic mechanisms as for coronary and cerebral atherosclerosis. Arterial occlusive disease results in reduced blood flow, particularly to the calf muscles during exercise in patients with claudication, but with critical leg ischemia, blood flow is inadequate to meet the resting metabolic demands of the limb.

Case E (Part 2)

Mr. Sherman continues to smoke two packs a day and doesn't feel he is ready to stop. On exam his pulses are not palpable below the femoral artery and there is no hair on the lower half of his calves. His blood pressure and cholesterol are well controlled. You send a hemoglobin A_{1c} to the lab and order an ankle-brachial index.

He returns to your office 1 month later and the results of his ABI are 0.6 and 0.7 on the left and right, respectively. His hemoglobin A_{1c} was 9.2%. He continues to be able to walk one block. You discuss with him the risk factors for peripheral arterial disease and again recommend smoking cessation. You also increase the diabetic regimen he is on and speak with him about his diet. You suggest starting a supervised exercise program, but he is not interested at this time. He continues to deny rest pain, his feet are cool and white but there are no ulcers. You refer him to a vascular surgeon for evaluation.

Diagnostic Evaluation

Symptoms and Signs

Peripheral arterial disease is associated with two very characteristic types of limb symptoms: intermittent claudication and ischemic rest pain. The discomfort most commonly involves the calf or buttocks during walking exercise and is resolved within 10 minutes of rest. These patients commonly walk no more than two to three blocks (200 to 300 m) before they must stop to relieve the claudication pain. Patients with chronic critical limb ischemia often present with rest pain in the distal foot that occurs at night, and is relieved with dependency. Patients with more severe disease develop ischemic ulcers that are usually found at the distal points of the foot (toes, etc.) and are painful. In general, any patient with an open foot wound needs to have adequate arterial circulation confirmed by vascular studies. Figure 23.1 provides an approach to the evaluation and treatment of patients with proven PAD.

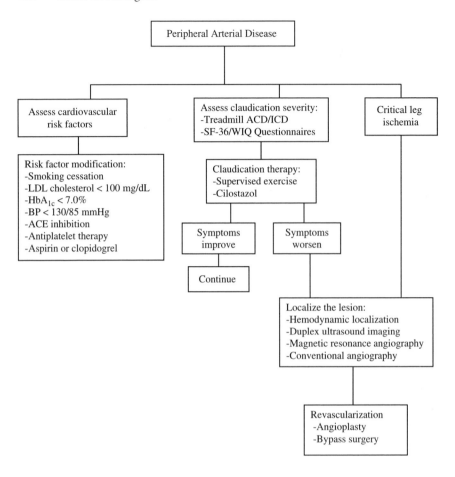

Hemodynamic Assessment

An ankle/brachial index (ABI) should be performed in patients suspected of having PAD. This would include persons at risk who are over the age of 70 years or younger patients between the ages of 50 and 69 years who smoke or have diabetes. In addition, patients with exertional leg symptoms should also be evaluated with an ABI. The ABI test can be performed in the office setting using a routine sphygmomanometer, and a handheld continuous-wave Doppler to determine the systolic blood pressure in the arms and posterior tibial and dorsalis pedis arteries of each ankle. The ABI calculation is based on the higher of the two arm pressures and the higher pressure of the two vessels in each ankle. There is not a single cutoff value to define an abnormal ABI, but a ratio ≤0.90 should be considered diagnostic for PAD (80); ABI values ≤0.40 are consistent with critical leg ischemia.

FIGURE 23.1. Evaluation and treatment of patients with proven peripheral arterial disease. All patients with peripheral arterial disease, regardless of symptom severity, should undergo risk factor modification to achieve the listed treatment goals and receive antiplatelet drug therapy with aspirin, but clopidogrel is an acceptable alternative drug. Angiotensin-converting-enzyme inhibitors should be considered because of the potential for prevention of ischemic events that is independent of blood pressure lowering.

A treadmill test to define the absolute claudication distance (ACD) and the initial claudication distance (ICD) can provide an objective assessment of the severity of claudication and response to therapy. The functional limitations of claudication and response to therapy can also be quantified by the physical function scales of the non–disease-specific Medical Outcomes Short Form-36 questionnaire (SF-36) and the disease-specific Walking Impairment Questionnaire (WIQ). Treatment of claudication should begin with exercise therapy or drugs such as cilostazol. Patients who do not improve and remain disabled, or who have worsening symptoms, should have additional localization of the occlusive lesions to plan endovascular or surgical intervention.

Noninvasive disease localization can be done with hemodynamic tests such as segmental limb pressures and/or pulse volume recordings. In addition, duplex ultrasound and magnetic resonance angiography (MRA) both have a high sensitivity and specificity for localization of lesions (with MRA having the highest sensitivity), but conventional angiography is still required in most patients prior to a surgical or angioplasty procedure. Patients with critical leg ischemia typically have an ankle/brachial index <0.40 and should initially be considered for localization of their occlusive disease in anticipation of the need for revascularization. (Hiatt WR, Nehler MR. Peripheral arterial disease. In: Cassel CK, Leipzig RM, Cohen HJ, et al., eds. Geriatric Medicine, 4th ed. New York: Springer, 2003:561–571.)

◀───

Functional Assessment

Patients with claudication have a severe limitation in exercise performance and walking ability. Thus, determining functional status is an important aspect of the overall evaluation of the patient with PAD. In patients with claudication, treadmill testing can be used to define the distance at which claudication pain begins (initial claudication distance) and the maximal walking distance. Claudication therapies typically increase both the initial and maximal walking distances (81).

Differential Diagnosis

The differential diagnosis in patients with leg symptoms includes PAD, diabetic sensory neuropathy, reflex sympathetic dystrophy, vasculitis, spinal stenosis, and arthritis. Claudication-like symptoms may also arise from spinal stenosis, which is due to osteophytic narrowing of the lumbar neurospinal canal. These symptoms include numbness and weakness in the lower extremity that is produced by standing or increasing lumbar lordosis rather than just ambulation. The symptoms are relieved not simply by rest, but also by sitting down or leaning forward to straighten out the lumbar spine. Patients with arthritis of the knee or hip may also have not only pain in the joint with ambulation, but also pain at rest or with weight bearing.

Case E (Part 3)

Mr. Sherman returns to your office 9 months later and explains that he missed his appointment with the vascular surgeon because his wife was in the hospital. He continues to smoke and says with all the stress currently, he has not been very good about his diet. He is finding it more difficult to walk except in the house. His left leg has been bothering him at night and he finds that when he hangs it off the side of the bed or stands up, the pain diminishes. He continues to be on aspirin and wonders about a medication (clopidogrel) he saw advertised on television that is supposed to help with leg pain. On exam his feet are cool with no sign of ulcerations or necrosis. You make an appointment for him to see the vascular surgeon again and give him a prescription for clopidogrel.

Management Considerations

Risk Factor Modification

Smoking Cessation

Several studies have suggested that smoking cessation decreases the risk of critical leg ischemia, and even reduces mortality in patients with PAD (82). All patients with PAD should be referred to a smoking-cessation program and prescribed nicotine replacement and antidepressants (83). A meta-analysis of several placebo controlled trials revealed cessation rates of 23% to 27% over 6 to 12 months using a nicotine patch as compared to placebo, where the quit rates ranged from 13% to 18% (84).

Adequate Glucose Control

Patients with diabetes should first undergo intensive blood glucose control to target a hemoglobin $A_{1c} < 7.0\%$. In addition to intensive blood sugar control, patients with atherosclerosis and diabetes also need aggressive risk factor modification. This may be particularly true in the treatment of hypertension, where an ACE inhibitor may be a preferable agent (85).

Cholesterol Management

Dietary restriction of cholesterol and saturated fats has only a modest effect on LDL cholesterol levels but a more substantial decrease in triglyceride levels, which is important in the management of PAD. The statin drugs have become a well-established means of reducing LDL cholesterol levels. The current recommendation for lipid therapy in the PAD population is to achieve an LDL cholesterol level <100 mg/dL and a triglyceride level <150 mg/dL (62).

Blood Pressure Control

All patients with PAD and hypertension should have aggressive lowering of their blood pressure according to the Joint National Committee VII guidelines (86). All classes of antihypertensive agents can be used in patients with PAD, including β-adrenergic blockers, which are safe for patients with claudication. In addition, β-adrenergic blockers are routinely used in the perioperative setting to decrease the risks of vascular surgery. The Heart Outcomes Prevention Evaluation Study demonstrated that ramipril was associated with a reduced risk for vascular death, nonfatal MI, or stroke in patients with PAD. This study suggests that ACE inhibitors may be important agents in reducing the risk of ischemic events in the PAD population (87).

Case E (Part 4)

Mr. Sherman finally sees the vascular surgeon, who recommends a magnetic resonance angiogram (MRA). The angiogram shows no lesion appropriate for angioplasty, but a good touch-down site for a femoral-popliteal vein graft bypass. In his preoperative testing, it is found that Mr. Sherman has an abnormal stress test, which shows a reversible ischemic lesion in the territory of the left anterior descending (LAD) artery. He is scheduled for catheterization and undergoes a successful angioplasty with a stent to his LAD. He is continued on his antiplatelet agent, clopidogrel.

Antiplatelet Therapy

The role of platelets in thrombus formation has led to many studies on the effectiveness of various antiplatelet agents, particularly aspirin, in the prevention of ischemic events. The meta-analysis by the Antiplatelet Trialists' Collaboration concluded that in patients with a history of MI or stroke, antiplatelet therapy reduced the risk of ischemic events by approximately 25% (88,89). In patients with PAD treated with bypass surgery, the Antiplatelet Trialists' Collaboration also found that antiplatelet therapy significantly promoted graft patency following vascular surgery (90).

The Clopidogrel vs. Aspirin for the Prevention of Ischemic Events (CAPRIE) trial demonstrated that PAD patients showed a 24% risk reduction on clopidogrel as compared to aspirin in terms of reducing risk for ischemic events (90).

Exercise Training

Exercise therapy for claudication had demonstrated efficacy in terms of improving exercise performance, quality of life, and functional capacity (91). Numerous types of exercise programs have been devised, but the most successful employ a supervised exercise setting. Patients should also undergo an exercise test to maximal claudication pain. The initial workload of the treadmill is set to a speed and grade that brings on claudication pain within 3 to 5 minutes. Patients walk at this work rate until they achieve claudication of moderate severity. They then rest until the claudication abates and then resume exercise. This repeated on-and-off form of exercise is continued throughout the supervised rehabilitation setting. On a weekly basis, patients should be reassessed as they are able to walk farther and farther at their chosen workload. This then necessitates an increase in speed or grade or both to allow patients to successfully work at harder and harder workloads. This scenario then induces a training benefit. The duration of an exercise program is 3 to 6 months.

Case E (Part 5)

Mr. Sherman has his bypass surgery. Two days postoperative he is found by his wife to be speaking incoherently. He is pulling at his hospital gown and his indwelling catheter. His urine grows *Enterococcus* sp. You order antibiotics and have his indwelling catheter removed. He recovers well and goes to a subacute rehabilitation unit for a month. He comes to see you 2 months later and announces that he has quit smoking. His left leg is completely pain free and his right leg bothers him only after walking two blocks. He finds he has been gradually able to increase the distance before the pain begins. He has been taking his diabetes medications but has not been checking his finger sticks. You check a hemoglobin A_{1c} and it is 7.2%.

Drug Therapy for Claudication

Cilostazol is currently the most effective drug for claudication. Approved in 1999, the primary action of cilostazol is to inhibit phosphodiesterase type 3, which results in vasodilation and inhibition of platelet aggregation, arterial thromboses, and vascular smooth muscle proliferation (91–93). In four trials of 1534 patients, cilostazol 100 mg twice daily improved both pain-free and maximal walking distance as compared with placebo (94–96). The most common side effects of cilostazol are headache, transient diarrhea, palpitations, and dizziness. Cilostazol should not be given to patients with claudication who also have heart failure.

Interventional Therapy for Claudication

The decision to proceed with interventional therapy for patients with claudication is typically based on lack of response to medical therapy and a suitable lesion for angioplasty or surgery. Angioplasty with or without stenting has been evaluated in both the iliac and femoral arteries. Although the initial technical success is high (>90% for both), the durability of angioplasty with stenting is far greater in the iliac vessels (97).

Surgery for claudication generally involves two operations, the aortofemoral bypass and the femoral above-knee popliteal bypass. Aortofemoral bypass has good patency in older patients (80% patent at 10 years) (98). However, these procedures have a 3% to 5% mortality risk and a 1% incidence of graft infection (99). Aortic surgery is a morbid operation that frequently takes months for an older patient to recover from completely. Femoral popliteal bypass is less durable, with patencies of 50% to 60% at 5 years (100,101). Operative mortality rates of up to 3% are typical when operating for claudication (102). In addition, femoral popliteal bypass is more likely to lead to limb threat following graft failure.

Interventional Therapy for Critical Leg Ischemia

The initial management of patients with critical leg ischemia involves pain relief including opioids. Patients with more severe disease, including ischemic ulceration or gangrene, also need wound care to control infection and prevention of further trauma to the extremity. Specific medical treatments for critical leg ischemia have been limited.

Definitive evaluation and management requires arteriography and revascularization, or primary amputation. Revascularization operations for critical limb ischemia use the patient's own veins (greater saphenous, lesser saphenous, and arm veins) as the optimal bypass conduit. Current 5-year patency rates for below-knee popliteal (distal anastomosis to modest-sized artery just below the knee) and tibial (distal anastomosis to smaller arteries at the calf level or below) bypass of 60% to 70% and 50% to 60%, respectively, have been reported by multiple centers (101). Limb salvage (prevention of amputation) rates of 80% or better for the same time interval are also the rule. This is due to success in second bypass surgeries when the first operation eventually fails. Operative mortality is 5% in most series, but may reach 10% in patients over 80 years of age (103). Hospital stays of 10 or more days are common due to slow healing, and frequent complications and comorbidities.

In patients who progress to amputation, below-knee amputations are performed in patients with ambulatory potential. However, despite many different techniques, there is no guaranteed method to ensure healing of below-knee amputations. Issues that complicate healing include poor circulation, chronic edema, and skin changes consistent with chronic venous disease. Importantly, half of all below-knee amputees who fail primary healing ultimately require above-knee amputation (104). Primary above-knee amputation is considered the best option for patients without any ambulatory potential (dementia, stroke, obesity, etc.).

More below-knee amputees achieve ambulation than above-knee amputees (105,106), although overall the number of major amputees who achieve meaningful independent ambulation is small. Initial rehabilitation can take up to 9 months or longer. Fifteen percent of amputees require contralateral amputation, and another 20% to 30% have died by 2 years (107,108).

General Principles

- Two thirds of health care expenditures for cardiovascular disease are for patients over 65 years of age.
- Fifty percent of resting electrocardiograms in the elderly will have some abnormality.
- Only one third of patients past age 85 years presenting with acute MI will experience chest pain.
- In the elderly patient presenting with shortness of breath, nausea/vomiting, change in mental status, and arm/neck pains, MI should be in the differential diagnosis.
- Diastolic dysfunction is common in the elderly and should be differentiated from systolic dysfunction, as the treatments are different.
- Warfarin reduces the incidence of stroke in patients with atrial fibrillation by up to 70%, and should be considered for all patients.
- Asymptomatic bradyarrhythmias usually do not need treatment.
- Patients with claudication can experience improvement in symptom burden and functionality by participating in a supervised walking exercise program.
- Patients with peripheral arterial disease should be considered candidates for secondary disease prevention strategies, with target goals similar to those with coronary artery disease.

- Aspirin should be considered as the primary antiplatelet agent for preventing ischemic events in PAD. Aspirin is also effective in maintaining vascular graft patency and may prevent thrombotic complications of PAD.
- Clopidogrel has Food and Drug Administration (FDA) approval for the prevention of ischemic events in PAD, and, although based on a subgroup analysis, clopidogrel may be more effective than aspirin in PAD patients.

Suggested Readings

Hiatt WR, Nehler MR. Peripheral arterial disease. In: Cassel CK, Leipzig RM, Cohen HJ, et al., eds. Geriatric Medicine, 4th ed. New York: Springer, 2003:561–571.

Wenger NK. Cardiovascular disease. In: Cassel CK, Leipzig RM, Cohen HJ, et al., eds. Geriatric Medicine, 4th ed. New York: Springer, 2003:509–543.

References

1. National Center for Health Statistics. Advance report of final mortality statistics, 1988. Monthly Vital Statistics Report, vol 39, No. 7 suppl. Hyattsville, MD: Public Health Service, 1990:p 1–48.
2. Mittelmark MB, Psaty BM, Rautaharju PM, et al. Prevalence of cardiovascular diseases among older adults: the Cardiovascular Health Study. Am J Epidemiol 1993;137:311–317.
3. Sollott SJ, Lakatta EG. Normal aging changes in the cardiovascular system. Cardiol Elderly 1993;1:349–358.
4. Lindroos M, Kupari M, Heikkilä J, et al. Prevalence of aortic valve abnormalities in the elderly: an echocardiographic study of a random population sample. J Am Coll Cardiol 1993;21:1220–1225.
5. Ooi WL, Barrett S, Hossain M, et al. Patterns of orthostatic blood pressure change an their clinical correlates in a frail, elderly population. JAMA 1997;277:1299–1304.
6. Newman AB, Siscovick DS, Manolio TA, et al., for the Cardiovascular Health Study (CHS) Collaborative Research Group. Ankle-arm index as a marker of atherosclerosis in the Cardiovascular Health Study. Circulation 1993;88:837–845.
7. Ingerslev J, Bjerregaard P. Prevalence and prognostic significance of cardiac arrhythmias detected by ambulatory electrocardiography in subjects 85 years of age. Eur Heart J 1986;7:570–575.
8. Iskandrian AS, Heo J, Decoskey D, et al. Use of exercise thallium-201 imaging for risk stratification of elderly patients with coronary artery disease. Am J Cardiol 1988;61:269–272.
9. Hilton TC, Shaw LJ, Chaitman BR, et al. Prognostic significance of exercise thallium-201 testing in patients aged ≥70 years with known or suspected coronary artery disease. Am J Cardiol 1992;69:45–50.

10. Lam JYT, Chaitman BR, Glaenzer M. Safety and diagnostic accuracy in dipyridamole-thallium imaging in the elderly. J Am Coll Cardiol 1988;11: 585–589.
11. Smith WM. Epidemiology of congestive heart failure. Am J Cardiol 1985;55:3A–8A.
12. McKee PA, Castelli WP, McNamara PM, et al. The natural history of congestive heart failure: the Framingham Study. N Engl J Med 1971;285: 1441–1446.
13. Moser M, Hebert PR. Prevention of disease progression, left ventricular hypertrophy and congestive heart failure in hypertension treatment trials. J Am Coll Cardiol 1996;27:1214–1218.
14. Konstam MA, Dracup K, Baker D, et al. Heart failure: evaluation and care of patients with left-ventricular systolic dysfunction. Clinical Practice Guideline No. 11. AHCPR Publication No. 94-0612. Rockville, MD: Agency for Health Care Policy and Research, Public Health Service, U.S. Department of Health and Human Services, June 1994.
15. Wong WF, Gold S, Fukuyama O, et al. Diastolic dysfunction in elderly patients with congestive heart failure. Am J Cardiol 1989;63:1526–1528.
16. The CONSENSUS Trial Study Group. Effects of enalapril on mortality in severe congestive heart failure: results of the Cooperative North Scandinavian Enalapril Survival Study (CONSENSUS). N Engl J Med 1987;316: 1429–1435.
17. The SOLVD Investigators. Effect of enalapril on survival in patients with reduced left ventricular ejection fractions and congestive heart failure. N Engl J Med 1991;325:293–302.
18. Cohn JN, Johnson G, Ziesche S, et al. A comparison of enalapril with hydralazine-isosorbide dinitrate in the treatment of chronic congestive heart failure. N Engl J Med 1991;325:303–310.
19. Chapman D, Wang T, Gheorghiade M. Therapeutic approaches to heart failure in elderly patients. Cardiol Elderly 1994;2:89–97.
20. De Bock V, Mets T, Romagnoli M, et al. Captopril treatment of chronic heart failure in the very old. J Gerontol 1994;49:M148–152.
21. Packer M, Bristow MR, Cohn JN, et al. The effect of carvedilol on morbidity and mortality in patients with chronic heart failure. N Engl J Med 1996;334: 1349–1355.
22. CIBIS-II Investigators and Committees. The Cardiac Insufficiency Bisoprolol Study II (CIBIS II): a randomized trial. Lancet 1999;353:9–13.
23. Effect of metoprolol CR/XL in chronic heart failure: Metoprolol CR/XL Randomised Intervention Trial in Congestive Heart Failure (MERIT-HF). Lancet 1999;353:2001–2007.
24. Pitt B, Zannad F, Remme WJ, et al. The effect of spironolactone on morbidity and mortality in patients with severe heart failure. Randomized Aldactone Evaluation Study Investigators. N Engl J Med 1999;341:709–717.
25. Packer M, Gheorghiade M, Young JB, et al. Withdrawal of digoxin from patients with chronic heart failure treated with angiotensin-converting-enzyme inhibitors. RADIANCE Study. N Engl J Med 1993;329:1–7.
26. The Digitalis Investigation Group. The effect of digoxin on mortality and morbidity in patients with heart failure. N Engl J Med 1997;336: 525–533.

27. Rich MW, Beckham V, Wittenberg C, et al. A multidisciplinary intervention to prevent the readmission of elderly patients with congestive heart failure. N Engl J Med 1995;333:1190–1195.

28. Rich MW, Gray DB, Beckham V, et al. Effect of a multidisciplinary intervention on medication compliance in elderly patients with congestive heart failure. Am J Med 1996;101:270–276.

29. Kornowski R, Zeeli D, Averbuch M, et al. Intensive home-care surveillance prevents hospitalization and improves morbidity rates among elderly patients with severe congestive heart failure. Am Heart J 1995;129:762–766.

30. Lipsitz LA, Wei JY, Rowe JW. Syncope in an elderly, institutionalized population: prevalence, incidence, and associated risk. Q J Med 1985;55:45–54.

31. Gordon M, Huang M, Gryfe CI. An evaluation of falls, syncope, and dizziness in prolonged ambulatory cardiographic monitoring in a geriatric institutional setting. J Am Geriatr Soc 1982;30:6–12.

32. Ryder KM, Benjamin EJ. Epidemiology and significance of atrial fibrillation. Am J Cardiol 1999;84:131R–138R.

33. Wolf PA, Abbott RD, Kannel WB. Atrial fibrillation: a major contributor to stroke in the elderly. Arch Intern Med 1987;147:1561–1564.

34. Furberg CD, Psaty BM, Manolio TA, et al., for the Cardiovascular Health Study (CHS) Collaborative Research Group. Prevalence of atrial fibrillation in elderly subjects (the Cardiovascular Health Study). Am J Cardiol 1994;74: 236–241.

35. Stroke Prevention in Atrial Fibrillation Investigators. Stroke prevention in atrial fibrillation study: final results. Circulation 1991;84:527–539.

36. Zado ES, Callans DJ, Gottlieb CD, et al. Efficacy and safety of catheter ablation in octogenarians. J Am Coll Cardiol 2000;35:458–462.

37. Shen W-K, Hayes DL, Hammill SC, et al. Survival and functional independence after implantation of a permanent pacemaker in octogenarians and nonagenarians. A population-based study. Ann Intern Med 1996;125: 476–480.

38. Panotopoulos PT, Axtell K, Anderson AJ, et al. Efficacy of the implantable cardioverter-defibrillator in the elderly. J Am Coll Cardiol 1997;29: 556–560.

39. Wenger NK, Furberg CD, Pitt E. Coronary Heart Disease in the Elderly. Working Conference on the Recognition and Management of Coronary Heart Disease in the Elderly, National Institutes of Health, Bethesda 1985. New York: Elsevier Science, 1986.

40. Marcus FI, Friday K, McCans J, et al. Age-related prognosis after acute myocardial infarction (the Multicenter Diltiazem Postinfarction trial). Am J Cardiol 1990;65:559–566.

41. Vaccarino V, Parsons L, Every NR, et al., for the National Registry of Myocardial Infarction 2 Participants. Sex-based differences in early mortality after myocardial infarction. N Engl J Med 1999;341:217–225.

42. Nadelmann J, Frishman WH, Ooi WL, et al. Prevalence, incidence and prognosis of recognized and unrecognized myocardial infarction in persons aged 75 years or older: The Bronx Aging Study. Am J Cardiol 1990;66: 533–537.

43. Solomon CG, Lee TH, Cook EF, et al., for the Chest Pain Study Group. Comparison of clinical presentation of acute myocardial infarction in patients

older than 65 years of age to younger patients: the Multicenter Chest Pain Study experience. Am J Cardiol 1989;63:772–776.

44. Forman DE, Bernal JLG, Wei JY. Management of acute myocardial infarction in the very elderly. Am J Med 1992;93:315–326.

45. ISIS-2 (Second International Study of Infarct Survival) Collaborative Group. Randomised trial of intravenous streptokinase, oral aspirin, both, or neither among 17,187 cases of suspected acute myocardial infarction: ISIS-2. Lancet 1988;2:349–360.

46. The First International Study of Infarct Survival (ISIS-I) Collaborative Group. Randomised trial of intravenous atenolol among 16,027 cases of suspected acute myocardial infarction. Lancet 1986;2:57–66.

47. Hjalmarson A, Elmfeldt D, Herlitz J, et al. Effect on mortality of metoprolol in acute myocardial infarction: A double-blind randomise trial. Lancet 1981; 2:823–827.

48. The MIAMI Trial Research Group. Metoprolol in acute myocardial infarction (MIAMI): a randomised placebo-controlled international trial. Eur Heart J 1985;6:199–226.

49. The International Collaborative Study Group. Reduction of infarct size with the early use of timolol in acute myocardial infarction. N Engl J Med 1984; 310:9–15.

50. The TIMI Study Group. Comparison of invasive and conservative strategies after treatment with intravenous tissue plasminogen activator in acute myocardial infarction: results of the Thrombolysis in Myocardial Infarction (TIMI) phase II trial. N Engl J Med 1989;320:618–627.

51. Held PH, Yusuf S, Furberg CD. Calcium channel blockers in acute myocardial infarction and unstable angina: an overview. BMJ 1989;299:1187–1192.

52. Majumdar SR, Gurwitz JH, Soumerai SB. Undertreatment of hyperlipidemia in the secondary prevention of coronary artery disease. J Gen Intern Med 1999;14:711–717.

53. Ryan TJ, Anderson JL, Antman EM, et al. ACC/AHA guidelines for the management of patients with acute myocardial infarction: a report of the American College of Cardiology/American Heart Association Task Force on Practice Guidelines (Committee on Management of Acute Myocardial Infarction). J Am Coll Cardiol 1996;28:1328–1428.

54. Chaitman BR, Thompson B, Wittry MD, et al. The use of tissue-type plasminogen activator for acute myocardial infarction in the elderly: Results from Thrombolysis in Myocardial Infarction Phase I, open label studies, and the Thrombolysis in Myocardial Infarction Phase II pilot study. J Am Coll Cardiol 1989;14:1159–1165.

55. The International Study Group. In-hospital mortality and clinical course of 20,891 patients with suspected acute myocardial infarction randomised between alteplase and streptokinase with or without heparin. Lancet 1990; 336:71–75.

56. Gruppo Italiano per lo Studio della Sopravvivenza nell'Infarto Miocardico. GISSI-2: a factorial randomised trial of alteplase versus streptokinase and heparin versus no heparin among 12 490 patients with acute myocardial infarction. Lancet 1990;336:65–71.

57. Gore JM, Sloan M, Price TR, et al. Intracerebral hemorrhage, cerebral infarction, and subdural hematoma after acute myocardial infarction and

thrombolytic therapy in the Thrombolysis in Myocardial Infarction Study: Thrombolysis in Myocardial Infarction, Phase II, pilot and clinical trial. Circulation 1991;83:448–459.

58. Noyez L, van der Werf T, Remmen GHJ, et al. Importance of the internal mammary artery for coronary bypass grafting in patients aged ≥70 years. Am J Cardiol 1995;75:734–736.

59. Eagle KA, Guyton RA, Davidoff R, et al. ACC/AHA guidelines for coronary artery bypass graft surgery: a report of the American College of Cardiology/American Heart Association Task Force on Practice Guidelines (Committee to Revise the 1991 Guidelines for Coronary Artery Bypass Graft Surgery). J Am Coll Cardiol 1999;34:1262–1347.

60. World Health Organization Study Group. Epidemiology and prevention of cardiovascular diseases in elderly people. WHO Technical Report Series 853. Geneva: World Health Organization, 1995.

61. Tervahauta M, Pekkanen J, Nissinen A. Risk factors of coronary heart disease and total mortality among elderly men with and without preexisting coronary heart disease: The Finnish Cohorts of the Seven Countries Study. J Am Coll Cardiol 1995;26:1623–1629.

62. The Expert Panel on Detection, Evaluation and Treatment of High Blood Cholesterol in Adults. Final Report of the Third Report of the National Cholesterol Education Program (NCEP) Expert Panel on Detection, Evaluation, and Treatment of High Blood Cholesterol in Adults (Adult Treatment Panel III). Circulation 2002;106(25):3143–3421.

63. Pacala JT, McBride PE, Grady SL, Management of older adults with hypercholesterolaemia. Drugs Aging 1994;4:366–378.

64. Santinga JT, Rosman HS, Rubenfire M, et al. Efficacy and safety of pravastatin in the long-term treatment of elderly patients with hypercholesterolemia. Am J Med 1994;96:509–515.

65. Hulley SB, Newman TB. Cholesterol in the elderly: Is it important? JAMA 1994;272:1372–1374.

66. Scandinavian Simvastatin Survival Study group. Randomised trial of cholesterol lowering in 4444 patients with coronary heart disease: the Scandinavian Simvastatin Survival Study (4S). Lancet 1994;344:1383–1389.

67. LaCroix AZ, Lang J, Scherr P, et al. Smoking and mortality among older men and women in three communities. N Engl J Med 1991;324:1619–1625.

68. Hermanson B, Omenn GS, Kronmal RA, et al., and Participants in the Coronary Artery Surgery Study. Beneficial six-year outcome of smoking cessation in older men and women with coronary artery disease. Results from the CASS Registry. N Engl J Med 1988;319:1365–1369.

69. Lavie CJ, Milani RV. Effects of cardiac rehabilitation programs on exercise capacity, coronary risk factors, behavioral characteristics, and quality of life in a large elderly cohort. Am J Cardiol 1995;76:177–179.

70. Hiatt WR, Hoag S, Hamman RF. Effect of diagnostic criteria on the prevalence of peripheral arterial disease. The San Luis Valley diabetes study. Circulation 1995;91:1472–1479.

71. Criqui MH, Langer RD, Fronek A, et al. Mortality over a period of 10 years in patients with peripheral arterial disease. N Engl J Med 1992;326:381–386.

72. Vogt MT, Cauley JA, Newman AB, Kuller LH, Hulley SB. Decreased ankle/ arm blood pressure index and mortality in elderly women. JAMA 1993;270: 465–469.
73. Newman AB, Tyrrell KS, Kuller LH. Mortality over four years in SHEP participants with a low ankle-arm index. J Am Geriatr Soc 1997;45: 1472–1478.
74. Leng GC, Fowkes FG, Lee AJ, et al. Use of ankle brachial pressure index to predict cardiovascular events and death: a cohort study. BMJ 1996;313: 1440–1444.
75. Leng GC, Lee AJ, Fowkes FG, et al. Incidence, natural history and cardio-vascular events in symptomatic and asymptomatic peripheral arterial disease in the general population. Int J Epidemiol 1996;25:1172–1181.
76. Murabito JM, D'Agostino RB, Silbershatz H, Wilson WF. Intermittent claudication. A risk profile from The Framingham Heart Study. Circulation 1997;96:44–49.
77. Quick CRG, Cotton LT. The measured effect of stopping smoking on inter-mittent claudication. Br J Surg 1982;69 (suppl):S24–S26.
78. Stewart CP. The influence of smoking on the level of lower limb amputation. Prosthet Orthot Int 1987;11:113–116.
79. Malinow MR, Kang SS, Taylor LM, et al. Prevalence of hyperhomocyst(e)inemia in patients with peripheral arterial occlusive disease. Circulation 1989;79: 1180–1188.
80. Carter SA. Clinical measurement of systolic pressures in limbs with arterial occlusive disease. JAMA 1969;207:1869–1874.
81. Hiatt WR, Hirsch AT, Regensteiner JG, Brass EP. Clinical trials for claudica-tion. Assessment of exercise performance, functional status, and clinical end points. Vascular Clinical Trialists. Circulation 1995;92:614–621.
82. Jonason T, Bergstrom R. Cessation of smoking in patients with intermittent claudication. Acta Med Scand 1987;221:253–260.
83. Jorenby DE, Leischow SJ, Nides MA, et al. A controlled trial of sustained-release bupropion, a nicotine patch, or both for smoking cessation. N Engl J Med 1999;340:685–691.
84. Joseph AM, Norman SM, Ferry LH, et al. The safety of transdermal nicotine as an aid to smoking cessation in patients with cardiac disease. N Engl J Med 1996;335:1792–1798.
85. Estacio RO, Jeffers BW, Hiatt WR, et al. The effect of nisoldipine as com-pared with enalapril on cardiovascular outcomes in patients with non-insulin-dependent diabetes and hypertension. N Engl J Med 1998;338:645–652.
86. Chobanian AV, Bakris GL, Black HR, et al. The seventh report of the Joint National Committee on prevention, detection, evaluation and treatment of high blood pressure; the JNC VII report. JAMA 2003:289(19):2560–2572.
87. The Heart Outcomes Prevention Evaluation Study Investigators. Effects of an angiotensin-converting-enzyme inhibitor, ramipril, on cardiovascular events in high-risk patients. N Engl J Med 2000;342:145–153.
88. Antiplatelet Trialists' Collaboration. Secondary prevention of vascular disease by prolonged antiplatelet treatment. Br Med J 1988;296:320–331.
89. Collaborative overview of randomised trials of antiplatelet therapy—I: Pre-vention of death, myocardial infarction, and stroke by prolonged antiplatelet

therapy in various categories of patients. Antiplatelet Trialists' Collaboration. BMJ 1994;308:81–106.

90. Collaborative overview of randomised trials of antiplatelet therapy—II: Maintenance of vascular graft or arterial patency by antiplatelet therapy. Antiplatelet Trialists' Collaboration. BMJ 1994;308:159–168.

91. Kohda N, Tani T, Nakayama S, et al. Effect of cilostazol, a phosphodiesterase III inhibitor, on experimental thrombosis in the porcine carotid artery. Thromb Res 1999;96:261–268.

92. Igawa T, Tani T, Chijiwa T, et al. Potentiation of anti-platelet aggregating activity of cilostazol with vascular endothelial cells. Thromb Res 1990;57: 617–623.

93. Tsuchikane E, Fukuhara A, Kobayashi T, et al. Impact of cilostazol on restenosis after percutaneous coronary balloon angioplasty. Circulation 1999;100: 21–26.

94. Beebe HG, Dawson DL, Cutler BS, et al. A new pharmacological treatment for intermittent claudication: results of a randomized, multicenter trial. Arch Intern Med 1999;159:2041–2050.

95. Money SR, Herd JA, Isaacsohn JL, et al. Effect of cilostazol on walking distances in patients with intermittent claudication caused by peripheral vascular disease. J Vasc Surg 1998;27:267–274.

96. Dawson DL, Cutler BS, Meissner MH, Strandness DEJ. Cilostazol has beneficial effects in treatment of intermittent claudication: results from a multicenter, randomized, prospective, double-blind trial. Circulation 1998;98: 678–686.

97. Wilson SE, Wolf GL, Cross AP. Percutaneous transluminal angioplasty versus operation for peripheral arteriosclerosis. J Vasc Surg 1989;9:1–8.

98. Poulias GE, Doundoulakis N, Prombonas E, et al. Aorto-femoral bypass and determinants of early success and late favourable outcome. Experience with 1000 consecutive cases. J Cardiovasc Surg 1992;33:664–678.

99. Lorentzen JE, Nielsen OM, Arendrup H, et al. Vascular graft infection: an analysis of sixty-two graft infections in 2411 consecutively implanted synthetic vascular grafts. Surgery 1985;98:81–86.

100. Veith FJ, Gupta SK, Ascer E, et al. Six-year prospective multicenter randomized comparison of autologous saphenous vein and expanded Polytetrafluoroethylene grafts in infrainguinal arterial reconstructions. J Vasc Surg 1986;3: 104–114.

101. Dalman RL, Taylor LM. Basic data related to infrainguinal revascularization procedures. Ann Vasc Surg 1990;4:309–312.

102. Samson RH, Veith FJ, Janko GS, Gupta SK, Scher LA. A modified classification and approach to the management of infections involving peripheral arterial prosthetic grafts. J Vasc Surg 1988;8:147–153.

103. Nehler MR, Moneta GL, Edwards JM, et al. Surgery for chronic lower extremity ischemia in patients eighty or more years of age: Operative results and assessment of postoperative independence. J Vasc Surg 1993;18: 618–626.

104. Tripses D, Pollak EW. Risk factors in healing of below-knee amputation. Appraisal of 64 amputations in patients with vascular disease. Am J Surg 1981;141:718–720.

105. Rigdon EE, Monajjem N, Rhodes RS. Criteria for selective utilization of the intensive care unit following carotid endarterectomy. Ann Vasc Surg 1997;11:20–27.
106. Gregg RO. Bypass or amputation? Concomitant review of bypass arterial grafting and major amputations. Am J Surg 1985;149:397–402.
107. Rush DS, Huston CC, Bivins BA, Hyde GL. Operative and late mortality rates of above-knee and below-knee amputations. Am Surg 1981;47:36–39.
108. Whitehouse FW, Jurgensen C, Block MA. The later life of the diabetic amputee: another look at the fate of the second leg. Diabetes 1968;17: 520–521.

24
Diabetes Mellitus

AUDREY K. CHUN

Learning Objectives

Upon completion of the chapter, the student will be able to:

1. Identify typical and atypical symptoms of diabetes mellitus in older adults.
2. Understand the laboratory evaluations necessary to confirm the diagnosis of diabetes mellitus.
3. Describe the pharmacologic and nonpharmacologic treatments available for the management of diabetes.

Case (Part 1)

Mr. H. is a 69-year-old man with a history of hypertension and hyperlipidemia who comes to your office with complaints of urinary incontinence. On further questioning, he admits to a 10-lb weight loss, polyuria, decreased vision, and numbness in his hands and feet. You suspect diabetes mellitus.

What are some of the risk factors for diabetes?

What are some of the age-associated changes that may be related to the diabetes?

General Considerations

Diabetes mellitus prevalence increases with age, and the numbers of older persons with diabetes are expected to grow as the elderly population increases in number. The National Health and Nutrition Examination

---

Material in this chapter is based on the following chapter in Cassel CK, Leipzig RM, Cohen HJ, Larson EB, Meier DE, eds. Geriatric Medicine: An Evidence-Based Approach, 4th ed. New York: Springer, 2003: Minaker KL. Treatment of Diabetes, pp. 681–694. Selections edited by Audrey K. Chun.

Survey (NHANES III) demonstrated that in the population over 65 years old, almost 18% to 20% have diabetes. Other abnormalities in carbohydrate metabolism observed included an additional 20% to 25% of older patients meeting the criteria for impaired glucose tolerance (IGT). The incidence of diabetes mellitus is approximately 2 per 1000 among those older than 45 and increases for those individuals greater than 75 years old (1). Prevalence is much higher in older Hispanics, African Americans, Native Indians, Scandinavians, Japanese, and Micronesians.

Individuals with diabetes mellitus who are older than 65 usually have type 2 diabetes mellitus. It accounts for only 5% to 10% newly diagnosed diabetes mellitus in late life (2). In addition, a small proportion of older individuals who initially have type 2 diabetes appear to become insulin dependent over time.

Age-Associated Changes Related to Glucose Metabolism

Glucose intolerance associated with aging itself may predispose to the development of overt diabetes mellitus. Glucose intolerance is present even in very healthy older individuals. Postprandial blood glucose increases by 5.3 mg/dL per decade after the age of 30 (3,4). Age-related changes in fasting blood glucose levels are 1 to 2 mg/dL (0.05 to 0.09 mM) per decade after age 30 (3,4).

Several factors appear to contribute to age-associated glucose homeostatic changes. Glucose absorption slows with increasing age, and hepatic glucose production shut down after food and glucose is delayed, most likely as a result of delayed insulin secretion (5,6). Other factors may contribute to glucose intolerance. Both the decline in lean body mass and the increase in body fat that accompany aging may contribute to insulin resistance (7). Reduced levels of physical activity and altered diet may cause these changes in body composition (8). Drugs commonly used by older individuals, including diuretics, tricyclic antidepressants, estrogen, sympathomimetics, glucocorticoids, niacin, and phenytoin, may adversely affect glucose metabolism. Stress states such as myocardial infarction, infection, burns, and surgery may also worsen glucose tolerance.

The reduction in glucose tolerance associated with aging is correlated with insulin resistance, obesity, hyperlipidemia, and hypertension. The pathogenesis of these associated and interrelated conditions is referred to as the metabolic syndrome or syndrome X. Although the pathogenesis is currently under detailed study, the emergence of insulin resistance as a central feature of diabetes mellitus in the elderly appears secure. (For further details on age-associated changes related to glucose metabolism, see Chapter 46: Treatment of Diabetes. In: Cassel CK, et al., eds. Geriatric Medicine, 4th ed., page 682.)

Pathogenesis/Risk Factors

Middle-aged and elderly people have a strong genetic predisposition to type 2 diabetes. The specific genes responsible have not been discovered. People with a family history of diabetes are more likely to develop the illness as they age. Elderly patients with peripheral insulin resistance and reduced glucose-induced insulin release are more likely to develop type 2 diabetes than those without (9).

Physiologic and environmental factors compound genetic predisposition. Lower testosterone levels in men (10) and higher testosterone levels in women (11) are risk factors for diabetes development. Elderly individuals who have a high intake of fat and sugar and a low intake of complex carbohydrates are more likely to develop diabetes (12). Physical inactivity and central fat distribution predispose to diabetes in the elderly (13). Unlike younger patients, fasting hepatic glucose production is normal in elderly patients with type 2 diabetes and they have specific alterations in carbohydrate metabolism. The primary metabolic defect in lean elderly subjects is an impairment in glucose-induced insulin release, whereas the primary abnormality in obese elderly subjects is resistance to insulin-mediated glucose disposal (14).

Diagnostic Evaluation

Symptoms and Signs

Diabetes may present for the first time in elderly individuals as a result of a fasting screening glucose level or concurrent with the presentation at the time of illness with a complication of illness, such as a myocardial infarction or stroke. Classic symptoms of polyuria or polydipsia are rarely present. Glucose is not spilled into the urine until the plasma glucose is markedly elevated, because the renal threshold for glucose increases with age. Polydipsia is also less common, because thirst is impaired. When symptoms are present, they are generally atypical (falls, failure to thrive, urinary incontinence, or delirium). Also, nonketotic hyperosmolar coma may be the first sign of diabetes in older individuals, particularly in older nursing home patients. This results from decreased access to water associated with osmotic diuresis, impaired thirst, and cognitive dysfunction.

Unusual clinical findings also develop in older patients with established diabetes. Malignant otitis externa is a necrotizing infection caused by *Pseudomonas*, occurring almost exclusively in elderly patients with diabetes. Renal papillary necrosis can occur in association with urinary tract infections. Diabetic amyotrophy causes asymmetric and painful weakness of the muscles of the pelvic girdle and thigh, and usually resolves spontaneously in a few months. It is most prevalent in older males. Diabetic neuropathic cachexia occurs in older patients with diabetes causing weight loss, depression, and painful peripheral neuropathy (15).

Case (Part 2)

On exam, Mr. H. is noted to have a blood pressure of 150/90 mm Hg and is obese. His visual acuity is 20/80 in both eyes and a symmetric sensory loss is noted in both hands and feet. Laboratory values reveal a fasting glucose of 200 mg/dL and 1+ glucose in the urine.

Does he meet diagnostic criteria for diabetes mellitus?
What other tests and evaluations would you order?
What type(s) of treatment would you recommend?

Laboratory Findings

The diagnosis of diabetes mellitus is made primarily through the findings of elevated glucoses on fasting laboratory samples, random glucoses during outpatient or inpatient care, and much less commonly now, after formal oral glucose tolerance testing (OGTT). In 1997, the American Diabetes Association (ADA) revised its diagnostic criteria to rely solely on a fasting plasma glucose value over 126 mg/dL (7.0 mmol/L), rather than on a fasting glucose over 140 mg/dL or a 2-hour oral glucose tolerance test plasma glucose value over 200 mg/dL, as had been recommended by the 1980–1985 World Health Organization (WHO) diagnostic criteria (16) and the ADA's 1979 criteria for diabetes (17). The new ADA criteria also recommended two other diagnostic classes. *Impaired fasting glucose* (IFG) is defined as a fasting plasma glucose between 110 mg/dL (6.1 mmol/L) and 126 mg/dL (7.0 mmol/L); *normal fasting glucose* is defined as a fasting plasma glucose less than 110 mg/dL. The OGTT is not recommended for routine diagnosis of glucose intolerance or diabetes.

The ADA 1997 criteria changed the incidence of diabetes by age, sex, and ethnicity, resulting in a significant increase in the number of individuals diagnosed with diabetes mellitus while perhaps excluding significant numbers of individuals who would have gained the diagnosis through post-challenge glucose elevations (18). Many of the reported studies show that the 1997 ADA diagnosis standards do not result in equal sensitivity for fasting and 2-hour glucose levels, especially in older individuals. Although the use of fasting plasma glucose alone for diabetes diagnosis may simplify testing, the WHO criteria would identify a much greater percentage of elderly subjects with diabetes or impaired glucose testing and move ahead the diagnosis by 5 to 8 years over the criteria based on fasting glucose levels. As diabetes prevention efforts increase, a move to a more sensitive bias in diagnosis may be needed. The majority of newly diagnosed diabetic patients (>90%) emerge from the population with IGT, no matter how it is defined, and are at higher risk for cardiovascular disorders.

Management Considerations

All older adults with diabetes mellitus should receive a standard basic care program regardless of the treatment goal chosen. These standards (19) include a complete history and physical examination to detect any complications of diabetes mellitus and any risk factors for complications (Table 24.1). A geriatric assessment, emphasizing a functional assessment, should be performed at the time of diagnosis. Skills in the basic activities of daily living (bathing, grooming, dressing, feeding, toileting, and transferring) and the instrumental activities of daily living (e.g., shopping, telephoning, finances, and housework) should be assessed. Social support systems and financial and insurance status often should also be assessed, by nursing and social work staff.

Laboratory evaluation at diagnosis includes determinations of fasting serum glucose level, glycosylated hemoglobin (to assess previous level of control and to be used as a baseline), fasting lipid profile, and serum creatinine; urinalysis with examination for proteinuria; and an electrocardiogram. Ophthalmologic evaluation at the time of diagnosis is recommended by the ADA for all patients with type 2 diabetes (20). This recommendation is particularly relevant for elderly patients who are at high risk for ocular diseases including cataract and glaucoma. Dietary assessment provides an initial dietary therapy for the diabetic patient.

Following evaluation, one of two levels of care can be recommended: symptom-preventing care or aggressive care. The patient and the primary caregiver make the decision jointly. Family members and consultants such as geriatricians, diabetologists, cardiologists, and nephrologists may be helpful. These consultants provide a clearer picture of the current medical condition and estimates of life expectancy.

TABLE 24.1. Minimum standards of care for older adults with diabetes mellitus

Initial evaluation
  Complete history and physical examination
  Geriatric assessment
  Laboratory examination: fasting blood glucose, glycosylated hemoglobin, fasting lipid
    profile, creatinine, urinalysis, electrocardiogram
  Ophthalmologic examination
  Dietary assessment
Continuing care
  Use of treatment as needed to meet target glucose levels: diet, oral agents, or insulin
  Assessment of blood glucose levels as frequently as needed to assure that treatment
    goals are being met
  Annual assessment for diabetes complications
  Annual review of geriatric assessment

Source: Minaker KL. Treatment of diabetes. In: Cassel CK, Leipzig RM, Cohen HJ, et al., eds. Geriatric Medicine, 4th ed. New York: Springer, 2003.

Symptom-Preventing Care

Symptom-preventing care is indicated for those individuals for whom the primary goal of treatment is avoidance of metabolic complications. The average glucose levels necessary to achieve this goal are approximately 200 mg/dL (11 mM) or the glucose level at which glycosuria is minimal. The elimination of glycosuria removes the risk of volume depletion and the risk of secondary problems related to hypotension and poor tissue perfusion. Hyperglycemic hyperosmolar nonketotic coma due to dehydration and glycosuria is the most dramatic expression of this phenomenon. Glycosuria also is associated with weight loss caused by the loss of calories in the urine. The resultant catabolic state leads to a loss of lean body tissue. The long-term consequences of poor nutrition include increased risk of infections.

Aggressive Care

Aggressive care has prevention of long-term complications as its goal. *Euglycemia* is defined as (1) a fasting glucose level lower than 115 mg/dL (6.4 mM), (2) a mean glucose level between 110 and 140 mg/dL (6 to 8 mM), and (3) normal levels of glycosylated hemoglobin. Prevention of long-term complications in type 1 diabetes patients results from this level of control. These benefits are believed to extrapolate to elderly patients with type 2 diabetes.

Aggressive management programs for older adults with diabetes require high levels of skill, commitment, and diabetes education. Standard diabetes therapy includes diet, exercise, and if necessary use of oral hypoglycemic agents or administration of insulin. Most older individuals are fully able to learn the complicated concepts and tasks required. Consequently, making the adjustments in lifestyle necessary for adherence to a good diabetes treatment program may at times be easier.

Case (Part 3)

You recommend medical therapy for Mr. H., but he desires a trial of diet and exercise prior to adding "more medicines that might hurt me." You agree to a trial and arrange for close follow-up. Additionally, you order an ophthalmologic evaluation, nutrition consult, and stress test prior to initiating his exercise regimen.

Is Mr. H.'s diabetes likely to be controlled with diet and exercise alone?

What factors may affect his ability to adhere to appropriate dietary therapy?

Diet

Diet alone has varying degrees of success. Elderly patients with diabetes are able to improve diabetes control with diet and weight loss (21). However, they may find it difficult to adhere to a strict dietary regimen and maintain weight loss. Older adults with mobility problems may find exercise to increase caloric expenditure impossible. If dramatic dietary restriction is employed in order to reduce weight, nutrient and vitamin deficiencies may develop. Aggressive dietary management cannot be recommended under these circumstances. Other considerations specific to older adults (22) may limit the effectiveness of dietary therapy (Table 24.2).

A diabetic diet is relatively high in carbohydrates (50% to 60% of total calories), low in fat (<30% of total calories from fat, with 10% saturated fat, 10% polyunsaturated fat, and 10% monosaturated fat), and moderate in protein (~20% of total calories). If malnourished or chronically ill, the elderly patient should increase protein and energy intake. Vitamin and mineral supplements are indicated when caloric intake falls below 1000 kilocalories per day.

Exercise

The role of formalized exercise programs in the management of diabetes mellitus remains controversial. The beneficial effects of exercise on glucose tolerance have been well documented (23,24). Its effectiveness in lowering plasma glucose levels is unclear. The effects of exercise on glucose tolerance are disappointingly transient, lessening within days of stopping an exercise program (25). Exercise for older adults with diabetes may pose additional problems. Perhaps four fifths of older men with newly diagnosed mild diabetes are unable to participate in a regular training program because of other diseases or treatments (26). Exercise for control of hyperglycemia may thus not be feasible for many older adults. These benefits and the risks of exercise in older adults (19) are outlined in Table 24.3.

TABLE 24.2. Dietary therapy: special considerations for older adults with diabetes

Financial difficulty
Difficulty with shopping because of transportation or mobility problems
Poor food-preparation skills (particularly elderly widowed men)
Ingrained dietary habits
Difficulty following dietary instruction because of impaired cognitive function
Decreased taste
Increased frequency of constipation

Source: Minaker KL. Treatment of diabetes. In: Cassel CK, Leipzig RM, Cohen HJ, et al., eds. Geriatric Medicine, 4th ed. New York: Springer, 2003.

TABLE 24.3. Potential benefits and risks of exercise for older adults with diabetes

Benefits	Risks
Improved exercise tolerance	Sudden cardiac death
Improved glucose tolerance	Foot and joint injuries
Improved maximal oxygen consumption	Hypoglycemia
Increased muscle strength	
Decreased blood pressure	
Decreased body fat and increased muscle mass	
Improved lipid profile	
Improved sense of well-being	

Source: Minaker KL. Treatment of diabetes. In: Cassel CK, Leipzig RM, Cohen HJ, et al., eds. Geriatric Medicine, 4th ed. New York: Springer, 2003.

Case (Part 4)

Mr. H. returns and has successfully lost 5 lb. However, his fasting glucose is 180 mg/dL and hemoglobin A_{1c} is 8.8%. He agrees to medical therapy.
   What medication(s) would you prescribe?

Oral Hypoglycemic Agents

Increasingly, therapy for type 2 diabetes builds on diet and exercise, and has become more mechanistically focused. Single or combination chemotherapy is used. Current best practices require a normal hemoglobin A_{1c}, certainly less than 7%. For those individuals in whom the demands of therapy are too great, medication side effects are too great, or access to monitoring is not possible, a reduction in expectations and greater complication rates will be higher. In addition to administration of insulin, medications currently available can promote insulin secretion, increase insulin sensitivity, or slow the digestion/processing of complex carbohydrates.

Agents Increasing Insulin Secretion

Sulfonylureas

First-generation agents such as chlorpropamide (Diabinese) are largely of historical interest. Because of chlorpropamide's very long half-life (up to 60 hours), risk of hypoglycemia, and production of hyponatremia from stimulation of excess antidiuretic hormone, it is rarely used today.

Second-generation agents in the sulfonylurea class have largely replaced chlorpropamide. Glipizide (Glucotrol and Glucotrol XL) and glyburide (Micronase, Glynase, and Diabeta) have been standards for many years. All, however, are associated with weight gain and hypoglycemia, and are of less utility with higher fasting glucose levels. These drugs rarely produce hyponatremia from central stimulation of antidiuretic hormone. Once fasting glucose levels rise above 200 mg/dL, insulin secretory reserve is very limited and these agents are less likely to be successful. As a general principle, dosing with second-generation agents should be initiated at the lowest end of the dosing range until individual susceptibility to hypoglycemia is known. Dosing is each morning, or twice a day.

Meglitinides

Repaglinide (Prandin) is an agent given before each meal, as it has a short half-life and is a shorter, more rapidly acting agent than classic sulfonylureas. It is therefore most useful when postprandial elevation of glucose dominates the clinical picture. Weight gain and hypoglycemia are shared side effects with sulfonylureas. However, in the treatment design for an individual experiencing between meal hypoglycemia while taking sulfonylureas, repaglinide is attractive.

D-Phenylalanine

Nateglinide (Starlix), which is a chemical derivative of the amino acid phenylalanine, has a similar profile and mode of action as repaglinide. Because of its very short action, it is most useful in early diabetes when fasting glucoses are only mildly elevated.

Case (Part 5)

You begin Mr. H. on glipizide 5 mg a day. On a subsequent visit, he reports fingerstick glucose levels ranging from 100 to 150 mg/dL. He expresses disappointment in a 5-lb weight gain despite adhering to a diet and exercise program. Repeat hemoglobin A_{1c} is 7.9%.
  Would you consider changing Mr. H.'s medications?

Agents Increasing Insulin Action

Because of the recognition of insulin resistance as a fundamental component of type 2 diabetes mellitus, agents increasing tissue sensitivity and responsiveness to endogenous insulin have become cornerstones of treatment. A very beneficial treatment side effect is the promotion of weight loss by these agents.

Metformin

Metformin (Glucophage, Glucophage XL) is given once or twice a day and assists altered diabetes physiology by improving insulin-mediated effects on the liver. This results in improvement in fasting hyperglycemia. On initiating treatment bloating, cramps, and diarrhea may result. There is still a rare risk of lactic acidosis in individuals with renal, cardiac, or liver failure or in individuals undergoing contrast studies where borderline renal function is already present. Because of this, it is suggested that metformin dosing be done in high-risk settings, such as hospitalization, dehydration, or planned radiologic studies. When creatinine clearance is low (serum creatinine >1.5 mg/dL), or there is advanced liver, cardiac, or pulmonary disease, this agent should be avoided. Creatinine levels greater than 1.5 are seen in approximately 5 percent of all elderly individuals.

Thiazolidinediones

Rosiglitazone (Avandia) and pioglitazone (Actos) are both once or twice per day medicines taken with food that specifically assist in insulin action on muscle and fat. They are useful alternatives to metformin. As with metformin, hypoglycemia is rare. However, monthly monitoring of liver function is required as approximately 10% of patients develop hepatic enzyme elevations, and rare fatal hepatitis has occurred. These drugs are much more expensive than sulfonylureas.

Agents Slowing Carbohydrate Processing in the Gut

α-Glucosidase Inhibitors

Acarbose (Precose) and miglitol (Glyset) both reduce postprandial increases in blood sugars by inhibiting the breakdown of dietary carbohydrate. These agents are taken with the first food intake of every meal. Although they are useful adjunctive therapy for more severe diabetes, acarbose and miglitol are helpful in impaired glucose tolerance and mild diabetes as well. High doses of bran have also been associated with improved glucose intolerance and have the additional benefit of lowering cholesterol. The common side effect of all these agents is gas, bloating, and diarrhea.

Case (Part 6)

You prescribe metformin 500 mg a day for Mr. H. in addition to the glipizide. When Mr. H. returns, he reports no additional weight gain and hemoglobin A_{1c} is 7%.

What are some of the reasons for combination therapy prior to initiation of insulin?

Combination Therapy

In recent times the use of drug combinations has increased in order to avoid or minimize insulin therapy and its inconvenience, hypoglycemia, weight gain, and possible acceleration of other atherogenesis. Several drug combinations have emerged, based on successful experience in combining drugs with complementary mechanisms of action.

Stepwise addition of agents is the practical approach. The most studied combination is sulfonylurea and insulin. Clearly some secretion of endogenous insulin must still be present. In this combination, insulin is given at night and sulfonylurea is given before each meal to produce insulin increments in the postprandial state. Insulin and metformin have been used in combination, with the goal of improving insulin action. Two oral hypoglycemics have been studied in combination—sulfonylurea and metformin. This is an attractive combination as the first produces insulin release, and is now able to stimulate tissues that have been sensitized by metformin.

Prevention

Diabetes mellitus affects more than 100 million individuals worldwide and because of known risk factors common to many individuals that can be manipulated, the development of type 2 diabetes may potentially be modifiable. A number of clinical trials have addressed this hypothesis through dietary modification, physical activity, and drug treatment. Although some studies indicate protection against diabetes development, conclusions remain limited due to study design problems with randomization, subject selection, or intervention intensity.

For further details on the prevention of diabetes, see Chapter 46: Treatment of Diabetes. In: Cassel CK, et al., Geriatric Medicine, 4th ed., page 690.

General Principles

- The prevalence of diabetes mellitus increases with age. Additionally, a number of conditions related to diabetes (e.g., hypertension, stroke, and neuropathy) are more prevalent in older diabetics than in younger adults with diabetes.
- Classic symptoms of diabetes may not be present in older adults. Presenting symptoms may include urinary incontinence, delirium, or falls.
- In 1997, the American Diabetes Association (ADA) revised its diagnostic criteria to rely solely on a fasting plasma glucose value over 126 mg/dL (7.0 mmol/L).

- Although current ADA guidelines do not require an oral glucose tolerance test for diagnosis of diabetes, glucose intolerance in older adults is still a risk factor for the complications associated with diabetes mellitus.
- Older adults may have several physical and social considerations that can affect adherence to the treatment of diabetes.

Suggested Readings

Expert Committee on the Diagnosis and Classification of Diabetes Mellitus. Follow-up report on the diagnosis and classification of diabetes mellitus. Diabetes Care 2003;26(11):3160–3107. *The International Expert Committee re-examined the classification and diagnostic criteria for diabetics.*

Lipson LG. Diabetes in the elderly: diagnosis, pathogenesis, and therapy. Am J Med 1986;80(Suppl 5A):10–21. *A rational approach for the maintenance of glucose homeostasis is presented for older patients with diabetes.*

Minaker KL. Treatment of diabetes. In: Cassel CK, Leipzig RM, Cohen HJ, et al., eds. Geriatric Medicine, 4th ed. New York: Springer, 2003:681–694.

Morrow LA, Halter JB. Treatment of diabetes mellitus in the elderly. In: Weir GC, ed. Joslin's Diabetes Mellitus, 13th ed. New York: Lea & Febiger, 1993. *A comprehensive review of the basic principles of the management of diabetes mellitus among older adults.*

References

1. Harris MI. Undiagnosed NIDDM: clinical and public health issues. Diabetes Care 1993;16:642–652.
2. Kilvert A, Fitzgerald MG, Wright AD, et al. Clinical characteristics and aetiological classification of insulin-dependent diabetes in the elderly. Q J Med 1986;60:865–872.
3. Wolf PA, D'Agostino RB, Belanger AJ, Kannel WB. Probability of stroke: a risk profile from the Framingham Study. Stroke 1991;22:312–318.
4. Elahi D, Muller DC. Carbohydrate metabolism in the elderly. Eur J Clin Nutr 2000;54:S112–S120.
5. Jackson RA, Blix PM, Matthews JA, et al. Influence of aging on glucose homeostasis. J Clin Endocrinol Metab 1982;55:840–848.
6. Jackson RA, Hawa MI, Roshania RD, et al. Influence of aging on hepatic and peripheral glucose metabolism in humans. Diabetes 1988;37:119–129.
7. Forbes GB, Reina JC. Adult lean body mass declines with age: some longitudinal observations. Metabolism 1977;19:653–663.
8. Sallis JF, Haskell WL, Wood PD, et al. Physical activity assessment methodology in the Five-City Project. Am J Epidemiol 1985;121:91–106.
9. Skarfors ET, Selinus KI, Lithell HO. Risk factors for developing non-insulin-dependent diabetes. A 10-year follow-up of men in Uppsala. Br Med J 1991;303:755–760.

10. Tibblin G, Adlerberth A, Lindstedt GB, Björntorp P. The pituitary-gonadal axis and health in elderly men. Diabetes 1996;45:1605–1609.

11. Goodman-Gruen D, Barrett-Connor E. Sex hormone-binding globulin and glucose tolerance in post-menopausal women. The Rancho Bernardo Study. Diabetes Care 1997;20:645–649.

12. Salmeron J, Asherio A, Rimm EB, Colditz GA, Spiegelman D, Jenkins DJ, et al. Dietary fiber, glycemic load, and risk of NIDDM in men. Diabetes Care 1997;20:545–550.

13. Lipton RB, Liao Y, Cao G, Cooper RS, McGee D. Determinants of incident non-insulin-dependent diabetes mellitus among blacks and whites in a national sample. The NHANES I Epidemiologic follow-up study. Am J Epidemol 1993;138:826–964.

14. Meneilly GS, Hards L, Tessier D, Elliott T, Tildesley H. NIDDM in the elderly. Diabetes Care 1996;19:1320–1325.

15. Ellenberg M. Diabetic neuropathic cachexia. Diabetes 1974;23:418–423.

16. World Health Organization. Diabetes Mellitus: Report of a WHO Study Group. Geneva: WHO, 1985.

17. National Diabetes Data Group. Classification and diagnosis of diabetes mellitus and other categories of glucose intolerance. Diabetes 1979;28: 1039–1057.

18. Alberti KG, Zimmet PZ. Definition, diagnosis and classification of diabetes mellitus and its complications. Part 1: diagnosis and classification of diabetes mellitus provisional report of a WHO consultation, Diabet Med 1998;15:539–553.

19. The Expert Committee on the Diagnosis and Classification of Diabetes Mellitus. Report of the expert committee on the diagnosis and classification of diabetes mellitus. Diabetes Care 1997;20:1183–1197.

20. Morrow LA, Halter JB. Treatment of diabetes mellitus in the elderly. In: Weir GC, ed. Joslin's Diabetes Mellitus, 13th ed. New York: Lea & Febiger, 1993.

21. American Diabetes Association. Standards of medical care for patients with diabetes mellitus. Diabetes Care 1989;12:365–368.

22. Reaven GM. Beneficial effect of moderate weight loss in older patients with non-insulin-dependent diabetes mellitus poorly controlled with insulin. J Am Geriatr Soc 1985;33:93–95.

23. Lipson LG. Diabetes in the elderly: diagnosis, pathogenesis, and therapy. Am J Med 1986;80(suppl 5A):10–21.

24. Holloszy JO, Schultz J, Kursnierkiewicz J, et al. Effects of exercise on glucose tolerance and insulin resistance. Brief review and some preliminary results. Acta Med Scand Suppl 1986;711:55–65.

25. Schneider SH, Amorosa LF, Khachadurian AK, et al. Studies on the mechanism of improved glucose control during regular exercise in type 2 (non-insulin-dependent) diabetes. Diabetologia 1984;26:355–360.

26. Skarfors ET, Wegener TA, Lithell H, et al. Physical training as treatment for type 2 (non-insulin-dependent) diabetes in elderly men. A feasibility study over 2 years. Diabetologia 1987;30:930–933.

25
Thyroid Disorders

AUDREY K. CHUN

Learning Objectives

Upon completion of the chapter, the student will be able to:

1. Identify the common and atypical presentations of thyroid disorders in older adults.
2. Interpret common tests used to evaluate thyroid disease.
3. Recognize the presentation of thyroid emergencies in older adults.
4. Consider basic concepts in the management of thyroid disorders.

Case A

Mrs. A. is a healthy 65-year-old woman who comes to you for her yearly exam. She denies any new problems but wonders if she should be screened for thyroid disease because her good friend is now taking thyroid replacement hormone. Review of systems reveals occasional constipation and fatigue. She denies decreased appetite, weight loss, palpitations, or depression. The physical exam is normal.

What changes occur in the thyroid with normal aging?
What tests are available to evaluate thyroid function?

General Considerations

Thyroid problems in the elderly are commonly encountered and are challenging to diagnose and treat. In the geriatric population, the prevalence of certain thyroid diseases (e.g., nodules, goiter, hypothyroidism) is high,

---

Material in this chapter is based on the following chapter in Cassel CK, Leipzig RM, Cohen HJ, Larson EB, Meier DE, eds. Geriatric Medicine: An Evidence-Based Approach, 4th ed. New York: Springer, 2003: Cooper DS. Thyroid Disorders, pp. 695–717. Selections edited by Audrey K. Chun.

and some thyroid disorders (e.g., hyperthyroidism), may have subtle or atypical presentations (1). In older patients with common nonthyroidal illnesses, thyroid function tests may be altered, making their interpretation all the more difficult. Finally, therapy may be more complex than in younger patients, due to the presence of underlying chronic illness, especially cardiac disease, and because of altered thyroid hormone metabolism.

Age-Associate Changes Related to Thyroid Anatomy and Function

During normal aging, atrophy and fibrosis of the thyroid occur. There is a corresponding reduction in thyroid weight, making palpation of the normal thyroid more difficult.

A number of studies have examined possible changes in thyroid function with advancing age. Most studies show little, if any, change in circulating thyroxine (T_4) or free T_4 levels in the blood, and the normal range for thyroid-stimulating hormone (TSH) should not differ between younger and older individuals. Possible alterations in serum triiodothyronine (T_3) concentrations are more controversial. The reported decline in serum T_3 noted by some investigators may be secondary to the presence of subtle or occult infirmities associated with aging, rather than the aging process itself.

Thyroid Function Testing

The many recent advances in the laboratory measurement of thyroid function have greatly simplified the evaluation of thyroid dysfunction. Even subtle forms of hypo- and hyperthyroidism can be diagnosed easily.

Measurement of Thyroid-Stimulating Hormone

The pituitary gland is exquisitely sensitive to changes in circulating thyroid hormone concentrations. Serum TSH levels, therefore, are elevated even in mild primary hypothyroidism and, theoretically, TSH levels should be low in virtually all forms of hyperthyroidism. Of course, the serum TSH level is inappropriately low in hypothyroid patients with pituitary or hypothalamic failure, and in the rare patient with a TSH-secreting pituitary adenoma causing hyperthyroidism, the TSH level is inappropriately elevated or normal.

Measurement of Thyroid Hormone Concentrations

Radioimmunoassays for T_4 and T_3 are routinely available with rapid turnaround times, but alterations in thyroxine-binding globulin (TBG) affect the total T_4 and T_3 concentrations without affecting circulating free thyroid

TABLE 25.1. Major causes of abnormal serum thyroxine (T_4) concentrations in elderly patients

Increased T_4	Decreased T_4
Hyperthyroidism	Hypothyroidism
Increased protein binding	TBG deficiency
TBG excess	Serious illness
Anti-T_4 antibodies	Anticonvulsant therapy
Abnormal binding proteins	
Acute illness (transient)	
Decreased T_4 catabolism	
Amiodarone	
High-dose propranolol	

TBG, thyroxine-binding globulin.
Source: Cooper DS. Thyroid disorders. In: Cassel CK, Leipzig RM, Cohen HJ, et al., eds. Geriatric Medicine, 4th ed. New York: Springer, 2003.

hormone concentrations. Thus, patients with TBG excess or deficiency have high or low T_4 and T_3 concentrations, respectively, but are clinically and biochemically euthyroid. Direct measurement of free T_4 has become more popular due to improved cost-effectiveness. It has rapidly replaced the free thyroxine index (FTI), which is the product of total T_4 and the T_3 resin uptake (T_3RU). The T_3RU is an indirect approximation of TBG binding capacity, and, when used in concert with the total T_4 concentration, it permits one to distinguish true thyroid disease from perturbations in TBG concentration. It is important not to confuse the T_3RU, which uses radioactive T_3 in vitro, with the direct assay of serum T_3 (the T_3 radioimmunoassay).

A low serum T_4 level is characteristic of hypothyroidism, while an elevated T_4 is seen in most patients with hyperthyroidism. However, other causes should be considered when evaluating an abnormal T_4 level (Table 25.1).

Radionuclide Evaluation of Thyroid Structure and Function

The thyroid gland traps iodide and other ions, permitting glandular morphology and function to be assessed with isotopes of iodine (^{123}I and ^{131}I) and technetium (^{99m}TcO$_4$). Technetium is used frequently to image the thyroid, because it is inexpensive and convenient (imaging after 20 minutes). But because it is trapped but not organized (unlike iodide), it cannot provide as much useful information about overall thyroid function as does iodide, with imaging after 6 to 24 hours. Although the 24-hour radioactive iodine uptake (RAIU) is of limited usefulness, thyroid scanning is helpful in determining the size and location of thyroid tissue and the functional nature of thyroid nodules. It is also invaluable in the diagnosis of functioning metastases from well-differentiated thyroid cancer.

Other Thyroid-Related Tests

Antithyroid antibodies are important in establishing the diagnosis of autoimmune thyroid disease. Antithyroglobulin antibodies are thought to be less specific than antithyroid peroxidase (anti-TPO antibodies). Thyroglobulin is released from the thyroid in a host of thyroid disorders, so it is not useful diagnostically. Its measurement is most crucial in the follow-up of patients with well-differentiated thyroid cancer. Thyroid needle biopsy and ultrasonography are discussed below (see Thyroid Goiter; for further details regarding these tests, see Chapter 47: Thyroid Disorders. In: Cassel CK, et al., eds. Geriatric Medicine, 4th ed., page 698).

Case B (Part 1)

Mrs. B. is a 72-year-old woman with a history of coronary artery disease who comes to your office with complaints of decreased appetite and weight loss. She denies any chest pain or palpitations. Her recent stress test, colonoscopy, and mammogram were all within normal limits. Physical exam reveals only borderline tachycardia with a heart rate of 95/min and a depressed affect. The exam is otherwise normal including palpation of the thyroid gland. You are concerned about the weight loss and order labs including a TSH. The TSH is reported as "undetectable."

What symptoms and signs of hyperthyroidism are common in older adults?

What are the possible reasons for the undetectable TSH level?

What treatment should be initiated?

Hyperthyroidism: General Considerations

Thyrotoxicosis is being recognized with increasing frequency in the elderly. Graves' disease is the most common cause of thyrotoxicosis in all age groups, but the proportion of patients with toxic multinodular goiter (Plummer's disease) increases with age. Because the prevalence of thyroid nodularity in general is higher in the elderly, some older patients with preexisting nontoxic nodules undoubtedly develop thyrotoxicosis due to Graves' disease, accounting for diagnostic difficulty. On the other hand, 20% to 50% of elderly thyrotoxic patients have nonpalpable thyroid glands, also making the diagnosis more obscure (2).

Diagnostic Evaluation

Symptoms and Signs

In contrast to the classic symptoms and signs of hyperthyroidism in younger individuals, elderly patients typically display few of the sympathomimetic features that are characteristic of the thyrotoxic state. Thus, the apt term *masked* or *apathetic thyrotoxicosis* has been applied to the elderly thyrotoxic patient who presents with depression, lethargy, weakness, and cachexia. Agitation and confusion (thyrotoxic encephalopathy) can mimic dementia (3). Unexplained weight loss, nervousness, palpitations, and tremulousness are present in well over half the patients, with weight loss occurring in up to 80% (3). Hyperthyroidism causes increased bone turnover, and the presence of what appears to be typical postmenopausal osteoporosis should prompt screening for hyperthyroidism.

It is well known that the cardiovascular system retains its sensitivity to thyroid hormone action in the elderly. This, coupled with a high prevalence of atherosclerotic coronary disease, probably is the explanation for palpitations, worsening angina, and, more rarely, symptoms of congestive heart failure. Atrial fibrillation, often with a relatively slow ventricular response (4), is the presenting feature in up to 20% of patients, and the development of atrial fibrillation should always prompt a thorough screen for thyrotoxicosis.

Laboratory Findings

In contrast to the ease with which the laboratory diagnosis of thyrotoxicosis is made in younger patients, thyroid function test interpretation in the elderly can be a vexing problem. Most truly hyperthyroid individuals have TSH levels that are below the limit of detection in a sensitive or a third-generation assay. Some euthyroid individuals with nontoxic multinodular goiter may have subclinical hyperthyroidism with normal T_4, free T_4, and T_3 levels, but with suppression of the hypothalamic pituitary axis (4). The TSH levels also may be low in hospitalized patients, and may be undetectable even in third-generation TSH assays in critically ill patients (5). However, such patients usually have low rather than high serum T_4 levels, and exclusion of central hypothyroidism is the diagnostic problem, rather than hyperthyroidism.

The 24-hour RAIU is normal in up to 30% of elderly patients with Graves' disease and in over two thirds of elderly individuals with toxic multinodular goiter (Plummer's disease), and is therefore often not helpful in ruling in hyperthyroidism. The measurement of serum T_3 and possibly free T_3 in patients with normal serum T_4 levels and low TSH levels should facilitate the laboratory evaluation and maximize diagnostic accuracy.

Differential Diagnosis

Before initiating a therapy for the thyrotoxic patient, the etiology of hyperthyroidism must be known. Graves' disease is the most frequent cause (in 50% to 70% of cases), followed by toxic multinodular goiter. Together, these two account for well over 95% of hyperthyroid patients.

Two uncommon forms of thyroiditis cause transient and self-limited hyperthyroidism, and are very uncommon in the elderly population. Subacute thyroiditis (De Quervain's) typically presents with severe anterior neck pain, fever, and general malaise and is thought to be viral in origin. Thyroid function test results are elevated due to release of stored hormone into the blood, but the 24-hour RAIU is low, because of damage to the thyroid gland as well as suppression of endogenous TSH by the high thyroid hormone levels. Painless ("silent") or lymphocytic thyroiditis, rare in the elderly, presents with thyrotoxicosis and small painless goiter (6). It can be extremely difficult to distinguish from Graves' disease by laboratory testing, except that, as in subacute thyroiditis, the 24-hour RAIU is very low.

Another diagnosis that should be considered in the elderly patient with thyrotoxicosis is the possibility of a TSH-secreting pituitary tumor. The hallmark is the presence of serum TSH levels that are inappropriate given the elevations in serum T_4 and T_3 levels (i.e., instead of being suppressed, TSH levels are normal or high).

Finally, iodine-induced thyrotoxicosis (*Jod-Basedow phenomenon*) occurs in individuals exposed to iodide or iodide-containing compounds who have an underlying multinodular goiter. The problem has become more common with the recent introduction of the antiarrhythmic amiodarone. There may be two types of amiodarone-induced thyrotoxicosis: one developing in patients with a preexisting multinodular goiter and a second, inflammatory type that resembles painless thyroiditis and may respond to steroid therapy, rather than to antithyroid drugs (7).

Management Considerations

The three treatments for hyperthyroidism are antithyroid drugs, radioactive iodine, and surgery. In elderly patients, surgery is rarely employed because of its attendant morbidity, unless a large toxic multinodular goiter is present and causing local symptoms (dysphagia and/or dyspnea). Additionally, in elderly patients, late complications of radioiodine are less relevant and the major goal is definitive therapy with permanent cure. Thus, radioiodine ablation is the treatment of choice for virtually all older thyrotoxic patients (8). A major concern of radioactive iodine therapy is the possible exacerbation of thyrotoxicosis after treatment, due to the release of preformed thyroid hormone into the circulation from radiation-induced thyroiditis. Following radioiodine therapy, patients must be followed up expectantly for the development of iatrogenic hypothyroidism. This complication occurs almost inevitably in patients with Graves' disease but is less common in toxic nodular goiter (9), presumably due to the failure of radioiodine to be concentrated in suppressed regions of the gland. The presence of a persistent goiter is a clinical clue that the hypothyroidism is likely to be transient, rather than permanent.

Antithyroid drugs (propylthiouracil and methimazole) cause fever, rash, and arthralgias in 1% to 5% of individuals. Agranulocytosis occurs in approximately one in 300 to 500 patients (usually in the first 2 months of treatment) and may be more common in elderly patients (10). Methimazole in low doses (<20mg/d) may pose less of a risk of agranulocytosis than propylthiouracil, and methimazole has the added advantage of being a once-a-day agent, which improves compliance. Patients beginning antithyroid drug therapy should be warned that if fever or oropharyngitis develops, the medication should be stopped immediately and the physician contacted.

The β-adrenergic blocking agents are an important adjunct in the management of thyrotoxicosis (11). Rapid and almost complete resolution of cardiac and neuromuscular symptoms can be accomplished with agents in this class. They do not normalize oxygen consumption or reverse the negative nitrogen balance that typifies the thyrotoxic state, and they should therefore not be used as sole therapy except in those rare patients with self-limited disease due to thyroiditis. These agents are extremely useful before and after antithyroid drug and radioiodine therapy, because euthyroidism generally is not attained for 1 to 2 months after antithyroid drugs are started or for up to 12 months after radioiodine.

Case B (Part 2)

Mrs. B. returns to you after missing her last several appointments. She is accompanied by her daughter, who states that Mrs. B. did not take her medications and missed the appointment with the endocrinologist. Her mother has been increasingly agitated over the last several days and appears to be short of breath. On exam, she is lethargic and dyspneic. Vital signs reveal blood pressure 100/50mmHg, heart rate = 120/min, respiration rate = 24/min, temperature = 39°C. Lung exam is significant for crackles in both lung fields and the heart sounds have an irregularly irregular rhythm. You admit her to the hospital immediately.

What is happening to Mrs. B.?

Severe Hyperthyroidism and Thyroid Storm

Thyroid storm is a state of decompensated thyrotoxicosis, defined by severe hypermetabolism, fever, neuropsychiatric changes, and, often, congestive heart failure. Thyroid function test results are no different in patients with thyroid storm than in those with less severe clinical disease. Rather, the ability to deal with the hypermetabolic state is compromised, often by the superimposed stress of acute illness (e.g., infection) or trauma (e.g., surgery). Therapy consists of fluid and electrolyte support, active cooling, and large doses of antithyroid drugs, iodide or iodinated contrast agents, and beta-blockers. Additionally, stress doses of glucocorticoids are usually employed. Due to the relatively more apathetic presentation of hyperthyroidism in elderly patients, they tend to have a better prognosis than younger patients in thyroid storm (12).

For those patients who are so severely ill with thyrotoxicosis that hospitalization is required, or if thyrotoxicosis occurs in the setting of severe medical illness (e.g., myocardial infarction), more rapid control of the disease is desirable. Large doses of antithyroid drugs are typically employed (e.g., 200 mg every 6 hours of propylthiouracil or 40 to 80 mg/d of methimazole as a single dose), which theoretically blocks thyroid hormone production completely. However, because thyroid hormone release is unaffected by antithyroid drugs, other agents must be employed to achieve an expeditious resolution of the thyrotoxic state. Traditionally, potassium iodide [as saturated solution of potassium iodide (SSKI), containing 35 mg of iodide per drop or Lugol's solution, containing 8 mg of iodide per drop] has been used for this purpose, because iodine is a potent inhibitor of thyroid hormone release. Doses range form 100 to 500 mg/d in divided doses; iodide should be given only after the patient has been started on antithyroid drugs.

More recently, the iodinated oral cholecystographic contrast agents sodium ipodate (Telepaque) and sodium iopanoate (Oragrafin) have been used in dosages of 1 to 2 g daily in divided doses. These compounds release free iodide into the circulation, which inhibits thyroid hormone secretion. They are also potent inhibitors of T_4 to T_3 conversion and rapidly lower serum T_3 levels toward normal.

The adrenergic blockers also are efficacious in reversing sympathomimetic symptoms and signs due to circulating thyroid hormone. For life-threatening tachyarrhythmias, 1 mg of propranolol hydrochloride can be given slowly intravenously, with the dose repeated every 5 minutes, or esmolol, a shorter-acting agent can be employed. For those patients in atrial fibrillation for whom beta-blockers are contraindicated, a calcium channel blocker such as diltiazem can be used (13).

Subclinical Hyperthyroidism

With the development of sensitive TSH assays came the ability to detect a more subtle form of thyroid dysfunction, in which the TSH levels are low or undetectable, but the T_4, free T_4, and T_3 levels are within normal limits. Patients with this constellation of laboratory results generally have few or no symptoms of hyperthyroidism, and may or may not have a palpable goiter on physical examination. Subclinical hyperthyroidism has been noted in 1% to 5% of older persons, with a higher frequency if those who are taking excessive quantities of thyroxine are included (14). This condition has been associated with a higher risk of overt hyperthyroidism, atrial fibrillation, and possible decreased bone density (15). Therefore, although treatment of elderly asymptomatic individuals with subclinical hyperthyroidism could be justified to protect the cardiovascular system or the skeleton, it remains controversial (15). Certainly, if subclinical hyperthyroidism is due to overzealous thyroxine replacement therapy, the dose of medication should be adjusted until the TSH levels are normal.

Case C

Mrs. C. is a 78-year-old woman with a long history of diabetes mellitus. She comes to your office with multiple complaints including fatigue, constipation, and weakness. These symptoms have progressed over the last several months. She denies cold intolerance or new edema. Physical exam reveals normal vital signs and a nonpalpable thyroid gland. Laboratory values reveal a TSH of 15 and a low free T_4.

What are the common physical manifestations of hypothyroidism in older adults?

What is the most common cause of hypothyroidism in older adults?

Hypothyroidism: General Considerations

Approximately 70% of hypothyroid patients are over age 50 years at the time of diagnosis (16). The prevalence of hypothyroidism in the population depends on how the condition is defined: if a low serum T_4 or free T_4 level is the criterion, approximately 0.5% of individuals (largely women) over age 65 years will be found to be overtly hypothyroid. If the more liberal definition of an elevated serum TSH level with or without a low T_4 level is employed, up to 17.5% of individuals over age 75 years will have mild hypothyroidism (17,18). This latter situation may be more appropriately termed "*subclinical hypothyroidism*," because serum T_4 and free T_4 levels are still within the broad range of normal (19).

Diagnostic Evaluation

Symptoms and Signs

The diagnosis of hypothyroidism is not difficult in a young patient with typical symptoms of fatigue, weight gain, dry skin, cold intolerance, and constipation. In elderly patients, however, these same complaints are attributed all too often to the aging process itself. The problem is further complicated by the insidious development of symptoms, often over a period of years, and by patients who present in an atypical manner or with no symptoms at all. Older hypothyroid patients were more likely to present with fatigue and weakness, and less likely to have cold intolerance, weight gain, paresthesiae, and muscle cramps compared to younger hypothyroid patients (20).

Certain findings on physical examination should alert the clinician to the possibility of hypothyroidism. Hypertension, for example, can be a presenting sign, as can bradycardia and, surprisingly, various tachyarrhythmias. Hypothermic patients always should be evaluated for hypothyroidism, hypoglycemia, and sepsis. Although nonpitting edema of the face and limbs is a hallmark of hypothyroidism, pitting edema also is frequently found, possibly due to a lowered glomerular filtration rate and decreased cardiac output. Frank congestive heart failure is unusual in hypothyroidism, and cardiomegaly more often is due to the presence of pericardial effusion; while the pericardial effusions in hypothyroidism are usually not hemodynamically significant, tamponade has been described. Pleural effusions and ascites also can be seen. Additionally, all patient with dementia should be evaluated for possible hypothyroidism.

Laboratory Findings

Hypothyroidism is perhaps the simplest thyroid functional abnormality to diagnose. The hallmark of primary hypothyroidism is a low serum free thyroxine index or free T_4, with concomitant elevation of the serum TSH. Measurement of T_3 is of little use in the diagnosis of hypothyroidism, because normal serum levels are often maintained until severe hypothyroidism supervenes.

Several pitfalls in the laboratory diagnosis of hypothyroidism warrant mention. First, some patients with secondary hypothyroidism (i.e., due to hypothalamic or pituitary disease with TSH deficiency) have low T_4 values with inappropriately low or normal serum TSH levels. In hypothalamic/pituitary disease, the pituitary may secrete a TSH molecule that is immunologically active in the radioimmunoassay but has lower than normal bioactivity. Thus, if hypothyroidism is suspected clinically and serum T_4 values are low, evaluation of hypothalamic and pituitary anatomy and function is indicated, even if the serum TSH level is normal. Generally, other hormonal deficits are present in this clinical circumstance such as adrenal insufficiency, low follicle-stimulating hormone (FSH) and luteinizing hormone (LH) in a postmenopausal woman, or hypogonadotropic hypogonadism in a man.

A second problem that confounds the diagnosis of hypothyroidism is severe illness (21). It may be extremely difficult to distinguish a critically ill patient with low T_4 and normal or low TSH levels from one with secondary hypothyroidism (see above). To further complicate matters, serum TSH levels occasionally rise during the recovery phase of illness, often to levels consistent with primary hypothyroidism. In this circumstance, repeating the TSH measurement after recovery is complete is the appropriate strategy.

Differential Diagnosis

The most common cause of hypothyroidism in the elderly is autoimmune thyroid failure (Hashimoto's thyroiditis, chronic lymphocytic thyroiditis). In parallel with the high prevalence of autoimmune thyroiditis in the elderly, the prevalence of antithyroid antibody positivity also rises with age (22). Over two thirds of patients with thyroid failure have antithyroid antibodies (23). Two types of antithyroid antibodies have been described in Hashimoto's thyroiditis: antimicrosomal (antithyroid peroxidase or anti-TPO antibodies) and antithyroglobulin. Antimicrosomal antibodies are highly specific for autoimmune thyroiditis. Antithyroglobulin antibodies, on the other hand, are not as specific for autoimmune thyroid disease, and their presence in the absence of antimicrosomal antibody is not sufficient to establish the diagnosis.

Iatrogenic hypothyroidism is an additional important, though less frequent, cause of thyroid failure. Radioiodine and surgical therapy for Graves' disease usually lead to permanent hypothyroidism. Additionally, several studies suggest that permanent hypothyroidism is a late phase in the evolution of drug-treated Graves' disease. Not surprisingly, external beam radiotherapy to the head and neck region also can cause late thyroid hypofunction. Lithium and iodine-containing medications can provoke hypothyroidism; this has become an increasing problem with the antiarrhythmic amiodarone, which is used widely in older patients. Finally, many patients with subacute or painless thyroiditis have mild transient hypothyroidism following hyperthyroidism, but this rarely requires therapy. Hypothalamic and pituitary disease are unusual causes of hypothyroidism.

Management Considerations

Once the diagnosis of primary hypothyroidism is made, therapy with thyroxine should be initiated. Patients with chronic fatigue or obesity who are not hypothyroid should never be treated with this drug. Thyroxine is generally well absorbed from the gastrointestinal tract, although the fractional absorption may decline slightly with age (24). Its long serum half-life produces nonfluctuating serum levels. Cholestyramine, sucralfate, aluminum hydroxide, and possibly ferrous sulfate and calcium supplements interfere with its absorption and should not be taken concurrently. As in healthy untreated individuals, much of the orally administered thyroxine is deiodinated to T_3, at a rate determined by the patient's clinical status (i.e., decreased in illness or starvation).

The dictum "start low, go slow" should be followed in elderly patients when initiating thyroxine therapy, because rapid increases in myocardial oxygen consumption theoretically could trigger or worsen angina. Therefore, it is best to be prudent and initiate treatment with doses of 25 to 50 μg/d, with monthly monitoring of thyroid function. The biochemical goal of therapy is the normalization of serum TSH levels in a sensitive TSH assay. The TSH level should not be below the normal range, which would suggest overreplacement. Even seemingly minor changes in dose can cause large changes in serum TSH values. Overreplacement is to be avoided, not only because of untoward cardiac effects but also because of convincing data in postmenopausal women showing that even mild asymptomatic iatrogenic hyperthyroidism can be associated with accelerated bone loss (25). The dose requirement may be higher in patients with malabsorption or in those taking anticonvulsants or amiodarone.

A large and potentially bewildering number of thyroid hormone preparations are available. They are traditionally classified as "synthetic" or "biologic." Synthetic thyroxine is the therapy of choice. The "biologic" thyroid hormone preparations include desiccated thyroid, derived from the thyroid glands of slaughterhouse animals. The generic biologic preparations are notorious for their lack of standardization. The proprietary preparations have better quality control but suffer from the same problem as liotrix and T_3, that is, they contain T_3, which is an undesirable drug for chronic replacement therapy. Most endocrinologists agree that the biologic preparations are of historical interest only. Patients who are taking them should be switched to synthetic thyroxine at doses of 0.8 μg/lb body weight per day.

Subclinical Hypothyroidism

Subclinical hypothyroidism is defined biochemically as normal serum T_4 and free T_4 levels with an elevated serum TSH level. It is one of the most common thyroid disorders among elderly persons, being present in up to 17.5% of women over age 60 years. Most patients have circulating antithyroid antibodies, suggesting that the condition is autoimmune in nature (26). Some patients have a history of Graves' disease, whereas others are taking drugs (lithium or iodide-containing compounds) that are known to inhibit thyroid function, especially in the presence of underlying autoimmune thyroid disease. Because of the high prevalence of subclinical hypothyroidism in elderly women, routine screening (every 5 years) of older individuals for hypothyroidism with a serum TSH determination has been recommended by the American Thyroid Association (27) and several other professional organizations, including the American College of Physicians (28).

A central question is whether patients with subclinical hypothyroidism, who are seemingly asymptomatic and appear to be suffering solely from a biochemical abnormality, should be treated. Although no definite answer can be provided at this time, one study indicated that patients with subclinical hypothyroidism do have subtle symptoms consistent with mild thyroid failure (29). Replacement therapy might be used as prophylaxis against overt hypothyroidism.

Myxedema Coma

Myxedema coma, like its hyperthyroid counterpart thyroid storm, results from the physiologic decompensation of a hypothyroid individual (30). Generally, there is a precipitating factor, most often an undiagnosed infection. Patients with myxedema coma are not necessarily comatose and can present with stupor, seizures, or psychotic manifestations. Myxedema coma is most often a disease of elderly hypothyroid individuals and generally occurs in the winter months.

The diagnosis of myxedema coma usually is difficult, although it is made easier if there is a history of thyroid disorder or a neck scar or proptosis on physical examination. Hypothermia is a frequent, but not invariable, manifestation; its absence should suggest an occult infection. If the diagnosis is considered, therapy should be initiated, because the mortality approaches 50%, even with treatment. Optimal management consists of scrupulous attention to the patient's pulmonary, cardiovascular, gastrointestinal, and renal status. Often intubation and ventilatory assistance are necessary because of carbon dioxide retention. Active warming is contraindicated, because severe hypotension may supervene. A search for infection and prompt treatment is mandatory. Hyponatremia is common, and free water must be administered judiciously. Sedatives and narcotics should be avoided because of the risk of further respiratory depression. Stress doses of glucocorticoids are usually given until adrenal insufficiency has been formally ruled out.

Thyroxine should be administered intravenously, because gastrointestinal absorption may be altered because of hypomotility. Initial doses of 0.3 to 0.5 mg have been traditionally recommended to replace the total body thyroid hormone pool, with daily doses of 0.1 mg thereafter.

Case D

Mrs. D. is a 72-year-old woman who comes to you for follow-up of her depression. On physical exam you palpate a single thyroid nodule. She denies any palpitations, fatigue, worsening depression, constipation, or weight loss/gain.

What is the significance of this exam finding?

What diagnostic tests should be ordered to work up this nodule?

Thyroid Nodules: General Considerations

Clinically significant nodules, that is, those that come to medical attention because they are palpable, are more prevalent in the elderly, with approximately 5% of adults having a palpable nodule in the Framingham study population. As would be expected, palpable nodules are also much more common in women than in men (6% vs. 2% in the Framingham study) (31). It is useful to distinguish clinically solitary nodules and so-called dominant nodules (nodules that are larger than the others that may be palpably present within the gland), because these have a greater likelihood of being malignant. Fortunately, malignancy is present in only about 10% of nodules, a frequency that is no higher and is perhaps lower than in younger patients with thyroid nodules. Given the low likelihood of malignancy, it is a challenge to diagnose and treat those nodules that are cancerous while at the same time avoiding unnecessary surgery in the 90% of patients who have benign disease.

Diagnostic Evaluation

Symptoms and Signs

Although a number of historical features (older age, male, rapid nodule growth, compressive symptoms) and physical findings (firm or rock-hard consistency, fixation to underlying neck structures, and cervical adenopathy) are important clues that suggest malignancy, there is considerable overlap in findings with benign nodules. Only a distinct minority of malignant nodules have a classic clinical presentation.

A history of head, neck, or upper thoracic radiation in childhood or adolescence is important to elicit. From the 1920s through the early 1960s, several million people received external irradiation for thymic enlargement, tonsillitis, mastoiditis, acne, and a host of other benign conditions. Many thousands of irradiated patients who are now in the geriatric population are at excess (three- to 10-fold) risk for the development of thyroid cancer, as well as benign nodular disease. In addition, it is becoming clear that radiation for malignancies that included the thyroid gland in the radiation port, for example, the mantle area for Hodgkin's disease, can also be associated with thyroid carcinoma. Thus, a history of radiation exposure warrants a prompt and definitive evaluation.

Laboratory Findings

Results of routine thyroid function tests are almost always normal, but are worth obtaining to find the rare patient with hyperthyroidism due to an autonomously functioning nodule, and to enable the diagnosis of hypothyroidism, which would suggest Hashimoto's thyroiditis as the underlying disease process.

Other blood tests should be used more selectively. A serum calcitonin determination should be obtained only if there is a family history of medullary thyroid carcinoma or other condition suggestive of multiple endocrine neoplasia syndrome type 2. Antithyroid antibody assays might be performed if the serum TSH level is elevated, suggesting Hashimoto's thyroiditis. Serum thyroglobulin levels are nonspecifically elevated in a host of thyroid diseases, and this determination is used mainly in the follow-up of patients with thyroid cancer.

An approach that is gaining wider acceptance is the performance of needle biopsy as the initial diagnostic step (32). Traditionally, after routine blood tests, thyroid scanning with radioiodine or technetium has been the next step in the workup of a thyroid nodule. Nodules that concentrate the radionuclide ("hot" nodules) are, for practical purposes, never malignant, and require no further evaluation other than to be sure that hyperthyroidism is not present. On the other hand, hypofunctioning nodules ("cold" nodules) require further evaluation with needle biopsy. However, it is not cost-effective, because at least 90% of all nodules are hypofunctioning. The advantage of needle biopsy as the next diagnostic step is that a scan is avoided in the 90% of patients who would require a biopsy. The disadvantage is that the 10% of patients with "hot" nodules undergo biopsy needlessly. On the other hand, the fine-needle aspiration biopsy is a relatively painless procedure with virtually no morbidity.

Thyroid ultrasonography can be a useful technique for monitoring the size of nodules, particularly those that are difficult to palpate, although it is being used with less frequency nowadays. Although purely cystic lesions are not malignant, pure cysts of the thyroid are rare. In fact, over 95% of nodules are either solid or complex (having solid and cystic components), the latter having the same clinical implications as a solid lesion. Thus, routine ultrasonography is not a cost-effective initial diagnostic test.

Fine-Needle Aspiration Biopsy of Thyroid Nodules

Thyroid needle biopsy, and more specifically, fine-needle aspiration biopsy, has revolutionized the care of patients with thyroid disease. Its diagnostic accuracy depends on the skill of the person performing the procedure, and, even more importantly, on the expertise of the cytopathologist who is interpreting the aspirate. For malignancy, the false-negative rate is low (<1% to 5%), although the specificity is only about 70% (if suspicious nodules are included). The positive predictive value approaches 99% in most series (32,33). Most series report that 60% to 70% of lesions are benign and 5% are malignant. About 25% are indeterminate or suspicious, and these include less well-differentiated benign follicular adenomas, Hürthle cell neoplasms, and follicular carcinoma. Only 15% of suspicious lesions prove to be malignant at the time of surgery (20).

Differential Diagnosis

Although most thyroid nodules are, in fact, benign tumors, any generalized thyroid disease can present as a thyroid nodule. Thus, the various forms of thyroiditis (subacute, Hashimoto's) are not infrequently asymmetric in their involvement and can mimic a solitary nodule. Other rare causes of an apparent thyroid nodule include congenital hemiagenesis of the opposite lobe of the thyroid, cystic hygromas, and teratomas. Thyroid cysts and neoplasms (benign follicular adenomas, colloid nodules, nodular adenomatous hyperplasia, and carcinomas) comprise the majority of all nodules, however. Although most forms of thyroid cancer (papillary, medullary, anaplastic) are easily diagnosed by means of biopsy, follicular lesions are notoriously difficult to evaluate cytopathologically. While the majority of follicular neoplasms are benign, it can be extremely difficult to distinguish a more atypical benign tumor from a minimally invasive follicular carcinoma. Hürthle cell tumors, a variety of follicular adenoma once thought to always be malignant, are usually benign. Rarely, thyroid nodules are due to metastatic spread of cancer to the thyroid gland.

Management Considerations

Although excision of all nodules would be simultaneously diagnostic and curative, surgery, particularly in the elderly, is associated with excess morbidity as well as great potential expense. If the nodule is benign, then no further diagnostic evaluation is necessary, although continued follow-up is important. Malignant nodules require surgery. If a nodule is suspicious cytologically, the next step would be a thyroid scan, if it had not been performed prior to the biopsy, because suspicious lesions can be benign functioning ("hot") follicular adenomas. If the nodule is "hot," then additional laboratory studies should be performed to rule out hyperthyroidism. If the suspicious nodule is "cold," then excision is generally recommended. An alternative approach would be a 3- to 6-month trial of suppression therapy with thyroxine. If the nodule fails to decrease in size, then surgery is indicated. If the nodule shrinks, then close follow-up with continued thyroxine therapy is reasonable.

Thyroid Goiter

Goiter, or a generalized enlargement of the thyroid, is a common problem in the elderly. A significant minority of goiters are caused by Hashimoto's thyroiditis, but most are idiopathic. Pathologically, most idiopathic multinodular goiters consist of areas of nodular adenomatous hyperplasia, interspersed with hemorrhagic cysts, fibrosis, and calcification.

Aside from the history and physical examination, routine thyroid function tests, including a serum T_3 or a high-sensitivity serum TSH determination, should be performed in all patients with goiter, because of the possibility of subtle thyrotoxicosis. Antithyroid antibodies (especially antithyroid peroxidase antibodies), are also helpful in diagnosing autoimmune thyroiditis, especially in patients whose goiter is diffuse and firm on palpation. Computed tomography or magnetic resonance imaging (MRI) of the neck and chest can be helpful in delineating the extent of the goiter in the thorax, or the degree of tracheal deviation or compression, but generally these procedures are unnecessary.

The central issues in the patient with a large goiter are (1) whether malignancy is present and (2) whether there is clinically significant compression of adjacent neck structures. Regarding malignancy, if there is any suggestion of a recently enlarging goiter or if there is a dominant nodule within a multinodular goiter, a biopsy should be performed. With respect to esophageal or tracheal compression, a history of dysphagia or dyspnea is usually obtained. It should be emphasized, however, that upper-airway compromise may be subtle or asymptomatic, or may present as "asthma" or wheezing. Pulmonary function testing, with evaluation of upper-airway function by means of flow-volume loops, should be performed in all patients with large goiters who have suggestive respiratory symptoms or evidence of tracheal compression, even in the absence of symptoms.

The indications for surgery in elderly patients with large goiters are more stringent than in younger individuals. Obviously, malignancy or significant esophageal, tracheal, or venacaval compression mandate surgery. Although thyroid surgery is generally well tolerated, even by octogenarians, there is no reason to remove a large asymptomatic goiter simply because it is there and may cause trouble in the future, especially if it is cytologically benign.

As indicated earlier, patients with nontoxic multinodular goiter are susceptible to iodine-induced thyrotoxicosis. Iodine-containing compounds, including iodinated contrast media, should be avoided, if possible, in such patients.

Thyroid Cancer

Thyroid cancer in elderly patients shares many features with that seen in younger patients, but there are dramatic differences as well. The histologic types (papillary, follicular, medullary, anaplastic, lymphoma) all occur, but with a shift in histologic type from the more indolent (papillary) to the more aggressive (Hürthle cell, medullary, anaplastic). Even within a histologic category, advanced age portends a far worse prognosis (34,35). (For further details on thyroid cancer, see Chapter 47: Thyroid Disorders. In: Cassel CK, et al., eds. Geriatric Medicine, 4th ed., page 712.)

General Principles

- Measurement of TSH and free T_4 should help the clinician accurately diagnose the majority of thyroid disorders.
- Hyperthyroidism in older adults may have atypical symptoms such as constipation, depression, lethargy, weakness, and cachexia. It is usually characterized by a low or undectable TSH and elevate free T_4.
- Hypothyroidism in older adults may also have an atypical presentation that is often incorrectly attributed to aging itself. Common symptoms include weakness and fatigue rather than the classic symptoms of cold intolerance, constipation, weight gain, and muscle cramps. Usually, TSH is elevated and free T_4 is low.
- Treatment for subclinical hypothyroidism and hyperthyroidism should be considered because of the higher risk of morbidity associated with these conditions.
- The histologic types of thyroid cancer (papillary, follicular, medullary, anaplastic, lymphoma) all occur in elderly patients but with a shift to the more aggressive (Hürthle cell, medullary, anaplastic) types. Advanced age portends a far worse prognosis.

Suggested Readings

Cooper DS. Thyroid disorders. In: Cassel CK, Leipzig RM, Cohen HJ, et al., eds. Geriatric Medicine, 4th ed. New York: Springer, 2003:695–717.

Franceschi C, Mariotti S, Chiovato L, et al. Thyroid autoimmunity and aging. Exp Gerontol 1998;33(6):535–541. *A discussion of the phenomenon of autoimmunity in aging and their biological and clinical significance in thyroid disorders and the aging process.*

Martin FR, Deam DR. Hyperthyroidism in elderly hospitalized patients. Med J Aust 1996;164:200–203. *A review of the clinical features and response to treatment of hyperthyroidism in the elderly hospitalized patients.*

Samuels MH. Subclinical thyroid disease in the elderly. Thyroid 1998;8:803–813. *A review of subclinical thyroid disease in the elderly in the advent of more sensitive assay for TSH. Prevalence, causes, potential risks and decisions to treat older adults are discussed.*

References

1. Mariotti S, Franceschi C, Cossarizza A, Pinchera A. The aging thyroid. Endocr Rev 1995;16:686–715.
2. Greenwood RM, Daly JG, Himsworth RL. Hyperthyroidism and the impalpable thyroid gland. Clin Endocrinol 1985;22:583–587.

3. Martin FR, Deam DR. Hyperthyroidism in elderly hospitalized patients. Med J Aust 1996;164:200–203.
4. Figge J, Leinung M, Goodman AD, et al. The clinical evaluation of patients with subclinical hyperthyroidism and free triiodothyronine (free T3) toxicosis. Am J Med 1994;96:229–234.
5. Wehmann RE, Gregerman RI, Burns WH, et al. Suppression of thyrotropin in the low-thyroxine state of severe nonthyroidal illness. N Engl J Med 1985;312:546–552.
6. Gordon M, Gryfe Cl. Hyperthyroidism with painless subacute thyroiditis in the elderly. JAMA 1981;246:2354–2355.
7. Newman CM, Price A, Davies DW, Gray TA, Weetman AP. Amiodarone and the thyroid: a practical guide to the management of thyroid dysfunction induced by amiodarone therapy. Heart 1998;79:121–127.
8. Solomon B, Glinoer D, Lagasse R, Wartofsky L. Current trends in the management of Graves' disease. J Clin Endocrinol Metab 1990;70:1518–1524.
9. Erickson D, Gharib H, Li Hongzhe, Van Heerden JA. Treatment of patients with toxic multinodular goiter. Thyroid 1998;8:277–282.
10. Cooper DS, Goldminz D, Levin AA, et al. Agranulocytosis associated with antithyroid drugs: effects of patient age and drug dose. Ann Intern Med 1983;98:26–29.
11. Geffner DL, Hershman JM. Beta-Adrenergic blockade for the treatment of hyperthyroidism. Am J Med 1992;93:61–68.
12. Nicoloff JT. Thyroid storm and myxedema coma. Med Clin North Am 1985;69:1005–1117.
13. Roti E, Montermini M, Roti S, et al. The effect of diltiazem, a calcium channel-blocking drug, on cardiac rate and rhythm in hyperthyroid patients. Arch Intern Med 1988;148:1919–1921.
14. Samuels MH. Subclinical thyroid disease in the elderly. Thyroid 1998;8:803–813.
15. Sawin CT, Geller A, Wolf PA, et al. Low serum thyrotropin concentrations as a risk factor for atrial fibrillation in older persons. N Engl J Med 1994;331:1249–1252.
16. Utiger R. Subclinical hyperthyroidism—just a low serum thyrotropin concentration, or something more? N Engl J Med 1994;331:1302–1303.
17. Davis PJ, Davis FM. Hypothyroidism in the elderly. Compr Ther 1984;10:17–23.
18. Canaris GJ, Manowitz NR, Mayor G, Ridgway EC. The Colorado thyroid disease prevalence study. Arch Intern Med 2000;160:526–534.
19. Lindeman RD, Schade DS, LaRue A, et al. Subclinical hypothyroidism in a biethnic, urban community. J Am Geriatr Soc 1999;47:703–709.
20. Gharib H, Goellner JR, Zinsmeister AR. Fine-needle aspiration biopsy of the thyroid: the problem of suspicious cytologic findings. Ann Intern Med 1984;101:25–28.
21. Docter R, Krenning EP, de Jong M, Hennemann G. The sick euthyroid syndrome: changes in thyroid hormone serum parameters and hormone metabolism. Clin Endocrinol 1993;39:499–518.
22. Mariotti S, Sansoni P, Barbesino G, et al. Thyroid and other organ-specific autoantibodies in healthy centenarians. Lancet 1992;339:1506–1508.

23. Sawin CT, Bigos ST, Land S, et al. The aging thyroid: relationship between elevated serum thyrotropin level and thyroid antibodies in elderly patients. Am J Med 1985;79:591–595.

24. Hays MT, Nielsen KRK. Human thyroxine absorption: age effects and methodological analyses. Thyroid 1994;4:55–58.

25. Stall GM, Harris S, Sokoll LJ, Dawson-Hughes B. Accelerated bone loss in hypothyroid patients overtreated with L-Thyroxine. Ann Intern Med 1990; 113:265–269.

26. Cooper DS, Halpern R, Wood LC, et al. L-thyroxine therapy in subclinical hypothyroidism. A double-blind, placebo-controlled trial. Ann Intern Med 1984;101:18–24.

27. Surks M, Chopra IJ, Mariash CN, Nicoloff JT, Solomon DH. American Thyroid Association guidelines for use of laboratory tests in thyroid disorders. JAMA 1990;263:1529–1532.

28. American College of Physicians. Screening for thyroid disease. Ann Intern Med 1998;129:141–143.

29. Rosenthal MJ, Hunt WC, Garry PJ, et al. Thyroid failure in the elderly: microsomal antibodies as discriminant for therapy. JAMA 1987;258:209–213.

30. Nicoloff JT, LoPresti JS. Myxedema coma: a form of decompensated hypothyroidism. Endocrinol Metab Clin NA 1993;22:279–290.

31. Vander JB, Gaston EA, Dawber TR. The significance of nontoxic thyroid nodules. Ann Intern Med 1968;69:537–540.

32. Mazzaferri EL. Management of a solitary thyroid nodule. N Engl J Med 1993;328:553–559.

33. Gharib H, Goellner JR. Fine-needle aspiration biopsy of the thyroid: an appraisal. Ann Intern Med 1993;118:282–289.

34. Hundahl SA, Fleming ID, Fremgen AM, Menck HR. A national cancer data base report on 53,856 cases of thyroid carcinoma treated in the U.S., 1985–1995. Cancer 1998;83:2638–2648.

35. Mazzaferri EL, Jhiang SM. Long-term impact of initial surgical and medical therapy on papillary and follicular thyroid cancer. Am J Med 1994;97: 418–428.

26
Anemia in the Elderly

Jennifer M. Hensley

Learning Objectives

Upon completion of the chapter, the student will be able to:

1. Identify the hematologic changes associated with aging.
2. Distinguish the initial workup for each of the different morphologic types of anemia.
3. Understand the diagnostic features and therapeutic options of common anemias in older adults.

Case A

Mr. Smith is a 90-year-old man with history of hypertension who comes to see you to review the results of his recent blood work. Everything is normal except for a mild anemia. Mr. Smith seems concerned with hearing the results. He asks, "Is a mild anemia normal for a 90-year-old?"

General Considerations

Although anemia is more prevalent as aging proceeds, it cannot be assumed to be due to aging alone. In the elderly as in young adults, discrete and identifiable diseases cause anemia. However, elderly persons can be considered to be more susceptible to anemia-inducing events because of an age-associated impairment of the marrow's ability to appropriately increase red cell production.

Material in this chapter is based on the following chapter in Cassel CK, Leipzig RM, Cohen HJ, Larson EB, Meier DE, eds. Geriatric Medicine: An Evidence-Based Approach, 4th ed. New York: Springer, 2003: Rothstein G. Hematologic Problems, pp. 819–833. Selections edited by Jennifer M. Hensley.

Definition and Prevalence

Anemia is defined as the decrease in red blood cells (RBCs) or hemoglobin (Hgb) resulting from blood loss, impaired production of RBCs, or RBC destruction. The prevalence of anemia in the elderly is greater than that in young adults, ranging from 5% to 51%, with the lowest prevalence in community-dwelling elderly who consider themselves healthy, intermediate values for prevalence among those enrolled in clinics for health care, and the greatest prevalence among the oldest old who are hospitalized (1–4). This correlation of age-associated anemia and health status supports the concept that anemia is a consequence of disease in the elderly and not due to age alone.

Age-Associated Changes in the Hematopoietic System

The bone marrow is the site of production for circulating RBCs, granulocytes, and platelets. As aging proceeds, the marrow becomes increasingly localized to the axial skeleton. However, in nondiseased elderly persons, the total number of marrow cells in the body is not decreased; it is similar to that of healthy young adults (5). Consequently, clinical examination of the marrow (the myeloid/erythroid ratio, maturation of cell lines, karyotypic analysis, and presence and distribution of stainable iron) of older persons does not differ from that of normal young adults.

The concentrations of red cells, platelets, and leukocytes in the blood of healthy older persons do not differ from those of young adults. The prevalence of anemia is increased in populations of community-dwelling, clinic-visiting, and hospitalized elderly. However, anemia is not a consequence of age. Indeed, the distribution of hematocrit values for elderly patients falls roughly into two populations: one that is in the anemic range, and another that overlaps with the distribution for normal young adults (1). This supports the concept that older persons develop anemia due to underlying disease. Indeed, careful diagnostic testing of elderly anemic subjects reveals one or more identifiable causes for the anemia in at least 80% of cases (1).

In steady state and during periods of increased demand, blood cell production is regulated by erythropoietin and a variety of cytokine stimulators, as well as being under the influence of endocrine hormones such as thyroxine and corticosteroids. During aging, steady-state regulation of the marrow appears normal, as evidenced by normal numbers of marrow precursors (5–8). During periods of increased hematopoietic demand, the hematopoietic response of the elderly is dysregulated. In elderly persons, deficiency of erythropoietin is a frequent contributing or causative factor and the administration of recombinant erythropoietin is effective in reversing at least some of the anemias in elderly persons due to erythropoietin deficiency (9). The marrow precursors of elderly persons show a similar defect, with paradoxical reductions in the concentrations of progenitor cells for granulocytes, as well as red cells (10). The age-associated paradoxical reduction in marrow cells during infection and anemia is not yet understood, but it can be speculated that the dysregulated production of cytokines, such as interleukin-10 (IL-10) (11,12), which induces programmed cell death (apoptosis), may account for it (13).

Case B (Part 1)

Mrs. Johnson is an 80-year-old woman with history of osteoarthritis who comes to see you for a routine visit. She tells you that for several weeks she has felt tired despite getting a good night's sleep. She is easily fatigued and takes frequent naps. She is no longer able to do her housework and she has not left the house for over a week.

Diagnostic Considerations

The etiology of anemia should be established to identify the pathologic process responsible for the anemia, to determine the appropriate therapeutic approach for the anemia, and to provide prognostic information. The task of diagnosis is simplified by the consideration that anemia can be categorized kinetically: as being due to *decreased production* of red cells, *increased destruction* of red cells, *loss of red cells* (bleeding), or *ineffective erythropoiesis.*

Symptoms and Signs

The clinical presentation of anemia depends on the degree of anemia, the underlying cause, and the presence of comorbid conditions. Often, anemia in the elderly is associated with such nonspecific symptoms as fatigue, functional decline, and weakness, and is only discovered by laboratory survey. Importantly, the fatigue and poor quality of life associated with anemia respond to correction of the anemia even when serious underlying conditions such as malignancy are unresponsive to treatment. When anemia is a consequence of malignancy such as myeloma, the dominant presenting symptoms may be those associated with the underlying neoplasm, such as bone pain, symptoms of uremia, or even confusion due to hypercalcemia. When anemia is associated with newly developed postural hypotension, increasing dyspnea, or increasing angina, this may indicate that the anemia has developed acutely, is severe, or is associated with acute bleeding and intravascular volume loss.

Laboratory Findings

The utilization of the various laboratory tests for the diagnosis of anemia requires an understanding of the strategies and pitfalls of their interpretation. The various laboratory tests that can be used to place anemia in one of these kinetic categories are shown in Table 26.1, as are disorders associated with each kinetic category.

Complete Blood Count

In addition to the basic tests in Table 26.1, the complete blood count (CBC) should include a measure of the *mean corpuscular volume* (MCV). In this way, the anemias may be characterized morphologically as normocytic, microcytic, or macrocytic. The morphologic categories of anemia are shown in Table 26.2, along with diseases associated with them.

TABLE 26.1. The kinetic categories of anemia, laboratory tests that support them, and disorders associated with them

Kinetic category of anemia	Laboratory tests	Corresponding disorders
Decreased Red cell production	Reticulocyte count* (reduced) Marrow cellularity (reduced) Marrow myeloid/erythroid ratio (increased)	Iron deficiency, anemia of chronic disease, megaloblastic anemias, protein/calorie malnutrition, endocrine diseases, erythropoietin deficiency, marrow infiltrative diseases, aplastic anemia, anemia secondary to chemotherapy
Increased Red cell destruction	Indirect bilirubin* (increased) LDH (increased)	Hemolytic anemias, bleeding into closed body spaces, paroxysmal nocturnal hemoglobinuria
Loss Of red cells	History of bleeding* Stool guaiac (positive)*	GI blood loss, surgical blood loss, bleeding diatheses
Ineffective erythropoiesis	Reticulocyte count* (reduced) Indirect bilirubin* (increased) LDH (increased) Marrow myeloid/erythroid ratio (increased)	Myelodysplastic syndromes, megaloblastic anemia

*Denotes tests useful for screening purposes.
LDH, lactate dehydrogenase.
Source: Rothstein G. Hematologic problems. In: Cassel CK, Leipzig RM, Cohen HJ, et al., eds. Geriatric Medicine, 4th ed. New York: Springer, 2003.

TABLE 26.2. The morphologic categories of anemia and selected corresponding disorders

Morphologic category	Disorders
Microcytic	Iron deficiency
	Anemia of chronic disease
	Thalassemia, hemoglobin E disease
	Spherocytic hemolytic anemias
Macrocytic	Megaloblastic anemia (B_{12} and/or folate deficiency, antimetabolites)
	Liver disease with target cells
	Greatly increased numbers of reticulocytes
Normocytic	Renal failure
	Erythropoietin deficiency
	Endocrine disorders
	Anemia of chronic disease
	Protein/calorie malnutrition
	Infiltrative diseases of the marrow
	Aplastic anemia
	Anemia secondary to chemotherapy
	Polymyalgia rheumatica

Source: Rothstein G. Hematologic problems. In: Cassel CK, Leipzig RM, Cohen HJ, et al., eds. Geriatric Medicine, 4th ed. New York: Springer, 2003.

Reticulocyte Count

Laboratory reports for reticulocyte count are expressed as percents, or the number of reticulocytes (young red cells) per 100 red cells in the blood smear preparation. The normal range is from 0.8% to 2.5% in men and 0.8% to 4.1% in women if anemia is not present. However, anemia is expected to stimulate increased production of reticulocytes. In anemic subjects, an adjusted reticulocyte percentage should be calculated by multiplying a patient's raw laboratory reticulocyte percent by the ratio of the patient's hematocrit to an average normal hematocrit value, such as 45%.

$$\text{Corrected reticulocyte \%} = \text{Uncorrected reticulocyte \%} \times \frac{\text{Patient hematocrit (\%)}}{45}$$

Serum Folate

Measurements of serum folate should be conducted before patients are fed in-hospital, because single feedings of foods rich in folic acid may raise folate levels into the normal range. Measurements of red cell folate content provide a better estimate of folate status for the preceding months. Folic acid deficiency is most frequently due to decreased dietary intake, although deficiency can also occur because of intestinal malabsorption and because of blockage of absorption by such drugs as anticonvulsants and sulfasalazine.

Serum Vitamin B$_{12}$

Serum levels of vitamin B$_{12}$ may also be difficult to interpret. Some reports have suggested that concentrations of less than 100 pg/mL are necessary for establishing the diagnosis B$_{12}$-deficient anemia. However, more recent studies suggest that levels of greater than 100 pg/mL are found in over one third of subjects with pernicious anemia (2). Other investigators suggest that even levels of B$_{12}$ in the low normal range may be associated with the central nervous system changes of B$_{12}$ deficiency, so that measurements of methylmalonic acid may be indicated when B$_{12}$ is in the low normal range (200–300 pg/mL) (5,14,15). Vitamin B$_{12}$ is plentiful in animal products and is stored in considerable quantity, so that strict vegetarian (vegan) diets appear necessary to cause deficiency states based on reduced dietary intake. More frequently, B$_{12}$ deficiency is based on defective absorption, either because of deficiency of gastric-produced intrinsic factor needed for B$_{12}$ absorption, or due to intestinal mucosal atrophy or removal of the jejunum. The Schilling test can be used to assess the mechanism of B$_{12}$ malabsorption but is relatively insensitive as a diagnostic tool for the deficiency state, so that normal Schilling test results do not exclude the diagnosis of B$_{12}$ deficiency.

Serum Erythropoietin

Measurements of erythropoietin must be interpreted in light of the degree of anemia that is present. In the presence of anemia, erythropoietin production should be increased and circulating levels should rise. Unfortunately, the response of serum erythropoietin to varying degrees of anemia has not been clearly defined and varies among laboratories. However, serum erythropoietin is expected to rise to levels above those described as normal for nonanemic individuals, and many laboratories can supply at least partially complete data for relationship of erythropoietin levels to various degrees of anemia. If such data are not available, a practical approach would be to expect erythropoietin levels in patients with moderate or severe anemia to rise to at least fivefold the upper limit of the laboratory's normal range.

Differential Diagnosis

A practical approach is to begin with the morphologic classification of the anemia and then proceed through additional selected tests to identify the etiology. Note that the values for MCV may differ among laboratories, and values specific for each laboratory should be used.

Case B (Part 2)

Upon further review of Mrs. Johnson's history, you discover that she has been taking ibuprofen regularly for her osteoarthritis. She often has symptoms of bloating, retrosternal burning, and occasional nausea. She has been taking antacids to relieve her symptoms three to four times a week. She denies any problems with constipation and has not noted any changes in the character of her stool. On physical exam, Mrs. Johnson appears pale, but her vital signs are stable. The rest of her exam was normal except for having brown stools that were positive on Hemoccult testing. Labs are significant for CBC: white blood count (WBC) = 5.0×10^9/L, Hgb = 9 g/dL, hematocrit (Hct) = 27%, platelets = 300,000, MCV = 75 fL, red blood cell distribution width (RDW) = 16%.

Microcytic Anemias (MCV <80 fL)

The most common diagnoses are iron deficiency, the anemia of chronic disorders, and thalassemia. First, iron status should be defined:

- *Initial laboratory tests*: Serum iron, serum total iron-binding capacity (TIBC), percent of transferrin saturation, serum ferritin. Optional: Marrow for stainable iron if the serum tests do not clearly define iron status.
- *Interpretation and course of action*: Reduced serum iron, increased TIBC, and greatly reduced percent of transferrin saturation establish the diagnosis of iron deficiency. When those results are ambiguous, staining of the marrow for iron represents the "gold standard" for evaluation of iron stores. When iron stores are depleted, stainable marrow iron is absent. The diagnosis of iron deficiency dictates an effort to identify the source of iron loss (bleeding) and to proceed with iron replacement therapy.

Reduced serum iron, decreased or normal TIBC, mildly decreased percent of transferrin saturation, normal or increased ferritin, the presence of stainable iron in the marrow, and the presence of an active inflammatory disease suggest the anemia of chronic disease. Approximately 30% of patients with the anemia of chronic disease have microcytic red cells, so the absence of microcytosis does not exclude this diagnosis (16). The anemia of chronic disease may respond partially or completely to effective treatment of the underlying inflammatory condition (17), and in some cases erythropoietin administration may be indicated to improve quality of life, even if the underlying condition is not responsive to treatments directed against it (18).

Case C

Mr. Gordon is a 65-year-old man with diabetes, hypertension, and hypothyroidism. His wife accompanies him for an urgent visit after a fall. He was walking to the kitchen when he tripped over a rug and fell forward. According to him he has fallen three times in the past 6 months. His wife has noticed that he has an unsteady gait and at times is forgetful. Upon further review of symptoms, he has noted a loss of appetite, occasional nausea, and a 10-pound weight loss.

On his neurologic examination he was noted to have a decreased position and vibration sense of the lower extremities. However, muscle power and gait were normal. His labs were significant for: WBC = 4.0×10^9/L, Hgb = 11 g/dL, Hct = 33%, MCV = 100 fL, RDW = 18%, reticulocyte count 2%, vitamin B_{12} level <100 pg/mL.

Macrocytic Anemias (MCV >100 fL)

In general, the diagnoses comprising this category can be divided into those caused by *impaired DNA synthesis* (megaloblastic anemias), *increased reticulocytes, alterations of the RBC membrane* due to liver disease, or more rarely, *hemoglobinopathy*. The anemias of myelodysplastic disorders usually are also macrocytic. The etiology usually can be identified as follows:

- *Initial laboratory tests*: Reticulocyte count, indirect bilirubin.
- *Interpretation and course of action*: An increased reticulocyte count signifies increased RBC production in response to either blood loss or hemolytic anemia. In the absence of an elevated bilirubin, blood loss is most likely and the source of blood loss should be identified. If the bilirubin is also elevated, hemolytic anemia should be suspected.

If reticulocyte number is normal or reduced, proceed to examination of blood and bone marrow for megaloblastic changes.

- *Interpretation and course of action*:
  - If megaloblastic changes are found in the marrow, this confirms the diagnosis of megaloblastic anemia. Serum vitamin B_{12} and folic acid concentrations should be measured. If a deficient value is found, therapy should be instituted to correct the deficiency. If antimetabolite therapy has been administered, this should be considered the cause of the anemia.
  - If the marrow is not megaloblastic, the blood smear should be examined for the presence of target cells, which may signal the presence of liver disease, hypothyroidism, or rarely, an inherited hemoglobinopathy such as hemoglobin C disease.

Case D

Mrs. Gleason is a 75-year-old woman with a history of osteoarthritis and osteoporosis who is seeing you for follow-up of her arthritic pain. For several months she has been complaining of increased pain and morning stiffness in her shoulders and neck that are unresponsive to her usual acetaminophen and celecoxib. Now she is having trouble combing her hair or putting on a coat. In addition to the pain, she has been feeling tired and weak. At night she often feels warm and diaphoretic. Physical exam reveals little evidence of swelling or tenderness of proximal joints that could account for Mrs. Gleason's symptoms. Labs taken at this visit revealed the following: WBC = 4.0 × 10^9/L, Hgb = 10 g/dL, Hct = 30%, platelets = 230,000, RDW = 14%, MCV = 85 fL, reticulocyte count 1%, erythrocyte sedimentation rate (ESR) 45 mm/h.

Normocytic Anemias (MCV 81–100 fL)

This morphologic category includes a wide variety of etiologies including posthemorrhagic anemias or hemolytic anemias without extensive reticulocytosis, conditions in which marrow cell production is impaired (e.g., aplastic anemia, infiltrative diseases of the marrow, anemia due to decreased erythropoietin production, the anemia of protein/calorie malnutrition, and most examples of the anemia of chronic disease). A useful initial procedure is to perform a reticulocyte count:

- *Initial laboratory test*: Reticulocyte count.
- *Interpretation and course of action*: An increased reticulocyte count reflects an increase in RBC production, and should prompt consideration of the diagnoses of hemolytic anemia or posthemorrhagic anemia. A history of blood loss should be sought, and tests that can reflect increased red cell destruction should be obtained [indirect bilirubin, lactose dehydrogenase (LDH)]. If evidence of hemolysis is found, the differential diagnosis should include autoimmune causes with or without underlying malignancy, and oxidant sensitivity due to glucose-6-phosphate dehydrogenase deficiency. It should also be noted that bleeding into closed body spaces, such as retroperitoneally, can yield kinetic and morphologic laboratory results that are indistinguishable from those of hemolytic anemia.

A normal or reduced reticulocyte count should prompt the consideration of hepatic, or endocrine disorders. If these screening surveys are negative:

- Microscopic examination of the peripheral blood, bone marrow aspirate and biopsy, serum iron, TIBC, transferrin saturation, and ferritin.

- *Interpretation and course of action*: Examination of the blood and bone marrow are frequently sufficient to establish or exclude the diagnoses of leukemia, myeloma, myelofibrosis, myelodysplasia, or infiltration of the marrow with metastases. Submission of aspirated marrow cells for karyotypic analysis may be useful in differentiating certain of the above etiologies. Iron studies that reveal a reduced serum iron, decreased TIBC, a modest decrease in the percent of transferrin saturation, and normal or elevated ferritin are consistent with the diagnosis of the anemia of chronic disease, in which normocytic RBC are found in approximately 70% of cases (17).

Case B (Part 3)

Mrs. Johnson is here for a follow-up 6 weeks after her diagnosis of iron deficiency anemia. Since her last visit she was seen by the gastroenterologist and underwent an upper gastrointestinal endoscopy that showed gastritis and a duodenal ulcer. She was started on a proton pump inhibitor and iron replacement, and her ibuprofen was discontinued. During this visit she is very happy because her fatigue has vanished. She is able to leave the house again and resume her social activities. She just wants to know how long she needs to continue taking the iron, because it makes her constipated.

Management Considerations

The goal in treating anemia is to increase or completely restore the circulating red cells to normal levels. The appropriate strategies for increasing the red cell mass should be specifically directed by the urgency of the need for treatment and the underlying cause of the anemia. Some remediable causes of anemia, their key laboratory findings and treatment, are displayed in Table 26.3.

Correction of Deficiencies of Substrates for Red Cell Production

This strategy represents the ideal for management of anemia. A diagnostic process clearly identifies a deficiency of iron, folic acid, vitamin B_{12}, or protein/calories, and administration of the appropriate substrate corrects the anemia. Usually a response to therapy can be observed within 4 weeks of initiating therapy, and the anemia is repaired in 3 months or less.

TABLE 26.3. Some remediable causes of anemia, their key laboratory results, and treatment

Etiology	Laboratory results	Treatment and other interventions/studies
Iron deficiency	Microcytic RBC Reduced serum iron Increased TIBC Reduced Tf saturation Reticulocytes not increased	Identify source of iron loss and correct. Give oral iron 3 months, repeat iron studies. Intravenous iron only if iron cannot be given orally.
Anemia of chronic disease	Normo- or microcytic RBC Reduced serum iron Reduced TIBC Reduced Tf saturation Reticulocytes not increased	Identify underlying inflammatory disease. Apply remedy to underlying disease when available. May be responsive to erythropoietin administration.
B_{12}, folate-deficient anemia	Macrocytic RBC Hypersegmented PMN on blood smear Reduced B_{12} or folic acid Megaloblastic changes on bone marrow exam Reticulocytes not increased	Evaluate diet for sources of B_{12}, folic acid. Rule out malabsorption. Administer B_{12} or folate for replacement. Track response with reticulocyte counts, Hct/Hgb. B_{12} replacement must be for lifetime.
Protein/calorie-deficient anemia	Normocytic RBC Reduced lymphocyte count Reduced serum albumin Reduced serum transferrin	Restoration of protein/calorie nutrition restores the hematocrit to normal.

Tf, transferrin; TIBC, total iron-binding capacity, RBC, red blood cell; PMN, polymorphonuclear; Hct, hematocrit; Hg-b, hemoglobin.
Source: Rothstein G. Hematologic problems. In: Cassel CK, Leipzig RM, Cohen HJ, et al., eds. Geriatric Medicine, 4th ed. New York: Springer, 2003.

Iron

When iron therapy is needed, oral administration is the preferred route, and the gluconate, sulfate, or fumarate salts of iron are all effective. The iron should be administered *with meals* to avoid gastrointestinal side effects, and therapy is continued for 3 to 6 months after the anemia is resolved to ensure replacement of iron stores. If taken as directed, oral iron therapy is almost always effective in treating iron deficiency, although treatment failures may be encountered because of patients who do not comply with therapy. Parenteral iron therapy may be necessary in patients who are unable to tolerate oral iron, patients who are noncompliant with oral therapy, situations in which bleeding continues at a rate that exceeds the ability of oral iron to compensate for loss, patients with malabsorption of oral iron, dialysis patients unable to maintain adequate iron by oral intake, and in those who repeatedly and very frequently donate large amounts of blood. Iron-dextran is the preferred preparation for parenteral use, and is usually administered intravenously because repeated intramuscular injections are painful and cause staining of the skin at the site of injection. It should be recognized that iron-dextran may cause hypersensitivity reactions.

Vitamin B_{12}

Vitamin B_{12} can be administered either intramuscularly, monthly at a dose of 1000 μg, or orally, in large doses of 1000 mg/day, even for treatment of pernicious anemia due to intrinsic factor deficiency (19).

Folic Acid

Folic acid is also administered orally, and daily doses of 1 mg/day provide a generous excess above minimum daily requirement of 50 to 100 μg/day. It should be noted, however, that large doses of folic acid are capable of reversing the anemia of B_{12} deficiency while permitting the neurologic consequences of pernicious anemia to advance. Consequently, therapeutic trials with folic acid are potentially dangerous and therapy should be directed in a focused manner only after the specific deficiency state has been identified. In some patients, the response to vitamin B_{12} or folate may appear to fail before the anemia is repaired. In such cases, the explanation may be that existing iron stores have been exhausted by utilization for new red cell production. Iron status, therefore, should be evaluated, and if iron is deficient, its cause should be identified and replacement therapy instituted.

Case D (Part 2)

Mrs. Gleason returns to your office for a follow-up visit after being diagnosed with polymyalgia rheumatica. For one month she has been on prednisone 20 mg daily. Her symptoms of polymyalgia and morning stiffness resolved after a few days of treatment. Repeat CBC at this visit shows an improvement in her hemoglobin.

Treatment of Underlying Conditions

Some anemias are partially or completely resolved when therapy is directed toward underlying etiologic conditions. A noteworthy example is the anemia associated with polymyalgia rheumatica (PMR), which resolves when corticosteroid treatment of PMR is successful. Similarly, replacement of thyroid hormone in hypothyroidism induces resolution of the associated anemia, unless it is due to the B_{12} deficiency related to associated gastric autoimmunity (20). However, the response may be sluggish, requiring 3 to 12 months before the anemia resolves (21). The anemia associated with myeloma is also resolved by chemotherapeutic measures that induce remission of the malignancy, but may also respond to erythropoietin.

Growth Factors and Erythropoietin

An important characteristic of the hematopoietic progenitors of the elderly is the preservation of their responsiveness to hematopoietic stimulators. With the availability of recombinant growth factors and erythropoietin, an evolving strategy for the treatment of anemia is the use of these agents to directly drive erythropoiesis. For example, it is now clear that in myelodysplastic syndromes (MDS), prolonged administration of a combination of the hematopoietic stimulator, recombinant granulocyte colony-stimulating factor (G-CSF), and erythropoietin can increase the hematocrits of individuals with these disorders (22).

Transfusion

Transfusion is associated with significant risks, such as volume overload, immunologic transfusion reactions, and the unintended infusion of infectious agents, such as transfusion-associated hepatitis, Epstein-Barr virus, and human immunodeficiency virus. Consequently, transfusion should not be given simply because a patient's hemoglobin or hematocrit has reached an arbitrary level. Indications for transfusion include acute blood loss with symptoms of hypovolemia, progressive symptoms of decreased oxygen delivery such as angina or increasing confusion, or symptomatic anemia that is refractory to nontransfusion therapy. When transfusion is used to treat refractory anemia without loss of blood volume, concentrated red cells should be used to avoid volume overload. However, even when restoration of blood volume is indicated, blood banks may supply only concentrated red cells rather than whole blood. In such cases, concentrated red cells may be given together with crystalloid or synthetic plasma volume expanders. The infusion of plasma or albumin appears unnecessary except when volume loss has exceeded 50% of total blood volume (23). When blood transfusion is urgent, it should be given together with measures to ensure restoration of the blood volume.

General Principles

- The prevalence of anemia increases with age. This is due to a combination of age-associated impairment of the marrow's ability to appropriately increase red cell production and the increased frequency of comorbidity in the elderly and not due to age alone.

- Symptoms of anemia in the elderly are often nonspecific and can be evidenced in functional decline and weakness. Quality of life can be affected even with hemoglobin levels of 11 g/dL.
- A practical approach to diagnosing the anemia is to classify the anemia morphologically as microcytic, macrocytic, or normocytic. Then proceed through additional selected tests to identify the etiology.
- The initial laboratory workup for microcytic anemia are serum iron, serum TIBC, percent of transferrin saturation, and serum ferritin.
- The initial laboratory tests for macrocytic and normocytic anemia include the reticulocyte count and indirect bilirubin.
- Management of anemia in the elderly is directed at identifying the cause and treating any underlying conditions and resultant deficiencies.

Suggested Reading

Rothstein G. Hematologic problems. In: Cassel CK, Leipzig RM, Cohen HJ, et al., eds. Geriatric Medicine, 4th ed. New York: Springer, 2003:819–834.

References

1. Baraldi-Junkins CA, Beck AC, Rothstein G. Hematopoiesis and cytokines. Relevance to cancer and aging. Hematol Oncol Clin North Am 2000;14:45.
2. Dallman PR, Yip R, Johnson C: Prevalence and causes of anemia in the United States, 1976 to 1980. Am J Clin Nutr 1984;39:437.
3. Lipschitz DA, Mitchell CO, Thompson C. The anemia of senescence. Am J Hematol 1981;11:47.
4. Timiras ML, Brownstein H. Prevalence of anemia and correlation of hemoglobin with age in a geriatric screening clinic population. J Am Geriatr Soc 1987;35:639.
5. Lipschitz DA, Udupa KB, Milton KY, et al. Effect of age on Hematopoiesis in man. Blood 1981;27:547.
6. Boggs DR, Patrene K. Hematopoiesis and aging. III: Anemia and a blunted erythropoietic response to hemorrhage in aged mice. Am J Hematol 1985; 19:327.
7. Rothstein G, Christensen RD, Neilsen GR. Kinetic evaluation of pool sizes and proliferative response in bacterially challenged aged mice. Blood 1987; 70:1836.
8. Udupa KB, Lipschitz DA: Erythropoiesis in the aged mouse: I. Response to stimulation in vivo. J Lab Clin Med 1984;103:574.
9. Cella D, Bron D. The effect of Epoietin alfa on quality of life in anemic cancer patients. Cancer Pract 1999;7:177.
10. Buchanan JJP, Peters CA, Rasmussen C, et al. Impaired expression of hematopoietic growth factors: a candidate mechanism for the hematopoietic defect of aging. Exp Gerontol 1996;31:135.

11. Ershler WB, Sun WH, Binkley N, et al. Interleukin-6 and aging: blood levels and mononuclear cell production increase with advancing age and in vitro production is modifiable by dietary restriction. Lymphokine Cytokine Res 1993;4:225.

12. Cohen HJ, Pieper CF, Harris T, et al. The association of plasma IL-6 levels with functional disability in the elderly. J Gerontol [A] Biol Sci Med Sci 1997;52:201.

13. Lopatin U, Yao X, Willams RK, et al. Increases in circulating and lymphoid tissue interleukin-10 in autoimmune lymphoproliferative syndrome are associated with disease expression. Blood 2001;97:3161.

14. Rasmussen K, Vyberg B, Pedersen KO, et al. Methylmalonic acid in renal insufficiency: evidence of accumulation and implications for diagnosis of cobalamin deficiency. Clin Chem 1990;36:1523.

15. Allen RH, Stabler SP, Savage DG, et al. Diagnosis of cobalamin deficiency; I. Usefulness of serum methylmalonic acid and total homocysteine concentrations. Am J Hematol 1990;34:90.

16. Beutler E, Fairbanks VF. The effects of iron deficiency. In: Jacobs A, Worwood M, eds. Iron in Biochemistry and Medicine, vol 2. New York: Academic Press, 1980.

17. Cartwright GE, Wintrobe MM. The anemia of infection. Adv Intern Med 1952;35:165.

18. Mantovani L, Lentini G, Hentschel B, et al. Treatment of anemia in myelodysplastic syndromes with prolonged administration of recombinant human granulocyte colony-stimulating factor and erythropoietin. Br J Haematol 2000;109:367.

19. Kuzminski AM, Del Giacco EF, Allen RH, et al. Effective treatment of cobalamin deficiency with oral cobalamin. Blood 1998;92:1191.

20. Tudhope GR, Wilson GM. Anaemia in hypothyroidism. QJ Med 1960;29:513.

21. Bomford R. Anemia in myxoedema. QJ Med 1938;7:495.

22. Shank WA Jr, Balducci L. Recombinant hemopoietic growth factors: comparative hemopoietic response in younger and older subjects. J Am Geriatr Soc 1992;40:151.

23. Adamson J, Hillman RS. Blood volume and plasma protein replacement following acute blood loss in normal man. JAMA 1968;205:609.

27
Benign Prostatic Hyperplasia

Hans L. Stöhrer

Learning Objectives

Upon completion of the chapter, the student will be able to:

1. Describe the epidemiology of benign prostatic hyperplasia (BPH) and lower urinary tract symptoms (LUTS) in older men.
2. Describe age-related changes of the prostate, and pathophysiology of BPH and LUTS.
3. Describe typical symptoms and signs of LUTS.
4. List steps in diagnostic evaluation of LUTS.
5. Discuss utility of urodynamic testing, and when to refer to a urologist.
6. List four main treatment approaches recommended for BPH, and discuss general treatment considerations.
7. Discuss pharmacology, dosage, and side effects of medications for treatment of BPH.

Case (Part 1)

Mr. P. is a 75-year-old self-employed clinical psychologist who sees you for an annual examination. You are evaluating his hypertension, hyperlipidemia, and arthritis, when he begins to tell you about symptoms of urinary frequency, straining, and nocturia. Though he has had these symptoms for a couple of years, he never mentioned them to you before. Lately, however, the symptoms have become more bothersome, interfering with his psychology practice by interrupting client visits and disrupting his sleep at night.

How common are his symptoms among older men?

What can you tell him about his condition?

Material in this chapter is based on the following chapter in Cassel CK, Leipzig RM, Cohen HJ, Larson EB, Meier DE, eds. Geriatric Medicine: An Evidence-Based Approach, 4th ed. New York: Springer, 2003: DuBeau CE. Benign Prostatic Hyperplasia, pp. 755–768. Selections edited by Hans L. Stöhrer.

TABLE 27.1. Terms used to describe prostate changes and symptoms (1–4)

Benign prostatic hyperplasia (BPH)
- Defined by histology
- Occurs in nearly all older men

Benign prostate enlargement (BPE)
- Defined by digital rectal exam, cystoscopy, MRI, or weight of tissue resected at TURP
- Occurs in only half of older men

Bladder outlet obstruction (BOO)
- Defined by urodynamic testing
- Demonstrated urodynamically in only two-thirds of symptomatic men with prostate enlargement.

Lower urinary tract symptoms (LUTS)
- Refer to the general term of "prostatism" symptoms
- Occur in only half of men with prostate enlargement

TURP, transurethral resection of prostate; MRI, magnetic resonance imaging
Source: Data from Schäfer W, Rubben H, Noppeney R, Deutz F-J. Obstructed and unobstructed prostatic obstruction: a plea for urodynamic objectivation of bladder outflow obstruction in benign prostatic hyperplasia. World J Urol 1989;6:198–203. Coolsaet BLRA, van Venrooij GEPM, Blok C. Prostatism: rationalization of urodynamic testing. World J Urol 1984;2:216–221. Abrams P. In support of pressure-flow studies for evaluating men with lower urinary tract symptoms. Urology 1994;44:153–155. Isaacs JT, Coffey DS. Etiology and disease process of benign prostatic hyperplasia. Prostate Suppl 1989;2:33–50.

General Considerations

Prostate symptoms are a common feature of aging for many men. Although the term *benign prostatic hyperplasia* often is used synonymously for *prostate enlargement, bladder outlet obstruction,* and *associated urinary tract symptoms*, these terms are not equivalent. Table 27.1 describes and defines these terms. Benign prostatic hyperplasia increases with age and occurs in 80% of men by age 80 (5). The symptoms are usually moderate-severe in 28–35% of older men (6), most prevalent in the seventh decade, and one fourth of men over 80 years of age receive treatment.

Age-Related Changes of the Prostate and Lower Urinary Tract

Histologic BPH develops early—in the third decade. The volume of hyperplasia increases significantly with age (3,7), but the change in prostate volume over time is highly variable among men in longitudinal studies (8). Aside from age, the other major predictor of volume increase is baseline prostate-specific antigen (PSA): levels >2 ng/mL predict subsequent prostate growth, while a third of men with PSA <2 ng/mL have prostate shrinkage (9).

Similar to the variability between men over time in prostate size, the evolution of prostate symptoms over time is also highly variable. Clinical natural history studies and placebo arms of treatment trials demonstrate that symptomatic progression is not inevitable, and urinary retention occurs in only a minority. [For further details on the natural history of benign prostatic enlargement (BPE) and LUTS progression, see Chapter 51: Benign Prostatic Hyperplasia. In: Cassel CK, et al., eds. Geriatric Medicine, 4th ed., page 756.]

Pathophysiology of Benign Prostatic Hyperplasia and Lower Urinary Tract Symptoms

Hyperplasia occurs when prostate cell proliferation outpaces programmed cell death (apoptosis). The mechanisms of BPH are androgen-dependent, complex, and incompletely understood. Sex hormones (especially dihydrotestosterone, produced by 5α-reduction of testosterone within the prostate) and aging are necessary to develop hyperplasia. Factors promoting BPH include age, androgens, androgen-independent factors (inflammatory infiltrates, autocrine cytokine growth factors), and neuroendocrine cell products.

The presence in a man of BPH, BPE, and LUTS is not necessarily equivalent. This divergent prevalence reflects the variable effect of pathophysiologic changes in BPH (Table 27.2). For example, BPH can cause mechanical occlusion of the prostatic urethra, but urethral compression and bladder outlet obstruction (BOO) are not universal with BPH. Benign prostatic hyperplasia–related BOO is also associated with several changes in bladder detrusor muscle structure and function (Table 27.2).

TABLE 27.2. Pathophysiologic changes in benign prostatic hyperplasia (BPH) and in bladder structure and function (10–14)

BPH
- Predominant fibromuscular stromal hyperplasia
  - Stromal prostates smaller, more symptomatic
  - Less responsive to prostatectomy
- BPH nodules in periurethral prostate zones
  - Predispose to mechanical occlusion of the prostatic urethra
- Fibroelastic composition of the prostate capsule
  - Alters prostate compliance and decreases urethral patency
- Increased number of alpha (α1C) adrenergic receptors
  - Mediate prostate smooth muscle contraction

Bladder
- Increased connective tissue infiltration
- Smooth muscle hypertrophy
- Decreased autonomic nerves
- Conversion from β-adrenergic (inhibitory) to α-adrenergic (stimulatory) responsiveness
- Increased uninhibited contractions (detrusor instability)

Source: Data from Dørflinger T, England DM, Madsen PO, Bruskewitz RC. Urodynamic and histological correlates of benign prostatic hyperplasia. J Urol 1988;140:1487–1490. Hinman F Jr. Point of view: capsular influence on benign prostatic hypertrophy. Urology 1986;28:347–350. Chapple CR, Burt RP, Andersson PO, Greengrass P, Wyllie M, Marshall I. Alphal–adrenoreceptor subtypes in the human prostate. Br J Urol 1994;74:585–589. Chapple CR, Smith D. The pathophysiological changes in the bladder obstructed by benign prostatic hyperplasia. Br J Urol 1994;73:117–123. Elbadawi A, Yalla SV, Resnick NM. Structural basis of geriatric voiding dysfunction. IV. Bladder outlet obstruction. J Urol 1993;150:1681–1695.

> **Case (Part 2)**
>
> Mr. P. appears relieved to know that his symptoms are not unusual among men his age. However, he still appears anxious. He is more concerned about his urinary symptoms and their impact on his daily activities than his other medical conditions, including osteoarthritis.
>
> How bothersome are his symptoms? How can you assess them?
>
> What further questions in the history should you ask him?
>
> What components of the physical exam and other tests should you recommend?

Diagnostic Evaluation

The recommended steps in the diagnostic evaluation of LUTS are outlined in Table 27.3. The first step in the evaluation of LUTS should always be to consider factors other than the prostate that can cause these symptoms. These factors include age-related lower urinary tract changes (atrophic urethritis), medications, fecal impaction, congestive heart failure, and neurologic disease (spinal stenosis, spinal cord injury, autonomic neuropathy such as diabetes).

It is important to remember that the prostate is not always the cause of LUTS in older men, regardless of the presence of prostate enlargement. The evaluation of older men with LUTS is similar to that of any older person with urine voiding dysfunction. (For further details, see Chapter 63: Urinary Incontinence. In: Cassel CK, et al., eds. Geriatric Medicine, 4th ed., page 938.)

Symptoms and Signs

The most common clinical manifestations of BPH are listed in Table 27.4. Typical symptoms and signs of LUTS include "obstructive" (hesitancy,

TABLE 27.3. Recommended steps in diagnostic evaluation of LUTS (15)

- History and relevant review of systems
- Symptom severity (i.e., American Urological Association symptom index)
- Medication review
- 48-hour voiding diary
- Physical exam, especially digital rectal exam (DRE)
- Postvoid residual urine volume (PVR)
- Urinalysis (to exclude hematuria or signs of infection)
- Serum creatinine (to exclude renal failure)
- Urodynamic testing (for complex cases)
- Prostate-specific antigen (PSA) testing (after discussion of risks/benefits)

Source: Adapted from AUA Practice Guidelines Committee (2003). AUA guideline on management of benign prostatic hyperplasia (2003). Chapter 1: Diagnosis and treatment recommendations. J Urol 2003;170:530–547.

TABLE 27.4. Manifestations of BPH-related lower urinary tract symptoms (LUTS)

Common	Less common	Review of systems
Urgency	Hematuria	Hematuria
Frequency	Urinary retention	Pelvic pain
Nocturia		Previous episodes of urinary retention
Hesitancy		Cardiac symptoms (regarding possible
Weak urine flow		congestive heart failure)
Interrupted stream		Bowel and sexual function (as clues to
Postvoid dribbling		potential sacral and pelvic neuropathies)
Sense of incomplete		Type and amount of fluid intake
emptying		Sleep disturbance
		Hematuria

weak urine flow, interrupted stream, postvoid dribbling, sense of incomplete emptying), and "irritative" symptoms (urgency, frequency, nocturia). Many men are asymptomatic, even if they have BPE and BOO. Less frequent manifestations include hematuria (from prostatic varices) and urinary retention.

In completing the medical history and review of systems, inquire about additional symptoms. All medications, including nonprescription drugs, should be reviewed, to look for causes of urinary retention (anticholinergics) and excess urine output (diuretics). A 48-hour voiding diary is also useful to clarify the possible role of fluids and urine volume in causing symptoms, especially nocturia.

Symptom bother often drives the decision to initiate therapy. Indices such as the American Urological Association (AUA) symptom score (Table 27.5) can be used to quantify voiding symptom severity and overall bother, and to follow these symptoms longitudinally. Symptoms are classified by score: mild, 0–7 points; moderate, 8–19 points; and severe, 20–35 points (15,21).

Physical Examination

The physical exam is important to search for nonurologic causes of LUTS, and to assess the prostate for size and signs of carcinoma. The digital rectal exam (DRE) is done to assess prostate consistency, nodularity, and size; to assess rectal tone; and to exclude fecal impaction. A prostate with BPH feels rubbery and enlarged. Presence of prostate nodules, induration, or rock-hard consistency is suggestive of carcinoma. Prostate size is considered important for choosing between transurethral and open surgical approaches, but it is not predictive of surgical outcome (16). Prostate size, however, should not be considered to decide on active treatment, because

TABLE 27.5. The American Urological Association symptom index (21)

	Not at all	Less than 1 time in 5	Less than half the time	About half the time	More than half the time	Almost always
1. Over the past month or so, how often have you had a sensation of not emptying your bladder completely after you finished urinating?	0	1	2	3	4	5
2. Over the past month or so, how often have you had to urinate again less than 2 hours after you finished urinating?	0	1	2	3	4	5
3. Over the past month or so, how often have you found you stopped and started again several times when you urinated?	0	1	2	3	4	5
4. Over the past month or so, how often have you found it difficult to postpone urination?	0	1	2	3	4	5
5. Over the past month or so, how often have you had a weak urinary stream?	0	1	2	3	4	5
6. Over the past month or so, how often have you had to push or strain to begin urination?	0	1	2	3	4	5
7. Over the last month, how many times did you most typically get up to urinate from the time you went to bed at night until the time you got up in the morning? 0 = none, 1 = 1 time, 2 = 2 times, 3 = 3 times, 4 = 4 times, 5 = 5 times or more.						

AUA symptom score = sum of questions 1–7.
Mild symptoms: 0–7 points; moderate symptoms: 8–19 points; severe symptoms: 20–35 points.
Source: Reprinted from Barry MJ, Fowler FJ Jr, O'Leary MP, et al. The American Urological Association symptom index for benign prostatic hyperplasia. J Urol 1992;148:1549–1557, with permission from Lippincott, Williams, & Wilkins.

it does not correlate with symptom severity, predict BOO, or predict treatment outcomes (17,18). Furthermore, prostate sizing by DRE is inaccurate and poorly reproducible, even by specialists (19).

Postvoid Residual Volume

The postvoid residual urine volume (PVR) should be checked in men with moderate-severe symptoms, coexistent neurologic disease, impaired renal function, or taking bladder suppressant medications. It is measured at the bedside by urethral catheterization or, less invasively (to avoid risk of infection), by ultrasound. A convenient bedside ultrasound used by urologists is called the bladder scanner; it digitally measures and displays the estimated PVR.

TABLE 27.6. Measurement of postvoid residual volume (PVR)

- Indications for checking PVR
  - Moderate-severe symptoms
  - Urinary retention
  - Coexistent neurologic disease
  - Impaired renal function
  - Taking bladder-suppressant medications
- How to measure PVR
  - Ask patient to void fully in his usual way, in a private area
  - Check by urethral catheterization ("straight catheter")
  - Or by ultrasound
- Elevated PVR
  - Roughly >100 cc
  - Due to bladder underactivity or obstruction
  - If elevated, consider
    - Indwelling catheter
    - Intermittent catheterization
    - Urologic consultation

Elevated PVR is considered roughly greater than 100 cc. This could be due to either detrusor underactivity or obstruction (20). Inability to pass a urethral catheter is not diagnostic of obstruction, because it is usually due to sphincter spasm from patient discomfort or anxiety. Guidelines for measurement of PVR are presented in Table 27.6.

Case (Part 3)

Mr. P. mentions that one of his friends had similar symptoms, and underwent urodynamic testing. He wants to know if he also needs this test.

Mr. P. returns for a follow-up visit. Through one of his friends at work, he met a urologist, who recommended urodynamic testing.

Does this patient require urodynamic testing? When is it indicated?

Urodynamic Evaluation

Urodynamic testing, when done by a trained urologist, can provide important functional and anatomic information about the bladder, bladder outlet, and urethral sphincter (Table 27.7). A student or physician can best learn about the utility of this procedure by observing with a urologist. Elements of urodynamic testing include urine free flow rate (Q) measured by electric uroflowmeter; pressure-flow studies that measure dynamic detrusor and urethral pressures; voiding cystourethrography; and cystoscopy, which is

TABLE 27.7. Indications for urodynamic testing

- To clarify differential diagnosis of LUTS
- To exclude types of lower urinary tract dysfunction that do not require surgical treatment (e.g., detrusor hyperactivity with impaired contractility) in a patient interested in and a candidate for surgical treatment
- When empiric treatment for BPH-related LUTS fails
- In the presence of neurologic disease (especially spinal cord injury)

used to evaluate intravesical pathology such as tumors, stones, or marked trabeculation, as well as prostate size, length, and median lobe enlargement. (For further details on the elements of urodynamic testing and their interpretation, see Chapter 51: Benign Prostatic Hyperplasia. In: Cassel CK, et al., eds. Geriatric Medicine, 4th ed., page 759.)

Prostate-Specific Antigen Testing

Screening for prostate cancer with prostate-specific antigen (PSA) should be considered in the evaluation of older men with LUTS, if the patient would be a candidate for curative treatment of localized cancer with radical prostatectomy or radiation therapy, or if a prostate cancer diagnosis would modify his management. Initial studies suggest that PSA level also may predict the progression of BPH-related LUTS (9). (For further details on PSA screening, see Chapter 8: Prevention and Chemoprophylaxis in the Elderly, page 117.)

Case (Part 4)

Your initial evaluation of Mr. P. reveals the following information: his stated symptoms, without prior episodes of retention or hematuria; his medications, which include a thiazide diuretic for hypertension, simvastatin for hyperlipidemia, and acetaminophen for arthritis pain; on exam the prostate is smooth, rubbery, and enlarged prostate; there are no signs of complicating conditions. You instruct him to keep a 48-hour voiding diary and bring it at the next visit.

What treatment options should you discuss?

How should you frame the discussion of treatment options?

Management Considerations

Treatment of BPH-related LUTS should always be patient-centered (15), and guided by symptom severity and bother, patient preferences, and potential treatment outcomes. The four main treatment approaches recom-

TABLE 27.8. Main treatment approaches for BPH-related LUTS

Watchful waiting
Behavioral approaches
Active monitoring
Medication
α-Adrenergic blockers
5α-reductase inhibitors
Phytotherapy
Antiandrogens
Surgery
Transurethral resection of prostate (TURP)
Transurethral incision of prostate (TUIP)
Open prostatectomy
Alternative procedures
Laser prostatectomy
Transurethral microwave thermotherapy (TUMT)
Transurethral needle ablation (TUNA)
Urethral stent placement
Balloon dilatation
Indwelling catheter

mended for BPH-related LUTS include watchful waiting, medication, surgery, and alternative procedures (Table 27.8).

The Decision to Treat

The Agency for Health Care Policy and Research (AHCPR) guidelines recommend that men with mild symptoms be treated with watchful waiting and lifestyle changes, while men with moderate to severe symptoms be offered the full range of treatment options.

Patient preferences should be elicited, and the clinical situation and comorbidities should be considered. For example, in frail institutionalized men, catheter removal may be the treatment goal, and side effects intolerable in younger men (such as impotence) may be less problematic. Time to treatment effect varies significantly among interventions (from days with surgery to months with finasteride). "Low-cost" medications can result in significant cost burden if treatment is long-term, requires frequent monitoring, or results in side effects.

Lifestyle Changes

Behavioral approaches can decrease LUTS and its impact for some men. Initial approaches include bladder retraining and unhurried voiding without straining to completely empty the bladder (22). Diuretic beverages with caffeine or alcohol should be avoided. If nocturia is bothersome, evening fluid intake should be avoided, and an afternoon diuretic can be considered for preemptive diuresis in men with large nocturnal fluid shifts.

Watchful Waiting

The repeated observation of marked symptom improvement without specific therapy has established watchful waiting as sound management. Men appropriate for watchful waiting are those with mild to moderate symptoms, who can be followed reliably, and have no evidence of retention (e.g., elevated PVR). Patients should be followed yearly to monitor symptoms, renal function, and possibly PVR and PSA level. They should be counseled to avoid medications that may precipitate urinary retention (e.g., over-the-counter "cold" tablets containing α-agonists), and monitored carefully if anticholinergic or calcium channel blocking drugs are prescribed.

Case (Part 5)

Mr. P.'s AUA symptom score is 20, equivalent to severe symptoms.
   What are the mechanisms, dosage, and side effects of medications for treatment of BPH? Which medication would you recommend first?
   When is surgery indicated? How will you describe the risks and benefits of surgery versus watchful waiting to Mr. P.?

Medical Therapy

α-Adrenergic Blockers

α_1-Adrenergic blockers reduce BPH-related LUTS by decreasing smooth muscle contractility in the prostate capsule, stroma, and urethra. Most commonly used are prazosin (Minipress) 1 to 2 mg twice a day, the longer-acting terazosin (Hytrin) 2 to 5 mg daily, and doxazosin (Cardura) 4 to 8 mg daily, and the α_1-selective tamsulosin (Flomax) 0.4 mg daily (Table 27.9). α-Blockers reduce symptoms by 30% to 40% over placebo in 50% to 70% of moderately symptomatic men (23). Time to effect is 2 to 4 weeks, compared with 3 to 6 months for finasteride (24). Common side effects include dizziness (up to 19%), orthostatic hypotension, asthenia, and headache; and retrograde ejaculation with tamsulosin (4–14%). Side effects are avoided by slow titration from low starting doses at bedtime. Although α-blockers are approved for treatment of hypertension, they are not recommended as first-line agents.

TABLE 27.9. Medications commonly used to treat BPH-related LUTS

Mechanism	Medication	Dosage	Side effects
α₁-Adrenergic blocker	Terazosin (Hytrin)	2–5 mg daily	Dizziness, orthostatic
	Doxazosin (Cardura)	4–8 mg daily	hypotension, asthenia,
	Prazosin (Minipress)	1–2 mg twice/day	and headache; and
	Alfuzosin (Uroxatral)	10 mg daily	retrograde ejaculation
α₁-selective blocker	Tamsulosin (Flomax)	0.4 mg daily	Retrograde ejaculation
5α-reductase inhibitor	Finasteride (Proscar)	5–10 mg daily	Sexual dysfunction, gynecomastia

5α-Reductase Inhibitors

Finasteride (Proscar) shrinks the prostate gland by blocking 5α-reduction of testosterone to dihydrotestosterone, the steroid sustaining prostate growth. Standard dosage of 5 mg daily decreases prostate volume by up to 30% in one third of men at 12 months and reduces symptoms by 25% in two thirds of men at 1 year (26). Time to effect may require up to 10 months. Sustained effect requires lifetime use, because prostate growth resumes once finasteride is stopped. Finasteride decreases PSA levels by up to 40% to 60% after 1 year in one third of men (27); this may make monitoring for prostate cancer difficult. Common side effects include adverse sexual effects, including decreased libido (3%), decreased ejaculation (3%), impotence (3–4%), and gynecomastia (0.4%) (28).

Phytotherapy

Plant-derived compounds are widely used as over-the-counter treatment for BPH. Though studies of these agents are methodologically flawed, meta-analyses suggest they are efficacious. Best studied is *Serenoa repens* or saw palmetto; compared to placebo, it improves urinary symptoms [risk ratio 1.75; 95% confidence interval (CI) 1.21–2.54], decreases nocturia, and increases flow rate (29–31). Other agents shown to be efficacious include β-sitosterols and cernilton (rye grass pollen) (32,33). These agents have few to no reported side effects, but long-term data are lacking.

Antiandrogens

Luteinizing hormone–releasing hormone (LHRH) agonists or androgen receptor inhibitors such as leuprolide cause medical castration and result in prostate shrinkage (34). Such agents may facilitate removal of indwelling catheters in frail older men with BOO (35). Time to effect may be 12 months. Like finasteride, these agents decrease PSA levels and must be continued indefinitely to maintain prostate reduction. Side effects include impotence, weight gain, and hot flashes (LHRH agonists and cyproterone acetate) and diarrhea and gynecomastia (flutamide).

Surgery

Transurethral Resection of Prostate

Transurethral resection of prostate (TURP) is the gold standard of BPH treatment because it has the highest rate of symptom improvement—generally 80% to 88% (36). Absolute indications for TURP are severe obstructive symptoms, acute urinary retention, hydronephrosis, recurrent urinary infections or hematuria, and obstructive renal failure. Sexual dysfunction following TURP is a concern for many men. Impotence occurs in 14% to 40% of men, with higher rates in older men (37); 74% develop retrograde ejaculation (15), a concern only if conception is desired. Urinary incontinence occurs in approximately 5%.

The major complications of TURP are bleeding requiring transfusion, urinary retention, and infection; rarer is *"TURP syndrome,"* severe hyponatremia due to systemic absorption of hypotonic bladder irrigation fluid used intraoperatively. Men over age 80 have higher rates of perioperative mortality (2–3% vs. <0.5% in younger men) (38), but in selected robust older men, TURP can be done as an outpatient procedure. In frail patients with small prostates, general or spinal anesthesia can be avoided and TURP performed with sedation and local prostate anesthesia (39).

Open Prostatectomy

Larger prostates require longer TURP resection times, with increased risk of TURP syndrome and complications of anesthesia. Open prostatectomy by abdominal or perineal approach is recommended for men with prostates greater than 60 g. In practice, open procedures account for fewer than 5% of surgeries, because many surgeons prefer to perform an "incomplete" TURP rather than risk the greater morbidity of open surgery (40).

Prostate Incision

If the prostate is small (less than 30 g), prostatotomy or transurethral incision of the prostate (TUIP) provides similar efficacy to TURP with a technically simpler procedure, shorter operation time, and the potential for using local anesthesia (41). Additional advantages of TUIP include lower rates of bleeding complications and postoperative retrograde ejaculation. For the higher risk older man with BOO and a small prostate for whom noninvasive management has failed or is not optimal, TUIP may be a safe and effective alternative to TURP.

Laser Prostatectomy

Several laser systems currently are used to cause prostate vaporization and coagulation necrosis. Randomized trials show outcomes for laser vs. TURP are equal at 1 year (42–44). Advantages of laser therapy include shorter hospital stay, fewer blood transfusions, and urethral strictures (45). Disadvantages include variable results depending on system used (46), longer catheterization, more infections, and side effects including impotence, retrograde ejaculation, increased urgency and frequency for several weeks, incontinence, and stricture.

Microwave Hyperthermia

Transurethral microwave thermotherapy (TUMT) has shown variable symptom improvement in controlled trials (45). Many patients require further therapy for their symptoms (46). Compared with terazosin, TUMT provided less symptom relief at 2 weeks, but was better at 6 months (47).

Other Approaches

Transurethral needle ablation (TUNA) is less efficacious in symptom relief than TURP at 1 year, but results in no retrograde ejaculation and less bleeding (48). Wire urethral stents may restore spontaneous voiding in frail men with retention who are not surgical candidates or for whom indwelling catheters are undesirable. Complications of stents include encrustation, infection, urinary incontinence, and retention.

General Principles

* Prostate symptoms are a common feature of aging for many men, with moderate to severe symptoms occurring in one third of older men. Prostate size and associated symptoms do not progress inevitably in most men, but vary over time.
* Benign prostatic hyperplasia, prostate enlargement, bladder outlet obstruction, and associated urinary tract symptoms are not equivalent; they have variable pathophysiologic causes and effects.
* Benign prostatic hyperplasia–related LUTS is associated with a variety of changes in the prostate, urethra, and bladder. It is important to remember that the prostate is not always the cause of LUTS in older men, regardless of the presence of prostate enlargement.
* Diagnostic evaluation should include the history and relevant review of systems, an measurement of symptom severity (e.g., AUA symptom index), medication review, digital rectal exam, urinalysis, and serum creatinine.
* The four main treatment approaches recommended for BPH-related LUTS include watchful waiting, medication, surgery, and alternative procedures.

- Men with mild symptoms (AUA Sympton Score ≤ 7) should be treated with watchful waiting and lifestyle changes, whereas men with moderate to severe symptoms (AUA Sympton Score ≥ 8) should be offered the full range of treatment options including watchful waiting, medical, minimally invasive, or surgical therapies.
- Medications used to treat BPH include α_1-adrenergic blockers and 5α-reductase inhibitors or a combination of both formen with demonstrable prostatic enlargement.
- Transurethral resection of prostate is the gold standard of BPH treatment, but is not indicated in most patients; complications include sexual dysfunction, bleeding, and infection.

Suggested Readings

Barry MJ, Fowler FJ Jr, O'Leary MP, et al. The American Urological Association symptom index for benign prostatic hyperplasia. J Urol 1992;148:1549–1557. *The AUA symptom index is clinically sensible, reliable, valid and responsive. It is practical for use in practice and for inclusion in research protocols.*

DuBeau CE. Benign prostatic hyperplasia. In: Cassel CK, Leipzig RM, Cohen HJ, et al., eds. Geriatric Medicine, 4th ed. New York: Springer, 2003:755–768.

AUA Practice Guidelines Committee (2003). AUA guideline on management of benign prostatic hyperplasia (2003). Chapter 1: Diagnosis and treatment recommendations. J Urol 203;170:530–547. *A comprehensive review of the identification and management of BPH. It includes an intensive review of the randomized trials addressing the different treatment approaches.*

References

1. Schäfer W, Rubben H, Noppeney R, Deutz F-J. Obstructed and unobstructed prostatic obstruction: a plea for urodynamic objectivation of bladder outflow obstruction in benign prostatic hyperplasia. World J Urol 1989;6:198–203.
2. Coolsaet BLRA, van Venrooij GEPM, Blok C. Prostatism: rationalization of urodynamic testing. World J Urol 1984;2:216–221.
3. Abrams P. In support of pressure-flow studies for evaluating men with lower urinary tract symptoms. Urology 1994;44:153–155.
4. Isaacs JT, Coffey DS. Etiology and disease process of benign prostatic hyperplasia. Prostate Suppl 1989;2:33–50.
5. Berry SJ, Coffey DS, Walsh PC, Ewing LL. The development of human benign prostatic hyperplasia with age. J Urol 1984;132:474–479.
6. Chute CG, Panser LA, Girman CJ, et al. The prevalence of prostatism: a population-based survey of urinary symptoms. J Urol 1993;150:85–89.
7. Partin AW, Oesterling JE, Epstein JI, Horton R, Walsh PC. Influence of age and endocrine factors on the volume of benign prostatic hyperplasia. J Urol 1991;145:405–409.
8. Watanabe H. Natural history of benign prostatic hypertrophy. Ultrasound Med Biol 1986;12:567–571.

9. Roehrborn CG, Boyle P, Bergner D, et al. Serum prostate-specific antigen and prostate volume predict long-term changes in symptoms and flow rate: results of a 4-year, randomized trial comparing finasteride versus placebo. Urology 1999;54:662–669.

10. Dørflinger T, England DM, Madsen PO, Bruskewitz RC. Urodynamic and histological correlates of benign prostatic hyperplasia. J Urol 1988;140:1487–1490.

11. Hinman F Jr. Point of view: capsular influence on benign prostatic hypertrophy. Urology 1986;28:347–350.

12. Chapple CR, Burt RP, Andersson PO, Greengrass P, Wyllie M, Marshall I. Alpha$_1$–adrenoreceptor subtypes in the human prostate. Br J Urol 1994;74:585–589.

13. Chapple CR, Smith D. The pathophysiological changes in the bladder obstructed by benign prostatic hyperplasia. Br J Urol 1994;73:117–123.

14. Elbadawi A, Yalla SV, Resnick NM. Structural basis of geriatric voiding dysfunction. IV. Bladder outlet obstruction. J Urol 1993;150:1681–1695.

15. AUA Practice Guidelines Committee (2003). AUA guideline on management of benign prostatic hyperplasia (2003). Chapter 1: Diagnosis and treatment recommendations. J Urol 203;170:530–547.

16. Bruskewitz RC, Larsen EH, Madsen PO, et al. 3 year followup of urinary symptoms after transurethral resection of the prostate. J Urol 1986;136:613–615.

17. Jensen KM-E, Bruskewitz RC, Iversen P, Madsen PO. Significance of prostatic weight in prostatism. Urol Int 1983;38:173–178.

18. Andersen JT, Nordling J. Prostatism II. The correlation between cystourethroscopic, cystometric, and urodynamic findings. Scand J Urol Nephrol 1980;14:23–27.

19. Meyhoff HH, Hald T. Are doctors able to assess prostatic size? Scand J Urol Nephrol 1978;12:219–221.

20. Coolsaet B, Blok C. Detrusor properties related to prostatism. Neurourol Urodynam 1986;5:435–447.

21. Barry MJ, Fowler FJ Jr, O'Leary MP, et al. The American Urological Association symptom index for benign prostatic hyperplasia. J Urol 1992;148:1549–1557.

22. Root MT. Living with benign prostatic hypertrophy [letter]. N Engl J Med 1979;301:52.

23. Djavan B, Marberger M. A meta-analysis on the efficacy and tolerability of alpha1–adrenoceptor antagonists in patients with lower urinary tract symptoms suggestive of benign prostatic obstruction. Eur Urol 1999;36:1–13.

24. Kirby RS, McConnell JD. Fast Facts-Benign Prostatic Hyperplasia, 2nd ed. Oxford, UK: Health Press, 1997:29.

25. Lee M. Tamulosin for the treatment of benign prostatic hypertrophy. Ann Pharmacother 2000;34:188–199.

26. Gormley GJ, Stoner E, Bruskewitz RC, et al. The effect of finasteride in men with benign prostatic hyperplasia. N Engl J Med 1992;327:1185–1191.

27. Gormley GJ, Ng J, Cook T, Stoner E, Guess H, Walsh P. Effect of finasteride on prostate-specific antigen density. Urology 1994;43:53–59.

28. McConnell JD, Bruskewitz R, Walsh P, et al. The effect of finasteride on the risk of acute urinary retention and the need for surgical treatment among men

with benign prostatic hyperplasia. Finasteride Long-Term Efficacy and Safety Study Group. N Engl J Med 1998;338:557–563.

29. Wilt T, Ishani A, Stark G, Mac Donald R, Mulrow C, Lau J. Serenoa repens for benign prostatic hyperplasia (Cochrane Review). In: The Cochrane Library, issue 3. Oxford: Update Software, 2000.

30. Boyle P, Robertson C, Lowe F, Roehrborn C. Meta-analysis of clinical trials of permixon in the treatment of symptomatic benign prostatic hyperplasia. Urology 2000;55:533–539.

31. Wilt TJ, MacDonald R, Ishani A. Beta-sitosterols for the treatment of benign prostatic hyperplasia: a systematic review. BJU Int 1999;83:976–983; see also: Wilt T, Ishani A, MacDonald R, Stark G, Mulrow C, Lau J. Beta-sitosterols for benign prostatic hyperplasia (Cochrane Review). In: The Cochrane Library, issue 3. Oxford: Update Software, 2000.

32. MacDonald R, Ishani A, Rutks I, Wilt TJ. A systematic review of Cernilton for the treatment of benign prostatic hyperplasia. BJU Int 2000;85:836–841; see also: Wilt T, Ishani A, MacDonald R, Ishani A, Rutks I, Stark G. Cernilton for benign prostatic hyperplasia (Cochrane Review). In: The Cochrane Library, issue 3. Oxford: Update Software, 2000.

33. McConnell JD. Medical management of benign prostatic hyperplasia with androgen suppression. Prostate Suppl 1990;3:49–59.

34. Eri LM, Tveter KJ. A prospective, placebo-controlled study of the luteinizing hormone-releasing hormone agonist leuprolide as treatment for patients with benign prostatic hyperplasia. J Urol 1993;150:359–364.

35. Jenkins BJ, Sharma P, Badenoch DF, Fowler CG, Blandy JP. Ethics, logistics and a trial of transurethral versus open prostatectomy. Br J Urol 1992;69: 372–374.

36. Libman E, Fichten CS. Prostatectomy and sexual function. Urology 1987;29: 467–478.

37. Mebust WK, Holtgrewe HL, Cockett ATK, et al. Transurethral prostatectomy: immediate and postoperative complications. A cooperative study of 13 participating institutions evaluating 3,885 patients. J Urol 1989;141:243–247.

38. Birch BR, Gelister JS, Parker CJ, Chave H, Miller RA. Transurethral resection of prostate under sedation and local anesthesia (sedoanalgesia). Urology 1991;38:113–118.

39. Neal DE. Prostatectomy: an open or closed case. Br J Urol 1990;66:449–454.

40. Orandi A. Transurethral incision of the prostate (TUIP): 646 cases in 15 years—a chronological appraisal. Br J Urol 1985;57:703–707.

41. Donovan JL, Peters TJ, Neal DE, et al. A randomized trial comparing transurethral resection of the prostate, laser therapy and conservative management for lower urinary tract symptoms associated with benign prostatic enlargement: the ClasP study. J Urol 2000;164:65–70.

42. Carter A, Sells H, Speakman M, Ewings P, MacDonagh R, O'Boyle P. A prospective randomized controlled trial of hybrid laser treatment or transurethral section of the prostate, with a 1-year follow-up. BJU Int 1999;83: 254–259.

43. Carter A, Sells H, Speakman M, Ewings P, O'Boyle P, MacDonagh R. Quality of life changes following KTP/Nd:YAG laser treatment of the prostate and TURP. Eur Urol 1999;36:92–98.

44. Jones JW, Carter A, Ewings P, O'Boyle PJ. An MRSA outbreak in a urology ward and its association with Nd:YAG coagulation laser treatment of the prostate. J Hosp Infect 1999;41:39–44.

45. Ogden CW, Reddy P, Johnson H, Ramsay JW, Carter SS. Sham versus transurethral microwave thermotherapy in patients with symptoms of benign prostatic bladder outflow obstruction. Lancet 1993;341:14–17.

46. Bdesha AS, Bunce CJ, Kelleher JP, Snell ME, Vukusic J, Witherow RO. Transurethral microwave treatment for benign prostatic hypertrophy: a randomised controlled clinical trail. BMJ 1993;306:1293–1296.

47. Brehmer M, Wiskell H, Kinn A. Sham treatment compared with 30 or 60 min of thermotherapy for benign prostatic hyperplasia: a randomized study. BJU Int 1999;84:292a–296.

48. Bruskewitz R, Issa M, Roehrborn C, et al. A prospective, randomized 1-year clinical trial comparing transurethral needle ablation to transurethral resection of the prostate for the treatment of symptomatic benign prostatic hyperplasia. J Urol 1998;159:1588–1594.

28
Erectile Dysfunction

Hans L. Stöhrer

Learning Objectives

Upon completion of the chapter, the student will be able to:

1. Describe the prevalence of erectile dysfunction (ED) and its impact on quality of life in older men.
2. Describe the age-related changes in male sexuality.
3. Understand the pathophysiology of ED.
4. Describe recommended diagnostic evaluation of ED.
5. Enumerate the five main treatment options for ED, and discuss the risks and benefits of each.

Case (Part 1)

Mr. C. is a 69-year-old retired postal worker. He has diabetes type 2 managed with oral hypoglycemics, mild diabetic retinopathy, and chronic intermittent low back pain. You have treated him for the past 3 years. At the end of a routine office visit at the end of a busy day, he looks at you anxiously, then says, "Doc, isn't there anything you can do? My sex life has been almost nonexistent."

What are some age-related changes in sexuality?

How prevalent is erectile dysfunction in the older population?

How prevalent is erectile dysfunction in diabetics?

Material in this chapter is based on the following chapter in Cassel CK, Leipzig RM, Cohen HJ, Larson EB, Meier DE, eds. Geriatric Medicine: An Evidence-Based Approach, 4th ed. New York: Springer, 2003: Mulligan T, Siddiqi W. Changes in Male Sexuality, pp. 719–726. Selections edited by Hans L. Stöhrer.

General Considerations

Sexuality remains an important issue in the older population. At the same time, sexual dysfunction increases in prevalence with age, and is associated with impaired quality of life. Despite a decreased ability to achieve an erection, there clearly is continued sexual desire. The term *erectile dysfunction* (ED) refers to the inability to achieve an erection, according to a National Institutes of Health (NIH) consensus panel (1). Erectile dysfunction in the aged is primarily due to age-associated chronic disease rather than normal, healthy aging. An estimated 10 million to 30 million American men are affected, with 52% prevalence in men aged 40 to 70 years; 41% of complete erectile failure cases occur in men aged 60 to 79 years, and 100% of incomplete erection cases occur in men >70 years (2).

Age-Associated Changes in Male Sexuality

As men proceed through life, there is a clear change in their sexuality. Table 28.1 outlines age-associated changes in sexual behavior. Causes of these age-associated changes are multifactorial, including organic and social factors. For further details, see Chapter 48: Changes in Male Sexuality. In: Cassel Ck et al., eds; Geriatric Medicine, 4th ed, page 719.

Pathophysiology of Erectile Dysfunction

The most common causes of ED in older men are vascular disease, neurologic disease, and medications. Erectile dysfunction is extremely common in diabetics. The prevalence of psychogenic ED, on the other hand, inversely correlates with age. Rarer causes of ED include hypogonadism,

TABLE 28.1. Age-associated changes in sexual behavior (3–7)

Decrease in frequency of sexual intercourse
- 95% of men aged 46–50 years have intercourse weekly, but only 28% of men aged 66–71 years have weekly intercourse
- Decline in sexual activity associated with declining health, not simply advancing age

Cessation of sexual intercourse attributed by men to loss of erectile function, decreased libido, and medical illness

Increase in expressions of intimacy (kissing, hugging, caressing, oral sex, or masturbation) without intercourse

Libido varies much less with advancing age
- Serum free-testosterone correlates with sexual desire and arousal in healthy older population

Four stages of sexual response (excitement, plateau, orgasm, and resolution) change with aging

Source: Data from Pfeiffer E, Verwoerdt A, Wang HS. Sexual behavior in aged men and women. Arch Gen Psychiatr 1968;19:753–758. Mulligan T, Retchin SM, Chinchilli VM, et al. The role of aging and chronic disease in sexual dysfunction. J Am Geriatr Soc 1988;36:520–524. Kaiser FE. Sexuality in the elderly. Urol Clin North Am 1996;23:99–109. Masters W, Johnson V. Human Sexual Response. Boston: Little, Brown, 1970. Rowland DL, Greenleaf WJ, Dorfman LJ, Davidson JM. Aging and sexual function in men. Arch Sex Behav 1993;22:545–557.

hyperprolactinemia, hypothyroidism, hyperthyroidism, chronic alcoholism, and chronic obstructive lung disease.

Vascular Disease

The most common etiology of ED in aged men is vascular disease, accounting for 68% of men with organic ED. The risk of ED increases with the number of vascular risk factors (diabetes mellitus, smoking, hyperlipidemia, and hypertension); 100% of men with three or more risk factors had ED in one study. Two mechanisms, *arterial insufficiency* and *venous leakage*, account for ED in vascular disease. Atherosclerotic arterial occlusive disease decreases perfusion pressure and arterial flow to the lacunar spaces necessary to achieve a rigid erection. Ischemia also results in replacement of smooth muscle by connective tissue, which results in impaired cavernosal expandability. Venous leakage, excessive outflow through the subtunical venules, prevents the development of high pressure within the corpora cavernosa necessary for a rigid erection. It is caused by an increased number of venous outflow channels, decreased compliance of trabeculae with inability to compress the subtunical venules, and insufficient relaxation of trabecular smooth muscle.

Neurologic Disease

Neurologic disease accounts for the second most common cause of ED in older men. It results from disorders of the parasympathetic sacral spinal cord or peripheral efferent autonomic fibers to the penis, which impair penile smooth muscle relaxation and prevent the vasodilation needed for erection. Common neurologic causes of ED in older men include autonomic dysfunction from diabetes mellitus, stroke, or Parkinson's disease, and injury to autonomic nerves from radical prostatectomy or proctocolectomy.

Diabetes Mellitus

The prevalence of ED in diabetes mellitus is as high as 75%. More than 50% of male diabetic patients have ED within 10 years of diagnosis; for some it is the presenting symptom. Though the etiology of diabetic ED is multifactorial, the major cause in older diabetic men is vascular disease; autonomic neuropathy is more important in younger patients (8). Other mechanisms of diabetic ED may include impairment in both autonomic and endothelium-dependent mechanisms for relaxation of smooth muscle, impaired penile cholinergic nerve synthesis with decreased ability to relax trabecular smooth muscle, and inactivation of endothelium-derived nitric oxide by advanced glycosylation end products (AGE) (9).

Testosterone Level

The role of androgens in erection is controversial. Androgen receptors have been demonstrated in sacral parasympathetic nuclei and hypothalamic and limbic system neurons. Libido is related to testosterone levels. In hypogonadal men there is a dose-related response to androgen treatment and the frequency of nocturnal erection and coitus. Studies suggest erections from direct penile stimulation may be androgen-independent, and response to fantasy androgen-dependent.

Drug-Induced Erectile Dysfunction

Many commonly used medications are associated with ED, with a reported 25% incidence of drug-induced ED in the outpatient population (10), but supportive data are often subjective and based on weak methodology, and the mechanisms of drug-induced ED are uncertain. Antihypertensive medications, especially beta-blockers, clonidine, and thiazide diuretics, may decrease perfusion pressure to the erectile bodies. Medications such as antidepressants, antipsychotics, and antihistamines (including cimetidine and ranitidine) have anticholinergic effects that may block parasympathetic-mediated penile artery vasodilation and trabecular smooth muscle relaxation. Antipsychotic medications cause sedation, elevation of serum prolactin level, and have anticholinergic or central antidopaminergic effects.

Psychogenic Erectile Dysfunction

The prevalence of psychogenic ED correlates inversely with age, with reported prevalence of only 9% in an aged male veteran population (11). Psychogenic ED may occur via increased sympathetic stimuli to the sacral cord, inhibiting the parasympathetic dilator nerves to the penis. Common causes include performance anxiety, relationship conflicts, sexual inhibition, history of childhood sexual abuse, and fear of sexually transmitted diseases. A classic psychogenic cause in older men is the "widower's syndrome," where the older man involved in a new relationship feels guilt and develops ED as a defense against perceived unfaithfulness to his dead spouse.

Other Factors in Erectile Dysfunction

In addition to hypogonadism, other endocrine abnormalities are rare causes of ED (12). Hyperprolactinemia decreases serum testosterone concentration due to inhibition of gonadotropin-releasing hormone secretion. Hypothyroidism may also cause ED via elevated prolactin and low testosterone levels. Hyperthyroidism is more associated with a decline in libido than with ED. Chronic alcoholism can cause ED via toxicity at the hypothalamic-pituitary-gonadal levels, or peripheral and autonomic neuropathy. Severe chronic obstructive lung disease with hypoxia suppresses the hypothalamic-pituitary-gonadal axis.

Case (Part 2)

You ask Mr. C. to return soon for a follow-up visit to discuss his concerns further.
What issues should you explore at the next visit?
What should you look for on physical exam?
What lab tests should you consider ordering?

Diagnostic Evaluation

Initial evaluation should include a sexual, psychosocial, and medical history, medication review, focused physical exam, and limited diagnostic tests (Table 28.2).

The sexual history should clarify whether a problem exists in arousal, erection, penetration, or orgasmic failure. It should inquire about the onset and duration of erectile dysfunction, presence of erection during sleep or with masturbation, and the presence of libido. It can explore the circumstances of sexual activity and which methods have been tried.

The psychosocial history explores the patient's emotions or fears associated with sexual activity, relationship with his partner, the partner's health, and living situation. History of alcohol or substance abuse should also be sought.

The medical history seeks risk factors for ED. Vascular risk factors include diabetes mellitus, smoking, hyperlipidemia, hypertension, as well as the presence of known vascular disease. Neurogenic risk factors include diabetes mellitus, stroke, Parkinson's disease, alcoholism, and pelvic or spinal injury or surgery. Medications must be reviewed, including nonprescription and herbal products, and especially whether the patient takes any nitrates.

The physical exam should search for signs of vascular disease (absent peripheral pulses, femoral bruits), neurologic disease (penile or peripheral neuropathy), penile plaques, hypogonadism (testicular atrophy, gynecomastia), and evidence of undiagnosed thyroid disease.

Few laboratory-based tests are essential, but many authors recommend blood glucose, testosterone, and cholesterol, and some recommend a diagnostic penile injection of a vasoactive medication (13).

TABLE 28.2. Recommended steps in diagnostic evaluation of erectile dysfunction (ED) (13,14)

Sexual history
- Clarify where the problem exists in stage of sexual response
- Onset abrupt vs. gradual (psychogenic or adverse drug vs. organic etiology)
- Presence of erection during sleep or with masturbation (psychogenic vs. organic etiology)
- Presence of libido (hypogonadism)
- Circumstances and methods of sexual activity tried

Psychosocial history
- Emotions or fears associated with sexual activity
- Relationship with partner
- Partner's health
- Living situation
- Alcohol or substance abuse

Medical history
- Vascular risk factors (diabetes mellitus, smoking, hyperlipidemia, and hypertension)
- Neurogenic risk factors (diabetes mellitus, stroke, Parkinson's disease, alcoholism, pelvic or spinal injury or surgery)
- Other chronic disease (severe chronic obstructive pulmonary disease, alcoholism)

Medication review
- Antihypertensives, antidepressants, antipsychotics, antihistamines, nitrates

Physical exam
- Peripheral pulses, femoral bruits
- Penile or peripheral neuropathy
- Testicular atrophy, gynecomastia
- Penile plaques
- Evidence of undiagnosed thyroid disease

Laboratory tests (optional)
- Blood glucose, cholesterol
- Testosterone, prolactin, luteinizing hormone
- Thyroid-stimulating hormone

Diagnostic penile injection of vasoactive medication. (optional)

Source: Data from Johnson III AR, Jarow JP. Is routine endocrine testing of impotent men necessary? J Urol 1992;147:1542–1543. Godschalk MF, Sison A, Mulligan T. Management of erectile dysfunction by the geriatrician. J Am Geriatr Soc 1997;45:1240–1246.

Case (Part 3)

Your evaluation of Mr. C. reveals a gradual onset of erectile dysfunction over the past couple of years; there is no erection with manual stimulation or during sleep; and no new medications have been prescribed recently. On exam there is evidence of retinopathy and decreased vibration and position sense in the feet. You consider decreasing Mr. C.'s angiotensin-converting enzyme (ACE)-inhibitor, but decide to continue it because of its beneficial effects in disease progression.

What treatment options should you discuss with your patient?

What risks should be considered in prescribing sildenafil?

Management Considerations

There are currently several effective treatment approaches for ED. Treatment should be individualized, considering the cause of ED, patient preference, and cost.

Sildenafil (Viagra) is the first available oral therapy. It is a phosphodiesterase inhibitor that blocks cyclic guanosine monophosphate (cGMP) degradation. It is effective in 65% of men with organic erectile dysfunction, but has limited effectiveness in men with advanced vascular disease. The most common side effects include headache, flushing, and dyspepsia, occurring in 6% to 18%. The initial dose should be 50 mg, reduced to 25 mg if side effects occur, or increased to 100 mg if necessary. Each dose costs about $9. Concurrent use of sildenafil and nitrates can be fatal. If a man who has taken sildenafil has an ischemic cardiac event, nitrates should not be prescribed within 24 hours. A consensus statement from the American College of Cardiology/American Heart Association also urged caution in men with coronary ischemia, congestive heart failure, and low blood pressure as well as those taking a multidrug antihypertensive regimen (15). In 2003, the newer oral medications, vardenafil (Levitra) and tadalafil (Cialis) were approved by the Food and Drug Administration (FDA) for erectile dysfunction (16) (Table 28.3).

Penile injection therapy with alprostadil (prostaglandin E_1), papaverine, or phentolamine is used to induce erection. These drugs, when injected into the corpora cavernosa, induce relaxation of smooth muscle, causing blood engorgement, compression of the emissary veins, and an erection within a few minutes after injection. Men can be trained to inject vasoactive medications into one corporal body; cross-circulation allows medication to diffuse into the contralateral side. Side effects include penile pain and bruising, fibrosis, and priapism. Alternatively, prostaglandin E_1 can be administered intraurethrally using MUSE (medicated urethral system for erection).

Several mechanical devices have been developed that utilize vacuum pressure to increase arterial inflow and occlusive rings to impede venous outflow from the corpora cavernosa. Mechanical dexterity is required to use these devices. Efficacy is reported to be 67%, and satisfaction with vacuum-assisted erections has varied between 25% and 49%. The cost per device is $200 to $400.

Surgical penile implants remain a viable option for men who do not respond to sildenafil and find penile injection, urethral, or vacuum therapy unacceptable. Side effects include those of anesthesia, infection, and mechanical failure necessitating surgical removal and reimplantation of a new prosthesis. The cost per implant is approximately $5000.

Testosterone supplementation should be reserved for men diagnosed with hypogonadism. In men with normal gonadal function, androgen therapy enhances sexual interest without enhancing erectile capacity.

TABLE 28.3. Current oral phosphodiesterase inhibitors type 5 (PDE-5) used for erectile dysfunction (17)

	Sildenafil (Viagra)	Vardenafil (Levitra)	Tadalafil (Cialis)
Initial dose	50mg, titrated up to 100mg or down to 25mg based on efficacy and tolerability, no more than once daily	10mg titrated up to 20mg or down to 5mg based on efficacy and tolerability, no more than once daily	10mg titrated up to 20mg or down to 5mg based on efficacy and tolerability, no more than once daily
Mean terminal half-life	About 4 hours	About 4 hours	About 17.5 hours
Duration of action	Up to 4 hours	Up to 4 hours	Up to 36 hours
Selectivity	10-fold more potent for PDE5 than for PDE6 (present in the retina); more than 700-fold more potent for PDE5 than for PDE11	15-fold more potent for PDE5 than for PDE6; more than 300-fold more potent for PDE5 than for PDE11	700-fold more potent for PDE5 than for PDE6; 14-fold more potent for PDE5 than for PDE11A1 (in skeletal muscle)
Use with α-blockers	50- or 100-mg doses should not be taken within 4 hours of α-blocker administration; a 25-mg dose may be taken at any time	Contraindicated	Contraindicated except with tamsulosin 0.4mg once daily
Use with congenital or acquired QT prolongation or with class Ia or III antiarrhythmic drugs	No special precautions	Should be avoided	No special precautions recommended
Use in renal insufficiency	Dose decreased to 25mg not more than once daily in severe renal failure (creatinine clearance <30mL/minute); limited experience in patients on hemodialysis	No dose adjustment recommended; not yet evaluated in patients on dialysis	Dose decreased to 5mg not more than once daily in moderate or severe renal insufficiency (creatinine clearance <30mL/minute); no data available in patients on dialysis
Use in age >65 years	Initial dose decreased to 25mg	Initial dose decreased to 5mg	No dose adjustment is warranted on the basis of age alone
Effect of food	High-fat meals decrease maximum plasma concentration by 29% and delay time to maximum plasma concentration by 60 minutes	High-fat meals decrease maximum plasma concentration by 18% to 50%; can be taken with or without food	Rate and extent of absorption are not affected by food; may be taken without regard to food
Effect of alcohol	Sildenafil 50mg did not potentiate the hypotensive effect of alcohol, with mean maximum blood alcohol level of 0.08%	Vardenafil 20mg did not potentiate the hypotensive effect of alcohol when given with alcohol 0.5g/kg (equivalent to about 40mL of absolute alcohol in a 70-kg person); plasma levels of alcohol and vardenafil were not altered when given simultaneously	Postural hypotension and dizziness may occur with coadministration of tadalafil 20mg with alcohol 0.7g/kg but not with 0.6g/kg; plasma levels of alcohol and tadalafil were not altered when given simultaneously

Source: Data from Mikhail N. Management of erectile dysfunction by the primary care physician. Cleve Clin J Med 2005;72(4):293–294,296–297,301–305.

General Principles

---

* Erectile dysfunction increases in prevalence with age, and is associated with impaired quality of life.
* Despite a decreased ability to achieve an erection, there clearly is continued sexual desire, and an increase in expressions of intimacy without intercourse. The most common causes of ED in older men are vascular disease, neurologic disease, and medications.
* The prevalence of psychogenic ED inversely correlates with age.
* Rarer causes of ED include hypogonadism, hyperprolactinemia, hypothyroidism, hyperthyroidism, chronic alcoholism, and chronic obstructive lung disease.
* Initial evaluation should include a sexual, psychosocial, and medical history, focused physical exam, and limited diagnostic tests.
* The effective treatment approaches currently for ED include sildenafil, vardenafil, tadalafil, penile injection therapy, mechanical devices, surgical implants, and in select cases, testosterone supplementation.

Suggested Readings

Cheitlin MD, Hutter AM Jr, Brindis RG, et al. Use of sildenafil (Viagra) in patients with cardiovascular disease. Circulation 1999;99:168–177. *A review of the first oral therapy for erectile dysfunction of varying etiology.*

Mulligan T, Siddiqi W. Changes in male sexuality. In: Cassel CK, Leipzig RM, Cohen HJ, et al., eds. Geriatric Medicine, 4th ed. New York: Springer, 2003: 719–726.

NIH Consensus Conference. Impotence. JAMA 1993;270:83–90. *A comprehensive review of erectile dysfunction albeit prior to the advent of oral therapy.*

References

1. NIH Consensus Conference. Impotence. JAMA 1993;270:83–90.
2. Feldman HA, Goldstein I, Hatzichristou DG, et al. Impotence and its medical and psychosocial correlates: results of the Massachusetts male aging study. J Urol 1994;151:54–61.
3. Pfeiffer E, Verwoerdt A, Wang HS. Sexual behavior in aged men and women. Arch Gen Psychiatr 1968;19:753–758.
4. Mulligan T, Retchin SM, Chinchilli VM, et al. The role of aging and chronic disease in sexual dysfunction. J Am Geriatr Soc 1988;36:520–524.
5. Kaiser FE. Sexuality in the elderly. Urol Clin North Am 1996;23:99–109.
6. Masters W, Johnson V. Human Sexual Response. Boston: Little, Brown, 1970.
7. Rowland DL, Greenleaf WJ, Dorfman LJ, Davidson JM. Aging and sexual function in men. Arch Sex Behav 1993;22:545–557.

8. Nehra A, Azadzoi KM, Moreland RB, et al. Cavernosal expandability is an erectile tissue mechanical property which predicts trabecular histology in an animal model of vasculogenic erectile dysfunction. J Urol 1998;59:2229–2236.

9. Morley JE, Kaiser FE. Sexual function with advancing age. Med Clin North Am 1989;73:1483–1495.

10. Hogan M, Cerami A, Bucala R. Advanced glycosylation endproducts block the antiproliferative effect of nitric oxide. J Clin Invest 1992;90:1110–1115.

11. Slag MF, Morley JE, Elson MK, et al. Impotence in medical clinic outpatients. JAMA 1983;249:1736–1740.

12. Mulligan T, Katz PG. Why aged men become impotent. Arch Intern Med 1989;149:1365–1366.

13. Johnson III AR, Jarow JP. Is routine endocrine testing of impotent men necessary? J Urol 1992;147:1542–1543.

14. Godschalk MF, Sison A, Mulligan T. Management of erectile dysfunction by the geriatrician. J Am Geriatr Soc 1997;45:1240–1246.

15. Cheitlin MD, Hutter AM Jr, Brindis RG, et al. Use of sildenafil (Viagra) in patients with cardiovascular disease. Circulation 1999;99:168–177 [erratum, Circulation 1999;100:2389].

16. Keating GM, Scott LJ. Vardenafil: a review of its use in erectile dysfunction. Drugs 2003;63(23):2673–2703.

17. Mikhail N. Management of erectile dysfunction by the primary care physician. Cleve Clin J Med 2005;72(4):293–294,296–297,301–305.

29
Urinary Incontinence

EILEEN H. CALLAHAN

Learning Objectives

Upon completion of the chapter, the student will be able to:

1. Diagnose urinary incontinence among older adults.
2. Differentiate the different types of urinary incontinence.
3. Develop and implement a plan of care for a patient with urinary incontinence.
4. Manage the symptoms of urinary incontinence.

Case (Part 1)

S.K. is a 76-year-old woman who reports that she often has "accidents" when she cannot make it to the bathroom in time. Even though this problem has bothered her for quite some time, she has not told you because she thought that it was part of "getting older." She sheepishly admits that her solution is to wear diapers.

.General Considerations

Urinary incontinence poses a major problem for the elderly, afflicting 15% to 30% of older people living at home, one third of those in acute-care settings, and at least half of those in nursing homes (1). It is more common in women. It predisposes to rashes, pressure ulcers, urinary tract infections, urosepsis, falls, and fractures (1–3). Frequently, urinary incontinence

---

Material in this chapter is based on the following chapters in Cassel CK, Leipzig RM, Cohen HJ, Larson EB, Meier DE, eds. Geriatric Medicine: An Evidence-Based Approach, 4th ed. New York: Springer, 2003: Timmons MC. Gynecologic and Urologic Problems of Older Women, pp. 737–754. Resnick NM. Urinary Incontinence, pp. 931–955. Selections edited by Eileen H. Callahan.

is not diagnosed because it is overlooked by the primary care physician and not discussed by patients (4,5). It is also associated with embarrassment, stigmatization, isolation, depression, and risk of institutionalization (1), as well as caregiver burden and depression (6). Finally, it costs more than $26 billion to manage in the United States in 1995 (7), exceeding the amount devoted to dialysis and coronary artery bypass surgery combined (7).

Age-Related Changes and Urinary Incontinence

Age-related changes, coupled with the increased likelihood that an older person will encounter an additional pathologic, physiologic, or pharmacologic insult, explains why the elderly are so likely to become incontinent. Incontinence in an older person is often due to reversible conditions outside the lower urinary tract. Furthermore, treatment of these precipitating factors alone may be enough to restore continence, even in cases where there is coexisting urinary tract dysfunction (Tables 29.1 and 29.2).

Case (Part 2)

S.K. tells you that she has had diabetes mellitus for many years. On review of systems, she says that her leg usually swells up and she frequently gets up approximately three times at night to urinate. Her medications include furosemide 20 mg daily, multivitamins 1 tablet daily, and glyburide 2.5 mg daily.

TABLE 29.1. Age-related changes in the female urogenital tract

External genitalia	Vagina	Urethra and bladder
• Thinning and graying of pubic hair • Shrunken, wrinkled appearance of labia majora • Dryness and paleness of the labia minora. • Erythema in the periurethral tissues • Clitoris prominent secondary to androgen predominance in a hypoestrogenic woman	• Vaginal atrophy inevitable in women w/o estrogen supplementation after menopause. • Changes can be reversed with estrogen therapy • Coitally active women have better preservation of the vagina and decreased degree of vaginal atrophy	• With aging and progressive hypoestrogenism, urethral functional length and maximal urethral closure pressure decrease • Urethral mucosa and bladder mucosa have estrogen-receptors; also subject to estrogen-deprivation atrophy

Source: Adapted from Timmons MC. Gynecologic and Urologic Problems of Older Women. In: Cassel CK, Leipzig RM, Cohen HJ, et al., eds. Geriatric Medicine, 4th ed. New York: Springer, 2003:737–754.

TABLE 29.2. Age-related changes that may predispose
to incontinence

- Bladder capacity and contractility decrease
- Bladder residual volume increases
- Involuntary detrusor contractions common
- Urine excretion at night increases, causing nocturia
- Estrogen decreases
- Prostate enlarges in men
- Urethral length decreases (in women)

Differential Diagnosis

Acute/Transient Incontinence

Because of their frequency, reversibility, and association with morbidity,
transient causes of incontinence should be diligently sought in every older
patient in all settings. These seven reversible causes can be recalled using
the mnemonic DIAPERS (Table 29.3) as follows:

Delirium

Incontinence may be an associated symptom that abates once the underlying cause of confusion is identified and treated. The patient needs medical
rather than bladder management (6).

Infection

Infection causes transient incontinence when dysuria and urgency are so
prominent that the older person is unable to reach the toilet before voiding.
Because illness can present atypically in older patients, incontinence is
occasionally the only atypical symptom of a urinary tract infection. Asymptomatic bacteriuria, which is much more common in the elderly, however,
does not cause incontinence. If asymptomatic bacteriuria is found on the
initial evaluation, it should be treated and the subsequent symptoms
recorded in the patient's record to prevent future futile therapy.

TABLE 29.3. Causes of transient incontinence (38)

Delirium
Infection
Atrophic urethritis/vaginitis
Pharmaceuticals
Excessive urine output (diabetes, hypercalcemia)
Restricted mobility
Stool impaction

Source: Adapted with permission from Resnick NM. Urinary Incontinence in the Elderly.
Medical Grand Rounds, vol 3. New York: Plenum, 1984. Reprinted as appears in Resnick
NM. Urinary Incontinence in Cassel CK, Leipzig RM, Cohen HJ, et al., eds. Geriatric
Medicine, 4th ed. New York: Springer, 2003.

Atrophic Urethritis/Vaginitis

This pathology frequently causes lower urinary tract symptoms, including incontinence usually associated with urgency or a sense of "scalding" dysuria, mimicking a urinary tract infection. In demented individuals, atrophic vaginitis may present as agitation. Atrophic vaginitis also can exacerbate or even cause stress incontinence. This responds to low-dose estrogen (e.g., 0.3–0.6 mg conjugated estrogen/day, orally or vaginally) (1).

Pharmaceuticals

Anticholinergic agents are used often by older people either by prescription or over-the-counter (OTC) (e.g., tricyclic antidepressants, antihistamines). They cause or contribute to incontinence in several ways: provoke urinary retention; induce subclinical retention; increase residual volume; decrease mobility and precipitate confusion; and intensify dry mouth, and the resultant increased fluid intake contributes to incontinence. Attempts should be made to discontinue anticholinergic agents, or to substitute ones with less anticholinergic effect.

Because the proximal urethra, prostate, and prostatic capsule all contain α-adrenergic receptors, urethral tone can be increased by α-*adrenergic agonists* and decreased by α-*antagonists*. α-Agonists include antihistamines and decongestants (e.g., pseudoephedrine). α-Antagonists include antihypertensive medications (e.g., prazosin, terazosin). Because older individuals often fail to mention nonprescription agents to a physician, urinary retention due to the use of OTC decongestants, antihistamines, or hypnotics should be ruled out. In older women, α-adrenergic antagonists (many antihypertensives) may induce stress incontinence by blocking receptors at the bladder neck (7). Before considering other interventions in these situations, one should substitute an alternative agent and reevaluate.

Calcium channel blockers may cause relaxation of the smooth muscle tissue in the detrusor. This leads to an increase in residual volume and occasionally even provokes overflow incontinence, particularly in obstructed men with coexisting detrusor weakness. The dihydropyridine class of these agents (e.g., nifedipine, nicardipine, isradipine, nimodipine) also can cause peripheral edema, which may exacerbate nocturia and nocturnal incontinence.

Angiotensin-converting enzyme inhibitors (ACEIs) can induce a chronic cough. Because the risk of this side effect increases with age, these agents may exacerbate what otherwise would be minimal stress incontinence in older women.

Excessive Urine Output

Conditions resulting in increased urine output include excessive fluid intake, diuretics, metabolic abnormalities (e.g., uncontrolled diabetes mellitus, which leads to glucosuria, and multiple myeloma with hypercalciuria) and disorders associated with fluid retention. Excessive output is a likely contributor when incontinence is associated with nocturia.

Restricted Mobility

Immobility can result from numerous treatable conditions including arthritis, deconditioning, spinal stenosis, stroke, foot problems, or being restrained in a bed or chair (8).

Stool Impaction

Impaction causes urinary incontinence in two ways: by urethral obstruction leading to overflow incontinence, and by bladder stimulation that causes "urge" symptoms.

Case (Part 3)

S.K. recently began having difficulty sleeping, so she bought an over-the-counter sleeping aid. Her sleep improved initially, but she then complained of a frequent "hangover" sensation. She realized that she was having more difficulty with her incontinence and ended up using more diaper pads.

Chronic/Persistent ("Established") Incontinence

If incontinence persists after transient and functional cause have been addressed, the urinary tract causes of incontinence should be considered. The lower urinary tract can malfunction in only four ways. Two involve the bladder, and two involve the outlet: The bladder either contracts when it should not (detrusor overactivity) or fails to contract when or as well as it should (detrusor underactivity). Alternatively, outlet resistance is high when it should be low (obstruction), or low when it should be high (outlet incompetence).

Detrusor Overactivity

Detrusor overactivity (DO) is the most common form of urinary incontinence in elderly individuals of either sex. Symptoms and characteristics of DO include increased spontaneous activity of detrusor smooth muscle, moderate to large leakage, and nocturnal frequency and incontinence. Sacral sensation and reflexes are preserved and voluntary control of the anal sphincter is intact. In the elderly there are multiple causes of DO: dementia, cervical disk disease or spondylosis, Parkinson's disease, stroke, subclinical urethral obstruction or sphincter incompetence, and age itself. Postvoid residual urine volume (PVR) is generally low. Residual volume in excess of 50 mL suggests outlet obstruction, detrusor hyperactivity with impaired contractility (DHIC), pooling of urine in a woman with a cystocele, Parkinson's disease, or spinal cord injury.

Stress Incontinence

Stress incontinence is the second most common cause of incontinence in older women. Causes include the following: (1) Urethral hypermobility due to pelvic muscle laxity: Proximal urethra and bladder neck "herniate" through the urogenital diaphragm when abdominal pressure increases. This causes unequal transmission of abdominal pressure to the bladder and urethra. The hallmark of the diagnosis is leakage that, in the absence of bladder distention, occurs *coincident* with the stress maneuver (e.g., cough, sneezing). (2) Intrinsic sphincter deficiency or type 3 stress incontinence (9,10): Afflicted women usually leak with even trivial stress maneuvers (e.g., walking) and may note continuous seepage when standing quietly. It is usually due to operative trauma, but milder forms also occur in older women, resulting only from urethral atrophy superimposed on the age-related decline in urethral pressure. (3) Urethral instability, a rare cause of stress incontinence in older women, in which the sphincter paradoxically relaxes in the absence of apparent detrusor contraction. (4) Sphincter damage following prostatectomy.

Incontinence Secondary to Outlet Obstruction

This is the second most common cause of incontinence in older men, although most obstructed men are not incontinent. If due to neurologic disease, obstruction is invariably associated with a spinal cord lesion. More commonly, obstruction results from prostatic enlargement, prostate carcinoma, or urethral stricture. Such men present with hesitancy, incomplete voiding sensation, postvoid dribbling, urge incontinence, diminished and interrupted flow, and a need to strain to void. Because symptoms, ease of catheterization, and palpated prostate size correlate poorly with obstruction—and PVR is insufficiently specific—obstruction is difficult to exclude without further testing.

Anatomic obstruction is rare in women, and is usually due not to stricture, but to kinking associated with a large cystocele or to obstruction following bladder neck suspension. Rarely, bladder neck obstruction or a bladder calculus is the cause.

Incontinence Secondary to Detrusor Underactivity

Detrusor underactivity, the source of 5% to 10% of incontinence in older persons, may be caused by mechanical injury to the nerves supplying the bladder (e.g., disk compression or tumor involvement) or by the autonomic neuropathy of diabetes, vitamin B_{12} deficiency, Parkinson's disease, alcoholism, vincristine therapy, or tabes dorsalis. Alternatively, the detrusor may be replaced by fibrosis and connective tissue, as occurs in men with chronic outlet obstruction, so that even when the obstruction is removed, the bladder fails to empty normally. Detrusor weakness in women is generally idiopathic; instead of fibrosis, the detrusor displays degeneration of both muscle cells and axons, without accompanying regeneration (11).

A mild degree of bladder weakness occurs commonly in older individuals. Although insufficient to cause incontinence, it can complicate treatment of other causes (see Management Considerations, below). However, when severe enough to cause leakage, detrusor underactivity is associated with overflow incontinence. Other presenting complaints include many of the same symptoms of outlet obstruction described earlier. Leakage of small amounts occurs frequently throughout the day and night. If the problem is neurologically mediated, perineal sensation, sacral reflexes, and anal sphincter control are frequently impaired.

Functional Incontinence

The causes of chronic geriatric incontinence generally lie *within* the urinary tract. The exception is functional incontinence, which is attributed to causes outside the urinary tract, such as deficits of cognition and mobility, environmental demands, and medical factors. The term *functional incontinence* implies that urinary tract function is normal. However, a diagnosis of functional incontinence does not rule out transient, that is, reversible, causes of incontinence, and functionally impaired individuals may benefit from targeted therapy. These factors are important to keep in mind because small improvements in each may markedly ameliorate both incontinence and functional status.

Diagnostic Evaluation

Symptoms and Signs

Elicit a detailed description of the incontinence, focusing on its onset, frequency, severity, pattern, precipitants, palliating features, and the following associated symptoms and conditions.

Urge

Although the clinical type of incontinence most often associated with detrusor overactivity (DO) is urge incontinence, urge is neither a sensitive nor a specific symptom. It is absent in 20% of older patients with detrusor overactivity, and the figure is higher in demented patients (12). Urge is also reported commonly by patients with stress incontinence, outlet obstruction, and overflow incontinence.

Urinary Frequency

Similar to the situation for urgency, other symptoms ascribed to DO also can be misleading unless explored carefully. *Urinary frequency* (more than seven diurnal voids) is common (13–15), and may be due to voiding habit, preemptive urination to avoid leakage, overflow incontinence, sensory urgency, a stable but poorly compliant bladder, excessive urine production, depression, anxiety, or social reasons (16). Conversely, incontinent individuals may severely restrict their fluid intake so that even in the presence of DO they do not void frequently.

Nocturia

It is essential that nocturia be defined (e.g., two episodes may be normal for the individual who sleeps 10 hours but not for one who sleeps 4 hours), and then approached systematically. There are three general reasons for nocturia: excessive urine output, sleep-related difficulties, and urinary tract dysfunction. These causes can be differentiated by careful questioning and examination of a voiding diary that includes voided volumes. Individuals with intrinsic sphincter deficiency, especially those who also have a poorly compliant bladder, may report leaking only at night if they allow their bladder to fill to a volume greater than their weakened outlet can withstand. Whatever the cause, the nocturnal component of incontinence is generally remediable.

Voiding Record

Kept by the patient or caregiver for 48 to 72 hours, the voiding diary records the time of each void and incontinent episode. No attempt is made to alter voiding pattern or fluid intake. To record voided volumes at home, individuals use a large-mouth container. Information regarding the volume voided provides an index of functional bladder capacity and, together with the pattern of voiding and leakage, can suggest the cause of leakage. [For further details on the void diary, see Chapter 63: Urinary incontinence, In: Cassel CK, et al., eds, Geriatric Medicine, 4th ed., page 940.]

Physical Examination

A comprehensive physical examination is essential to detect transient causes, comorbid disease, and functional impairment (Table 29.4).

Rectal Examination

One should assess the tone of the rectal sphincter, because the same sacral roots (S2–S4) innervate both the external urethral and the anal sphincters. The patient should be asked to volitionally contract and relax the anal sphincter. Because abdominal straining may mimic sphincter contraction,

TABLE 29.4. Comprehensive evaluation of the incontinent elderly patient (39)

History
   Type (urge, reflex, stress, overflow, or mixed)
   Frequency, severity, duration
   Pattern (diurnal, nocturnal, or both; also e.g., after taking medications)
   Associated symptoms (straining to void, incomplete emptying, dysuria, hematuria,
      suprapubic/perineal discomfort)
   Alteration in bowel habit/sexual function
   Other relevant factors (cancer, diabetes, acute illness, neurologic disease, urinary tract
      infections, and pelvic or lower urinary tract surgery or radiation therapy)
   Medications, including nonprescription agents
   Functional assessment (mobility, manual dexterity, mentation, motivation)
Physical examination
   Identify other medical conditions (e.g., orthostatic hypotension, congestive heart
      failure, peripheral edema)
   Test for stress-induced leakage when bladder is full, but not during abrupt urgency
   Observe/listen to void for force, continuity, straining
   Palpate for bladder distention after voiding
   Pelvic examination (atrophic vaginitis or urethritis; pelvic muscle laxity; pelvic mass)
   Rectal examination (skin irritation; resting tone and voluntary control of anal
      sphincter; prostate nodules; fecal impaction (*Note*: ease of catheterization and
      prostate size correlate poorly with presence or absence of urethral obstruction)
   Neurologic examination (mental status and affect, mobility, and elemental examination,
      including sacral reflexes and perineal sensation)
Laboratory investigation
   Voiding record (incontinence chart)
   *Metabolic survey (measurement of electrolytes, calcium, glucose, and urea nitrogen)
   Measurement of postvoiding residual volume (PVR) by catheterization or portable
      ultrasound
   Urinalysis and culture
   *Renal ultrasound for men whose residual urine exceeds 100–200 mL
   *Urine cytology for patients with sterile hematuria, suprapubic/perineal pain, or
      unexplained new onset or worsening of incontinence
   *Uroflowmetry for men in whom urethral obstruction is suspected
   *Cystoscopy for patients with hematuria, suspected lower urinary tract pathology (e.g.,
      bladder fistula, stone, or tumor; urethral diverticulum), or need for surgery; cannot
      diagnose obstruction
   *Urodynamic evaluation when the risk of empiric therapy exceeds the benefit, when
      empiric therapy has failed or might be improved by more precise assessment, or when
      surgery would be clinically appropriate if a correctable condition were found

*Tests indicated only for selected individuals, as described.
Source: Resnick NM, Yalla SV. Management of urinary incontinence in the elderly. N Engl
J Med 1985;313:800–805. Copyright 1985, Massachusetts Medical Society. All rights
reserved.

place a hand on the patient's abdomen to check for it. Many neurologically
unimpaired elderly patients are unable to volitionally contract their sphincter, but if they can, it is evidence against a cord lesion. When the perineum
is relaxed, one can assess motor innervation further by testing the anal
wink (S4–S5) and bulbocavernosus reflexes (S2–S4). In an older person,
however, the absence of these reflexes is not necessarily pathologic, nor
does their presence exclude an underactive detrusor (due to a diabetic
neuropathy, for example). Finally, afferent supply is assessed by testing
perineal sensation.

Pelvic Muscle Examination

This examination is done for the assessment of pelvic muscle laxity in women that may be caused by a cystocele, rectocele, enterocele, or uterine prolapse. One accomplishes this by removing one blade of the vaginal speculum (or using a "tongue blade"), and sequentially placing the remaining blade on the anterior and posterior vaginal walls and asking the patient to cough. If bulging of the anterior wall is detected when the posterior wall is stabilized, a cystocele is present. If bulging of the posterior wall is detected, a rectocele or enterocele is present. Although the extent of pelvic muscle laxity may be underestimated if one checks in only the supine position, the presence of laxity can usually be determined in any position. It is important to realize, however, that the presence or absence of pelvic muscle laxity reveals little about the cause of an individual's leakage. Detrusor overactivity may exist in addition to a cystocele, and stress incontinence may exist in the absence of a cystocele.

Stress Testing and Postvoid Residual Measurement

Stress testing is important for incontinent women. Optimally, it is performed when the bladder is full and the patient is relaxed (check gluteal folds to corroborate) and in as close to the upright position as possible. The cough or strain should be vigorous and *single*, so that one can determine whether leakage coincides with the increase in abdominal pressure or follows it. Stress-related leakage can be missed if any of these conditions is not met.

Immediate/instantaneous leakage is typical of stress incontinence, whereas delayed leakage is associated with stress-induced DO. *To be useful diagnostically, leakage must replicate the symptom for which help is sought,* because many older women have incidental but not bothersome leakage of a few drops. The test should not be performed if the patient has an abrupt urge to void, because this is usually due to an involuntary detrusor contraction that will lead to a falsely positive stress test. Falsely negative tests occur when the patient fails to cough vigorously or fails to relax the perineal muscles, the bladder is not full, or the test is performed in the upright position in a woman with a large cystocele (which kinks the urethra). If performed correctly, the stress test is reasonably sensitive and quite specific (>90%) (17–19).

Following the stress test, the patient is asked to void into a receptacle and the postvoid residual (PVR) is measured. Optimally, the PVR is measured within 5 minutes of voiding. Measuring it after an intentional void is better than after an incontinent episode, because many patients are able to partially suppress the involuntary contraction during the episode and more than the true PVR remains. The PVR is also spuriously high if measurement is delayed (especially if the patient's fluid intake was high or included caffeine), the patient was inhibited during voiding, or there is discomfort due to urethral inflammation or infection. It is spuriously low if the patient augmented voiding by straining (most important in women), if the catheter is withdrawn too quickly, and if the woman has a cystocele that allows urine to "puddle" beneath the catheter's reach. Of note, relying on the ease of catheterization to establish the presence of obstruction can be misleading, because difficult catheter passage may be caused by urethral tortuosity, a "false passage," or catheter-induced spasm of the distal sphincter, whereas catheter passage may be easy in even obstructed men (20). If the stress test was negative but the history suggests stress incontinence *and* the combined volume of the void and PVR is <200 mL, the bladder should be filled with sterile fluid so that the stress test can be repeated at an adequate volume. There is no need to repeat a well-performed positive stress test or to repeat it in a woman whose history is negative for stress-related leakage; the sensitivity of the history for stress incontinence—unlike its specificity—exceeds 90%, making the likelihood of stress incontinence remote in this situation.

Laboratory Findings

One should check the blood urea nitrogen (BUN), creatinine, urinalysis, and PVR in all patients. Urine culture should be obtained in those with dysuria or an abnormal urinalysis. Serum sodium, glucose, and calcium should be measured in patients with confusion. If the voiding record suggests polyuria, serum glucose and calcium should be determined. Sterile hematuria suggests partially or recently treated bacteriuria, malignancy, calculus, or tuberculosis (21–23).

Urodynamic Studies

Urodynamic studies are useful when diagnostic uncertainty may affect therapy, and when empiric therapy has failed, or other approaches would be tried. They consist of a battery of tests that characterize bladder and urethral function during both the filling and voiding phases of the micturition cycle. Optimally, bladder, urethral, and rectal pressures are measured simultaneously and during both phases of the cycle. Concurrent fluoroscopic monitoring is extremely helpful for the elderly patient, because pressure monitoring alone may miss involuntary contractions, obstruction, and stress incontinence. Because conditions that closely mimic obstruction and stress incontinence are so common in the elderly, urodynamic corroboration of the diagnosis is strongly recommended if surgery will be performed.

Radiographic Evaluation

Optimally, the radiographic and urodynamic evaluations are performed simultaneously, allowing correlation of visual and manometric information. If this is not feasible, substantial information can still be gleaned from cystography. *Voiding* films allow one to check for outlet obstruction. Postvoiding residual volume also can be assessed radiographically. However, a low volume does not exclude a weak bladder if the patient augmented voiding by straining or by multiple voids before the film was obtained.

Management Considerations

Urge Incontinence

Nonpharmacologic Management

Simple measures include adjusting the timing or amount of fluid excretion or providing a bedside commode or urinal, and are often successful. Behavioral therapy includes bladder training regimens, which will extend the voiding interval (24–27). For cognitively impaired patients, try "prompted voiding." Asked every 2 hours whether they need to void, patients are escorted to the toilet if the response is affirmative. Use positive verbal reinforcement; avoid negative comments. A voiding record can be provide helpful information.

Pharmacologic Management

Drugs augment behavioral intervention but do not supplant it, because they generally do not abolish involuntary contractions. Timed toileting or bladder retraining, in conjunction with a bladder relaxant, is thus especially useful for older adults who have little warning before detrusor contraction (28). Table 29.5 provides information on drugs used to treat DO.

Adjunctive Measures

Pads and special undergarments are invaluable if incontinence proves refractory. For bedridden individuals, a launderable bed pad may be preferable; for those with a stroke, a diaper or pants that can be opened using the good hand may be preferred. For ambulatory patients with large volumes of incontinence, wood pulp–containing products are usually superior to ones containing polymer gel. Optimal products for men and women differ because of the location of the target zone of the urinary loss. Finally, the choice of product is influenced by the presence of fecal incontinence.

A condom catheter can be helpful for men, but it is associated with skin breakdown, bacteriuria, and decreased motivation to become dry (29–32); it is not feasible for the older man with a small or retracted penis. External collecting devices have been devised for institutionalized women. Whether they will adhere adequately in more active women remains to be determined. Indwelling urethral catheters are not recommended for detrusor overactivity because they usually exacerbate it.

TABLE 29.5. Bladder relaxant medications used to treat urge incontinence[a] (40)

Medication class, name, and dosage	Comments
Smooth muscle relaxant Flavoxate 300–800mg daily (100–200mg po tid-qid)[b]	Has not proved effective in placebo-controlled trials.
Calcium channel blocker Diltiazem 90–270mg daily (30–90mg po qd-tid) Nifedipine 30–90mg daily (10–30mg po qd-tid)	No controlled trial data. Most useful for the patient with another indication for the drug (e.g., hypertension, angina pectoris, or abnormalities of cardiac diastolic relaxation).
Combination smooth muscle relaxant and anticholinergic Oxybutynin IR 7.5–20mg daily (2.5–5mg po tid-qid)[c] Oxybutynin XL 5–30mg daily (given once daily) Tolterodine 2mg twice daily Dicyclomine 30–90mg daily (10–30mg po tid)	Both oxybutynin and tolterodine have proven effective in rigorous controlled trials when used continuously; less controlled data are available for dicyclomine but efficacy appears to be similar. Because immediate release oxybutynin and dicyclomine have a rapid onset of action, they can be tried prophylactically if incontinence occurs at predictable times.
Tricyclic antidepressants[d] Doxepin 25–75mg daily (10–25mg po qd-tid) Imipramine 25–100mg daily (10–25mg po qd-qid)	May be particularly helpful in women with coexistent stress incontinence. Orthostatic hypotension often precludes their use, but a tricyclic antidepressant may be preferred for a depressed incontinent patient without orthostatic hypotension.

[a] All drugs should be started at the lowest dose and increased slowly until encountering maximum benefit or intolerable side effects. All are given in divided doses, except the antidepressants and long-acting forms of oxybutynin and tolterodine, which may be given as a single daily dose.
[b] Some uncontrolled reports suggest that doses up to 1200mg/d may be effective with tolerable side effects; efficacy has not been supported by randomized controlled trials at any dose.
[c] May also be applied intravesically in patients who can use intermittent catheterization.
[d] May give as single daily dose of 25–100mg after determining the optimal dose.
IR, immediate release; XL, extended release.
Source: Reprinted from Resnick NM. Urinary incontinence. Lancet 1995;346:94–99, with permission from Elsevier.

Stress Incontinence

Nonpharmacologic Management

Urethral hypermobility may be improved by weight loss if the patient is obese, by postural maneuvers (33), by therapy of precipitating conditions, and (rarely) by insertion of a pessary (34,35). Adjusting fluid excretion and voiding intervals to keep bladder volume low are also helpful. However, if the incontinence threshold is less than 150 to 200mL, this strategy is generally not alone sufficient.

Pelvic muscle (Kegel) exercises can decrease incontinence substantially for women. Proven regimens involve 30 to 200 contractions/day for up to 10 seconds at a time. Exercises must be pursued indefinitely. Efficacy is limited for severe incontinence because only 10% to 25% of women become fully continent, and many older women are unable or unmotivated to follow such regimens. Adding vaginal cones, biofeedback, or electrical stimulation likely enhances efficacy but their marginal benefit is unclear. Many devices other than pessaries have been developed to contain leakage for women. Most are applied as a "cap" over the urethral meatus. However, application of such devices, especially in older women with atrophic mucosal, can be quite problematic. For men, prostheses such as condom catheters or penile clamps may be useful, but most require substantial cognitive capacity and manual dexterity and are often poorly tolerated. Penile sheaths (e.g., McGuire prosthesis or adhesive underwear liners) are also an alternative for men. As discussed above, pads and undergarments are used as adjunctive measures. However, in these cases, polymer gel pads are frequently successful because the gel can more readily absorb the smaller amount of leakage. Some products can be flushed down the toilet, a convenient feature for ambulatory individuals.

Pharmacologic Management

α-Adrenergic agonists, such as phenylpropanolamine (PPA) or pseudo-ephedrine, may be added and are often beneficial for women, especially when administered with estrogen. Pseudoephedrine and estrogen may also work for women with sphincter deficiency. Unfortunately, PPA—the agent for which most data are available—was withdrawn from the American market, owing to reports of a very small risk of stroke. Imipramine, with beneficial effects on the bladder and the outlet, is a reasonable alternative for patients with evidence of both stress and urge incontinence.

Surgical Intervention

If urethral hypermobility is confirmed, surgical correction is successful in the majority of selected elderly patients. If sphincter incompetence is diagnosed instead, it can be corrected with a different procedure (pubovaginal sling), but the morbidity is higher and precipitation of chronic retention is more likely than with correction of urethral hyper-mobility. The influence of coincident DO on outcome in older women has been inadequately investigated for either type of stress incontinence. Other treatments for sphincter incompetence include periurethral bulking injections (e.g., bovine collagen) and insertion of an artificial sphincter. Each is effective in selected cases, but reported experience with these approaches in individuals over age 75 is still limited, and so is long-term follow-up.

Outlet Obstruction

Nonpharmacologic Management

In the absence of urinary retention, modification of fluid excretion and voiding habits may be effective.

Pharmacologic Management

α-Adrenergic antagonists (e.g., terazosin, prazosin) are useful and generally well tolerated, except for men with diastolic dysfunction or significant aortic stenosis, in whom these agents should be used with more caution. Tamsulosin may be better tolerated than less specific α-blocking agents, but definitive clinical data are still not available (36). Finasteride, a 5α-reductase inhibitor, is another alternative, but fewer men appear to benefit, the effect is more modest, and the benefit is more delayed (37).

Surgical Intervention

Surgical techniques that now permit resection under local anesthesia have made surgery increasingly feasible for this population. Less extensive resection often suffices for frail elderly men, in whom recurrence of symptoms with adenoma regrowth years later is often not an issue. In women, if a large cystocele is the problem, surgical correction is usually required and should include bladder neck suspension if urethral hypermobility is also present. Bladder neck obstruction is also corrected easily, in even the frailest patient. Distal urethral stenosis can be dilated and treated with estrogen. If meatal stenosis is present, more extensive intervention may be necessary; alternatively, dilation can be repeated at fairly frequent intervals.

Underactive Detrusor

The management of detrusor underactivity is directed at reducing the residual volume, eliminating hydronephrosis (if present), and preventing urosepsis.

The first step is to use indwelling or intermittent catheterization to decompress the bladder for up to a month (at least 7 to 14 days) while reversing potential contributors to impaired detrusor function (fecal impaction and medications). If an indwelling catheter has been inserted, it then should be withdrawn. If decompression does not fully restore bladder function, augmented voiding techniques such as double voiding and implementation of the Credé (application of suprapubic pressure during voiding) or Valsalva maneuver may help if the patient is able to initiate a detrusor contraction or if there is coexistent stress incontinence, especially in a woman.

Pharmacologic Management

Bethanechol (40–200 mg/day in divided doses) is occasionally useful in a patient whose bladder contracts poorly because of treatment with anticholinergic agents that cannot be discontinued (e.g., tricyclic antidepressant). Evidence for bethanechol's efficacy is equivocal at best, and residual volume should be monitored to assess its effect.

Catheterization

If after decompression the detrusor is acontractile, the interventions described above are apt to be fruitless, and the patient should be started on intermittent or indwelling catheterization.

Intermittent Catheterization

A condom catheter is contraindicated in the setting of retention. For individuals at home, intermittent self-catheterization is preferable and requires only clean, rather than sterile, catheter insertion. Catheters are cleaned daily, allowed to air dry at night, sterilized periodically, and may be reused repeatedly. Antibiotic or methenamine prophylaxis against urinary tract infection is probably warranted if the individual gets more than an occasional symptomatic infection or has an abnormal heart valve. Intermittent catheterization in this setting is generally painless, safe, inexpensive, and effective, and allows individuals to carry on with their usual daily activities. If used in an institutional setting, sterile rather than clean technique should be employed until studies document the safety of the latter.

Indwelling Catheterization

Unfortunately, despite the benefits and proven feasibility of intermittent catheterization, most elderly individuals choose indwelling catheterization instead. Complications of chronic indwelling catheterization include renal inflammation and chronic pyelonephritis, bladder and urethral erosions, bladder stones and cancer, as well as urosepsis. When indicated, indwelling catheters can be extremely effective, but their use should be restricted. They are indicated in the acutely ill patient to monitor fluid balance, in the patient with a nonhealing pressure ulcer, for temporary bladder decompression in patients with acute urinary retention, and in the patient with overflow incontinence refractory to other measures. Even in long-term care facilities, they are probably indicated for only 1% to 2% of patients. However, patient preference and values are also important. Thus, an indwelling catheter may also be justified for a cognitively intact patient who is willing to accept the risk in return for the security and convenience the catheter can provide.

General Principles

- Although both providers and older patients often neglect incontinence or dismiss it as a normal part of growing older, it is abnormal at any age.
- Incontinence in an older person is often due to reversible conditions (factors) outside the lower urinary tract. Treatment of these precipitating factors alone may be enough to restore continence.
- The seven acute/transient causes of urinary incontinence can be recalled by using the mnemonic DIAPERS: delirium, infection, atrophic urethritis/vaginitis, pharmaceuticals, excessive urine output, restricted mobility, stool impaction.
- There are four basic causes of chronic/persistent urinary incontinence; two involve the bladder, and two involve the outlet. The bladder either contracts when it should not (detrusor overactivity) or fails to contract when or as well as it should (detrusor underactivity). Alternatively, outlet resistance is high when it should be low (obstruction), or low when it should be high (outlet incompetence).

Suggested Readings

Fantl JA, Newman DK, Colling J. Urinary Incontinence in Adults: Acute and Chronic Management. Clinical Practice Guideline, No. 2, 1996 Update, AHCPR Pub. No. 96–0682. Rockville, MD: U.S. Department of Health and Human Services. Public Health Service, Agency for Health Care Policy and Research, March 1996. *A comprehensive review of the care of the older adult with urinary incontinence.*

Resnick NM. Urinary incontinence. In: Cassel CK, Leipzig RM, Cohen HJ, et al., eds. Geriatric Medicine, 4th ed. New York: Springer, 2003:931–956.

Timmons MC. Gynecologic and urologic problems of older women. In: Cassel CK, Leipzig RM, Cohen HJ, et al., eds. Geriatric Medicine, 4th ed. New York: Springer, 2003:737–754.

References

1. Fantl JA, Newman DK, Colling J. Urinary Incontinence in Adults: Acute and Chronic Management. Clinical Practice Guideline, No. 2, 1996 Update, AHCPR Pub. No. 96–0682. Rockville, MD: U.S. Department of Health and Human Services. Public Health Service, Agency for Health Care Policy and Research, March 1996.
2. Tromp AM, Smit JH, Deeg DJH, Bouter LM, Lips P. Predictors for falls and fractures in the Longitudinal Aging Study Amsterdam. J Bone Miner Res 1998;13:1932–1939.

3. Brown JS, Vittinghoff E, Wyman JF, et al. Urinary incontinence: does it increase risk for falls and fractures? J Am Geriatr Soc 2000;48:721–725.

4. Branch LG, Walker LA, Wetle TT, DuBeau CE, Resnick NM.: Urinary incontinence knowledge among community-dwelling people 65 years of age and older. J Am Geriatr Soc 1994;42:1257–1262.

5. Cohen SJ, Robinson D, Dugan E, et al. Communication between older adults and their physicians about urinary incontinence. J Gerontol 1999;54A: M34–M37.

6. Resnick NM. Voiding dysfunction in the elderly. In: Yalla SV, McGuire EJ, Elbadawi A, Blaivas JG, eds. Neurourology and Urodynamics: Principles and Practice. New York: Macmillan, 1988:303–330.

7. Resnick NM. Geriatric medicine. In: Kasper DL, Braunweld B, Fauci A, Jameson JL, eds. Harrison's Principles of Internal Medicine. New York: McGraw-Hill, 2005.

8. Marshall HJ, Beevers DG. α-Adrenoceptor blocking drugs and female urinary incontinence: prevalence and reversibility. Br J Clin Pharmacol 1996;42: 507–509.

9. McGuire EJ. Urinary Incontinence. New York: Grune and Stratton, 1981.

10. Blaivas JG, Olsson CA. Stress incontinence: classification and surgical approach. J Urol 1988;139:727–731.

11. Elbadawi A, Yalla SV, Resnick NM. Structural basis of geriatric voiding dysfunction. II. Aging detrusor: normal vs. impaired contractility. J Urol 1993;150:1657–1667.

12. Resnick NM, Yalla SV, Laurino E. The pathophysiology and clinical correlates of established urinary incontinence in frail elderly. N Engl J Med 1989;320:1–7.

13. Resnick NM. Voiding dysfunction in the elderly. In: Yalla SV, McGuire EJ, Elbadawi A, Blaivas JG, eds. Neurourology and Urodynamics: Principles and Practice. New York: Macmillan, 1988:303–330.

14. Brocklehurst JC, Dillane JB, Griffiths L, Fry J. The prevalence and symptomatology of urinary infection in an aged population. Gerontol Clin 1968;10: 242–253.

15. Diokno AC, Brock BM, Brown M, Herzog AR. Prevalence of urinary incontinence and other urological symptoms in the non-institutionalized elderly. J Urol 1986;136:1022–1025.

16. Resnick NM. Noninvasive diagnosis of the patient with complex incontinence. Gerontology 1990;36(suppl 2):8–18.

17. Hilton P, Stanton SL. Algorithmic method for assessing urinary incontinence in elderly women. BMJ 1981;282:940–942.

18. Diokno AC. Diagnostic categories of incontinence and the role of urodynamic testing. J Am Geriatr Soc 1990;38:300–305.

19. Kong TK, Morris JA, Robinson JM, Brocklehurst JC. Predicting urodynamic dysfunction from clinical features in incontinent elderly women. Age Ageing 1990;19:257–263.

20. Klarskov P, Andersen JT, Asmussen CF, et al. Symptoms and signs predictive of the voiding pattern after acute urinary retention in men. Scand J Urol Nephrol 1987;21:23–28.

21. DuBeau CE, Resnick NM. Evaluation of the causes and severity of geriatric incontinence: a critical appraisal. Urol Clin North Am 1991;18:243–256.

22. Resnick NM. Initial evaluation of the incontinent patient. J Am Geriatr Soc 1990;38:311–316.
23. Resnick NM, Ouslander JG, eds. National Institutes of Health consensus development conference on urinary incontinence. J Am Geriatr Soc 1990;38:263–386.
24. Fantl JA, Wyman JF, McClish DK. Efficacy of bladder training in older women with urinary incontinence. JAMA 1991;265:609–613.
25. Burgio KL, Locher JL, Goode PS, et al. Behavioral vs drug treatment for urge urinary incontinence in older women: a randomized controlled trial. JAMA 1998;280:1995–2000.
26. Berghmans LCM, Hendriks HJM, DeBie RA, Van Waalwijk Van Doorn ESC, Bo K, Van Kerrebroeck PHEV. Conservative treatment of urge urinary incontinence in women: a systematic review of randomized clinical trials. BJU Int 2000;85:254–263.
27. Payne CK. Behavioral therapy for overactive bladder. Urology 2000;55(5A): 3–6.
28. Wagg A, Malone-Lee J. The management of urinary incontinence in the elderly. Br J Urol 1998;82(suppl 1):11–17.
29. Ouslander JG, Schnelle JF. Incontinence in the nursing home. Ann Intern Med 1995;122:438–449.
30. Ouslander JG. Intractable incontinence in the elderly. BJU Int 2000;85(suppl 3):72–78.
31. Johnson ET. The condom catheter: urinary tract infection and other complications. South Med J 1983;76:579–582.
32. Jayachandran S, Moopan UMM, Kim H. Complications from external (condom) urinary drainage devices. Urology 1985;25:31–34.
33. Norton PA, Baker JE. Postural changes can reduce leakage in women with stress urinary incontinence. Obstet Gynecol 1994;84:770–774.
34. Suarez GM, Baum NH, Jacobs J. Use of standard contraceptive diaphragm in management of stress urinary incontinence. Urology 1991;37:119–122.
35. Zeitlin MP, Lebherz TB. Pessaries in the geriatric patient. J Am Geriatr Soc 1992;40:635–639.
36. Mann RD, Biswas P, Freemantle S, Pearce G, Wilton L. The pharmacovigilance of tamsulosin: event data on 12484 patients. BJU Int 2000;85: 446–450.
37. Gormley GJ, Stoner E, Bruskewitz RC, et al. The effect of finasteride in men with benign prostatic hyperplasia. N Engl J Med 1992;327:1185–1191.
38. Resnick NM. Urinary Incontinence in the Elderly. Medical Grand Rounds, vol 3. New York: Plenum, 1984.
39. Resnick NM, Yalla SV. Management of urinary incontinence in the elderly. N Engl J Med 1985;313:800–805.
40. Resnick NM. Urinary incontinence. Lancet 1995;346:94–99.

30
Pressure Ulcers

R. MORGAN BAIN

Learning Objectives

Upon completion of the chapter, the student will be able to:

1. Identify the risk factors that contribute to the development of pressure ulcers.
2. Describe the staging of pressure ulcers.
3. Describe the other possibilities of chronic ulcers among older adults.
4. Understand the principles of the management and prevention of pressure ulcers.

Case (Part 1)

Mrs. K. is an 86-year-old widowed Caucasian woman who lives alone in her three-story home. She has a medical history of hypertension, hypercholesterolemia, and hypothyroidism, which are well controlled with medications. She has been a lifelong smoker, but has cut down to a few cigarettes per day at present. Last month, during a regular office visit, her daughter was complaining about Mrs. K.'s memory problems. A subsequent workup showed a Mini–Mental State Exam (MMSE) score of 18 and no evidence for reversible causes of dementia. A head computed tomography (CT) scan did not show any signs of ischemic changes. A diagnosis of probable Alzheimer's disease was made.

What are Mrs. K.'s risks for developing a chronic ulcer?

Material in this chapter is based on the following chapter in Cassel CK, Leipzig RM, Cohen HJ, Larson EB, Meier DE, eds. Geriatric Medicine: An Evidence-Based Approach, 4th ed. New York: Springer, 2003: Thomas DR. Management of Chronic Wounds, pp. 967–977. Selections edited by R. Morgan Bain.

General Considerations

Pressure ulcers occur across the spectrum of care. The reported overall prevalence of pressure ulcers was 10.1% (range 1.4% to 36.4%), with the sacrum and heels the most common sites among hospitalized patients.

Pressure ulcers have been associated with over a fourfold increase in mortality rates in both acute and long-term care settings. Death has been reported to occur during acute hospitalization in 67% of patients who develop a pressure ulcer compared to 15% of at-risk patients without pressure ulcers (1). Patients who develop a new pressure ulcer within 6 weeks after hospitalization are three times as likely to die as patients not developing a pressure ulcer (2). In long-term-care settings, development of a pressure ulcer within 3 months among newly admitted patients was associated with a 92% mortality rate, compared to a mortality rate of 4% among residents who did not subsequently develop a pressure ulcer (3). Despite this association with death rates, it is not clear if pressure ulcers contribute to increased mortality or are mainly a marker for increased frailty. The severity of the pressure ulcer has not correlated with an increased mortality risk.

Age-Related Changes in Skin Integrity

The elderly account for most pressure ulcers, with about 70% of all ulcers occurring in patients over the age of 70 years. In elderly patients the incidence of pressure ulcers may be due to associated changes of aging. With aging, local blood supply to the skin decreases, epithelial layers flatten and thin, subcutaneous fat decreases, and collagen fibers lose elasticity. Cutaneous pain sensitivity decreases after age 50, perhaps leading to failure to shift weight appropriately. These changes in aging skin and resultant lowered tolerance to hypoxia may enhance pressure ulcer development. In addition, the response to treatment in older patients may be confounded by comorbid disease.

Pathophysiology

Chronic wounds, including pressure ulcers, fail to proceed through an orderly and timely process to produce anatomic or functional integrity (4). Normally, fibroblasts and epithelial cells grow rapidly in skin tissue cultures, covering 80% of in vitro surfaces within the first 3 days. In contrast, biopsy specimens from pressure ulcers usually do not grow until much later, covering only 70% of surfaces by 14 days (5). The lack of hemorrhage in chronic wounds interferes with bringing wound healing factors into contact with tissue. Platelet release and fibrinolytic activity are diminished.

Finally, these wounds contain complex polymicrobial colonizations that are poorly understood (6). The result is slow healing. Thus, treatment of these chronic wounds extends over months to years.

Diagnostic Evaluation

Differentiation of pressure ulcers from other chronic ulcers is imperative, because the management of each wound type differs substantially. Most often the diagnosis of ulcer type is made by wound location, wound appearance, and the presence of pain. The sites of occurrence among the various kinds of chronic wounds overlap, but careful history and physical examination usually establishes the correct etiology. Adequate tissue perfusion with blood is important for healing of all types of wounds, particularly on the extremities. Examination of pulses and an ankle-brachial blood pressure index (See Chapter 22: Hypertension, page 23: Cardiovascular and Peripheral Arterial Diseases, page 422) can assess healing adequacy. An ankle-brachial index below 0.7 is abnormal, and an index below 0.4 is associated with a poor likelihood of healing. Pressure ulcers are the visible evidence of pathologic changes in dermal blood flow caused by pressure. The most common sites of occurrence are found on the sacrum, posterior heels, and trochanteric areas.

Diabetic ulcers are often caused by recurrent pressure in neuropathic extremities and may be complicated by diminished blood flow in small and larger vessels. These ulcers frequently occur at sites on the foot subjected to pressure, especially over the plantar aspect of the foot and metatarsal heads. Diabetic ulcers often coexist with arterial ischemic ulcers, due to macrovascular and microvascular complications of the diabetic state.

Arterial ischemic ulcers usually occur in areas not necessarily subjected to pressure and result from decreased blood flow to that area. Ischemic ulcers typically occur distally to the impaired blood supply and frequently are painful, particularly with leg elevation. Microemboli from infection or cholesterol plaques can cause the sudden onset of pain and discoloration in the distal extremity (7,8).

Venous stasis ulcers develop in the lower extremities due to incompetent valves in the veins. Typically, they occur on the lateral aspect of the calf. Edema may or may not be present, but hyperpigmentation changes are usually present when the condition is chronic.

Case (Part 2)

On her way to the bathroom last week, Mrs. K. fell and fractured her right femur, which required open reduction and internal fixation (ORIF) at her local hospital. On postoperative day 3, the day-shift nurse noticed a new sacral pressure ulcer measuring 3 cm × 3 cm × 2 cm, stage III.

There was scant exudate, without any eschar or foul odor. Mrs. K.'s stage III pressure ulcer was treated with moistened gauze and hydrogel film.

How do you stage pressure ulcers?

If the wound was completely covered by an eschar, what stage would it be?

Clinical Staging of Pressure Ulcers

Several scales have been proposed for assessing the severity of pressure ulcers. The most common staging, recommended by the National Pressure Ulcer Task Force and Omnibus Budget Reconciliation Act (OBRA) nursing home guidelines, derives from a modification of the Shea scale (9). Under this schematic, pressure ulcers are divided into four clinical stages (Table 30.1).

The first response of the epidermis to pressure is hyperemia. Blanchable erythema happens when capillary refilling occurs after gentle pressure is applied to the area. Nonblanchable erythema exists when pressure of a finger in the reddened area does not produce a blanching or capillary refilling. A *stage I* pressure ulcer is defined by nonblanchable erythema of the

TABLE 30.1. National Pressure Ulcer Advisory Panel (NPUAP) staging system

Stage	Description
I	Pressure ulcer is an observable pressure-related alteration of intact skin whose indicators as compared to an adjacent or opposite area on the body may include changes in one or more of the following: skin temperature (warmth or coolness), tissue consistency (firm or boggy feel), and/or sensation (pain, itching). The ulcer appears as a defined area of persistent redness *in lightly pigmented skin*, whereas *in darker skin tones*, the ulcer may appear with persistent red, blue, or purple hues.*
II	Partial-thickness skin loss involving epidermis, dermis, or both. The ulcer is superficial and presents clinically as an abrasion, blister, or shallow crater.
III	Full-thickness skin loss involving damage to, or necrosis of, subcutaneous tissue that may extend down to, but not through, underlying fascia. The ulcer presents clinically as a deep crater with or without undermining of adjacent tissue.
IV	Full-thickness skin loss with extensive destruction, tissue necrosis, or damage to muscle, bone, or supporting structures (e.g., tendon, joint, capsule). Undermining and sinus tracts also may be associated with Stage IV pressure ulcers.

*In 1998, the NPUAP Task Force on Darkly Pigmented Skin and Stage I Pressure Ulcers drafted a new definition for stage I pressure ulcers. The NPUAP has not changed the definition of stage II to IV pressure ulcers.
Source: Data from National Pressure Ulcer Advisory Panel (NPUAP) website: http://www.npuap.org.

intact skin. Nonblanchable erythema is believed to indicate extravasation of blood from the capillaries. A stage I pressure ulcer always understates the underlying damage because the epidermis is the last tissue to show ischemic injury. *Stage II* ulcers extend through the epidermis or dermis. The ulcer is superficial and presents clinically as an abrasion, blister, or shallow crater. *Stage III* pressure ulcers are full-thickness skin loss involving damage or necroses of subcutaneous tissue that may extend down to, but not through, underlying fascia. The ulcer presents clinically as a deep crater with or without undermining of adjacent tissue. *Stage IV* pressure ulcers are full-thickness wounds with extensive destruction, tissue necrosis, or damage to muscle, bone, or supporting structures. Because of the cone-shaped pressure gradient, undermining and sinus tracts may be associated with stage IV pressure ulcers.

This staging system for pressure ulcers has several limitations. The primary difficulty lies in the inability of defining the progression between stages. Because pressure ulcers develop over time, a wound may seem to progress from stage I to stage IV as a result of the initial injury rather than subsequent injuries. Healing from stage IV does not progress through stage III to stage I, but rather heals by contraction and scar tissue formation. Thus, improvement or deterioration between clinical stages cannot be determined. Diagnosing stage I pressure ulcers in darkly pigmented skin is problematic. Stage III and stage IV ulcers cannot be accurately determined until all the eschar is removed. Other staging systems that include descriptions of exudates, necrotic material, or eschar have been suggested to monitor healing of pressure ulcers but benefits over the Shea scale have not been demonstrated.

It is important to note that description of ulcers by the staging system pertains only to wounds caused by pressure. Wounds created by vascular compromise, diabetes, or other causes are described as being either *partial-thickness* or *full-thickness ulcers*.

Case (Part 3)

Mrs. K. became confused during hospitalization and missed a few days of physical therapy, remaining in bed during this time. Upon reexamining the wound on postoperative day 7, it had extended to 5 cm × 6 cm × 3 cm with increased drainage of pus and a thick film of fibrin. The wound required surgical debridement of the fibrin layer. It was treated with topical antibiotics and filled with moist gauze and covered with hydrogel film.

Besides hydrogels, what other occlusive dressings are used in pressure ulcer management?

Management Considerations

Chronic wounds, particularly pressure ulcers, represent complex clinical problems for which no gold standard for prevention or treatment has yet been established. Local wound treatment is directed to providing an optimum wound environment and improving host factors. In practice guidelines for the treatment of pressure ulcers published by the Agency for Health Care Policy and Research, approximately 85 specific recommendations were made based on a careful literature review (10). Of the 85 recommendations, only 14 were validated by the literature as being of benefit. The remaining recommendations were made using expert opinion.

Pain Management

A primary goal of wound assessment should be to relieve pain. Except in neurologically impaired patients, pressure ulcers may be painful. Relief of pressure results in pain relief. A decrease in wound pain with occlusive dressings has been noted in donor sites and venous stasis ulcers (11,12), but studies in pressure ulcers have been limited. Analgesics should be used when pain assessment reveals discomfort. Principles of pain therapy should be incorporated into management of pressure ulcers (see Chapter 32: Principles of Pain Management, page 573).

Nutrition

One of the most important reversible host factors contributing to wound healing is nutritional status. Several studies suggest that dietary intake, especially of protein, is important in healing pressure ulcers. Greater healing of pressure ulcers has been reported with a higher protein intake irrespective of positive nitrogen balance (13).

An optimum dietary protein intake in patients with pressure ulcers is unknown, but may be much higher than current adult recommendations of 0.8 g/kg/day. Half of chronically ill elderly persons are unable to maintain nitrogen balance at this level (14). A reasonable protein requirement is 1.2 to 1.5 g/kg/day (15).

The deficiency of several vitamins and minerals has significant effects on wound healing. However, supplementation to accelerate wound healing is controversial. High doses of vitamin C have not been shown to accelerate wound healing (16).

Dressings

Moist wound healing allows experimentally induced wounds to resurface up to 40% faster than air-exposed wounds (17–19). The concept of a moist wound environment led to development of occlusive dressings. The term *occlusive* describes the lessened ability of a dressing to transmit moisture vapor from a wound to the external atmosphere. In chronic wounds such as pressure ulcers, occlusion has been shown to reduce wound pain (20,21), enhance autolytic debridement (22,23), and prevent bacterial contamination (24,25).

Wound exudate in pressure ulcers has been found to be an excellent medium for fibroblast stimulation (26). Removal of this medium by aggressive scrubbing or drying has been shown to be detrimental. Wound fluid is thought to contain a variety of growth factors such as interleukin-1, epidermal growth factor, and platelet-derived growth factor-β, which may enhance healing (27). Wound fluid under occlusive dressings may also increase bacterial overgrowth, stimulating epidermal migration.

Any therapy that dehydrates the wound such as dry gauze, heat lamps, air exposure, or liquid antacids, is detrimental to wound healing (28–31). Several types of topical wound treatments can promote more rapid epidermal resurfacing while others can delay wound healing (Table 30.2).

Occlusive dressings can be divided into broad categories of polymer films, polymer foams, hydrogels, hydrocolloids, alginates, and biomembranes. Each has several advantages and disadvantages. No single agent is perfect. The choice of a particular agent depends on the clinical circumstances. The available agents differ in their properties of permeability to water vapor and wound protection. Understanding these differences is the key to planning for wound management in a particular patient. Comparative qualities among available agents are shown in Table 30.3 (32,33).

TABLE 30.2. Agents that promote and delay epidermal resurfacing (47)

Promote epidermal resurfacing
　DuoDerm
　Blisterfilm
　Benzoyl peroxide (20%)
　Bacitracin zinc
　Silvadene
　Neosporin
　Polysporin
　J&J first-aid cream
　Bioclusive
　Op-Site
Delay epidermal resurfacing
　Neomycin sulfate
　Dakin's solution (1%)
　Hibiclens
　Hydrogen peroxide (3%)
　Povidone iodine solution
　Wet to dry gauze
　Liquid detergent
　Furacin
　Triamcinolone acetonide (0.1%)

Source: Reprinted from Alvarez O. Moist environment: matching the dressing to the wound. Ostomy/Wound Manage 1988;12:64–83, with permission from HMP Communications.

TABLE 30.3. Comparison of occlusive wound dressings (48,49)

	Moist saline gauze	Polymer films	Polymer foams	Hydrogels	Hydrocolloids	Alginates, granules	Biomembranes
Pain relief	+	+	+	+	+	±	+
Maceration of surrounding skin	±	±	−	−	−	−	−
O₂ permeable	+	+	+	+	−	+	+
H₂O permeable	+	+	+	+	−	+	+
Absorbent	+	−	+	+	±	+	−
Damage to epithelial cells	±	+	−	−	−	−	−
Transparent	−	+	−	−	−	−	−
Resistant to bacteria	−	−	−	−	+	−	+
Ease of application	+	−	+	+	+	+	−

Source: Data from Helfman T, Ovington L, Falanga V. Occlusive dressings and wound healing. Clin Dermatol 1994;12:121–127. Witkowski JA, Parish LC. Cutaneous ulcer therapy. Int J Dermatol 1986;25:420–426.

All of the occlusive dressings offer pain relief. Only absorbing granules or polymers fail to reduce pain. Polymer films are impermeable to liquid but permeable to both gas and moisture vapor. Because of low permeability to water vapor, these dressings are not dehydrating to the wound. Nonpermeable polymers such as polyvinylidene and polyethylene can be macerating to normal skin, which inhibits wound healing. Polymer films are not absorptive and may leak, particularly when the wound is highly exudative. Most films have an adhesive backing that may remove epithelial cells when the dressing is changed. Polymer films do not eliminate dead space and do not absorb exudate.

Hydrogels are three-layer hydrophilic polymers that are insoluble in water but absorb aqueous solutions. They are poor bacterial barriers and are nonadherent to the wound. Because of their high specific heat, these dressings are cooling to the skin, aiding in pain control and reducing inflammation. Most of these dressings require a secondary dressing to secure them to the wound.

Hydrocolloid dressings are complex dressings similar to ostomy barrier products. They are impermeable to moisture vapor and gases and are highly adherent to the skin. Their adhesiveness to surrounding skin is higher than some surgical tapes, but they are nonadherent to wound tissue and do not damage epithelialization of the wound. The adhesive barrier is frequently overcome in highly exudative wounds. Hydrocolloid dressings cannot be used over tendons or on wounds with eschar formation. Several of these dressings include a foam-padding layer that may reduce pressure to the wound.

Only the hydrocolloid and biomembranes offer bacterial resistance. The biomembranes are very expensive and not readily available. Hydrocolloid dressings theoretically have a disadvantage because of impermeability to oxygen. These dressings could be problematic in wounds contaminated by anaerobes, but this effect has not been demonstrated clinically. The agents differ in the ease of application. This difference is important in pressure ulcers in unusual locations, or when considering for home care. Dressings should be left in place until wound fluid is leaking from the sides, a period of days to 3 weeks.

Alginates are complex polysaccharide dressings that are highly absorbent in exudative wounds. This high absorbency is particularly suited to exudative wounds. Alginates are nonadherent to the wound, but if the wound is allowed to dry, damage to the epithelial tissue may occur with removal.

Saline-soaked gauze that is not allowed to dry is an effective wound dressing. When moist saline gauze has been compared to occlusive-type dressings, healing of pressure ulcers has been similar with both dressings (34–36). The use of occlusive-type dressings has been shown to be more cost-effective than traditional dressings, primarily due to a decrease in nursing time for dressing changes.

Debridement

Necrotic debris increases the possibility of bacterial infection and delays wound healing (37). The preferred method of debriding the pressure ulcer remains controversial. Options include mechanical debridement with gauze dressings, sharp surgical debridement, autolytic debridement with occlusive dressings, or application of exogenous enzymes. Surgical sharp debridement produces the most rapid removal of necrotic debris and is indicated in the presence of clinical wound infection. Mechanical debridement can be easily accomplished by letting the saline gauze dressing dry before removal. Remoistening of gauze dressings in an attempt to reduce pain can defeat the debridement effect. Aggressive surgical or mechanical debridement can damage healthy tissue or fail to completely clean the wound.

Thin portions of eschar can be removed by occlusion under a semipermeable dressing. Both autolytic and enzymatic debridement requires periods of several days to several weeks to achieve results. Enzymatic debridement can dissolve necrotic debris, but whether it harms healthy tissue is debated. Penetration of enzymatic agents is limited in eschar and requires either softening by autolysis or cross-hatching by sharp incision prior to application.

Pressure-Relieving Devices

Pressure-relieving devices have a therapeutic role in treating pressure ulcers. This therapy is successful in the acute hospital and in some nursing home studies, but is very expensive. When patients with pressure ulcers in an acute hospital setting were randomized to air-fluidized therapy or a vinyl alternating air mattress, patients treated on air-fluidized beds had a decrease in ulcer size over a mean of 15 days. However, there was no difference in the number of ulcers showing a size reduction of at least 50%. The cost was estimated at an additional $80 per day (38).

Surgical Management

Nowhere does the difference in pressure ulcers among younger spinal cord injury patients and elderly patients become so pronounced as in discussing surgical management. Surgical closure of pressure ulcers results in a more rapid resolution of the wound. The chief problems are the frequent recurrence of ulcers and the inability of the frail patient to tolerate the procedure.

The efficacy of surgical repair of pressure ulcers is high in the short-term but the efficacy for long-term management has been questioned, even in younger patients (39). (For further details on the surgical management of pressure ulcers, see Chapter 65: Management of Chronic Wounds. In: Cassel CK, et al., eds. Geriatric Medicine, 4th ed., page 973.)

Case (Part 4)

Mrs. K.'s condition improved and she was transferred to a subacute rehabilitation facility for continued physical therapy. Two months later, her sacral wound eventually healed after diligent care by the nursing staff. Due to Mrs. K.'s moderate dementia and her decline in activities of daily living (ADLs), it was deemed unsafe for her to return to her home and it was planned for her to go to a long-term-care facility.

What can be done to prevent further pressure ulcers from occurring while in the nursing home?

Bacteremia and Sepsis from Pressure Ulcers

The incidence of bacteremia from pressure ulcers is about 1.7 per 10,000 hospital discharges (40). However, sepsis is a serious complication of pressure ulcers and a frequent cause of death. The bacteremia occurring with pressure ulcers is likely to be polymicrobial.

Osteomyelitis is a frequent complication of pressure ulcers and diabetic ulcers, reported in 38% of patients who have infected pressure ulcers (41) and in 61% of foot infections in diabetic patients (42). Plain radiographs are unable to differentiate true osteomyelitis from pressure changes to bone (43). Computed tomography may be more useful than radionuclide studies, with a specificity of 90%, although the sensitivity is only 10% (44). A needle biopsy of bone is the most useful single test, with a sensitivity of 73% and a specificity of 96% (45), and should be used whenever osteomyelitis must be excluded.

Prevention

Pressure ulcers are extremely difficult to heal. Once developed, this type of chronic wound is very resistant to any known medical therapy. Estimates of complete healing for pressure ulcers have been placed as low as 10%. Thus, prevention offers the best opportunity for management. Whether or not pressure ulcers are preventable remains controversial. Furthermore, pressure ulcers often occur in terminally ill patients where the goals of care may not include prevention of pressure ulcers. In orthopedic patients the necessity for immobilization may preclude turning or the use of pressure-relieving devices.

For most patients the opportunity to prevent pressure ulcers occurs early in the course of the illness. Intermittent relief of pressure is the goal of pressure ulcer management. If the patient is bed-bound, he or she should be repositioned every 2 hours. This will also prevent the formation of ulcers over bony prominences, such as the trochanters and lateral malleoli. When repositioning the patient, it is important to maintain the back at a 30-degree angle from the support surface with a wedge or foam cushion in order to keep weight directly off the trochanters or sacrum.

Patients who are in seated positions should be repositioned flat at regular intervals to avoid shear forces or have special foam, air, gel, or combination cushions to lower the risk of new ulcers. Those who can do so should be taught to reposition themselves every 15 minutes. Doughnut-type cushions should not be used because they can decrease blood supply to the area.

Other strategies for prevention includes recognizing the risk, improving nutritional status, avoiding excessive bed rest, and preserving the integrity of the skin (46). Interventions for reducing the risk of pressure ulcers are listed in Table 30.4.

General Principles

- Chronic wounds i.e., pressure ulcers, diabetic ulcers, arterial ischemic ulcers and venous stasis ulcers, are a significant source of morbidity and mortality across the spectrum of health care. Understanding the etiology of chronic wounds is vital because it dictates treatment options.
- A *stage I* pressure ulcer is defined by nonblanchable erythema of the intact skin. *Stage II* ulcers extend through the epidermis or dermis. *Stage III* pressure ulcers are full-thickness skin loss involving damage or necroses of subcutaneous tissue that may extend down to, but not through, underlying fascia. *Stage IV* pressure ulcers are full-thickness wounds with extensive destruction, tissue necrosis, or damage to muscle, bone, or supporting structures. Only pressure ulcers are described using this staging system.
- The hallmark for treating and preventing pressure ulcers is identifying patients at risk and reducing forces that cause pressure to susceptible areas.

TABLE 30.4. Interventions to reduce the risk of pressure ulcers (50)

Risk factor	Intervention	Comments
Reduced mobility and activity	If possible, teach resident to change positions frequently Place resident on pressure-reducing mattress/bed and chair cushion Implement turning/repositioning schedule Assess resident position (alignment, stability, pressure redistribution) and potential pressure points, including devices (eg, catheters)	If possible, regularly lower head of bed/back of chair <30 degree angle Keep written records of turning/ repositioning schedule Pay particular attention to heels and elbows and use pillows to position/elevate
Shear and friction (secondary to reduced mobility/activity)	Position resident to avoid "sliding" in bed (eg, keep head of bed at lowest degree of elevation) Use lifting devices to help move/reposition resident	A trapeze may help residents who are able to assist with repositioning
Nutritional/hydration deficit	Develop nutritional care plan Encourage increased dietary intake (particularly protein) Monitor fluid intake/output Multivitamin may be appropriate	Involuntary weight loss, poor dietary intake, and/or low albumin or prealbumin levels are common signs of malnutrition
Skin exposed to moisture	Establish bladder/bowel program and/or select absorbent products that wick moisture away from skin Gently cleanse and dry skin after each incontinence episode Apply skin barrier products Consider temporary use of fecal management system or urinary catheter	Urinary/fecal incontinence can cause dermatitis and skin breakdown Use pH-balanced cleansers and avoid friction

Source: Adapted from Pressure Ulcer Prevention and Care: Incorporating New Federal Guidelines for Assessment, Documentation, Treatment, and Prevention. Ostomy/Wound Management, April 2005, used with permission.

Suggested Readings

Bergstrom N, Bennett MA, Carlson CE, et al. Treatment of Pressure Ulcers. Clinical Practice Guideline No. 15. AHCPR Publication No. 95-0652. Rockville, MD: U.S. Department of Health and Human Services. Public health Service, Agency for Health Care Policy and Research, December 1994. *A comprehensive review on the recognition and management of pressure ulcers.*
Thomas DR. Management of chronic wounds. In: Cassel CK, Leipzig RM, Cohen HJ, et al., eds. Geriatric Medicine, 4th ed. New York: Springer, 2003:967–978.

References

1. Allman RM, Laprade CA, Noel LB, et al. Pressure sores among hospitalized patients. Ann Intern Med 1986;105:337–342.
2. Berlowitz DR, Wilking SVB. The short-term outcome of pressure sores. J Am Geriatr Soc 1990;38:748–752.
3. Bergstrom N, Braden B. A prospective study of pressure sore risk among institutionalized elderly. J Am Geriatr Soc 1992;40:747–758.
4. Lazarus GS, Cooper DM, Knighton DR, et al. Definitions and guidelines for assessment of wounds and evaluation of healing. Arch Dermatol 1994;130; 489–493.
5. Seiler WO, Stahelin HB, Zolliker R, et al. Impaired migration of epidermal cells from decubitus ulcers in cell culture: a cause of protracted wound healing? Am J Clin Pathol 1989;92:430–434.
6. Baxter CR. Immunologic reactions in chronic wounds. Am J Surg 1994; 167:12S–14S.
7. Coffman JD. Atheromatous embolism. Vasc Med 1996;1:267–273.
8. O'Keefe ST, Woods BB, Reslin DJ. Blue toe syndrome: causes and management. Arch Intern Med 1992;152:2197–2202.
9. National Pressure Ulcer Advisory Panel. Pressure ulcers: incidence, economics, risk assessment. Consensus development conference statement. Decubitus 1989;2:24–28.
10. Bergstrom N, Bennett MA, Carlson CE, et al. Treatment of Pressure Ulcers. Clinical Practice Guideline No. 15. AHCPR Publication No. 95-0652. Rockville, MD: U.S. Department of Health and Human Services. Public Health Service, Agency for Health Care Policy and Research, December 1994.
11. Handfield-Jones SE, Grattan CEH, Simpson RA, et al. Comparison of hydrocolloid dressing and paraffin gauze in the treatment of venous ulcers. Br J Dermatol 1988;118:425–427.
12. Nemeth AJ, Eaglstein WH, Taylor JR, et al. Faster healing and less pain in skin biopsy sites treated with an occlusive dressing. Arch Dermatol 1991;127: 1679–1683.
13. Chernoff RS, Milton KY, Lipschitz DA. The effect of very high-protein liquid formula (Replete) on decubitus ulcer healing in long-term tube-fed institutionalized patients. Investigators Final Report 1990. J Am Dietetic Assoc 1990; 90(9):A-130.

14. Gersovitz M, Motil K, Munro HN, et al. Human protein requirements: assessment of the adequacy of the current Recommended Dietary Allowance for dietary protein in elderly men and women. Am J Clin Nutr 1982;35:6–14.

15. Long CL, Nelson KM, Akin JM Jr, et al. A physiologic bases for the provision of fuel mixtures in normal and stressed patients. J Trauma 1990;30:1077–1086.

16. Vilter RW. Nutritional aspects of ascorbic acid: uses and abuses. West J Med 1980;133:485.

17. Eaglstein WH, Mertz PM. New method for assessing epidermal wound healing. The effects of triamcinolone acetonide and polyethylene film occlusion. J Invest Dermatol 1978;71:382–384.

18. Odland G. The fine structure of the interrelationship of cells in the human epidermis. J Biophys Biochem Cytol 1958;4:529–535.

19. Winter GD. Formation of scab and the rate of epithelialization of superficial wounds in the skin of the young domestic pig. Nature 1962;193:293–294.

20. Eaglstein WH. Experiences with biosynthetic dressings. J Am Acad Dermatol 1985;12:434–440.

21. May SR. Physiology, immunology and clinical efficacy of an adherent polyurethane wound dressing Op-site. In: Wise DL, ed. Burn Wound Coverings, vol 2. Boca Raton, FL: CRC Press, 1984:53–78.

22. Freidman S, Su DWP. Hydrocolloid occlusive dressing management of leg ulcers. Arch Dermatol 1984;120:1329–1336.

23. Kaufman C, Hirshowitz B. Treatment of chronic leg ulcers with Opsite. Chir Plastica 1983;7:211–215.

24. Buchan IA. Clinical and laboratory investigation of the compositions and properties of human skin wound exudate under semi-permeable dressings. Burns 1981;7:326–334.

25. Mertz RM, Marshall DA, Eaglstein WH. Occlusive wound dressings to prevent bacterial invasion and wound infection. J Am Acad Dermatol 1985;12:662–668.

26. Sporr M, Roberts A. Peptide growth factors and inflammation, tissue repair and cancer. J Clin Invest 1986;78:329–332.

27. Lawrence WT, Diegelmann RF. Growth factors in wound healing. Clin Dermatol 1994;12:157–169.

28. Fowler E, Goupil D. Comparison of the wet-to-dry dressing and a copolymer starch in the management of derided pressure sores. J Enterostomal Ther 1984;11:22–25.

29. Gorse GJ, Messner RL. Improved pressure sore healing with hydrocolloid dressings. Arch Dermatol 1987;123:766–771.

30. Kurzuk-Howard G, Simpson L, Palmieri A. Decubitus ulcer care: a comparative study. West J Nurs Res 1985;7:58–79.

31. Sebern MD. Pressure ulcer management in home health care: efficacy and cost effectiveness of moisture vapor permeable dressing. Arch Phys Med Rehabil 1986;67:726–729.

32. Helfman T, Ovington L, Falanga V. Occlusive dressings and wound healing. Clin Dermatol 1994;12:121–127.

33. Witkowski JA, Parish LC. Cutaneous ulcer therapy. Internat J Dermatol 1986;25:420–426.

34. Alm A, Hornmark AM, Fall PA, et al. Care of pressure sores: a controlled study of the use of a hydrocolloid dressing compared with wet saline gauze compresses. Acta Derm Venereol 1989;149(suppl):142–148.

35. Colwell JC, Foreman MD, Trotter JP. A comparison of the efficacy and cost-effectiveness of two methods of managing pressure ulcers. Decubitus 1992; 6:28–36.

36. Xakellis GC, Chrischilles EA. Hydrocolloid versus saline gauze dressings in treating pressure ulcers: a cost-effective analysis. Arch Phys Med Rehabil 1992;73:463–469.

37. Constantine BE, Bolton LL. A wound model for ischemic ulcers in the guinea pig. Arch Dermatol Res 1986;278:429–431.

38. Allman RM, Walker JM, Hart MK, et al. Air-fluidized beds or conventional therapy for pressure sores: a randomized trial. Ann Intern Med 1987;107: 641–648.

39. Evans GRD, Dufresne CR, Manson PN. Surgical correction of pressure ulcers in an urban center: Is it efficacious? Advances Wound Care 1994;7:40–46.

40. Byran CS, Dew CE, Reynolds KL. Bacteremia associated with decubitus ulcers. Arch Intern Med 1983;143:2093–2095.

41. Sugarman B, Hawes S, Musher DM, et al. Osteomyelitis beneath pressure sores. Arch Intern Med 1983:143:683–688.

42. Grayson MI, Gibbons GW, Habershaw GM, et al. Use of ampicillin/sulbactam versus imipenem/cilastine in the treatment of limb-threatening foot infections in diabetic patients. Clin Infect Dis 1994;18:683–693.

43. Thornhill-Joyness M, Gonzales G, Stewart CA, et al. Osteomyelitis associated with pressure ulcers. Arch Phys Med Rehab 1986;67:314–318.

44. Firooznia H, Rafii M, Golimbu C, et al. Computed tomography of pressure ulcers, pelvic abscess, and osteomyelitis in patients with spinal cord injury. Arch Phys Med Rehabil 1982;63:545–548.

45. Lewis VL, Bailey MH, Pulawski G, et al. The diagnosis of osteomyelitis in patients with pressure sores. Plast Reconstr Surg 1988;81:229–323.

46. Thomas DR. Pressure Ulcers. In: Cassel CK, Cohen HJ, Larson EB, et al., eds. Geriatric Medicine, 3rd ed. New York: Springer, 1997:767–785.

47. Alvarez O. Moist environment: matching the dressing to the wound. Ostomy/ Wound Manage 1988;12:64–83.

48. Helfman T, Ovington L, Falanga V. Occlusive dressings and wound healing. Clin Dermatol 1994;12:121–127.

49. Witkowski JA, Parish LC. Cutaneous ulcer therapy. Int J Dermatol 1986; 25:420–426.

50. Pressure Ulcer Prevention and Care: Incorporating New Federal Guidelines for Assessment, Documentation, Treatment, and Prevention. Ostomy/Wound Management, April 2005.

31
Overview of Palliative Care and Non-Pain Symptom Management

RAINIER P. SORIANO

Learning Objectives

Upon completion of the chapter, the student will be able to:

1. Define palliative care and differentiate it from hospice care.
2. Enumerate and understand the general rules of good doctor–patient communication including communicating bad news and advance care planning.
3. Identify and treat nonpain symptoms including dyspnea, cough, nausea and vomiting, constipation, diarrhea, bowel obstruction, mouth symptoms, skin symptoms, odor, and spiritual distress.
4. Understand the Medicare hospice benefit.

Case (Part 1)

Mrs. Greenwald is a 68-year-old woman who returns to your primary care office to go over test results. You saw Mrs. Greenwald for the first time last week. She has not had a regular physician for 4 years. She came in to see you for back pain, which had gradually been increasing over the last month. She also has some left hip pain, which is making it difficult for her to sleep at night.

Mrs. Greenwald has a history of stage 2 breast cancer, treated 5 years ago with a right mastectomy plus radiation and chemotherapy. There was no evidence of residual tumor after the treatment. Because of this

---

Material in this chapter is based on the following chapters in Cassel CK, Leipzig RM, Cohen HJ, Larson EB, Meier DE, eds. Geriatric Medicine: An Evidence-Based Approach, 4th ed. New York: Springer, 2003: Meier DE. Old Age and Care Near the End of Life, pp. 281–285. Tulsky JA. Doctor-Patient Communication Issues, pp. 287–297. Goodlin S. Care Near the End of Life, pp. 299–309. Carney MT, Meier DE. Sources of Suffering in the Elderly, pp. 311–321. Selections edited by Rainier P. Soriano.

history, you ordered additional tests and a total body bone scan. You told her that you wanted to make sure the cancer did not come back. She also has rheumatoid arthritis, but otherwise has no significant medical problems.

Last week you asked her if she had any questions about diagnostic tests, and she had none at the time. She did make it clear, however, that she is the kind of person who likes to know everything that is going on with her health.

You told her that you want her to return in a week to review the bone scan results.

General Considerations

Palliative care is interdisciplinary medical care focused on the relief of suffering and achievement of the best possible quality of life for patients and for their family caregivers. It involves (1) formal symptom assessment and treatment; (2) aid with decision-making and establishing goals of care; (3) practical and moral support for patients and their family caregivers; (4) mobilization of community supports and resources to ensure a secure and safe living environment; and (5) collaborative models of care (hospital, home, nursing home, hospice) for persons living with serious, complex, and eventually terminal illnesses.

General Rules of Good Communication

A central goal of palliative care is to meet the disparate needs of patients and families. Everyone defines a good death differently (1). Good communication is indispensable to uncovering these needs through empathic exploration and individually negotiated goals of care. Good communication skills provide the pathway to excellent care for elderly persons. The fundamentals of such communication are listening, attending to patients' emotional needs, and achieving a shared understanding of the concerns at hand. Specific tasks such as delivering bad news, discussing advance care planning, helping patients through the transition to hospice care, and responding to bereavement require using these skills to ensure that patients' concerns are elicited and addressed, that they are informed, and that they feel supported.

Advance Preparation

A little effort spent on advance preparation can have a tremendous impact on the quality of the encounter with the elderly patient. Whenever possible, important medical information, particularly bad or sad news, should be delivered during a scheduled meeting. This allows patients to prepare themselves for the type of information they will hear and to make sure that appropriate family members or friends are present. It also allows the physician to allocate the necessary time to the encounter. Communication best occurs face to face, particularly with elderly patients. Telephones accentuate physical communication difficulties, such as hearing loss and speech problems. There is no opportunity to employ the benefits of nonverbal communication. And, if the topic is emotionally threatening, it is more difficult to ensure the patient's safety at the other end of the telephone.

One also needs to approach all such conversations prepared with basic medical information and anticipating the most likely questions regarding treatment options, prognosis, and resources for support and guidance. Finally, to the extent possible, such conversations are best held when both the physician and patient are well rested.

Sensory Issues and Control of the Environment

When speaking with older adults, choose a quiet, private room with good lighting to enhance the patient's ability to comprehend. The physician should sit at eye level and within reach of the patient. If possible, one's pager or cellular phone should be turned off, or at least on a quiet mode, and one should avoid interruptions. As presbycusis first affects higher sound frequencies, it is helpful to speak slowly in a clear, loud, low voice. If the patient wears hearing assistive devices, these devices should be in place.

Increasingly, we encounter patients with limited English proficiency. One must absolutely employ the assistance of an interpreter in such settings. However, it is equally important to avoid using family members as interpreters. Not only does this run the risk of faulty translation or reinterpretation of the physician's statements, but it also places family members into the uncomfortable position of being the physician's and patient's spokesperson. Most hospitals and health care facilities in regions with high numbers of immigrants employ professional translators or maintain lists of language skills among facility staff members.

The Role of Affect in Communication

Most difficulties in communication are the result of inattention to affect. *Affect* refers to the feelings and emotions associated with the content of the conversation. Feelings such as anger, guilt, frustration, sadness, and fear modify our ability to hear, to communicate, and to make decisions.

It is important, as well, that physicians be attentive to their own affect. When caring for dying patients, physicians are likely to experience many emotions. These include guilt ("If only I'd convinced him to get that screening colonoscopy"), impotence ("There's nothing I can do for her . . ."), failure ("I messed up. I'm a bad doctor"), loss ("I'm really going to miss this person"), resentment ("This patient is going to keep me in the hospital all night"), and fear ("I know they're going to sue me"). Such feelings, although normal and common, can affect one's ability to interact successfully with the patient.

Emotion-Handling Skills

The primary goal of emotion handling is to convey a sense of empathy. *Empathy* is the sense that "I could be you" and is what patients are usually feeling when they comment about a physician that really cared for them (2). Robert Smith has created a useful mnemonic to recall four basic techniques to use when confronted by patient emotions, NURS: name, understand, respect, and support (3). This discussion adds a final E for explore (Table 31.1). *Naming* the emotion serves to acknowledge the feeling and to demonstrate that it is a legitimate area for discussion. Expressing a sense of *understanding* normalizes the patient's emotion and conveys empathy. *Respect* reminds us to praise patients and families for what they are doing and how they are managing with a difficult situation. *Support* is essential to helping people in distress not feel alone. Finally, patients will frequently make statements that deserve further *exploration*. (For further details on emotion-handling skills, see Chapter 25: Doctor–Patient Communication Issues. In: Cassel CK, et al., eds. Geriatric Medicine, 4th ed., page 289.)

TABLE 31.1. Useful basic techniques on emotion handling skills (5)

NURSE-ing an emotion	Sample statements
Name the emotion	"Many people would feel angry if that happened to them. I wonder if you ever feel that way?"
Understand the emotion	"Although I've never shared your experience, I do understand that this has been a really hard time for you."
Respect or praise the patient	"I am so impressed with how you've continued to provide excellent care for your mother as her dementia has progressed."
Support the patient	"We will send an RN to your home to check in on you for a couple of days, and if you'd like, I could ask the chaplain to pay you a visit."
Explore what underlies the emotion	"Tell me more."

Source: Reprinted from Fischer GS, Tulsky JA, Arnold RM. Communicating a poor prognosis. In: Portenoy RK, Bruera E, eds. Topics in Palliative Care, vol 5. New York: Oxford University Press, 2000, with permission.

Case (Part 2)

Mrs. Greenwald comes into the exam room. She appears anxious and still complaining of the back pain, which has been increasing in severity since the last time you have seen her. She starts asking if you already have the results of the bone scan. You nod your head and say, "We have the test results back, and I am afraid they don't look good." Mrs. Greenwald stares at you and says, "Oh no, what is it?" You then say, "The results showed unequivocally that your cancer has returned and has spread to your back."

Communicating Bad News

Communicating bad news draws upon the skills discussed previously. Many protocols exist for the delivery of bad news; however, the behaviors tend to be grouped into several key domains that include preparation, content of message, dealing with patient responses, and ending the encounter (Table 31.2) (4,5). The primary elements of preparation (getting the setting right, getting needed information) have been addressed above.

TABLE 31.2. Key elements of delivering bad news (5)

Preparation
    Find out what patient knows and believes
    Find out what patient wants to know
    Suggest a supportive person accompany the patient
    Learn about the patient's condition
    Arrange the encounter in a private place with enough time
Content
    Get to the point quickly
    Fire "warning shot" (e.g., "I have bad news")
    State the news clearly, simply, and sensitively
    Allow silence
    Avoid false reassurance
    Make truthful, hopeful statements
    Provide information in small chunks
Handle patient's reactions
    Inquire about meaning of the condition for the patient
NURSE (name, understand, respect, support, explore) expressed emotions
    Assure continued support
Wrap-up
    Set up a meeting within the next few days
    Offer to talk to relatives/friends
    Suggest that patients write down questions
Provide a written appointment and contact information and how to be reached in emergencies
    Assess suicidality

Source: Reprinted from Fischer GS, Tulsky JA, Arnold RM. Communicating a poor prognosis. In: Portenoy RK, Bruera E, eds. Topics in Palliative Care, vol 5. New York: Oxford University Press, 2000, with permission.

Content of Message

Knowledge of what the patient already knows or believes is extremely valuable to have prior to revealing bad news to a patient (5). This allows the physician to begin his or her explanation from the patient's perspective, aligning oneself with the patient and making communication more efficient and effective. The time that a test is ordered is a good time to assess this. One might ask, "Is there anything that you are particularly concerned about?" If the patient mentions a serious illness that might be present, the physician can follow up by asking what the patient's specific fears and concerns are.

When prepared to deliver the content of the message, the physician should begin by firing a brief "warning shot" and then stating the news in clear and direct terms. One should avoid spending any time "beating around the bush" prior to sharing the news. Perhaps most important is what follows this exchange. The clinician should remain silent and allow the patient an opportunity for the news to sink in. One can strike an empathic stance, maintain comfortable eye contact, and perhaps use a nonverbal gesture, such as reaching out and touching the patient's hand. However, silence is imperative to allow the patient an opportunity to process the information, formulate a response, and experience his or her emotions. The clinician who feels uncomfortable during this silent phase needs to appreciate that the discomfort is rarely shared by the patient, who is engrossed in thought about the meaning of the news and thoughts about the future. Furthermore, very little that is said by the physician at this time will be remembered by the patient, so it is best not to say anything at all. If the patient makes no verbal response after, perhaps, two minutes, it can be useful to check in: "I just told you some pretty serious news. Do you feel comfortable sharing your thoughts about this?"

Case (Part 3)

Upon hearing the news, Mrs. Greenwald starts crying. You hand her a box of tissues and place your hand gently on her shoulder. She starts saying out loud, "Why me? I thought I have been cured before after the chemotherapy and radiotherapy. Now it has come back again." You do not say a word at this point and you just let her talk.

Dealing with the Response

The remainder of the conversation should be spent primarily dealing with the patient's response. This includes using the skills of the NURSE mnemonic to legitimize and empathize with the patient's experience. It is also important to explore the meaning the news has for the patient and to achieve a shared understanding of the disease and its implications.

When effective treatment is available, this fact should be explained. When the treatment options are poor, hope may be found by alleviating patients' worst fears. Doctors may reassure patients that they will not be abandoned during their illness, that the doctor will remain available if things get worse, that everything will be done to maintain the patient's comfort, and that the doctor will continue to watch for new treatment developments (6). Often people find hope and strength from their religious or spiritual beliefs, from having their individuality respected, from meaningful relationships with others, and from finding meaning in their lives (7). Exploring these resources with the patient over time may help to foster realistic hope. Although physicians may have a desire to make an overly reassuring statement to the patient right after revealing the diagnosis, hopeful statements that are truthful and that are made after taking the time to explore the patient's concerns first are more likely to be accepted by the patient (8).

Ending the Encounter

The clinician must end the encounter in a way that leaves the patient feeling supported and with some sense of hope. Support can be provided through meeting the patient's immediate health needs and risks. One must treat pain and palliate other symptoms. Patients should be asked how they plan to cope with the news, and if their response raises any concerns about suicide, this should be asked about directly and addressed. One should try to minimize aloneness through statements of non-abandonment and referral to other resources, such as support groups, counselors, or pastoral care.

Lastly, one should provide a specific follow-up plan: "I'd like you to keep a list of questions so I can answer them for you on our next visit this Tuesday. We'll talk about all your options again at that time. Okay? And please feel free to call me." A legibly written phone number and date and time for the next appointment will provide concrete evidence of the ongoing connection to the physician and help a distressed patient to remember the plan. The physician needs to remember that the goal of this conversation is not to leave a happy patient. That is rarely possible (or even desirable) after delivering bad news. Instead, one hopes to leave a patient who feels supported and cared for and who can look forward to a specific plan of action.

Case (Part 4)

Mrs. Greenwald then turns to you and says, "I know I'm going to get better. I know that this new chemotherapy I have heard about in the news that they are offering at the university will make the difference." You then say to her, "I wish that there was a treatment that would make this cancer go away. It's hard to come to terms with this, but unfortunately I don't believe it would help you overcome your cancer." She then says, "I was afraid you might say that. What do we do now?" You then say, "There's a lot that we can do. Let's talk about what goals are most important for you right now."

Advance Care Planning

Discussions about advance care planning encompass many goals. These include preparing for death and dying, exercising control, relieving burdens placed on loved ones, helping patients make decisions consistent with their values, and leaving patients feeling supported and understood (9).

The first step in preparing to discuss advance care plans is deciding on the appropriate goals for the discussion. What one hopes to accomplish varies depending on the clinical situation (10). Advance care planning includes many different tasks: informing the patient, eliciting preferences, identifying a surrogate decision maker, and providing emotional support. Frequently, one cannot accomplish all of this in one conversation, and focusing on the goals of the discussion allows the physician to tailor the encounter. Advance care planning is completed as a process over time that allows patients and providers an opportunity for thoughtful reflection and interaction with others.

It is possible that the greatest communication challenges face physicians and patients as they discuss progression of disease, the transition from a primary focus on life-prolonging therapy to a primary focus on palliation and the referral for hospice care. Such times of transition involve the recognition of loss, redefinition of self-concept and social role, and great emotional stress. Patients are likely to feel sadness, anger, and denial. Physicians frequently have difficulty with such discussions because they feel a sense of failure or are worried that patients will feel abandoned or that they will be overcome in the conversation by anxiety or despair (5).

As a general rule, it is important for physicians to employ behaviors that promote the sharing of concerns by patients, and avoid behaviors such as reassurance that inhibit such sharing. See Table 31.3 for useful open-ended

TABLE 31.3. Open-ended questions to initiate conversations about dying (12)

"What concerns you most about your illness?"
"How is treatment going for you (your family)?"
"As you think about your illness, what is the best and the worst that might happen?"
"What has been most difficult about this illness for you?"
"What are your hopes (your expectations, your fears) for the future?"
"As you think about the future, what is most important to you (what matters the most to you)?"

Source: Reprinted from Lo B, Quill T, Tulsky J. Discussing palliative care with patients. Ann Intern Med 1999;130:744–749, with permission from American College of Physicians.

questions with which one can initiate such conversations. (For further details on the process of advance care planning, see Chapter 25: Doctor-Patient Communication Issues. In: Cassel CK, et al., eds. Geriatric Medicine, 4th ed., page 291.)

Dreaded Questions

Finally, it is useful to consider several of the questions that many physicians find most difficult to answer. Responding to such questions draws upon the many skills described in this chapter, and it is useful to keep several additional points in mind (11). Check the reason for the question (e.g., "Why do you ask that now?"), show interest in the patient's ideas, and empathize with his or her concerns. It is also important to be prepared to admit that you don't know. Having anticipated replies can be useful and several examples follow (12):

How Long Do I Have to Live?

Patient: *How long do I have to live?*
Doctor: *I wonder if it is frightening not knowing what will happen next, or when.*

This response acknowledges that underlying such a question is tremendous emotion, most likely fear. It will be important for the physician to give a factual response to this question. However, the patient will not be prepared to hear this response until the doctor has addressed his or her emotional concerns. The suggested answer above allows patients to speak about their fears and worries. When the physician needs to use a more factual response, the following is a way of being honest while maintaining hope:

Doctor: *On average, a person in your situation lives 3 to 4 months, but some people have much less time, and others may live longer. I would now take care of any practical or family matters that you wish to have completed before you die but continue to hope that you are one of the lucky people who gets a bit more time.*

Does This Mean You Are Giving Up on Him?

Family: *Does this mean you're giving up on him?*
Doctor: *Absolutely not. But tell me, what do you mean by giving up?*

Suggesting that a patient receive palliative care risks conveying a sense of abandonment. Physicians must be emphatic that palliative care and hospice are active forms of care that meet patients' varying goals at the end of life. However, further exploration of a patient's or family's concerns about abandonment are important to understanding their perceptions and attitudes toward care at the end of life.

Are You Telling Me That I Am Going to Die?

Patient: *Are you telling me that I am going to die?*
Doctor: *I wish that were not the case, but it is likely in the near future. I am also asking, how would you want to spend the remaining time if it were limited?*

This wish statement helps the physician identify with the patient's loss. The third sentence above is an attempt by the physician to reframe the patient's understanding of the situation. He has acknowledged that the patient is dying, but now he seeks to understand what the patient's goals might be in light of this new information. Creating new goals in this way provides an outlet for the patient's hope.

Bereavement

Caring for elderly patients means caring for bereaved patients. The loss of spouses, siblings, other family members, and close friends is extremely common among older persons. Patients ought to be encouraged to tell their stories of loss, including describing details of the days and weeks around the death of their loved one. Similarly, patients benefit by recalling earlier positive memories of the person. Physicians can explore how the patient has responded to the grief ("How have things been different for you since your husband died?"), and identify the patient's social support and coping resources ("Has anyone been particularly helpful to you recently?" "What helps you get through the day?"). Lastly, one should not overlook the frequently enormous practical ramifications of loss, such as financial difficulties or the possible loss of a home and transportation.

Non-Pain Symptom Control

Formal Assessment

Symptom control is an essential component of medical care. For most patients, physical pain is only one of several sources of distress. Symptom relief encompasses physical, psychological, social, and spiritual aspects of suffering. Physical aspects of pain cannot be effectively treated in isolation from the emotional and spiritual components that contribute to it, nor can these sources of suffering be addressed adequately when patients are in physical distress. The various components of suffering must be addressed simultaneously.

Distressing symptoms include dyspnea, cough, nausea and vomiting, constipation, diarrhea, bowel obstruction, mouth symptoms, skin symptoms, odors, and suffering caused by spiritual distress. (Pain Management is discussed in Chapter 32: Principles of Pain Management, page 573.)

Dyspnea

Dyspnea is a subjective sensation of shortness of breath (13) that is described in 70% of cancer patients during the last 6 weeks of life and in 50% to 70% of patients dying from other illnesses (14). It is a common symptom associated with pneumonia, congestive heart failure exacerbations, and chronic obstructive pulmonary disease—all illnesses common to elderly people. Nevertheless, dyspnea may be a subjective symptom that may not match any objective signs of respiratory function (13), and its management can be challenging. It is important to diagnose and treat the underlying reversible causes of dyspnea when possible. When therapy specific to the underlying cause is unavailable or ineffective, several techniques may alleviate breathlessness. Simple techniques include pursed lip breathing and diaphragmatic breathing, leaning forward with arms on a table, cool air ventilation (fan or open window), and nasal oxygen. Opiates have been shown in numerous studies to be highly effective in the amelioration of dyspnea (15,16). Along with treating the underlying cause, steroids and oxygen therapy may be of benefit. A list of some medications and dosages to alleviate refractory dyspnea can be found in Table 31.4 (17).

Cough

Cough is a normal but complex physiological mechanism that protects the airways and lungs by removing mucus and foreign matter from the larynx,

TABLE 31.4. Dyspnea drug treatment (17)

- Morphine 2.5–5 mg po q 4 hours while awake (opiate naïve patient)
- Morphine infusion 0.5 mg per hour, titrate to relief of respiratory distress. Once dose requirement established, switch to long-acting opiate or fentanyl patch.
- Nebulized morphine or hydromorphone:
    Injectable morphine 2.5–0 mg in 2 cc NS
    or
    Injectable hydromorphone 0.25–1 mg in 2 cc NS
    With or without
        Albuterol 0.083% (3 cc)
    With or without
        Solu-Medrol 10 mg
- Corticosteroids:
    Dexamethasone 16 mg initial, then
        8 mg bid × 2 days, then 4 mg bid × 2 days, then 2 mg bid
    Prednisone pulse
        40 mg po bid × 5–7 days
- Oxygen

NS, normal saline.
Source: Reprinted from Stegman MB. Non-pain symptoms. In: Stegman MB, ed. Hope Hospice Pain and Symptom Control in Palliative Medicine, Part 6. Fort Myers, Hospice Resources, 1997;6.1–6.38, with permission from Hospice Resources.

trachea, and bronchi. Cough is under both voluntary and involuntary control (18). Management of cough should be determined by the type and the cause of the cough, as well as the patient's general condition and likely diagnosis. When possible, the aim should be to reverse or ameliorate the cause, combined with appropriate symptomatic measures. Exacerbating factors should be defined, and simple measures such as a change in posture can be very helpful. Breathlessness can trigger cough and vice versa. Persistent cough can also precipitate vomiting, exhaustion, chest or abdominal pain, rib fracture, syncope, and insomnia.

Cough suppressants are usually used to manage dry cough. The most effective antitussive agents are the opioids. Codeine is a mild antitussive, whereas other opioids (morphine, oxycodone, hydrocodone, hydromorphone) have a more pronounced effect. Methadone can be particularly effective at night, but due to its prolonged half-life, the risk of accumulation exists. Other useful measures include decongestants, antihistamines, and corticosteroids.

Case (Part 5)

You decide to start Mrs. Greenwald with some oxycodone for pain control. You tell her some of the possible adverse effects of the opioids. You tell her that she may have episodes of nausea and vomiting. You say that this adverse effect usually goes away after a couple of days and also could be treated with antiemetics if it becomes worse. You also tell her about the possibility of constipation and gave her a prescription for a stool softener and a laxative. You ask her to fill the prescription and start taking them.

Mrs. Greenwald asks, "Why do I have to start taking the stool softener and laxative when I don't even have any constipation yet. Shouldn't I just take it when I have problems moving my bowels? Also, shouldn't it go away once my body gets used to these pain medications?"

Nausea and Vomiting

Nausea and vomiting are present in up to 62% of cancer patients (19). There are multiple potential causes for both nausea and vomiting, yet symptomatic relief is relatively easy to achieve with the appropriate use of medications. A thorough assessment is crucial to understanding the underlying etiology and, in turn, providing the most beneficial form of treatment.

There are two organ systems that are particularly important in nausea and vomiting: the central nervous system and the gastrointestinal system (20). The gastric lining, the chemoreceptor trigger zone in the base of the fourth ventricle, the vestibular apparatus, and the cortex are all involved in the physiology of nausea. Stimulation of the vomiting center from one or more of these areas is mediated through the neurotransmitters serotonin, dopamine, acetylcholine, and histamine. Serotonin seems to be important in the gastric lining and central nervous system, whereas acetylcholine and histamine are important in the vestibular apparatus. Cortical responses are mediated both via neurotransmitters, as well as through learned responses (e.g., nausea related to anxiety).

Table 31.5 lists the major causes of nausea and vomiting, classified by the mechanism's principal site of action. Dopamine-mediated nausea is probably the most common form of nausea, and the most frequently targeted for initial symptom management. These medications are phenothiazines or butyrophenone neuroleptics (metoclopramide, prochlorperazine) and have the potential to cause drowsiness and extrapyramidal symptoms. Haloperidol is a highly effective antinausea agent and may be less sedating. Antihistamines such as diphenhydramine can be used to control nausea, but may cause sedation. Antihistamines also have anticholinergic properties covering two mechanisms of nausea. Serotonin has been implicated in chemotherapy-associated nausea. Serotonin blockers can be effective but expensive. Other agents are listed in Table 31.6.

Nausea can also be due to a slow gastric/intestinal motility, "squashed" stomach syndrome due to mechanical compression of the stomach, or constipation, and thus prokinetic agents such as metoclopramide should be

TABLE 31.5. Management of nausea/vomiting (21)

Etiology	Pathophysiology	Therapy
Metastases		
Cerebral	Increased intracranial pressure Direct chemoreceptor trigger zone	Steroids, mannitol, Antidopamine, antihistamine
Liver	Toxin buildup	Antidopamine, antihistamine
Meningeal irritation	Increased intracranial pressure	Steroids
Movement	Vestibular stimulation	Antiacetylcholine
Mentation (e.g., anxiety)	Cortical	Anxiolytics
Medications		
Opioids	Chemoreceptor trigger zone, vestibular effect, gastrointestinal tract	Antidopamine, antiacetylcholine, prokinetic agents, stimulant cathartics
Chemotherapy	Chemoreceptor trigger zone, gastrointestinal tract	Antiserotonin, antidopamine, steroids
Others	Chemoreceptors	Antidopamine, antihistamine
Mucosal irritation		
NSAIDs	Gastrointestinal tract	Cytoprotective agents, antacids
Hyperacidity		
Gastroesophageal reflux		
Mechanical obstruction		
Intraluminal	Constipation, obstipation	Manage constipation
Extraluminal	Tumor, fibrotic stricture	Surgery, manage fluids, steroids, octreotide, scopolamine
Motility		
Opioids, ileus, other meds	Gastrointestinal tract	Prokinetic agents, stimulant laxatives
Metabolic		
Hypercalcemia	Chemoreceptor trigger zone	Antidopamine, antihistamine, rehydration, steroids
Hyponatremia		
Hepatic/renal failure		
Microbes		
Local irritation	Gastrointestinal tract antifungals, antacids	Antibacterials, antivirals
Systemic sepsis	Chemoreceptor trigger zone	Antidopamine, antihistamine, antibacterials, antivirals, antifungals
Myocardial		
Ischemia	Vagal stimulation	Oxygen, opioids, anti dopamine, anti histamine, anxiolytics
Congestive heart failure	Cortical, chemoreceptor trigger zone	

Source: Reprinted from Emanuel LL, von Gunten CF, Ferris FD, eds. The Education in Palliative and End-of-life Care (EPEC) Curriculum: Copyright 1999, The EPEC Project, The Robert Wood Johnson Foundation, with permission.

TABLE 31.6. Medications for nausea and vomiting (17)

- Oral medications:
  Dexamethasone 2–8 mg q 6–12 hours
  Diphenhydramine (Benadryl) 25–50 mg q 4–6 hours
  Haloperidol (Haldol) 0.5–5 mg q 6–8 hours
  Hydroxyzine (Atarax) 25–50 mg tid-qid
  Hyoscyamine (Levsin) 0.125–0.25 sublingual q 4 hours
  Lorazepam 1–2 mg q 2–4 hours
  Marinol 2.5–10 mg bid, tid
  Meclizine (Antivert) 12.5–25 mg bid-qid
  Metoclopramide (Reglan) 10–40 mg qid
  Ondansetron (Zofran) 8 mg po tid-qid
  Prochlorperazine (Compazine) 5–10 mg q 4–6 hours
  Prochlorperazine (Compazine) SR 10–15 mg bid
  Promethazine (Phenergan) 12.5–225 mg tid-qid
  Thiethylperazine (Torecan) 10 mg qd-tid
  Trimethobenzamide (Tigan) 250 mg tid-qid
- Suppositories:
  Prochlorperazine (Compazine) 25 mg q 6 hours
  Promethazine (Phenergan) 12.5, 25, 50 mg tid-qid
  Trimethobenzamide (Tigan) 200 mg tid-qid
- Continuous infusion:
  Dexamethasone 8–100 mg/24 hour
  Haloperidol 2.5–10 mg/24 hours
  Hyoscyamine (Levsin) 1–2 mg/24 hours
  Scopolamine 0.8–20 mg/24 hours
  Metoclopramide (Reglan) 20–80 mg/24 hour
  Ondansetron 0.45 mg/kg/24 hours
- IV medications:
  Dexamethasone 2–8 mg q 4–6 hours
  Diphenhydramine (Benadryl) 25–50 mg q 6 hours
  Dronabinol 5 mg/m^2 q 4 hours; max. 6 doses/day
  Granisetron (Kytril) 10 µg/kg qd
  Haloperidol 0.5–2 mg q 4–6 hours
  Lorazepam 1–2 mg q 6–8 hours
  Metoclopramide (Reglan) 10–20 mg q 6 hours
  Ondansetron 4–8 mg q 8 hours
  Prochlorperazine (Compazine) 5–10 mg q 4–6 hours

Source: Reprinted from Stegman MB. Non-pain symptoms. In: Stegman MB, ed. Hope Hospice Pain and Symptom Control in Palliative Medicine, Part 6. Fort Myers, Hospice Resources, 1997;6.1–6.38, with permission from Hospice Resources.

considered as therapeutic modalities. Hyperacidity and mucosal erosion may be associated with significant nausea. Consider the use of antacids, H2 blockers, proton-pump inhibitors, and misoprostol.

Constipation

Constipation can be defined as the passage of small hard feces infrequently and with difficulty (22). Constipation is a common complaint among elderly patients. Risk factors include immobility, depression, female sex, and polypharmacy (23–27). Constipation also tends to be associated with illnesses or conditions such as diabetes mellitus, hypothyroidism, diverticular disease, irritable bowel syndrome, and hemorrhoids (Table 31.7) (28).

Inquiry should be made about the frequency and consistency of stools, nausea, vomiting, abdominal pain, distention and discomfort, mobility, diet, and any other symptoms (22). As with any symptom, evaluation of a reversible cause is initial and paramount. A plain x-ray can be useful. Invasive evaluation with colonoscopy should be considered in difficult, refractory, or complicated cases. Nevertheless, many medications can contribute to constipation. First and foremost are opioid agents; many other medications, including beta-blockers, calcium-channel blockers, anticholinergic agents, and diuretics, are also contributors (21) (Table 31.8).

Constipation is a universal side effect of opioid analgesic therapy, especially in the terminally ill and elderly. This can lead to serious, if not life-threatening, complications, including bowel obstruction, ulceration, perforation, and delirium. Prevention of constipation must be accomplished by using stool softeners, rectal suppositories, laxatives, and hyperosmotic agents, prior to and during opiate therapy (29). A multiple agent bowel regimen must be begun coincident with the initiation of opiates. Table 31.10

TABLE 31.7. Constipation causes and/or risk factors (22)

Idiopathic
    Dietary factors—low residue, poor nutrition
    Motility disturbances—colonic inertia or spasm
    Sedentary living, weakness
    Depression
    Poor fluid intake
    Confusion
    Inability to reach the toilet
    Change in setting, travel
Structural abnormalities
    Anorectal disorders—fissures, thrombosed hemorrhoids
    Strictures
    Tumors
    Adhesions
Endocrine/metabolic
    Hypercalcemia
    Hypokalemia
    Hypothyroidism
Neurogenic
    Cerebrovascular events
    Spinal cord tumors
    Trauma
Smooth muscle/connective tissue disorders
    Amyloidosis
    Scleroderma

Source: Reprinted from Fallon M, O'Neill B. ABC of palliative care: constipation and diarrhea. BMJ 1997;315:1293–1296, with permission from the BMJ Publishing Group.

TABLE 31.8. Drugs/medications commonly associated with constipation (22)

Antacids—aluminum, and calcium containing compounds
Antihistamines
Anticholinergics
Antidepressants
Barium sulfate
Beta-blocking agents
Calcium channel blockers
Calcium supplements
Cholestyramine
Cytotoxic agents
Iron supplements
Narcotics
Nonsteroidal antiinflammatory drugs
Neuroleptics
Sympathomimetics—pseudoephedrine

Source: Reprinted from Fallon M, O'Neill B. ABC of palliative care: constipation and diarrhea. BMJ 1997;315:1293–1296, with permission from the BMJ Publishing Group.

describes a seven-step suggested bowel regimen to avoid constipation in a patient receiving opioid therapy (30). This regimen could also be utilized for anyone complaining of constipation once intestinal obstruction is ruled out. Operative management of severe constipation may be required in refractory cases.

Fecal impaction is stool impacted in the intestines often causing "overflow" diarrhea. This must be treated from below utilizing digital

TABLE 31.9. Bowel regimen

With few exceptions all patients on opioid therapy need an individualized bowel regimen. Start with the step 1 regimen. When an effective regimen is found it must be continued for the duration of the opioid therapy. If fecal impaction is present or suspected, rectal evacuation must occur (before any laxative agents are given orally), using digital disimpaction, enemas, high colonic enemas, and bisacodyl suppositories (2–4 at a time).

Step 1: Docusate 100mg tid plus senna 1 tab q d or bid
Step 2: Docusate 100mg tid plus senna 2 tab bid, plus bisacodyl rectal suppository 1–2 after breakfast
Step 3: Docusate 100mg tid plus senna 3 tab bid, plus bisacodyl suppository 3–4 after breakfast
Step 4: Docusate 100mg tid, senna 4 tab bid plus lactulose or milk of magnesia or polyethylene glycol powder or sorbitol 15–30cc bid, plus bisacodyl suppository 3–4 after breakfast
Step 5: Sodium phosphate or oil retention enema; if no results add a high colonic tap water enema*, and continue until results

* High colonic enemas are given by warming 2-L bags of saline or water to body temperature, hanging bag at ceiling level, and infusing rectally over 30–60 minutes. May repeat continuously or until results.
Source: Mount Sinai Pain Card. New York: Lilian and Benjamin Hertzberg Palliative Care Institute, Mount Sinai Medical Center.

disimpaction and rectal laxatives (rectal suppositories, and/or enemas) before any forms of oral treatment are used (22).

Various forms of laxatives exist. Rectal laxatives are available as suppositories or enemas. Table 31.10 lists stimulant, osmotic, and detergent laxatives, along with prokinetic agents, lubricant stimulants, and large-volume enemas. Clinicians should dose escalate a particular modality to a maximum therapeutic dose.

Polyethylene glycol solution (Golytely) or powder (Miralax) is often used as a pre-colonoscopic regimen but may be an effective means to treat constipation. It offers advantages over other laxatives in that it may cause less cramping. Mineral oil, as it may predispose to aspiration pneumonitis in people with swallowing problems, is usually avoided in the elderly.

TABLE 31.10. Treatments for constipation

Stimulant Laxatives—irritate the bowel and increase peristaltic activity
- Prune juice, 120–240 ml qd or bid
- Senna, two po q hs, titrate to effect (up to 9 or more per day)
- Casanthranol, two po q hs, titrate to effect (up to 9 or more per day)
- Bisacodyl, 5 mg po, pr q hs, titrate to effect

Osmotic Laxatives—draw water into the bowel lumen, increase overall stool volume
- Lactulose 30 ml (sorbitol is cheaper alternative) po q 4–6 hours, then titrate
- Milk of magnesia, 1–2 tablespoons 1–3 times per day
- Magnesium citrate, 1–2 bottles prn
- Polyethylene glycol solution (Golytely) or powder (Miralax)

Detergent Laxatives (stool softeners)—increase water content in stool by facilitating the dissolution of fat
- Sodium docusate, 1–2 po q d—bid, titrate to effect
- Calcium docusate, 1–2 po q d—bid, titrate to effect
- Phosphosoda enema prn

Prokinetic agents—stimulate the bowel's myenteric plexus, and increase peristaltic activity and stool movement
- Metoclopramide, 10–20 mg po q 6 hours

Lubricant stimulants- lubricate the stool and irritate the bowel, increasing peristaltic activity and stool movement
- Glycerin suppositories
- Oils—mineral, peanut

Large-volume enemas—soften stool by increasing its water content, distend the colon and induce peristalsis
- Warm water (addition of soap suds irritates bowel wall to induce peristalsis, however, too much soap suds may damage the bowel wall)

High Colonic Enemas
- Utilize gravity to bring fluid to more proximal parts of bowel. Uses 2 liter bags of water or saline warmed to body temperature, hang on intravenous pole at ceiling level and run in over, 30 minutes, repeat q 1 hour.

Source: Adapted from Emanuel LL. von Gunten CF, Ferris FD. The Education for Physicians on End-of-Life (EPEC) Curriculum. Chicago: Institute for Ethics at the American Medical Association, 1999.

Diarrhea

Diarrhea, potentially due to fecal impaction, antibiotic-associated colitis, gastrointestinal bleeding, malabsorption, medications, or even stress, is a particularly distressing and exhausting symptom (22). A general approach is to determine the patient's normal bowel habits. Once diarrhea is confirmed, the underlying cause must be evaluated and treated if possible. Initial therapy for transient or mild diarrhea may respond to attapulgite or bismuth salts (22). For persistent and bothersome diarrhea, kaolin-pectin of psyllium, loperamide, or tincture of opium may be effective. Octreotide is also an effective means of reducing gastrointestinal secretions (31).

Bowel Obstruction

Symptoms of bowel obstruction include anorexia, confusion, abdominal distention, nausea and vomiting, constipation, and pain. Obstruction may be the presenting symptom that heralds the diagnosis of cancer or may occur later in the course of disease. Bowel obstruction can be caused by multiple and often coexisting etiologies, including intraluminal obstruction, infiltration of the bowel wall, external compression of the lumen, dysmotility, fecal impaction, and intraabdominal adhesions. The prevalence of bowel obstruction is as high as 40% in bowel and pelvic cancers. Gastrointestinal obstruction can be particularly challenging to palliate if the cause of the obstruction cannot be removed. Therefore, investigation of the underlying cause of the obstruction is the first step in alleviating the distress. Furthermore, aggressive measures to prevent or treat constipation and impaction as above may be necessary. Treatment of bowel obstruction may involve the surgical relief of obstruction, nasogastric suction, and pharmacologic measures. Colicky or cramping pain may respond to dicyclomine, opiates (parenteral or rectal), and warm soaks to the abdomen. The obstruction and associated nausea and vomiting may respond to metoclopramide, haloperidol, or dexamethasone. Parenteral octreotide is also useful in this setting to decrease the volume of bowel secretions (31).

Mouth Symptoms

Patients' oral problems can be kept to a minimum by good hydration, brushing the teeth with a fluoride toothpaste twice daily, and daily observation of the oral mucosa. Oral problems can reduce intake of food and fluid due to altered taste, pain, and difficulty swallowing. The first step is managing local problems. Key questions to ask concerning mouth care include the following: Is the mouth dry? Is infection present? Is the mouth dirty? Is the mouth painful? Are oral ulcerations present?

Dry Mouth

The presence of saliva is hardly ever noticed, but the lack of it can seriously damage the quality of life for those experiencing a sensation of oral dryness. Xerostomia describes the subjective complaint of dry mouth. Xerostomia may have both salivary and nonsalivary causes (32). More than 50% of elderly people have been reported to have noticed oral dryness (32–35). Table 31.12 lists medications that have the potential to reduce salivary flow rates.

Almost all forms of xerostomia require symptomatic therapy irrespective of etiology. The goal of therapy is to moisten the oral mucosa, and the best, simplest aid is to sip water frequently. However, several mouth moisteners or artificial salivas have been designed that contain mucin and may be preferred by patients (36,37). Pilocarpine tablets (Salagen) may be used (5 to 10 mg q 8 hours) if the above measures fail. Side effects may include nausea, diarrhea, urinary frequency, and dizziness.

Oral Ulcers/Mucositis

Oral infection can be due to multiple etiologies. Aphthous ulcers are common and can be helped by topical corticosteroids or tetracycline mouthwash. Oral candidiasis usually presents as adherent white plaques but can also present as erythema or angular cheilitis. Nystatin suspension is the usual treatment, but a 5-day course of oral ketoconazole 200 mg can be used as well. Severe viral infection (herpes simplex or zoster) will need acyclovir 200 mg every 4 hours for 5 days. Malignant ulcers are often asso-

TABLE 31.11. Medications that have potential to reduce salivary flow rate

---

Anticholinergic agents
Medications with anticholinergic effects
    Antiarrhythmics
    Antihypertensives
    Antihistamines
    Antidepressants
    Antipsychotics
    Monoamine oxidase (MAO) inhibitors
    Opiates
Psychotropic agents
    Benzodiazepines
Medications causing changes in fluid and electrolyte balance
    Diuretics
Antineoplastic agents
    Interleukin-2

Source: Reprinted from Narhi TO, Meurman JH, Ainamo A. Xerostomia and hyposalivation: causes, consequences and treatment in the elderly. Drugs Aging 1999;15(2):103–116, with permission from Adis International.

TABLE 31.12. Local measures for oral problems (42)

Dry mouth
- Semifrozen fruit juice
- Frequent sips of cold water or water sprays
- Petroleum jelly rubbed on lips

Dirty mouth
- Regular brushing with soft toothbrush and toothpaste
- Pineapple chunks
- Cider and soda mouthwash

Infected mouth
- Topical corticosteroids—betamethasone 0.5 mg in 5 mL water as mouthwash or triamcinolone in carmellose paste
- Tetracycline mouthwash, 250 mg every 8 hours (one capful dissolved in 5 mL water)

Painful mouth
- Coating agents—sucralfate suspension as mouthwash, carmellose paste, carbenoxolone
- Topical anesthesia—benzydamine mouthwash, choline salicylate, Mucasine, lozenges containing local anesthetics

Source: Reprinted from Regnard C, Allport S, Stephenson L. ABC of palliative care: mouth care, skin care, and lymphoedema. Br Med J 1997;315:1002–1005, with permission from the BMJ Publishing Group.

ciated with anaerobic bacteria and may respond to metronidazole 400 to 500 mg orally or rectally every 12 hours or as a topical gel (38). See Table 31.12 for other local measures.

Pressure Ulcers

Pressure ulcers are due to immobility, moisture, friction, shear (sliding movement), and pressure. Prevention and treatment require reduction in pressure (frequent turning and repositioning, foam or low-pressure mattresses), maintaining dryness and cleanliness, avoidance of shear, and friction. Patients at risk of pressure sores should be monitored regularly with daily visual inspection of pressure areas. How a patient moves or is moved by caregivers needs to be assessed and monitored. Even with regular turning and careful lifting and positioning, special pressure surfaces or mattresses are sometimes needed (38).

Pressure ulcer management should be consistent with goals of care. If overall maintenance or improvement of function is the goal and the prognosis is weeks to months, then treat the ulcer with expected management guidelines. If the prognosis is limited, then the intent is to optimize quality of life (see Chapter 30: Pressure Ulcers, page 531).

Foul-Smelling Wounds

Odors may be very distressing to patients, families, and caregivers, and may lead to poor quality care, as even professional caregivers avoid sickening smells. Odors are usually due to anaerobic infections or poor hygiene.

Treat superficial infections with topical metronidazole or silver sulfadiazine (21). For soft tissue infections, add systemic metronidazole to topical management.

To control odors, place open kitty litter or activated charcoal in a pan under the patient's bed, provide adequate room ventilation, place an open cup of vinegar in the room, or burn a candle. Special charcoal-impregnated dressings placed over the odorous wound may also be helpful (21).

Spiritual Suffering

Patients who are living with life-threatening illness are frequently distressed by hopelessness, meaninglessness, remorse, anxiety, being worried, and disruption of personal identity (38). These worries are universal and may result from past, present, or future concerns, independent of religious background or beliefs (39). Facing a life-threatening illness brings to surface questions about what life is all about (40). People may suffer from an inability to find meaning in this last chapter of their lives: from an abbreviated future, from an inability to deal meaningfully with family and loved ones at their final opportunity, from anger about being ill, and from isolation due to the reluctance of the healthy to broach the subject of dying (40,41). These are all spiritual issues.

Physicians are participants in their patient's lives and have a distinctive role and responsibility to minimize patient and family suffering. Patients and families should be afforded the opportunity to explore issues relating to the nature of death and issues of afterlife (39). Discussion of religious or spiritual beliefs might enhance physician–patient understanding and communication.

The Medicare Hospice Benefit

The Medicare hospice benefit, available through certified visiting nurse agencies, allows patients to elect palliative care rather than usual (life-prolonging) care under Medicare Part A. Patients must sign a consent form (drafted by each agency) to enroll in hospice care. The patient's attending physician and hospice medical director must sign a statement that life expectancy is 6 months or less, though hospice care may be recertified and provided indefinitely once a patient has enrolled. The National Hospice and Palliative Care Organization published guidelines for estimating prognosis in noncancer illnesses, though some Medicare intermediaries unfortunately apply these as criteria to determine the appropriateness of hospice referral and reimbursement.

The hospice benefit provides home care to meet patients' needs and covers the cost of all palliative medications (except a $5 co–pay per medication), durable medical equipment, and any treatments and medical services (except for a 5% deductible) pertaining to the patient's terminal illness. Acute hospital stays are minimized (usually limited to periods of up to 5 days for acute symptom management or respite for caregivers). The continuous care level benefit provides intensive hospice services for a minimum of 8 and up to 24 hours per day for brief periods. Intravenous medications, transfusions, artificial nutrition, radiation therapy, chemotherapy, and dobutamine infusions and other treatments may be provided in hospice care when the treatment is intended to palliate symptoms. In practice, such treatments are too expensive for all except for large hospice agencies to cover, given their Medicare per diem reimbursement of approximately $102 per day. (Reimbursement rates are higher for continuous care and for inpatient stays.) Hospice care under the Medicare benefit may be provided to patients residing in nursing homes when the daily nursing home care is paid for privately or by Medicaid. Medicaid reimburses hospice care in 43 states and Washington, D.C. An individual may revoke hospice care, and return to usual Medicare coverage at any time.

General Principles

- Palliative care is interdisciplinary medical care focused on the relief of suffering and achievement of the best possible quality of life for patients and for their family caregivers.
- Good communication skills provide the pathway to excellent care for elderly persons. The fundamentals of such communication are listening, attending to patients' emotional needs, and achieving a shared understanding of the concerns at hand.
- The behaviors for communicating bad news tend to be grouped into several key domains that include preparation, content of message, dealing with patient responses, and ending the encounter.
- Symptom control is an essential component of medical care. Distressing symptoms include dyspnea, cough, nausea and vomiting, constipation, diarrhea, bowel obstruction, mouth symptoms, skin symptoms, odors, and suffering caused by spiritual distress.
- The Medicare hospice benefit allows patients to elect palliative care rather than usual life-prolonging care under Medicare Part A. The patient's attending physician and hospice medical director must sign a statement that life expectancy is 6 months or less.
- The hospice benefit provides home care to meet patients' needs and covers the cost of all palliative medications, durable medical equipment, and any treatments and medical services pertaining to the patient's terminal illness.

Suggested Readings

Carney MT, Meier DE. Sources of suffering in the elderly. In: Cassel CK, Leipzig RM, Cohen HJ, et al., eds. Geriatric Medicine, 4th ed. New York: Springer, 2003:311–322.

Goodlin S. Care near the end of life. In: Cassel CK, Leipzig RM, Cohen HJ, et al., eds. Geriatric Medicine, 4th ed. New York: Springer, 2003:299–310.

Meier DE. Old age and care near the end of life. In: Cassel CK, Leipzig RM, Cohen HJ, et al., eds. Geriatric Medicine, 4th ed. New York: Springer, 2003:281–286.

Tulsky JA. Doctor-patient communication issues. In: Cassel CK, Leipzig RM, Cohen HJ, et al., eds. Geriatric Medicine, 4th ed. New York: Springer, 2003:287–298.

References

1. Steinhauser KE, Christakis NA, Clipp EC, McNeilly M, McIntyre L, Tulsky JA. Factors considered important at the end of life by patients, family, physicians, and other care providers. JAMA 2000;284:2476–2482.
2. Spiro HM. What is empathy and can it be taught? In: Spiro HM, ed. Empathy and Practice of Medicine: Beyond Pills and the Scalpel. New Haven: Yale University Press, 1993:7–14.
3. Smith RC, Hoppe RB. The patient's story: integrating the patient- and physician-centered approaches to interviewing. Ann Intern Med 1991;115:470–477.
4. Ptacek JT, Eberhardt TL. Breaking bad news. A review of the literature. JAMA 1996;276:496–502.
5. Fischer GS, Tulsky JA, Arnold RM. Communicating a poor prognosis. In: Portenoy RK, Bruera E, eds. Topics in Palliative Care, vol 5. New York: Oxford University Press, 2000.
6. Carnes JW, Brownlee HJ Jr. The disclosure of the diagnosis of cancer. Med Clin North Am 1996;80:145–151.
7. Herth K. Fostering hope in terminally-ill people. J Adv Nurs 1990;15:1250–1259.
8. Buckman R. Breaking bad news: why is it still so difficult? Br Med J (Clin Res Ed) 1984;288:1597–1599.
9. Singer PA, Martin DK, Lavery JV, Thiel EC, Kelner M, Mendelssohn DC. Reconceptualizing advance care planning from the patient's perspective. Arch Intern Med 1998;158:879–884.
10. Teno JM, Lynn J. Putting advance-care planning into action. J Clin Ethics 1996;7:205–213.
11. Faulkner A. ABC of palliative care. Communication with patients, families, and other professionals. BMJ 1998;316:130–132.
12. Lo B, Quill T, Tulsky J. Discussing palliative care with patients. Ann Intern Med 1999;130:744–749.
13. Carrieri VK, Janson-Bjerklie S. The sensation of dyspnea: a review. Heart Lung 1984;13:436.

14. Hockely JM, Dunlop R, Davies RJ. Survey of distressing symptoms in dying patients and their families in hospital and their response to a symptom control team. BMJ 1988;296:1715–1717.
15. Bruera E, MacMillan K, Pither J, et al. Effects of morphine on the dyspnea of terminal cancer patients. J Pain Symptom Manage 1990;5:341.
16. Cohen MH, Anderson AJ, Krasnow SH, et al. Continuous infusion of morphine for severe dyspnea. South Med J 1991;84:229.
17. Stegman MB. Non-pain symptoms. In: Stegman MB, ed. Hope Hospice Pain and Symptom Control in Palliative Medicine, Part 6. Fort Myers, Hospice Resources, 1997:6.1–6.38.
18. Davis C. ABC of palliative care: breathlessness, cough, and other respiratory problems. BMJ 1997;315:931–934.
19. Reuben DB, Mor V. Nausea and vomiting in terminally ill cancer patients. Arch Intern Med 1986;146:2021–2023.
20. Baines MJ. ABC of palliative care: nausea, vomiting and intestinal obstruction. BMJ 1997;315:1148–1150.
21. Emanuel LL, von Gunten CF, Ferris FD. The Education for Physicians on End-of-Life Care (EPEC) curriculum. Chicago: Institute for Ethics at the American Medical Association, 1999.
22. Fallon M, O'Neill B. ABC of palliative care: constipation and diarrhea. BMJ 1997;315:1293–1296.
23. Donald IP, Smith RG, Cruikshank JG, Elton RA, Stoddard ME. A study of constipation in elderly living at home. Gerontology 1985;31:112–118.
24. Campbell AJ, Busby WJ, Horwath CC. Factors associated with constipation in a community based sample of people aged 70 years and over. J Epidemiol Community Health 1993;47:23–26.
25. Harari D, Gurwitz JH, Minaker KL. Constipation in the elderly. J Am Geriatr Soc 1993;41:1130–1140.
26. Stewart RB, Moore MT, Marks RG, Hale WE. Correlates of constipation in an ambulatory elderly population. Am J Gastroenterol 1992;87:859–864.
27. Whitehead WE, Drinkwater D, Chisken LJ, Heller BR, Shuster MM. Constipation in the elderly living at home: definition, prevalence and relationships to lifestyle and health status. J Am Geriatr Soc 1989;37:423–429.
28. Meiring PJ, Joubert G. Constipation in elderly patients attending a polyclinic. S Afr Med J 1998;88(7):888–890.
29. Physician's Desk Reference, 55th ed. Montvale, NJ: Medical Economics, 2001:991.
30. Mount Sinai Pain Card. New York: Lilian and Benjamin Hertzberg Palliative Care Institute, Mount Sinai Medical Center.
31. Muir JC, von Gunten CF. Antisecretory agents in gastrointestinal obstruction. Clin Geriatr Med 2000;16:327–334.
32. Fox PC, van der Ven PF, Sonies BC, et al. Xerostomia: evaluation of a symptom with increasing significance. J Am Dent Assoc 1985;110(4):519–525.
33. Sreebny LM, Valdini A. Xerostomia part i: relationship to other oral symptoms and salivary gland hypofunction. Oral Surg Oral Med Oral Pathol 1988;66(4):451–458.
34. Narhi TO. Prevalence of subjective feelings of dry mouth in the elderly. J Dent Res 1994;73(1):20–25.

35. Loesche WJ, Bromberg J, Terpenning MS, et al. Xerostomia, xerogenic medications and food avoidances in selected geriatric groups. J Am Geriatr Soc 1995;43(4):401–407.
36. Narhi TO, Meurman JH, Ainamo A. Xerostomia and hyposalivation: causes, consequences and treatment in the elderly. Drugs Aging 1999;15(2):103–116.
37. Visch LL, S-Gravenmade EJ, Panders AK, et al. A double-blind crossover trial of cmc- and mucin containing saliva substitutes. Int J Oral Maxillofac Surg 1986;15(4):393–400.
38. Cassell EJ. The nature of suffering and the goals of medicine. N Engl J Med 1982;306:639–645.
39. Fainsinger R, MacEachern T, Hanson J, et al. Symptom control during the last week of life on a palliative care unit. J Palliat Care 1991;7:5–11.
40. Hardwig J. Spiritual issues at the end of life: a call for discussion. Hastings Center Report. March–April 2000:28–30.
41. Pulschaski CM. Taking a spiritual history: FICA. Spirituality and Medicine Connection 1999;3:1.
42. Regnard C, Allport S, Stephenson L. ABC of palliative care: mouth care, skin care, and lymphoedema. Br Med J 1997;315:1002–1005.

32
Principles of Pain Management

R. Morgan Bain

Learning Objectives

Upon completion of the chapter, the student will be able to:

1. Understand the pathophysiology of pain.
2. Know the steps on how to obtain an adequate pain history.
3. Identify the different types of medications used for treating pain, and their indications and limitations.
4. Appreciate that pain is multifactorial and often requires multiple modalities of treatment for improvement.

Case (Part 1)

Mr. Peters is a 70-year-old man with a medical history of essential hypertension and hyperlipidemia for which he has been under your care for the past 7 years. He takes a diuretic medication for his hypertension and a hepatic hydroxymethylglutaryl coenzyme A (HMG-CoA) reductase inhibitor for his high cholesterol. He is married and has three adult children and seven grandchildren. He is a retired accountant and enjoys volunteering at his local hospital.

Mr. Peters has had complaints of pain in his left knee after playing tennis on occasion, which is relieved with acetaminophen. Generally, he has been in good health lately.

What are some potential causes of Mr. Peters' knee pain?

Material in this chapter is based on the following chapter in Cassel CK, Leipzig RM, Cohen HJ, Larson EB, Meier DE, eds. Geriatric Medicine: An Evidence-Based Approach, 4th ed. New York: Springer, 2003: Ferrell BA. Acute and Chronic Pain, pp. 323–342. Selections edited by R. Morgan Bain.

General Considerations

Pain is one of the most common symptoms of disease in older persons. Second only to symptoms of upper respiratory tract infections, it is one of the most common complaints in physicians' offices.

The approach to pain assessment and management is different in elderly versus younger persons (1). Older persons may underreport pain for a variety of reasons (2), despite functional impairment, psychological distress, and needless suffering related to pain. They often present with concurrent illnesses and multiple problems, making pain evaluation and treatment more difficult. Elderly persons have a higher incidence of side effects to medications and higher potential for complications and adverse events related to many treatment procedures. Despite these challenges, pain can be effectively managed in most elderly patients. Moreover, clinicians have an ethical and moral obligation to prevent needless suffering and provide effective pain relief, especially for those near the end of life (3).

Age-Associated Changes Related to Pain Perception

Age-related changes in pain perception have been a topic of interest for many years. Elderly persons have been observed to present with painless myocardial infarction and painless intraabdominal catastrophes. The extent to which these observations are attributable to age-related changes in pain perception remains uncertain (4,5). Table 32.1 summarizes anatomic and neurochemical changes associated with pain perception in aging. Unfortunately, most of these findings are not specific to pain, and changes in pain perception related to these findings remain poorly defined.

Acute Pain

Acute pain is often defined by its distinct onset, obvious cause, and short duration. Trauma, burns, infarction, and inflammation are examples of pathologic processes that can result in acute pain. Acute pain is often associated with autonomic nervous system signs including tachycardia, diaphoresis, or elevation in blood pressure (6). The presence of acute pain often indicates an acute injury or acute disease; and the intensity of acute pain often indicates the severity of injury or disease. Thus, acute pain should trigger an urgent search for an underlying cause that might be life threatening or require immediate intervention.

TABLE 32.1. Age-related changes in pain perception (4)

Component	Age-related change	Comments
Pain receptors	• 50% decrease in Pacini's corpuscles • 10–30% decrease in Meissner's/ Merkel's disks • Free nerve endings—no age change	Few studies largely limited to skin

Peripheral
nerves
	• Myelinated nerves
	—Decreased density
	—Increase abnormal/degenerating
	  fibers
	—Slower conduction velocity
	• Unmyelinated nerves
	—Decreased number of large fibers
	  (1.2–1.6 µm)
	—No change in small fibers (0.4 µm)
	—Substance P content decreased
		Evidence of change in pain
		function is lacking;
		findings are not specific
		to pain

Central nervous
system
	• Loss in dorsal horn neurons
	—Altered endogenous inhibition,
	  hyperalgesia
	• Loss of neurons in cortex, midbrain,
	  brainstem
	—18% loss in thalamus
	—Altered cerebral evoked responses
	—Decreased catecholamines,
	  acetylcholine,
	  GABA, 5-HT
	—Endogenous opioids—mixed changes
	—Neuropeptides—no change
		Findings not specific to
		pain

GABA, γ-aminobutyric acid; 5-HT, 5-hydroxytryptamine (serotonin), µm, micrometer.
Source: Adapted from Gibson SJ, Helme RD. Age differences in pain perception and report: a review of physiological, psychological, laboratory and clinical studies. Pain Rev 1995;2:111–137. Reprinted by permission of Sage Publications Ltd. Copyright 1995, SAGE Publications. Reprinted as appears in Ferrell BA. Acute and Chronic Pain, pp. 323–342. In: Cassel CK, Leipzig RM, Cohen HJ, et al., eds. Geriatric Medicine, 4th ed. New York: Springer, 2003.

Chronic Pain

Chronic pain is usually defined by its persistence beyond an expected time frame for healing. The International Association for the Study of Pain defines chronic pain as lasting more than 3 months (7). Intensity of chronic pain is often out of proportion to the observed pathology and often associated with prolonged functional impairment, both physical and psychological. Autonomic signs are often absent or exhausted. Underlying causes of chronic pain are often associated with chronic disease and are less curable (7).

Chronic pain is often more difficult to manage because the underlying cause is less remedial and many treatment strategies are short lived, difficult to maintain, or associated with long-term side effects. Chronic pain usually requires a multidimensional approach to treatment, including use of both analgesic drug and nondrug strategies, with attention to sensory, emotional, and behavioral components of the pain experience.

Case (Part 2)

Today, Mr. Peters presents to your office with complaints of pain in his left flank, which started a couple of days ago and is making it difficult to sleep or take a deep breath. His blood pressure is 145/90 mmHg, pulse 95/min, and he is afebrile. He appears to be in much discomfort and is holding his hand against his left chest. Upon examination of his chest, you notice a vesicular rash with crusting that appears in a dermatomal distribution on his left flank that does not cross the midline. You find out that Mr. Peters had an episode of chickenpox as a young child.
What is the most possible diagnosis?
What is the mechanism of Mr. Peters's pain?

Classification Based on Pathophysiology

The classification of pain by pathophysiologic mechanisms may help clinicians choose and target pain management strategies more effectively. The American Geriatrics Society Panel on Chronic Pain identified four basic pathophysiologic pain mechanisms that have important implications for choosing pain management strategies (Table 32.2) (8).

TABLE 32.2. Pain classification based on pathophysiology (8)

I. Nociceptive pain (somatic and visceral)
  a. Trauma (and burns)
  b. Ischemia
  c. Inflammation (e.g., infection, inflammatory diseases, arthritis)
  d. Mechanical deformity (e.g., tissue strain, swelling, tumor, physical distortion)
  e. Myalgias (e.g., myofascial pain syndromes)
II. Neuropathic pain
  a. Peripheral nerves
    i. Diabetic neuralgia
    ii. Viral neuralgia (e.g., postherpetic neuralgia)
    iii. Traumatic neuralgia (e.g., postsurgical neuralgia, phantom limb)
    iv. Trigeminal neuralgia
  b. Central nervous system
    i. Post-thalamic stroke pain
    ii. Myelopathic pain (e.g., multiple sclerosis)
  c. Sympathetic nervous system
    i. Reflex sympathetic dystrophy
    ii. Causalgia (e.g., complete regional pain syndromes)
III. Mixed or undetermined pathophysiology
  a. Chronic recurrent headaches
  b. Vasculopathic pain syndromes (e.g., vasculitic pain syndromes)
IV. Psychologically based pain syndromes (e.g., somatization disorders, hysterical reactions)

Source: Adapted from American Geriatric Society Panel on Chronic Pain in Older Persons. The management of chronic pain in older persons. J Am Geriatr Soc 1998;46:635–651, with permission from Blackwell Publishing Ltd. Reprinted as appears in Ferrell BA. Acute and Chronic Pain, pp. 323–342. In: Cassel CK, Leipzig RM, Cohen HJ, et al., eds. Geriatric Medicine, 4th ed. New York: Springer, 2003.

Nociceptive Pain

Pain problems that result largely from stimulation of pain receptors are called nociceptive pain (9). Nociceptive pain may arise from tissue injury, inflammation, or mechanical deformation. Examples include trauma, burns, infection, arthritis, ischemia, and tissue distortion. Pain from nociception usually responds well to common analgesic medications.

Neuropathic Pain

Neuropathic pain results from pathophysiologic processes that arise in the peripheral or central nervous system (10,11). Examples include diabetic neuralgia, postherpetic neuralgia, and posttraumatic neuralgia (postamputation or "phantom limb" pain). In contrast to nociceptive pain, neuropathic pain syndromes have been found to respond to nonconventional analgesic medications such as tricyclic antidepressants and anticonvulsant drugs.

Mixed Pain Syndrome

Mixed pain syndromes are often thought to have multiple or unknown pathophysiologic mechanisms. Treatment of these problems is more problematic and often unpredictable. Examples include recurrent headaches and some vasculitic syndromes.

Psychologically Based Pain Syndromes

Psychologically based pain syndromes are those with psychological factors that play a major role in the pain experience (12). Examples include somatoform disorders and conversion reactions. These patients may benefit from specific psychiatric intervention, but traditional pain strategies are probably not indicated.

Epidemiology

The precise incidence and prevalence of pain in older populations is not known. In general, the most common causes of pain in elderly persons is probably related to musculoskeletal disorders such as back pain and arthritis. Neuralgia is common, stemming from common diseases, such as diabetes or herpes zoster, and trauma, such as surgery, amputation, and other nerve injuries. Nighttime leg pain (e.g., cramps, restless legs) is also common, as is claudication. Cancer, although not as common as arthritis, is a cause of severe pain that is distressing to patients, families, and staff.

Pain is also common in nursing homes. It has been suggested that 45% to 80% of nursing home residents may have substantial pain (13). Many of these patients have multiple pain complaints and multiple potential sources of pain.

Pain is associated with a number of negative outcomes in elderly people. Depression, decreased socialization, sleep disturbance, impaired ambulation, and increased health care utilization and costs have all been associated with the presence of pain in older people. Older patients rely heavily on family and other caregivers near the end of life. For these patients and their caregivers, pain can be especially distressing. Pain can have a substantial impact on caregiver strain and caregiver attitudes (14).

Case (Part 3)

A diagnosis of herpes zoster (shingles) is made. Mr. Peters tells you that the pain is severe and that it is limiting his ability to dress himself as well as perform any of his household chores. He tried taking acetaminophen to help with the pain but it was ineffective.

What other questions are necessary to get an adequate pain history from Mr. Peters?

Diagnostic Evaluation

Symptoms and Signs

Assessment of pain should begin with a thorough history and physical examination to help establish a diagnosis of underlying disease and form a baseline description of pain experiences. The history should include questions to elicit the following: *when* the pain started; *what* events or illnesses coincided with the onset; *where* it hurts (location) and *how* it feels (character); *what* are the aggravating and relieving influences; and *what* treatments have been tried. Past medical and surgical history is important to identify coexisting disease and previous experience with pain and analgesic use. The review of systems should focus on the musculoskeletal and nervous system. Any history of trauma should be thoroughly investigated because falls, occult fractures, and other injuries are common in this age group. In this setting, care must be taken to avoid attributing acute pain to preexisting conditions. Complicating pain assessment is the fact that chronic pain does fluctuate with time. Injuries from minor trauma and acute disease, such as gout or calcium pyrophosphate crystal arthropathy, can be easily overlooked. Finally, many older persons do not use the word *pain* but may refer to their problems as "hurting," "aching," or some other description. It is important to probe for and identify pain in the patient's own words so that references for subsequent follow-up evaluations are clearly established (15).

A physical examination should confirm any suspicions suggested by the history. Because of the frequency with which problems are often identified, the physical exam should concentrate on the musculoskeletal and nervous systems. Tender points of inflammation, muscle spasm, and trigger points should be sought. Observation of abnormal posture, gait impairment, and limitations in range of motion may trigger a need for physical therapy and rehabilitation. Evidence of kyphosis, scoliosis, and abnormal joint alignments should be identified. A systematic neurologic exam is also important to identify potential sources of neuropathic pain. Focal muscle weakness, atrophy, abnormal reflexes, or sensory impairments may indicate peripheral or central nervous system injury.

It is important to assess functional status to identify self-care deficits and formulate treatment plans that maximize independence and quality of life. Functional status can also represent an important outcome measure of overall pain management. Functional status can be evaluated from information taken from the history and physical examination, as well as the use of one or several functional status scales validated in elderly people.

A brief psychological and social evaluation is also important. Depression, anxiety, social isolation, and disengagement are all common in patients with chronic pain. There is a significant association between chronic pain and depression, even when controlling for overall health and functional status. Therefore, assessment should include routine screening for depression. Psychological evaluation should also include consideration of anxiety and coping skills. Anxiety is common among patients with acute and chronic pain and requires extra time and frequent reassurance from health care providers. Chronic pain often requires effective coping skills for anxiety and other emotional feelings that can be learned (16). For those with significant psychiatric symptoms, referral for formal psychiatric evaluation and management may be required.

Case (Part 4)

On the Verbal 0–10 Scale, Mr. Peters rates his pain on his side as a 9/10 at present. After taking the acetaminophen, the pain in his side only decreased to 8/10. He says that the pain in his knee at its worse is usually a 4/10.

What are some other methods/scales for characterizing pain severity?

Pain Assessment Scales

Pain assessment is the most important part of pain management. Accurate pain assessment is important to identify the underlying source and associated physiologic pain mechanisms in order to choose the most effective treatment and maximize patient outcomes. Pain management is most effective when the underlying cause of pain has been identified and treated definitively. Inherent in pain assessment is the need to evaluate acute pain that may indicate life-threatening injury and distinguish this from exacerbations of chronic pain. For chronic pain in which the cause is not reversible or only partially treatable, a multidimensional or multidisciplinary evaluation may be required. Among those with cognitive impairment or difficulty reporting pain, other clinicians, family, and caregivers may be helpful in providing a more accurate description.

Pain scales can be grouped into multidimensional and unidimensional scales. In general, *multidimensional scales* with multiple items often provide more stable measurement and evaluation of pain in several domains. At the same time, multidimensional scales are often long, time-consuming, and can be difficult to score at the bedside, making them difficult to use in a busy clinical setting.

Unidimensional scales consist of a single item that usually relates to pain intensity alone. These scales are usually easy to administer and require little time or training to produce reasonably valid and reliable results. They have found widespread use in many clinical settings to monitor treatment effects and for quality assurance indicators. Table 32.3 describes some unidimensional scales that are commonly used. Unidimensional scales may be more useful in assessing pain at the moment while evaluating changes in pain reports over time, much the way vital signs are used. This is especially true for those with some cognitive impairment.

Case (Part 5)

After much discussion, Mr. Peters agrees to be admitted to the hospital for acute pain management. You feel that his pain is too severe for him to be effectively treated as an outpatient. You start him on acyclovir plus intravenous morphine. The morphine is to be administered around the clock every 4 hours with a PRN dose every hour as needed for breakthrough pain.

Would treating Mr. Peters's pain with a nonsteroidal antiinflammatory drug (NSAID) be a more appropriate first-line therapy than an opioid?

What are the common side effects of opioids?

TABLE 32.3. Unidimensional scales for pain measurement (38)

Scale	Description	Validity	Reliability	Advantages	Disadvantages	References
Visual analog	100-mm line; vertical or horizontal	Good	Fair	Continuous scale	Requires pencil and paper	Clinical Practice Guidelines (7,8,39)
Present pain intensity	6-point 0–5 scale with word descriptors (subscale of McGill Pain Questionnaire)	Good	Fair	Easy to understand, word anchors decrease clustering toward middle of scale	Usually requires visual cue	Melzack, 1975 (28,40)
Graphic pictures	Happy faces; others	Fair	Fair	Amusing	Requires vision and attention	Herr et al. (14,41)
Sloan Kettering pain card	7 words randomly distributed on a card	Good	Fair	Ease of administration	Requires visual cue	Ferrell et al. (13,42,43)
Verbal 0–10 Scale	"On a scale of 0 to 10, if 0 means no pain and 10 means the worst pain you can imagine, how much is your pain now?"	Good	Fair	Probably easiest to use	Requires hearing	Ferrell et al. (13,42)

Source: Adapted from Ferrell BA. Pain. In: Osterweil D, Brummel-Smith K, Beck JB, eds. Comprehensive Geriatric Assessment. New York: McGraw-Hill, 2000:390, with permission from The McGraw-Hill Companies. Reprinted as appears in Ferrell BA. Acute and Chronic Pain. In: Cassel CK, Leipzig RM, Cohen HJ, et al., eds. Geriatric Medicine, 4th ed. New York: Springer, 2003.

Management Considerations

Acute and Perioperative Pain Management

The treatment of acute pain relies largely on short-term use of analgesic medications and resolution of the underlying cause. The World Health Organization (WHO) recommends that the treatment of acute pain be based on the intensity of the pain (6,17). Pain of *mild intensity* usually responds to nonopioid drugs used alone or in combination with other physical and cognitive-behavioral interventions. Pain of *moderate intensity* often requires more intensive efforts, such as weak opioids or low doses of more potent opioid drugs. Many of these drugs are compounded with NSAIDs or acetaminophen to achieve enhanced relief, with only modest exposure to the side effects of opioids. *Severe pain* usually requires potent opioid analgesic medications given alone or in combination with other analgesic strategies. For severe trauma or postoperative pain, intermittent intravenous, continuous intravenous, or spinal anesthesia may provide faster and more continuous pain relief. Table 32.4 provides an outline of acute pain control options for mild, moderate, and severe pain.

Although initially designed as a stepwise approach to cancer pain management, the WHO approach has become an acceptable approach to all pain with a few caveats. First, it is important to remember that the model does not require that strong opioids be withheld until after other treatments have failed. When patients present with severe pain, they should be treated initially with strong medications. Second, when pain rapidly escalates from mild to severe, analgesia should be rapidly escalated to strong opioids, with or without other combined strategies. Third, adjuvant drugs and combined treatments should be used early for mild to moderate pain,

TABLE 32.4. Acute pain control options

Mild pain
* Administration of acetaminophen or NSAIDs
* Cognitive-behavioral strategies (relaxation, distraction, etc.)
* Physical agents (cold, heat, massage, etc.)
* Combined strategies

Moderate pain
* Low-dose or low-potency opioids
* Combinations of acetaminophen or NSAIDs with low-dose or low-potency opioids
* Combined strategies

Severe pain
* Potent opioid analgesics (intermittent or around the clock)
* Continuous infusions of opioid analgesics (e.g., PCA)
* Neural blockade (intermittent or continuous)
* Spinal anesthesia (e.g., epidural anesthesia, intermittent or continuous)
* Combined strategies

NSAID, nonsteroidal antiinflammatory drug; PCA, patient-controlled analgesia.
Source: Adapted from Acute Pain Management Guideline Panel. *Acute Pain Management: Operative Medical Procedures and Trauma. Clinical Practice Guideline.* AHCPR Pub 92-0032. Rockville, MD: Agency for Health Care Policy and Research, Public Health Service, U.S. Department of Health and Human Services; 1992. Reprinted as appears in Ferrell BA. Acute and Chronic Pain, pp. 323–342. In: Cassel CK, Leipzig RM, Cohen HJ, et al., eds. Geriatric Medicine, 4th ed. New York: Springer, 2003.

especially those of the neuropathic type. Finally, when patients present with acute pain, even though establishing a diagnosis is a priority, symptomatic pain treatment should be initiated while investigations are proceeding. It is rarely justified to defer analgesia until a diagnosis is made. In fact, a comfortable patient is better able to cooperate with diagnostic procedures.

Chronic Pain Management

Chronic pain management often requires a multimodal approach of drug and nondrug pain management strategies (8). Although analgesic medications are the most common strategy employed, the concurrent use of cognitive-behavioral therapy and other nondrug strategies may be helpful to reduce long-term reliance on medications alone.

In general, chronic pain is often more difficult to relieve than acute pain. Patients should be given an expectation of pain relief, but it is unrealistic to suggest or sustain an expectation of complete relief for some patients with chronic pain. The goals and trade-offs of possible therapies need to be discussed openly. Sometimes a period of trial and error should be anticipated when new medications are initiated and titration occurs. Review of medications, doses, use patterns, efficacy, and adverse effects should be a regular process of care (8). Ineffective drugs should be tapered and discontinued.

It is appropriate to consider economic issues and make balanced decisions while basic principles of pain assessment and treatment are followed. Health care professionals should be aware of the costs and financial barriers patients and families may encounter with the strategies often prescribed. These issues include limited Medicare reimbursement, limited formularies, delays in referrals in some managed care environments, delays from mail-order pharmacies, and limited availability of opioid medications in some pharmacies.

Case (Part 6)

After spending a week in the hospital to manage his acute pain, Mr. Peters was discharged. His lesions were clearing up and the pain had been substantially reduced. Upon repeat pain assessment, he rated the pain as 3/10 with occasional flares to 5/10. He was given a prescription for a combination analgesic to be taken every 4 hours as needed.

Four months later, despite regular office visits and continued use of analgesics, Mr. Peters states that the pain in his left flank is still persistent and bothersome.

What is the mechanism for his pain now?

What other types of medications may be helpful in treating the pain?

Pharmacologic Approach to Pain Management

Any patient who has pain that impairs functional status or quality of life is a candidate for analgesic drug therapy (8). Analgesic medications are safe and effective for elderly people. Dosing for most patients requires beginning with low doses with careful upward titration, including frequent reassessment for optimum pain relief and management of side effects.

The least invasive route of drug administration should be used. Some drugs can be administered from a variety of routes, such as subcutaneous, intravenous, transcutaneous, sublingual, and rectal. The oral route is preferable because of its convenience and relatively steady blood levels produced. Intravenous bolus provides the most rapid onset and shortest duration of action, which may require substantial labor, technical skill, and monitoring. Subcutaneous and intramuscular injection, although commonly used, has the disadvantages of wider fluctuations in absorption and rapid fall-off of action compared to oral routes. Transcutaneous, rectal, and sublingual routes are also more difficult to predict but may be essential for those with difficulty swallowing (8).

Timing of medications is also important. Fast-onset, short-acting analgesic drugs should be used for episodic pain on an as-needed schedule. For continuous pain, medications should be provided around the clock. In these situations, a steady-state analgesic blood level is more effective in maintaining comfort. Long-acting or sustained-release preparations should be used only for continuous pain. Most patients with continuous pain also need fast-onset short-acting drugs for breakthrough pain. *Breakthrough pain* includes (1) end-of-dose failure as the result of decreased blood levels of analgesic with concomitant increase in pain prior to the next scheduled dose; (2) incident pain, usually caused by activity that can be anticipated and pretreated; and (3) spontaneous pain, common with neuropathic pain that is often fleeting and difficult to predict (8).

Acetaminophen

Acetaminophen is the drug of choice for elderly persons with mild to moderate pain, especially that of osteoarthritis and other musculoskeletal problems (8). As an analgesic and antipyretic, acetaminophen acts in the central nervous system to reduce pain perception. Despite the lack of antiinflammatory activity, studies have shown that acetaminophen is as effective as ibuprofen for chronic osteoarthritis of the knee (18). Given in a dose of 650 to 1000 mg four times a day, it remains the safest analgesic medication compared to traditional NSAIDs and other analgesic drugs for most patients. Unfortunately, acetaminophen overdose can result in irreversible hepatic necrosis. Therefore, the maximum daily dose should never exceed 4000 mg per day (8).

Nonsteroidal Antiinflammatory Drugs

Nonsteroidal antiinflammatory drugs (NSAIDs) have analgesic activity both peripherally and centrally. They are potent inhibitors of prostaglandin synthesis, which have effects on inflammation, pain receptors, and nerve conduction, and may have central effects, as well (19).

Nonspecific inhibitors of cyclooxygenase (COX) enzymes (most older NSAIDs) are still appropriate for short-term use in inflammatory arthritic conditions such as gout, calcium pyrophosphate arthropathy, acute flare-ups of rheumatoid arthritis, and other inflammatory rheumatic conditions. They have also been reported to relieve the pain of headache, menstrual cramps, and other mild-to-moderate pain syndromes. These drugs can be used alone for mild-to-moderate pain or in combination with opioids for more severe pain. They have the advantage of being non–habit forming. Individual drugs in this class vary widely with respect to antiinflammatory activity, potency, analgesic properties, metabolism, excretion, and side-effect profiles. Moreover, it has been observed that failure of response to one NSAID may not predict the response to another. A disadvantage of NSAIDs is that, unlike opioids, they all demonstrate a ceiling effect, that is, a level at which increased dose results in no further increase in analgesia. A large number of NSAIDs are now available; however, there is no evidence to support a particular compound as the NSAID of choice. Several are available over-the-counter without a prescription. Table 32.5 lists selected NSAIDs for pain.

High-dose NSAIDs for long periods of time should be avoided in elderly patients (8). Of major concern is the high incidence of adverse reactions, including gastrointestinal bleeding (20), renal impairment (21), and bleeding diathesis from platelet dysfunction. The concomitant use of misoprostol, high-dose histamine-2 receptor antagonists, and proton pump inhibitors is only partially successful at reducing the risk of significant gastrointestinal bleeding associated with NSAID use (22–24). Also, the side-effect profiles of gastroprotective drugs in this population must be weighed against their limited benefits (25). For those with multiple medical problems, NSAIDs are associated with increased risk of drug–drug and drug–disease interactions; NSAIDs may interact with antihypertensive therapy (26). Thus, the relative risks and benefits of NSAIDs must be weighed carefully against other available treatments for older patients with chronic pain problems. For some patients, chronic opioid therapy, low-dose or intermittent corticosteroid therapy, or other nonanalgesic drug strategies may have fewer life-threatening risks compared to long-term NSAID use (8) (see Chapter 3: Geriatric Pharmacology and Drug Prescribing for Older Adults, page 39).

Opioid Analgesic Medications

Opioid analgesic medications act by blocking receptors in the central nervous system (brain and spinal cord), resulting in a decreased perception of pain. Selected opioid analgesic medications are listed in Table 32.6.

TABLE 32.5. Selected nonsteroidal antiinflammatory drugs for pain

Drug	Maximum dose	Description	Comments
Relafen (Nabumetone)	2000 mg/24h (q 24h dosing)	Partially Cox-2 selective; gastric toxicity may be less; occasionally requires q 12h dosing	Avoid maximum dose for prolonged periods
Aspirin	4000 mg/24h (q 4–6h dosing)	Prototype NSAID	Salicylate levels may be helpful in monitoring
Salsalate (Disalcid)	3000 mg/24h (q 6–8h dosing)	Hydrolyzed in small intestine to aspirin	Elderly may require dose adjustment downward to avoid salicylate toxicity; salicylate levels may be helpful in monitoring
Ibuprofen (Motrin by prescription; Advil, Nuprin, and others OTC)	2400 mg/24h (q 6–8h dosing)	Gastric, renal, and abnormal platelet function may be dose dependent; constipation, confusion, and headaches may be more common in older persons	Avoid high doses for prolonged periods of time
Diflunisal (Dolobid)	1000 mg/24h maximum dose Loading = 1000 mg then 500 q 12h; or 750 mg then 250 mg q 8h in small patients or frail elderly	Relatively good analgesic properties, but requires loading dose	Dose may need downward adjustment for small patients or frail elderly
Sulindac (Clinoril)	400 mg/24h (q 12h dosing)	Same as ibuprofen	Same as ibuprofen
Naproxen (Naprosyn by prescription: Aleve and others OTC)	1000 mg/24h (q 8–12h dosing)	Same as ibuprofen; may require a loading dose	Same as ibuprofen
Choline magnesium trisalicylate (Trilisate)	5500 mg/24h (q 12h dosing)	Lower effect on platelet function	Salicylate levels may be helpful to avoid toxicity
Indomethacin (Indocin)	200 mg/24h (q 8–12h dosing)	Extremely high toxicity in frail elderly; should be reserved for acute inflammatory conditions (e.g., gout, etc.)	Keep dose to a minimum (25 mg q 8h) and for short-term use only; avoid use for osteoarthritis or other noninflammatory problems
Ketorolac (Toradol)	IM: 120 mg/24h (30–60 mg loading dose; followed by half the loading dose (15–30 mg q 6h limited to not more than 5 days) PO: 60 mg/24h (q 6h dosing limited to not more that 14 days)	Substantial gastrointestinal toxicity as well as renal and platelet dysfunction; relatively high postoperative complications have been documented	Duration of treatment limited because of high toxicity; reduce dose in half for those<50 kg or >65 years of age

Note: Limited number of examples are provided. For comprehensive lists of other available NSAIDs and a host of brand names, clinicians should consult other sources.

COX, cyclooxygenase; IM, intramuscular injection; OTC, over-the-counter or available without prescription; PO, per oral route or by mouth.

Source: Ferrell BA. Acute and Chronic Pain. In: Cassel CK, Leipzig RM, Cohen HJ, et al., eds. Geriatric Medicine, 4th ed. New York: Springer, 2003.

Drug	Starting dose (oral)	Description	Comments
Morphine (Roxanol, MSIR)	30 mg (q 4 h dosing)	Short–intermediate half-life; older people are more sensitive than younger people to side effects	Titrate to comfort; continuous use for continuous pain; intermittent use for episodic pain; anticipate and prevent side effects
Codeine (plain codeine, Tylenol #3, other combinations with acetaminophen or NSAIDs)	30–60 mg (q 4–6 h dosing)	Acetaminophen or NSAIDs limit dose; constipation is a major issue	Begin bowel program early; do not exceed maximum dose for acetaminophen or NSAIDs
Hydrocodone (Vicoden, Lortab, others)	5–10 mg (q 3–4 h dosing)	Toxicity similar to morphine; acetaminophen or NSAID combinations limit maximum dose	Same as above
Oxycodone (Roxicodone, Oxy IR; or in combinations with acetaminophen or NSAIDs, such as Percocet, Tylox, Percodan, others)	20–30 mg (q 3–4 h dosing)	Toxicity similar to morphine; acetaminophen or NSAID combinations limit maximum dose; oxycodone is available generically as a single agent	Same as above
Hydromorphone (Dilaudid)	4 mg (q 3–4 h dosing)	Half-life may be shorter than morphine; toxicity similar to morphine	Similar to morphine
Sustained-release morphine (MS Contin, Oramorph, Kadian)	MS Contin: 30–60 mg (q 12 h dosing) Oramorph: 30–60 mg (q 12 h dosing) Kadian: 30–60 mg (q 24 h dosing)	Morphine sulfate in a wax matrix tablet or sprinkles; MS Contin and Oramorph should not be broken or crushed; Kadian capsules can be opened and sprinkled on food, but should not be crushed	Titrate dose slowly because of drug accumulation; rarely requires more frequent dosing than recommended on package insert; immediate release opioid analgesic often necessary for breakthrough pain
Sustained-release oxycodone (Oxycontin)	15–30 mg (q 12 h dosing)	Similar to sustained release morphine	Similar to sustained release morphine
Transderm fentanyl (Durgesic)	25-μg patch (q 72 h dosing)	Reservoir for drug is in the skin, not in the patch; equivalent dose compared to other opioids is not very predictable (see package insert); effective activity may exceed 72 hours in older patients	Drug reservoir is in skin, not patch; titrate slowly using immediate-release analgesics for breakthrough pain; peak effect of first dose may take 18–24 hours; not recommended for opioid naive patients
Fentanyl lozenge on an applicator stick	Rub on buccal mucosa until analgesia occurs, then discard	Short half-life; useful for acute and breakthrough pain when oral route is not possible	Absorbed via buccal mucosa, not effective orally

Note: Limited number of examples are provided. For comprehensive lists of other available opioids, clinicians should consult other sources.
Source: Ferrell BA. Acute and Chronic Pain. In: Cassel CK, Leipzig RM, Cohen HJ, et al., eds. Geriatric Medicine, 4th ed. New York: Springer, 2003.

Opioid drugs have no ceiling to their analgesic effects and have been shown to relieve all types of pain.

Opioid drugs have the potential to cause cognitive disturbances, nausea, respiratory depression, constipation, and habituation in older people. Drowsiness, performance-based measures of cognitive impairment, and respiratory depression associated with opioids should be anticipated when opioids are initiated and doses are escalated rapidly. Central nervous system effects are dose dependent and can be used to judge rate of dose escalations. If patients have unrelieved pain with little drowsiness or cognitive impairment, doses may be escalated. Tolerance usually develops in a few days to central nervous system side effects, at which time patients usually return to a fully alert status and baseline cognitive function. Until tolerance develops, patients should be instructed not to drive and to take precautions against falls or other accidents. But once tolerance to these effects has developed, patients can return to normal activities, including driving and other demanding tasks, despite high doses of opioid drugs. Constipation is a side effect of opioid drugs to which patients do not develop tolerance. The management of constipation must be preemptive and preventative and include increasing fluid intake, maintaining mobility, and regular use of cathartic medications. All patients require stool softeners and osmotic laxatives, such as milk of magnesia, lactulose, or sorbitol. For many patients, opioid-induced constipation also requires potent stimulant laxatives, such as senna or bisacodyl. It should be remembered that stimulants should not be used until impactions have been removed and obstruction has been ruled out.

Nausea also occasionally complicates opioid therapy. Nausea from opioid medications may result from several mechanisms and typically wanes as tolerance develops over several days to a week. Traditionally, antiemetics such as prochlorperazine, chlorpromazine, and antihistamines have been the mainstay of treatment for nausea in younger patients. Recently, low-dose haloperidol and metoclopramide have been used, anecdotally noting a lower side-effect profile compared to other neuroleptic drugs. It should be remembered that all of these agents have high side-effect profiles in elderly patients, including movement disorders, delirium, and anticholinergic effects. Thus, clinicians should choose antiemetic medications with the lowest side effects and continue to monitor patients frequently (8).

Case (Part 7)

You determine that Mr. Peters need pain medications for his postherpetic neuralgia. You talk to Mr. Peters about medication options when he stops you midsentence. He says, "I don't want to take any drug that would make me dependent on it for life. Those drugs are used by crack addicts so I don't want to do that!"

How do you explain to Mr. Peters about the concept of addiction, tolerance, and dependency?
What measures could you take to allay his concerns and fears?

Tolerance, Dependency, Addiction, and Pseudo-Addiction

It is important for clinicians who prescribe opioid analgesics to understand issues of tolerance, dependency, and addiction. *Tolerance* is defined by diminished effect of a drug associated with constant exposure to the drug over time. For opioid drugs, tolerance is difficult to predict. In general, tolerance to drowsiness and respiratory depression occurs much faster than tolerance to analgesic properties of the drug. Tolerance develops quickly to central nervous system side effects and to nausea and never develops to constipation.

Dependency is also a pharmacologic phenomenon associated with many drugs, including corticosteroids and beta-blockers. Dependency is present when patients experience uncomfortable side effects when the drug is withheld abruptly. Drug dependence requires constant exposure to the drug for at least several days. Symptoms associated with abrupt opioid withdrawal may include anorexia, restlessness, nausea, diaphoresis, tachycardia, mild hypertension, and mild fever. Worsening symptoms may including skin mottling, gooseflesh, and frank autonomic crisis. Fortunately, these symptoms can be completely prevented by tapering opioids over a few days. Opioid doses can be reduced every few days and safely discontinued within a week. It is important to remember that physiologic effects of opioid withdrawal are usually not life threatening compared to those common with alcohol, benzodiazepine, or barbiturate withdrawal (27).

Addiction is a psychiatric and behavioral problem and is defined in such terms. *Addictive behavior* is defined by compulsive drug use despite negative physical and social consequences (harm to self and others) and the craving for effects other than pain relief. Addicted patients often have erratic behavior that can be observed in a clinical setting in the form of selling, buying, and procuring drugs on the street and using medication by bizarre means such as crushing or dissolving tablets for self-IV administration. It is now clear that drug use alone is not the major factor in the development of addiction. Other medical, social, and economic factors play immense roles in addictive behavior (27). It is also important not to construe certain behaviors as necessarily addictive behaviors. Hoarding of medications, persistent or worsening pain complaints, frequent office visits, requests for dose escalations, and other behaviors associated with inadequately treated and unrelieved pain has been termed *"pseudo-addiction."* Laws, regulations, and unintentional behavior by prescribing clinicians may require patients to hoard medication and seek other physicians for additional help. In fact, true addiction is rare among patients taking opioid analgesic medications for medical reasons. This is not meant to imply that opioid drugs can be used indiscriminately, only that exaggerated fear of addiction and side effects do not justify failure to treat pain in elderly patients, especially those near the end of life (28).

Fear of addiction has been identified as a major barrier to pain management in elderly people (29). Unfortunately, fears by clinicians and patients have been overly influenced by social pressures to reduce illegal drug use among younger people and those who take narcotics for emotional rather than medical reasons. Regulation of controlled substances by state and federal authorities, as well as scrutiny of physician practices by state license boards, have intimidated many clinicians, who, as a result, may not prescribe potent analgesic medications, even for patients with severe pain near the end of life. This hesitancy to treat symptom distress may actually contribute to patients who seek suicide rather than endure inadequately managed pain. Clinicians have an obligation to provide comfort, pain relief, and dignity for patients.

Other Nonopioid Medications

A variety of other medications not formally classified as analgesics have been found to be helpful in certain specific pain problems. The term *adjuvant analgesic drugs*, although frequently used, is a misnomer in that some of these nonopioid drugs may be the primary pain-relieving pharmacologic intervention in certain cases. Table 32.7 provides some examples of nonopioid drugs that may help certain kinds of pain. The largest body of evidence available relates to the use of these drugs for neuropathic pain, such as diabetic neuropathies, postherpetic neuralgia, and trigeminal neuralgia. Tricyclic antidepressants, anticonvulsants, and local anesthetics are the most frequently used nonopioid analgesics for neuropathic conditions. Usually these agents work better in combination with other traditional drug and nondrug strategies in an effort to improve pain and keep other drug doses to a minimum. In general, nonopioid medications for neuropathic pain should be chosen according to lowest side effects. Treatment should usually start with lower doses than those recommended for younger patients, and doses should be escalated slowly based on known pharmacokinetics of individual drugs and appropriate knowledge of disease-specific treatment strategies. Unfortunately, most of the nonopioid medications for pain management have high side-effect profiles in elderly people. Thus, these medications often have to be monitored carefully.

Antidepressants have been the most widely studied class of nonopioid medications for pain. The mechanism of action for these drugs is not entirely known, but probably has to do with interruption of norepinephrine- and serotonin-mediated mechanisms in the brain (30). For neuropathic pain, the major effect of these drugs is not their mood-altering capacity, although this may also be helpful in those with concurrent major depression. More is known about tricyclic antidepressants than the other subclasses. Studies of the serotonin reuptake inhibitors, which may have lower side-effect profiles for elderly people, have had mixed reviews, and most have not been shown effective for pain management, with the exception of chronic headache and diabetic neuropathy (paroxetine) (30).

It has been known for many years that some medications with antiepileptic activity may relieve the pain of trigeminal neuralgia (*tic douloureux*) (31). Studies have shown that compounds such as diphenylhydantoin, carbamazepine, and valproic acid may also help diabetic neuralgia and other neuropathic pains in some patients. Of recent interest has been the effectiveness of gabapentin for treatment of diabetic neuralgia and postherpetic neuralgia (32,33). Clinical observations suggest that this agent has a significant analgesic effect on neuropathic pain with a much lower side-effect profile compared to other antiepileptic drugs and also most antidepressants.

Several local anesthetics have also been shown to relieve neuropathic pain when administrated systemically, in addition to their known local anesthetic effects. For example, lidocaine transdermal patches have been effective for treatment of neuropathic pain.

Anesthetic and Neurosurgical Approaches to Pain Management

A wide variety of anesthetic and neurosurgical approaches to pain are available, and some require highly specialized skills (34). Table 32.8 lists some common anesthesia and neurosurgical interventions for severe pain. (For further details on these techniques, refer to Chapter 28: Acute and Chronic Pain. In: Cassel CK, et al., eds. Geriatric Medicine, 4th ed., page 338.)

Case (Part 8)

A year later, after you treated Mr. Peters's postherpetic neuralgia with gabapentin and combination analgesics, he reports a pain level of 1–2/10 chronically. He is back to playing tennis regularly and his knee pain is rarely a problem now.

What are some of the nonpharmacologic methods that may help improve Mr. Peters's chronic pain syndrome?

Nondrug Strategies for Pain Management

Nondrug strategies, used alone or in combination with appropriate analgesic medications, should be an integral part of the care plan for most elderly patients with significant pain problems (Table 32.9). Nondrug

TABLE 32.7. Selected nonopioid medications for pain

Drug	Description	Comments
Antidepressants: amitriptyline, desipramine, nortriptyline, others	Older people are more sensitive to side effects, especially anticholinergic effects; desipramine, or nortriptyline are better choices than amitriptyline	Complete relief unusual; used best as adjunct to other strategies; start low and increase slowly every 3–5 days
Anticonvulsants: clonazepam, clonazepam, carbamazepine	Carbamazepine may cause leukopenia, thrombocytopenia and rarely aplastic anemia; clonazepam side effects may be similar to other benzodiazepines in the elderly	Start low and increase slowly; check blood counts on carbamazepine
Gabapentin (also an anticonvulsant) Neurontin	Less serious side effects than other anticonvulsants	Start with 100mg and titrate up slowly; t.i.d. dosing; monitor for idiosyncratic side effects such as ankle swelling, ataxia, etc.; effective dose reported 100–800mg q 8h
Antiarrhythmics mexiletine (Mexitil)	Common side effects include tremor, dizziness, paresthesias; rarely may cause blood dyscrasias and hepatic damage	Avoid use in patients with preexisting heart disease; start low and titrate slowly; monitor electrocardiograms; q 6–8h dosing
Local anesthetics Lidocaine (intravenous)	IV lidocaine associated with delirium	IV lidocaine may predict response to anticonvulsants and antiarrhythmics
Lidocaine transdermal patch (Lidoderm)	Transdermal patch has minimal systemic absorption	May apply up to 3 patches alternating 12-h intervals to improve pain, reduce denervation hypersensitivity, and decrease systemic absorption
Capsaicin	Capsaicin depletes nerve endings of substance P	May take 2 weeks to peak effect
Tramadol (Ultram)	Partial opioid and serotonin agonist; more of a norepinephrine antagonist; may cause drowsiness, nausea, vomiting, and constipation	Has ceiling effect; dose >300mg/24h usually not tolerated because of nausea; q 4–6h dosing

Muscle relaxants (baclofen, chlorzoxazone [Paraflex], cyclobenzaprine [Flexeril])	Sedation; anticholinergic effects; abrupt withdrawal of baclofen may cause central nervous system irritability	Mechanism of action not precisely known; monitor for sedation and anticholinergic effects; taper baclofen on discontinuation Poorly tolerated in older adults
Substance P inhibitors (capsaicin) available OTC; for topical use only	Burning pain during depletion of substance P may be intolerable by as many as 30% of patients; may take 14 days for maximum response; avoid eye contamination	Start with small doses; can be partially removed with vegetable oil
NMDA inhibitors Ketamine Dextromethorphan	N-methyl-D-aspartate antagonists (NMDA) Ketamine: potent anesthetic Dextromethorphan: common cough suppressant	Ketamine only available IV Both may cause delirium
Drugs for osteoporosis Calcitonin Bisphosphonates	Pain relief mechanisms unknown	Not effective on pain other than osteoporosis
Corticosteroids Prednisone Dexamethasone	Decrease inflammation in many tissues	Classic corticosteroid side effects limit overall usefulness in chronic pain

Note: Limited number of examples are provided. For comprehensive lists of other available medications for pain, clinicians should consult other sources.

Source: Ferrell BA. Acute and Chronic Pain. In: Cassel CK, Leipzig RM, Cohen HJ, et al., eds. Geriatric Medicine, 4th ed. New York: Springer, 2003.

TABLE 32.8. Anesthetic or neurosurgical pain management techniques

Procedure	Possible indications	Comments
Continuous infusion opioids (morphine, hydromorphone, fentanyl)	Perioperative pain; severe cancer pain when all oral route has failed	Subcutaneous infusions are usually well tolerated by patients in nursing homes or home care; IV infusions may require more skilled monitoring
Epidural analgesia (intermittent local anesthetics or opioids; or continuous opioids)	Perioperative pain; severe cancer pain when oral route has failed	Can be supplied by external or internally implanted pumps; does not avoid constipation and occasional delirium; serious complications are rare but can be devastating
Nerve blocks	Mononeuropathies, postherpetic neuralgia, intercostal nerve pain (postthoracotomy or postherpetic neuralgia)	Usually temporary relief limited to a few days or weeks
Intrathecal analgesia	Perioperative pain	Can cause respiratory depression
Stellate ganglia blockade	Sympathetically mediated pain of the upper extremity	Not to be confused with complex regional pain syndromes
Lumbar sympathetic blockade	Sympathetically mediated pain of the lower extremity, peripheral vascular disease	
Celiac plexus blockade	Severe pain from carcinoma of pancreas	Requires substantial skill
Neuroablation (permanent nerve destruction)	Severe recalcitrant mononeuropathic pain	May recur after several years
Cordotomy	Severe recalcitrant cancer pain	May not relieve all pain
Neurostimulation (dorsal column or thalamic)	Severe recalcitrant pain usually following thalamic stroke or spinal cord injury	Requires substantial skill

Source: Ferrell BA. Acute and Chronic Pain. In: Cassel CK, Leipzig RM, Cohen HJ, et al., eds. Geriatric Medicine, 4th ed. New York: Springer, 2003.

TABLE 32.9. Selected nondrug strategies for pain management

Intervention	Comments	Limitations
Education	Content should include basic knowledge about pain (diagnosis, treatment, complications, and prognosis), other available treatment options, and information about over-the-counter medications and self help strategies	May require substantial time
Exercise	Can be tailored for individual patient needs and lifestyle; moderate intensity exercise should be maintained for 30 minutes or more 3–4 times a week and continued indefinitely	Maintenance is critical and difficult to continue indefinitely
Cognitive-behavioral therapy	Should be conducted by a trained therapist	Requires substantial cognitive function
Physical modalities (heat, cold, and massage)	A variety of techniques are available for application	Heat and cold should be used with caution in those with cognitive impairment to avoid thermal injuries
Physical or occupational therapy	Should be conducted by a trained therapist	Not appropriate for maintenance therapy; can be expensive if not reimbursed
Chiropractic	Has been shown to be as effective as Mackenzie exercises for acute back pain	Potential spinal cord or nerve root impingement should be ruled out prior to any spinal manipulation
Acupuncture	Should be provided only by a qualified acupuncturist	Effects may be short lived and require repetitive treatments
Transcutaneous electrical nerve stimulation (TENS)	Should initially be applied and adjusted by an experienced professional	Effects are often short lived; clear placebo effects have been observed
Relaxation and distraction techniques	Therapeutic modalities require individual buy in and may require substantial training	Patients with cognitive impairment may not be good candidates

Source: Ferrell BA. Acute and Chronic Pain. In: Cassel CK, Leipzig RM, Cohen HJ, et al., eds. Geriatric Medicine, 4th ed. New York: Springer, 2003.

strategies for pain management encompass a broad range of treatments and physical modalities, many of which carry low risks for adverse effects. Used in combination with appropriate drug regimens, these interventions often enhance therapeutic effects while allowing medication doses to be kept low to prevent adverse drug effects (7).

Among the nondrug interventions, the importance of *patient education* cannot be overstated. Studies have shown that patient education programs alone significantly improve overall pain management (35,36). Such programs often include content about the nature of pain, how to use pain diaries and pain assessment instruments, how to use medications appropriately, and how to use self-help nondrug strategies. Whether conducted in groups or individually, education should be tailored for individual patient needs and level of understanding. Written materials and methods of reinforcement are important to the overall success of the program.

Physical exercise is important for most patients with pain. A program of exercise can be tailored to most patients' needs and is extremely important for rehabilitation and the maintenance of strength and endurance. Initial training for chronic pain patients usually requires 8 to 12 weeks with supervision by a professional who can focus on the needs of older people with musculoskeletal disorders. There is no evidence that one form of exercise is better than another, so programs can be tailored for the individual's needs, lifestyle, and preference. The intensity of exercise, along with frequency and duration, must be adjusted to avoid exacerbation of the underlying condition, while gradually increasing and later maintaining overall conditioning. It is important to remember that feeling better often gives rise to a false impression that the discipline of regular exercise is not necessary. Continued encouragement and reinforcement is often required. Unless complications arise, the program of exercise should be maintained indefinitely to prevent deconditioning and deterioration.

Psychological strategies have also been shown to be helpful for some with significant pain. *Cognitive therapies* are strategies aimed at altering belief systems and attitudes about pain and suffering. Cognitive therapies include various forms of distraction, relaxation, biofeedback, and hypnosis. Cognitive-behavioral therapy in its purest form includes a structured approach to teaching coping skills that might be used alone or in combination with analgesic medications and other nondrug strategies for pain control.

Finally, a variety of alternative therapies are also used by many patients. Many patients seek alternative medicine approaches with and without the knowledge or recommendation of their physician or other primary care provider. *Alternative medicine* approaches to chronic pain may include homeopathy, spiritual healing, or the growing market of vitamin, herbal, and natural remedies. Although there is little scientific evidence to support these strategies for pain control, it is important that health care providers not abandon or react to patients using these modalities, but rather educate both themselves and their patients about their benefits and risks (37).

General Principles

* Pain is a common complaint of patients in an office setting. Understanding its pathophysiology helps determine proper therapy and improve patient outcomes.
* Historically, multiple factors (fear of addiction and side effects, fear of litigation, poor history taking, etc.) have led to the underrecognition and inadequate treatment of pain. Clinicians have an ethical and moral obligation to prevent needless suffering and provide effective pain relief, especially to those near the end of life.
* A complete pain history is the foundation in differentiating acute from chronic pain and developing an appropriate management plan.
* Pain management should be guided by the World Health Organization recommendations for choosing the intensity of treatment based on the intensity of pain. Pain of *mild* intensity usually responds to nonopioid drugs used alone or in combination with other physical and cognitive-behavioral interventions. Pain of *moderate* intensity often requires low-dose opioids or combination analgesics. *Severe* pain requires potent opioid analgesics alone or in combination with other analgesic strategies.

Suggested Readings

Acute Pain Management Guideline Panel. Acute Pain Management: Post-operative or Medical Procedures and Trauma. Clinical Practice Guideline. AHCPR Pub. No. 92-0032. Rockville, MD: Agency for Health Care Policy and Research, Public Health Service, U.S. Department of Health and Human Services, February 1993. *A thorough review of current practices in acute pain management.*

American Geriatric Society Panel on Chronic Pain in Older Persons. The management of chronic pain in older persons. J Am Geriatr Soc 1998;46:635–651. *A comprehensive guide to the management of pain among older adults with special emphasis to non-pharmacologic measures as well as dosing recommendations of pain medications.*

Ferrell BA. Acute and chronic pain. In: Cassel CK, Leipzig RM, Cohen HJ, et al., eds. Geriatric Medicine, 4th ed. New York: Springer, 2003:323–342.

References

1. Ferrell BA. Overview of aging and pain. In: Ferrell BR, Ferrell BA, eds. Pain in the Elderly. Seattle: IASP Press, 1996:1–10.
2. Ferrell BA, Ferrell BR, Osterweil D. Pain in the nursing home. J Am Geriatr Soc 1990;38:409–414.
3. American Geriatric Society Ethics Committee. The care of dying patients: a position statement. J Am Geriatr Soc 1995;43:577–578.
4. Gibson SJ, Helme RD. Age differences in pain perception and report: a review of physiological, psychological, laboratory and clinical studies. Pain Rev 1995;2:111–137.

5. Gibson SJ, Helme RD. Age related differences in pain perception and report. Pain Reviews 1995;2:111–137.

6. Max MB, et al. Principles of Analgesic use in Treatment of Acute Pain and Cancer Pain, 4th ed. Glenview, IL: American Pain Society, 1999.

7. Acute Pain Management Guideline Panel. Acute Pain Management: Post-Operative or Medical Procedures and Trauma. Clinical Practice Guideline. AHCPR Pub. No. 92-0032. Rockville, MD: Agency for Health Care Policy and Research, Public Health Service, U.S. Department of Health and Human Services, February 1993.

8. American Geriatric Society Panel on Chronic Pain in Older Persons. The management of chronic pain in older persons. J Am Geriatr Soc 1998;46:635–651.

9. Myer RA, Campbell JN, Raja SN. Peripheral and neural mechanisms of nociception. In: Wall PD, Melzack R, eds. Textbook of Pain, 3rd ed. New York: Churchill Livingstone, 1994:13–44.

10. Bennett GF. Neuropathic pain. In: Wall PD, Melzack R, eds. Textbook of Pain, 3rd ed. New York: Churchill Livingstone, 1994:201–224.

11. Galer BS, Dworkin RH. A Clinical Guide to Neuropathic Pain. New York: McGraw-Hill, 2000:33–36.

12. Craig KD. Emotional aspects of pain. In: Wall PD, Melzack R, eds. Textbook of Pain, 3rd ed. New York: Churchill Livingstone, 1994:261–274.

13. Ferrell BA. Pain evaluation and management in the nursing home. Ann Intern Med 1995;123(9):681–687.

14. Herr KA, Mobily PR. Pain management in alternate care settings. In: Ferrell BR, Ferrell BA, eds. Pain in the Elderly. Seattle: IASP Press, 1996:101–109.

15. Nishikawa ST, Ferrell BA. Pain assessment in the elderly. Clin Geriatr Issues Long Term Care 1993;1:15–28.

16. Keefe FJ, Beaupre PM, Weiner DK, Siegler IC. Pain in older adults: A cognitive behavioral perspective. In: Ferrell BR, Ferrell BA, eds. Pain in the Elderly. Seattle: IASP Press, 1996:11–19.

17. World Health Organization. Cancer Pain Relief, 2nd ed. With a guide to opioid availability, cancer pain relief and palliative care: Report of the WHO Expert Committee (WHO Technical Report Series, No. 804). Geneva: WHO, 1996.

18. Bradley JD, Brandt KD, Katz BP, et al. Comparison of an anti-inflammatory dose of ibuprofen, an analgesic dose of ibuprofen and acetaminophen in treatment of patients with osteoarthritis of the knee. N Engl J Med 1991;325:87–91.

19. Roth SH. Merits and liabilities of NSAID therapy. Rheumatol Dis Clin North Am 1989;15:479–498.

20. Griffin MR, Piper JM, Daugherty JR, et al. Nonsteroidal anti-inflammatory drug use and increased for peptic ulcer disease in elderly persons. Ann Intern Med 1991;114:257–263.

21. Gurwitz JH, Avorn J, Ross-Degnan D, Sipsitz LA. Nonsteroidal anti-inflammatory drug associated azotemia in the very old. JAMA 1990;264:471–475.

22. Graham DY, White RH, Foreland LW, et al. Duodenal and gastric ulcer prevention with misoprostol in arthritis patients taking NSAIDs: Misoprostol Study Group. Ann Intern Med 1993;119:257–262.

23. Ehsanullah RS, Page MC, Tildesley G, Wood JR. Prevention of gastroduodenal damage induced by non-steroidal anti-inflammatory drugs: controlled trial of ranitidine. Br Med J 1988;297:1017–1021.

24. Taha As, Hudson N, Hawkey CJ, et al. Famotidine for the prevention of gastric and duodenal ulcers caused by nonsteroidal anti-inflammatory drugs. N Engl J Med 1996;334:1435–1449.
25. Stucki J, Hohannesson M, Liang MH. Use of misoprostyl in the elderly: Is the expense justified? Drugs Aging 1996;8:84–88.
26. Pope JE, Anderson JJ, Felson DT. A meta-analysis of the effects of nonsteroidal anti-inflammatory drugs on blood pressure. Arch Intern Med 1993;153: 477–484.
27. Jaffe JH. Drug addiction and drug abuse. In: Gilman AG, Goodman LS, Rall TW, Murad F, eds. Goodman and Gillman's The Pharmacological Basis of Therapeutics, 7th ed. New York: Macmillan, 1985:532–581.
28. Melzack R. The tragedy of needless pain. Sci Am 1990;262:27–33.
29. Portenoy RK. Opiate therapy for chronic noncancer pain: Can we get past the bias? Am Pain Soc Bull 1991;1:4–7.
30. Max MB. Antidepressants and analgesics. In: Fields HL, Leibeskind JC, eds. Progress in Pain Research and Management, vol 1. Seattle: IASP Press, 1994:229–246.
31. Swerdlow M. The use of local anesthetics for relief of chronic pain. Pain Clin 1988;2:3–6.
32. Backonja M, Beydoun A, Edwards KR, et al. Gabapentin for the symptomatic treatment of painful neuropathy in patients with diabetes mellitus: a randomized controlled trial. JAMA 1998;280(21):1831–1836.
33. Rowbotham M, Harden N, Stacey B, Bernstein P, Magnus-Miller L. Gabapentin for the treatment of postherpetic neuralgia: a randomized controlled trial. JAMA 1998;280(21):1837–1842.
34. Prager JP. Invasive modalities for the diagnosis and treatment of pain in the elderly. Clin Geriatr Med 1996;12(3):549–561.
35. Ferrell BR, Rhiner M, Ferrell BA. Development and implementation of a pain education program. Cancer 1993;72(11 suppl):3426–3432.
36. Rhiner M, Ferrell BR, Ferrell BA, Grant MM. A structured nondrug intervention program for cancer pain. Cancer Pract 1993;1:137–143.
37. Eisenberg, Kessler RC, Foster C, et al. Unconventional medicine in the United States: prevalence, costs and patterns of use. N Engl J Med 1993;328:246–252.
38. Ferrell BA. Pain. In: Osterweil D, Brummel-Smith K, Beck JB, eds. Comprehensive Geriatric Assessment. New York: McGraw-Hill, 2000:390.
39. Jocox A, Car DB, Payne R, et al. Management of Cancer Pain. Clinical Practice Guideline No. 9. AHCPR Publ 94-0592. Rockville, MD: Agency for Health Care Policy and Research, U.S. Department of Health and Human Services, Public Health Service; 1994.
40. Melzack R. The McGill Pain Questionnaire: major properties and scoring methods. Pain 1975;1:277–299.
41. Herr KA, Mobily PR, Kohour FJ, et al. Evaluation of the faces pain scale for use with the elderly. Clin J Pain 1998;14:1–10.
42. Ferrell BA, Ferrell BR, Rivera L. Pain in cognitively impaired nursing home patients. J Pain Symptom Manage 1995;10:391–598.
43. Fishman B, Pasternak S, Wallenstein SL, Houde RW, Holland JC, Foley KA. The Memorial Pain Assessment Card: a valid instrument for the evaluation of cancer pain. Cancer 1987;60(5):1151–1158.

Index